LEON DĂNĂILĂ

Functional Neuroanatomy of the Brain

Third Part

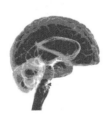

To Alexandra

To Alexandra

Faith, Tenacity and Genius

Also called the "Brain sculptor", appearing alongside Einstein among the 500 geniuses of the 21st century and one of the top 5000 personalities of the world, Academician Professor Doctor Leon Danaila is a famous neurosurgeon, considered the best in Europe, renowned and recognized at international level.

The law that he set as guide throughout his entire life, with dignity, passion and modesty, is summarized by the professor himself in these words: "I have faith that God helps the sick through me. God gave me a brain, He gave me hands, He gave me reason and I have to use them for the good of mankind. For the sick, poor things, I did everything for them..."

Living as an ascetic and learning as a perpetual student, he gives life and asks nothing in return. The professional activity of Professor Leon Danaila can be also translated in figures, many figures. For about half a century, his hand has performed over 40,000 surgeries in the country and abroad, rendering his fellow men new chance at life, rebuilding their body, but also their soul.

Convinced that "Life means the others" and "Our mission is to discover God's creation," Prof. Leon Danaila describes himself the legend of his life in a prayer-psalm that defines his existence:

"I have asked the Lord to give me strength

He gave me hardships that have made me stronger

I asked for wisdom

And He gave me problems that I had to solve

I asked for a rise

And He gave me a thoughtful brain and physical power to work

I asked for courage

And God gave me dangers that I had to face

I asked to be able to love

And the Good Lord gave me people in pain that I could help

He gave me nothing of what I asked for

But He gave me everything I needed

My prayer has been heard"

CONTENTS

FIRST PART

Chapter 1

HISTORY OF THE BRAIN AND MIND

Chapter 4

PONS

Chapter 5

MIDBRAIN

Chapter 8

DIENCEPHALON

SECOND PART

Chapter 9

THE BASAL GANGLIA

Chapter 10

LIMBIC LOBE AND LIMBIC SYSTEM

Chapter 11

HIPPOCAMPAL FORMATION

Chapter 12

AMYGDALA

Chapter 13

OLFACTORY SYSTEM

Chapter 14

GUSTATORY SYSTEM

Chapter 15

FRONTAL LOBES

Chapter 16

PARIETAL LOBE

Chapter 17

TEMPORAL LOBES

THIRD PART

Chapter 18
OCCIPITAL LOBE

Chapter 19

WHITE MATTER OF CEREBRAL HEMISPHERE

Chapter 20
CORPUS CALLOSUM

Chapter 21

CEREBRAL CORTEX

Chapter 23
CEREBRAL ASYMMETRY in nonhumans

Chapter 24

THE NEURAL BASIS OF CONSCIOUSNESS

Chronological and Professional Information

Biographical info

Academician Professor Dr. Leon Dănăilă had been born on the 1st of July 1933 in Darabani, Botoşani county, where he had attended the first four years of the elementary school. He had continued his education at "Grigore Ghica V.V." secondary school in from which he had graduated in 1952. In the same year, he had been admitted by competitive examination to attend the courses of the Faculty of Medicine in Iasi, from which he had graduated in 1958.

After graduating from the Faculty of Medicine in Iasi (1958), he had worked for 2 years as an intern in the hospital in Comăneşti (between 1958 and 1960) and then for one year in the Medical Dispensary in Darmanesti (between 1960 and 1961). In 1961, following the competitive examination he had enter into residency and had occupied the position of neurosurgery resident physician in the Neurosurgery Clinic of "Gh. Marinescu" Hospital in Bucharest where he continues to practice in the present.

Following the graduation of severe exams, as well as of competitive examinations, he had achieved in 1966 the qualification of specialist neurosurgery physician, and in he had been awarded the title of doctor of medicine with the doctoral thesis "Neuronomul Spinal [The Spinal Neurinoma]", in 1974 he had reached the qualification of 3rd degree head consultant neurosurgeon, in 1981 that of 2nd de gree head consultant neurosurgeon and had been appointed head of the VII vascular neurosurgery and microneurosurgery department. In 1972 he had graduated from the Faculty of Philosophy and Psychology in Bucharest after attending as a full-time student.

A graduate of the Faculty of Medicine in Iasi (1958) and of the Faculty of Philosophy and Psychology in Bucharest (1972), following the competitive examination which had been held in 1991, he had achieved the position of Professor of Neurosurgery in the Neurosurgery II Clinic of *"Carol Davila"* University of Medicine and Pharmacy in Bucharest, and in 1992 that of Professor in Psychoneurology at the Faculty of Psychology of *"Titu Maiorescu"* University in Bucharest.

Member of academies and international scientific organizations

He had become a full member of *The Romanian Academy* beginning with the 20th of December 2004, after being a corresponding member since the 24th of October 1997; full member of *The Academy of Medical Sciences of Romania* (1993); member of *The Romanian Academy of Sciences* (2004), member of the New York Academy of Sciences (1995), of The London Diplomatic Academy (2000), of

"L'Académie Centrale Européenne des Sciences, des Lettres et des Arts" and of The World Academy of Letters.

He is also a member of the following international scientific organizations: L'Union Medical Balkanique (1986), The European Association of Neurosurgical Societies (EANS) (1987), The International Society of Psycho-neuroendocrinology (1991), The International Psychogeriatric Association (1991), Société Française de Pharmacologie Clinique et Thérapeutique (1991), The Biomedical Optics Society (1992), The International Society for Optical Engineering (SPIE) (1992), The Balkan Society of Angiology and Vascular Surgery (1994), The World Federation of Neurosurgical Societies (WFNS) (1992), Société de Neurochirurgie de Langue Française (1996), The American Heart Association (1999); The European Medical Laser Association (1998); The International Stroke Society (Japan) (1999), The American Association for the Advancement of Science (2003), The European Society for Stereotactic and Functional Neurosurgery (2003), The Congress of Neurological Surgeons (2004), active honorary member of The National Association Against Corruption, Abuse and for The Promotion of Human Rights (2006), member of the "International Neuropsychologicaly Society" (2008), member of the "American Chemical Society" (2008), member of the „American Association For the Advancement of Science" (AAAS) (2014).

He sits on the board of directors of the following specialized medical journals: "The Romanian Journal of Reconstructive Microsurgery", "Romanian Neurosurgery", "The Romanian Journal of Neurology and Psychiatry", "National Medical Review" and "The Proceedings of the Romanian Academy", "Chirugia [Surgery]", "Medicina Moderna [The Modern Medicine]".

He is the chief editor of "The Romanian Journal of Neurosurgery" and Honorary President revue "Modern Medicine".

Patents, books and scientific papers

He is the owner of 18 invention patents and of 10 innovation patents.

He is the author of 46 specialized books and textbooks among which we mention:

- *Nerurinomul Spinal [The Spinal Neurinoma],* Doctoral thesis (1972);
- *Tratat de Neurologie [Textbook of Neurology],* Volume 1 - Editura Medicala (1979);
- *Tratat de Neurologie [Textbook of Neurology],* Volume II - Editura Medicala (1980);
- *Tratat de patologie chirurgicală [Textbook of Surgical Pathology],* Volume IV, Editura Medicala (1983);

- *Sistemul arterial aortic. Patologie şi tratament chirurgical [The Aortic Arterial System. Pathology and surgical treatment]*, Volume II, Editura Medicală (1983);
- *Psihoneurologie [Psychoneurology]*, Editura Academiei RSR (1983);
- *Bolile Vasculare ale Creierului şi Măduvei Spinării vol II. Bolile vasculare ischemice [Vascular Diseases of the Brain and Spinal Cord, Volume II -Ischemic Vascular Diseases]*, Part II, Editura Academiei RSR (1984);
- *Bolile Vasculare ale Creierului şi Măduvei Spinării vol. III Hematoamele Intracraniene şi Spinale [Vascular Diseases of the Brain and Spinal Cord, Volume III - Intracranial and Spinal Hematomas]*, Editura Academiei RSR (1985);
- *Romanian Neurosurgery,* Volume I, Editura Academiei RSR, 1986;
- *Romanian Neurosurgery,* Volume II, Editura Academiei RSR (1987);
- *Tromboembolismul Cardiovascular [The Cardiovascular Thromboembolism]*, Editura Ştiinţifică şi Enciclopedică (1987);
- *Ateroscleroza Cerebrală din Sistemul Carotidian [The Cerebral Atherosclerosis of the Carotid Arterial System]*, Editura Ştiinţifică şi Enciclopedică (1988);
- *Chirurgia Psihiatrică [Psychiatric Surgery]*, Editura Academiei RSR (1988);
- *Tratamentul Tumorilor Cerebrale [The Treatment of Cerebral Tumors]*, Editura Academiei Române (1993);
- *Maladia Alzheimer [Alzheimer's Disease]*, Editura Militară (1996);
- *Sculptură în creier [Sculpture in The Brain]*, Editura Du Style (1998);
- *Apoptoza [Apoptosis]*, Editura Academiei (1999);
- *Tratat de Neuropsihologie [Textbook of Neuropsychology]*, Editura Medicală (2000) (second edition 2002);
- *Actualităţi şi perspective în Neurochirurgie [New Developments and Perspectives in Neurosurgery]*, Editura Naţional (2000);
- *Atlas de patologie chirurgicală a creierului [Atlas of Surgical Pathology of the Brain]*, Editura Moonfal Press (2000);
- *Lasers in Neurosurgery*, Editura Academiei (2001);
- *Atlas of Surgical Pathology of the Brain*, Editura Moonfal Press (2001);
- *Vascularizaţia arterială şi venoasă a creierului [The Arterial and Venous Vascularization of the Brain]*, Editura Tipart Group (2001);
- *Sinteze Neurochirurgicale [Syntheses in Neurosurgery]*, Editura Ceres (2001);

- *Apoptoza [Apoptosis]* (revised and expanded second edition), Editura Academiei (2002);

- *Ateroscleroza cerebrală ischemică [Ischemic Cerebral Atherosclerosis]*, Editura Medicală (2004);

- *Atlas de patologie cerebro-vasculară [Atlas of Cerebrovascular Pathology]*, Editura Cartea Universitară Bucureşti (2005);

- *Programed Cell Death in the Vascular Diseases of the Brain*, Editura Cartea Universitară Bucureşti (2005);

- *Clinica şi morfopatologia proceselor expansive ale sistemului nervos central [The Clinical Presentation and the Morphopathology of the Expanding Processes of the Central Nervous System]*, Editura Cartea Universitară Bucureşti (2005);

- *Cerebrovascular Malformations*, an atlas of histopathology and ultrastructure, Editura Cartea Universitară Bucureşti (2005);

- *The Vascular Wall and the Intracerebral Hemorrhage,* an atlas of light and electron microscopy, Editura Cartea Universitară Bucureşti (2005),

- *Hemoragia Subarahnoidiană Anevrismală [The Aneurysmal Subarachnoid Hemorrhage],* Editura Cartea Universitară Bucureşti (2006);

- *The Interstitial Cells of the Human Brain*, Editura Cartea Universitară Bucureşti (2006);

- *Cerebral Vascular Occlusions*, an atlas of histopathology and ultrastructure - Editura Cartea Universitară Bucureşti (2006);

- *Tratat de Neuropsihologie [Textbook of Neuropsychology]*, Volume II - Editura Medicală (2006),

- *Patologia neurochirurgicală a hipofizei [Neurosurgical Pathology of the Pituitary Gland]*, Editura Didactică şi Pedagogică (2006);

- *Vasculogenesis, Angiogenesis and Vascular Tumorigenesis in the Brain,* an atlas of cerebrovascular cyto-histopathology, Editura Cartea Universitară Bucureşti (2007);

- *Vasculogenesis, Angiogenesis and Vascular Tumorigenesis in the Brain,* an atlas of cerebrovascular cyto-histopathology, second edition (2007),

- *Anevrismele cerebrale [Cerebral Aneurysms]*, Editura Academiei Române (2007);

- *Programmed Cell Death in the Brain, an atlas of light and electron microscopy*, Editura Cartea Universitară Bucureşti (2008, 2009);

- *The Interstitial Cells of the Human Brain - an atlas of light and electron microscopy,* Second Edition, Editura Cartea Universitară Bucureşti (2008);

- *Neuropsihologie [Neuropsychology],*Editura Renaissance (2008);

- *Malformaţiile vasculare cerebrale şi spinale [Vascular Cerebral and Spinal Malformations],* Editura Academiei Române (2010);

- *The Interstitial Cells of the Human Brain -an atlas of light and electron microscopy,* Third Edition, Editura Ars Academica (2010);

- *The Ultrastructure of the Dying Cells in the Brain - an atlas of transmission electron microscopy ,* Editura Ars Academica (2011);

- *Diagnosistic Techniques and Surgical Management of Brain Tumors,* Chapter 13,   Ed. INTECH (2011);

- *Functional Neuroanatomy of the Brain (3 volums),* Editura Didactică şi Pedagogică Bucureşti (2012);

- *Clinical Management and Evolving Novel Therapeutic Strategies for Patients with Brain Tumors,* Chapter 22, Ed. INTECH (2013);

- *The Cordocytes of the Human Brain - an atlas of transmission electron microscopy,* Editura Ars Academica (2014),

- *Normal and Pathological Cerebral Venous System* (2015), *Tratat de Neuropsihologie [Textbook of Neuropsychology],* Editura Medicală (2015).

He had been among the contributors in the publication of 3 other books:

- *Lichidul cefalo-rahidian [The Cerebrospinal Fluid],* Editura Didactică şi Pedagogică (1979);

- *Ghid de practică medicală [Guide for The Medical Practice]* Volume 1 - Editura Infomedica (1999);

- *Enciclopedie Medicală Românească - Secolul XX [Romanian Medical Encyclopedia - The 20th Century],* Editura Fundaţiei Medicale a Rinichiului (2001).

Out of the total of 45 published books, he had been the sole author of 6 books, the primary author of 27 books, joint author, but not the primary one, of 13 books and contributing author in 3 books. He had published and had presented 405 scientific papers, as follows: 140 published abroad and in Romanian journals with international circulation (in English language); 63 published in Romanian language in various Romanian medical journals; 71 communicated to various international congresses, and 131 communicated to symposia and congresses in Romania. His works are quoted by renowned scholars and researchers throughout the world.

He had attended more than 200 national and international scientific manifestations (congresses, conferences, symposia).

International specializations

He had studied neurosurgery for a year in New York as part of a Fulbright scholarship (1980-1981) and he had attended various specialization courses and experience exchange programs in Budapest (1978 and 1979), Delft (1981), Moscow (1982), Edinburgh (1990), Glasgow (1990), Dusseldorf (1991), Paris (1991), Bruxelles (1995).

During these specialized training programs, both in Europe and in The United States of America, as well as at the various international congresses, he had met directly and had exchanged professional opinions with the world's most important personalities in the field of neurosurgery.

Professional achievements

Due to these specializations and to the putting into practice of the most modern operative techniques, he had been successful in performing the most complex neurosurgical interventions and in reducing the operative mortality rates to percentages which were comparable to those achieved in the most renown neurosurgery clinics in the world. In this way, he had succeeded in reducing the operative mortality rates for the cases of acoustic neurinomas from 51% to 4%, while in the cases of intra-cerebral aneurysms, the rates had been reduced from 59% to 4%. These results are the consequence of a very well perfected operative technique, as well of the fact that he had introduced in 1979 the operating microscope and in 1894 the operative laser in the arsenal of the neurosurgical operating room in Romania.

Up to the present, he had performed more than 40,000 surgical interventions, out of which 27,000 using the operating microscope and 715 through the use of laser. The degree of difficulty of the surgical interventions (intracranial aneurisms - over 3,700, over 367 arteriovenous malformations, more than 400 acoustic neurinomas, over 300 tumors of the pituitary gland, more than 1300 meningiomas, brain stem tumors, spinal cord tumors, intraorbitary tumors, tumors of the skull base, intraventricular tumors, pineal gland tumors etc.), their large number, as well as the excellent postoperative results achieved through the significant reduction of the mortality rates (less than 4%) places him among the greatest neurosurgeons in the world.

Progresses and research of national and international importance
On a national level he had described and had published first in Romania:

- *Malformaţii arterio-venoase cu interesarea venei Galen [Arteriovenous Malformations with the Involvement of the Vein of Galen]*, in the national neurology journal Studii şi Cercetări de Neurologie 15, 1970;

- *Cisticercoza de ventricol IV [The Cysticercosis of the Fourth Ventricle]*, in the national neurology, psychiatry and neurosurgery journal Neurologia, Psihiatria, Neurochirurgia 15, 1970; *Encefalopatia paraneoplazică [The Paraneoplastic encephalopathy]* in the national neurology, psychiatry and neurosurgery journal Neurologia, Psihiatria, Neurochirurgia 15, 1970;

- *Peridurografia gazoasă în hernia de disc lombară [TheGas Peridurography in the Lumbar Disc Herniation]*, in the national oncology and radiology journal Oncologia şi Radiologia 9; 1970.

He had studied and had published first on an national level:

- *Correlations Between the Blood Group and the Incidence of Congenital Neurosurgical Diseases,* in Revue Roumaine de Neurologie 9, 1971;

- *Considerations on the Correlation Between the Blood Groups and the Incidence of Cerebral Tumors,* in Revue Roumaine de Neurologie 9, 1972;

- *Cranial and Orbital Epidermoid Tumors,* in Journal of Neurosurgical Sciences 19; 1975;

- *Cranial Vault Metastases,* in Revue Roumaine de Neurologie et de Psychiatrie 13, 1975;

- *Intraselar Abscesses,* Neurochirurgia 18, 1975; *Cerebral Dermoid Tumours,* Neurochirurgia 19; 1976;

- *Haematological Aspects of the Hypophyseal Tumors* in the Romanian journal Acta Neurochirurgica 37, 1977;

- *Anatomoclinical Aspects in Meningeal Carcinomatosis,* in Revue Roumaine de Neurologie et de Psychiatrie 15, 1977;

- *Cranial Eosinophilic Granuloma,* Neurochirurgia 20, 1977;

- *Monitoring Intracranial Pressure in Cat and Man,* in Revue Roumaine de Neurologie et de Psychiatrie 1, 1980.

He had introduced for the first time the operative laser (beginning with 1984) and the operating microscope (beginning with 1979) in the current neurosurgical practice and had published the first papers in these fields (the book -*Lasers in Neurosurgery,* 2001).

He had introduced and had been the first to publish in Romania and among the first authors on an international level to publish papers with regard to the conservative treatment of the primary intra-cerebral hematomas; see the paper *Surgical and conservative management of primary intra-cerebral hematoma* published in the national journal Romanian Journal of Gerontology and Geriatrics 7, 1986.

He is the only neurosurgeon in the country who had operated on the aneurysms of the vertebra-basilar arterial system beginning with 1985. The outcomes of these surgical interventions had been published in various medical papers in scientific journals such as: Romanian Neurosurgery 1, 3, 1992; Romanian Neurosurgery 11, 1992; Romanian Neurosurgery 2, 1993; Infomedica No. 4, 1994; Romanian Journal of Reconstructive Microsurgery, Volume 1, 1996; Chirurgia 107, 2012.

He had performed the first endarterectomies of the middle cerebral artery and of the carotid artery and he had published papers with reference to them in: *Revue Roumaine de Neurologie et de Psychiatrie* 23, 1985; *Romanian Journal of Neurology and Psychiatry* 31, 1993, as well as in the book *Ateroscleroza cerebrală ischemică [Ischaemic Cerebral Atherosclerosis], 2004.*

He had performed 476 extra-intracranial bypass interventions (see *Ateroscleroza cerebrală din sistemul carotidian [The Cerebral Atherosclerosis of the Carotid Arterial System],* 1988 and *Ateroscleroza cerebrală ischemică [Ischaemic Cerebral Atherosclerosis], 2004).*

He had investigated the apoptosis in glioblastomas, (the results had been presented at The 48th *Congres de la la Sociétés De Neurochirurgie de Langue Française,* 1998 and published under the titles of *In situ and Peripheral Mononuclear Cells' Apoptosis in Glioblastomas,* Romanian Neurosurgery 8, 35-43, 1999; *High Levels of sFas and PBMC Apoptosis Before and After Excision of Malignant Melanoma,.* Case report, Romanian Archives of Microbiology and Immunology 61, 267-273, 2002, as well as in the book *Apoptoza [Apoptosis]* (first edition in 1999, and second edition in 2002).

He had studied and had performed the first corpus calossotomies for the treatment of epilepsy and their results are mentioned in: *Tratat de Neuropsihologie [Textbook of Neuropsychology]* Volume I 2000; 2002; 2006 and in the scientific paper presented at the 8th International Child Neurology Congress in Ljubljana in 1998.

He had performed and published the results of the first cerebro-myo-synangioses and cerebro-arterio-synangioses (see *Ateroscleroza cerebrală [Cerebral Atherosclerosis],* 1988 and *Ateroscleroza cerebrală ischemică [Ischemic Cerebral Atherosclerosis], 2004).*

He had studied and had been the first to publish the results concerning the intracranial meningiomas induced by radiation (see *Romanian Neurosurgery New Series* 1, 1993). He had been the first to study and to treat cases of mycotic aneurysms (see *Romanian Neurosurgery New Series* 2, 1993).

He had performed the first studies of electronic microscopy in Alzheimer disease and the results had been published in 1996 his the book *Maladia Alzheimer [Alzheimer's Disease]*.

He had been the one who had applied for the first time in Romania the use of immunotherapy in cerebral tumors, and the results had been published in the book *Tratamentul tumorilor cerebrale [The Treatment of Cerebral Tumors]*, published in 1993 and in the scientific paper *Interleukin-2 Therapy of Malignant Brain Tumors (Glioblastoma Multiforme)* which had appeared in the journal Acta Neurochirurgica Moldávica 3; 22-27, 1995.

He had performed the first studies on the subject of psychosurgery, studies which had been published in the book *Chirurgia Psihiatrică [Psychiatric Surgery]* (1988).

He had studied the apoptosis of the cerebral tumors, and the results had been published in the book *Apoptoza [Apoptosis]*, the first edition published in 1999 and the second edition published in 2002. He had conducted the first research studies on the subject of photodynamic therapy of the cerebral tumors, and the results had been published and reported at various national and international congresses, as well as in the book *Lasers in Neurosurgery* published in 2001.

He had conducted histopathology studies the of the cerebral tumors, their results being included in the book *Atlas of Surgical Pathology of the Brain* published in 2001. In 2006, he had described the cortico-optico-falciform syndrome in the book *Psihologia Neurochirurgicala a hipofizei [The Neurosurgical Psychology of the Pituitary Gland]* (2006).

He had performed for the first time in the country a study on the subject of the role of the interactions between the two cerebral hemispheres in the integration of the speech system, the results being published in the journal *Revue roumaine des sciences sociales. Serie de psychologie* (1987); a study concerning the serological levels of the ICAM and ELAM adhesion molecules in astrocitomas and glioblastomas, published in *Romanian Journal of Neurology* (1997); a study concerning the serological levels of interleukin 6 and interleukin 2 in the adenomas of the pituitary gland (see *Romanian Journal of Neurology* 34, 1996); and a study on the subject of the neurosurgical stress and the immune function, whose results had been published in *Romanian Journal of Neurology and Psychiatry* in 1994.

On the 28th of May 2003, he had performed for the first time in Romania the translabyrinthine approach for the treatment of the acoustic neurinoma and the transmastoid approach of the glomus jugulare tumors. He had published the first case of intracerebral calcifying psammomatous pesudotumor in the scientific paper *Psammomatous Pseudotumoral Intracerebral Calcification: A case Report and Review of the Literature* which had appeared in Annals of Neurosurgery 5, 2005.

On an international level, he had described for the first time the *Logorrhea syndrome with hyperkinesia* (1972) in his diploma thesis for the graduation of the Faculty of Philosophy and Psychology and then in the international journal *European Neurology* (1977).

He had performed and had studied more than 1000 cerebral vascular biopsies using the operating microscope and their results had been published in the books: *Ateroscleroza Cerebrala din Sistemul Carotidian [The Cerebral Atherosclerosis of the Carotid Arterial System]* (1988); *Ateroscleroza cerebrala ischemica [Ischemic Cerebral Atherosclerosis] (2004); Atlas de patologie cerebro-vasculara [Atlas of Cerebrovascular Pathology]* (2005); *Programed Cell Death in the Vascular Diseases of the Brain* (2005); in the scholarly journals with international circulation *"Romanian Journal of Gerontology and Geriatrics"* (1986) and *"Proceedings of the Romanian Academy, Series B"* (2001; 2002, 2003) and presented at various internal and international congresses.

He had been the first neurosurgeon to perform on an international level the procedure of osseous plasty with autologous bone powder (Patent of invention No. 112951 of February 1998).

The distinction between the cerebral hematoma and the cerebral hemorrhage had been illustrated in the study with the title: *Cellular Mechanisms of Cerebral Vessels Breaking in Different Pathological Conditions. An Optic and Electron-optic Study,* published in Proceedings of the Romanian Academy, Series B 3, 147-151, 2003.

The introduction of the concept of "intimoma" or "myoma" in the classification of the intimal lesions found in atherosclerosis had been done in the scientific paper: *Smooth Muscle Migration and Proliferation in the Cerebral Arteries Lumen with Formation of a New Type of Arteriosclerosis Lesion* which had been published in the journal Proceedings of the Romanian Academy, Series B 1, 55-67, 2001 and included in the book *Ateroscleroza cerebrala ischemica [Ischemic Cerebral Atherosclerosis], 2004.*

The intimal sarcoma with the transmural migration of the tumoral cells had been described for the first time on an international level in the scientific paper - *The Histopathologic and Ultrastructural Study of an Intimal Intracranial Sarcoma with Transluminal Cell Migration* which had been published in the scientific journal Proceedings of the Romanian Academy, Series B 3, 165-170, 2002.

Professor Danaila Leon, had discovered a new cerebral cell named **cordocyte,** which had been brought to the attention of the world scientific community for the first time in 2006 at the Congress in Cape Town, in San Diego in 2009, in Los Angeles in 2011 and in the Romanian medical journal *Chirurgia* 106 (6) 723-730, 2011. For this project he collaborated a period of time with the biologist Viorel Pais (died in 2 July 2014).

XL

On an international level, he had also published the medical papers *Laser-induced Autofluorescence Measurement on Brain Tissues* in the journal The Anatomical Record, Volume 292; 213-222, 2009 and *Laser-induced Autofluorescence as a Possible Diagnostic Tool for use in Neurosurgery* in the book *Brain Tumors*, INTECH (Croatia) Chapter 13 pages 245-274, 2011, as well as *A Comparative Ultrastructural Study of a New Type of Autoschizis versus a Survival Cellular Mechanism that Involves Cell Membranes of Cerebral Arteries in Humans* published in Ultrastructural Pathology 36; 166-170, 2012, and *Contributions to the Understanding of the Neural Bases of the Consciousness* in *Brain Tumors* Chapter 22, pp 473-520, 2013.

Since 2007, he is a member in the Board of Directors of the three COST (European Cooperation in Science and Technology) European research programs: COST Action BM0605 - Consciousness; COST Action BM0601- NeuroMath; COST Action B30 -Neural Regeneration and Plasticity: NEREPLAS.

Organizational activities

Between 1994 and 1995 Professor Leon Danaila had been General Director of "Gheorghe Marinescu" Clinical Hospital in Bucharest, and beginning with 1995 and until 2004 he had been Deputy General Director of "Vlad Voiculescu" Institute of Cerebrovascular Diseases in Bucharest. He had managed to build, without any funding from the state budget, 16 hospital wards and a fully equipped operating room, fact which had greatly improved the medical care in the Neurosurgery II Clinic because it had made possible to double, or even triple, the daily number of surgical interventions. In 1981, he had established the first vascular neurosurgery and microneurosurgery department in the country which continues its existence in the present.

He had been the director of the Neurosurgery department of *"Carol Davila"* University of Medicine and Pharmacy in Bucharest (1992 - 2004) and the head of the Vascular Neurosurgery II Clinic of the *Institute of Cerebrovascular Diseases* (IBCV), position he had held since 1981.

He had been president at national level of the neurosurgery commission of the Ministry of Health (1990 - 2004) and the president at national level of the Ministry of Health Commission for the approval of the travel abroad of the entitled patients for the performance of neurosurgical treatment (1990 - 2004). He also holds the position of President at national level of the neurosurgery commission of the National Institute of Legal Medicine since 1996.

Since 1990, he had been scientific coordinator of Ph.D. programs for both Romanian and foreign Ph.D. candidates (Israel, Greece, Egypt). In this capacity, he had supervised the training of 16 Doctors of Medical Sciences. He had also coordinated a large number of graduation papers.

Orders and medals

He had been distinguished in the healthcare activity through the Order No. 117/ 1980.

He had been granted five awards of the Romanian Academy for the books *Tratamentul tumorilor cerebrale [The Treatment of Cerebral Tumors]* - 1995, *Apoptoza [Apoptosis]* -2001, *Atlas of Surgical Pathology of the Brain* - 2002, *Lasers in Neurosurgery* - 2003, *Malformații Vasculare Cerebrale și Spinale [Vascular Cerebral and Spinal Malformations]* - 2012, as well as the "Arthur Kreindler" award of The Romanian Academy of Sciences in 2012, for the book *"Neuroanatomy of the Brain"*.

He had been granted in 1996 the international *Romeo del Vivo* award by the Neurosurgery Deparment in Calabria, Italy.

He had been awarded a diploma by the Military Publishing House [Editura Militară] in 1976 and the *Medal of the Romanian Atheneum Society* in 1990, as well as the *Medal of Caritas Catholica Vlaanderen* - Belgium in 1995.

In 2009 he had been awarded the *Excellence Trophy for His Entire Career - Ten for Romania.*

By presidential decree, he had been awarded the ranks of *Officer of The National Order of Faithful Service* (1st of December 2000) and *The National Order of "Faithful Service" in rank of "Commodore"* (6th of April 2010).

He had also received *The Gold Medal* and the title of *Doctor honoris causa* of the "Ștefan cel Mare" University of Suceava (12th of April 2011).

He had been awarded *The Prize of The Academy of Medical Sciences for the Research - Innovation Activity in the Field of Medicine* (8th of December 2000).

He had been conferred *The Honorary Diploma of The "Titu Maiorescu" University* in Bucharest (18th of December 2000) and *The Diploma for Academic Excellence* of the "Carol Davila" University of Medicine and Pharmacy in Bucharest (December 2004), the *Top Physicians* award (31st of January 2008), *The Centenary Gold Medal of "Mărcuța Church",* the award *„Romanian Oscar for Excellence" the fifteenth edition,* 2012, *The "Excellence Diploma" for Outstanding Merits in the Entire Activity* issued by the Romanian College of Physicians (2013), *The Diploma of Excellence* awarded by The Romanian Academy of Sciences de Academia (29th of May 2013), *The Diploma of Excellence* awarded at the *"Leon Dănăilă - 80 years of age Jubilee Symposium"* by The Academy of Medical Sciences (12th of June 2013), *The Diploma of Excellence* awarded by the de "Ștefan Odobleja" Foundation in Drobeta Tunu-Severin (25th of October 2013), *The "Ștefan Odobleja" Diploma of Excellence* for the outstanding contribution to the medical research and practice, on the occasion of the re-establishment of the "Ștefan Odobleja" Academy (25th of October 2013).

He is elected in the *"Honorary List for the Romanian Award for Excellence and the Elites of the Last Millennium"* (December 2013^, *Secretary-General of the United Cultural Convention* - Cambridge, England (25th of September 2014), *The Diploma Excellentiae* of the "Carol Davila" University of Medicine and Pharmacy in Bucharest (2014), *The Diploma of Excellence* awarded by the Romanian Society of Criminology (2014), *"The personally engraved Worldwide Laureate"* Green marble award Cambridge England (IBC) (2014), *Diploma* (SSMB, „Days of Medical Education" 2015), where in 7 April he lectured to approximate 700 students, *The Diploma of Excellence* - UMF Targu Mures (2015), where in 23 April 2015 he lectured to approximate 1000 students in the National Theatre of Târgu Mureş, *"Excellence in Medicine"* Ministerul Sănătăţii 2015, *The Gold Medal* awarded by AOS (2015), *The Silver Medal* awarded by ASM (2015), with the occasion the eight decade from founded, *Honorary Medal* awarded by The "Titu Maiorescu" University (2015), occasion to reach a 25 years from it founded, *United Cultural Convention* - Secretary General.

He had also been conferred the title of Honorary Citizen of the town of Darabani (21st of May 1999), that of Honorary Citizen of the town of Dorohoi (18th of September 1999) and of Honorary Graduate of the "Grigore Ghica V.V." High School in Dorohoi (18th of September 1999).

He had been nominated as World Laureate by the American Biographical Institute in 1999, and in 2003, The World Nations Congress of ABI in the United States had awarded him the title of Senator.

In 2001 he had received the *Noble Prize* awarded by the "United Cultural Convention", and in 2002 he had been awarded the title of *Cavalier* conferred by the "Académie Européenne d'Informatisation"

(Updated 27th of May 2015)

XLIII

Foreword

As a neurosurgeon who has performed over 40 000 surgeries on the central and peripheral nervous system during my 50 years of continuous neurosurgical activity, I can comprehend the structural and functional complexity of the brain.

In order not to disturb the highly functional areas of the central nervous system, I was forced to get familiar with the details of the brain map, which, taking into consideration my experience, varies from individual to individual, and I can say that each person, healthy or sick, is unique.

I have been an assiduous reader of many books and papers in order to have a better documentation in this area, but I could not find any manual or book to contain relatively complete and up-to-date information on the anatomy and physiology of the brain. The existing neuroanatomy textbooks are not thorough enough, in my opinion, as they do not explain the morphological and neurophysiological complexity of white and grey matter.

That is why – and also because of practical reasons – I decided to gather information from books and recent papers and make a precise and complete synthesis of the structure and functions of the brain, the most complex system in the universe, without claiming originality. I carefully and respectfully quoted from the works of great neuroanatomists and I mentioned them in references.

So, this book is not written by a neuroanatomist, but it represents a textbook assembled by me as a neurosurgeon, as I have often had to deal with a variety of known or still unknown, normal or abnormal activities of the brain during my numerous years of activity.

To keep up with the vast literature in this research field, and with the investigations of the brain as a whole has been for me a real challenge or better said an impossible task, an unreachable goal.

The clinical pre- and post-op information has been of great help in understanding the basic scientific concepts and the way in which the central nervous system, especially the brain, operates and interacts in the presence of various internal and external harmful factors, or in abnormal, pathological situations.

The turmoil of my life as a neurosurgeon came with sacrifices, sleepless nights, but also with the great satisfaction of saving many lives, which has helped keeping my physical and moral tonus.

The struggle with the mentalities, with the hostility of people and especially that one of my colleagues sometimes brought me down, but never made me give up.

I have lived desolation and bitterness of painful defeats, but I have also won extremely tough battles with the diseases I fought. I considered neurosurgery to be a true religion to which I dedicated my entire life. I was selfish with myself but an offering person to the ones around me. I have worked a lot without receiving help from anyone and I became a well known name forgetting about my own life. I have always struggled to conquer centimetre by centimetre the way I had chosen in life. But, in order to study and write, I had to isolate myself from the surrounding reality and carry on with my existence in a rather symbolic way.

Patients, beginning with the adult, paediatric or elderly population admitted into the hospital with various cognitive disorders caused by cerebral tumours, vascular diseases, parasites, traumatisms, developmental or psychiatric disorders and degenerative diseases have always been thoroughly investigated and helped. The evaluation and diagnosis of their cognitive topography represented the starting point for an early rehabilitating treatment. In order to achieve this I carefully studied the neuropathology of different morbid entities as well as their consequences upon the highly functional activities of the cerebral cortex.

When I decided how to operate on a patient I have always considered the post-surgical quality of life. The main goal of neurosurgical operations was to re-establish patients' possibility of going back to school, to work, and their ability to carry on their own business, to drive and thus to have their own independence.

Publishing this book concurs with an enormous explosion of knowledge about the morphology and physiology of the central nervous system and its vast reciprocal connections and plasticity. Consequently, I found it hard to keep up with the multitude of works published during the past ten years about functional neuroimaging, neuropharmacology, computational modulation, rehabilitation methods, theories of thinking, of memory, attention, frontal functions, language etc., as well as the structures and the immense number of neural connections and columns that build them.

First, as a graduate of the Faculty of Psychology and then as a Professor in neuropsychology at the same university, I had to prove accurate knowledge about the central nervous system, its macroscopic, cellular and chemical architecture, primary and associative areas for sight, hearing, taste, motion, sensibility, visceral, endocrine and speech functions.

While psychology is the science that studies behavior, neuropsychology deals with its neural and neuronal determinants. Modern neuroimagistics make the scanning of healthy persons possible, clarifying the brain - behavior interrelationships. It also helps us to comprehend the normal cerebral processes which concern language, recognizing objects, attention, memory, thinking and control of movements.

These were the reasons that determined me for a period of 7 years, day by day, to gather the most significant and up-to-date information regarding the activity of all areas, structures, regions and cerebral connections – realizing, however, that I cannot exhaust all subjects.

This book, which includes an immense material, starts with the history of neuroscience, data and ideas referring to soul, mind and brain, the way they have been imagined and conceived by healers, witches and philosophers since old times.

XLV

Nevertheless, the book aims at revealing some basic and recent data about mind and brain, making them accessible to students, doctors, psychologists, biologists and all those interested in this vast topic and research field – the brain – who are studying by themselves.

The information included in the entire content of this book which comes from studies on animals, primates and humans is non-exhaustive. Critics, comments, corrections and suggestions from neuroanatomists, neurophysiologists, colleagues and all those who come in contact and use this book are welcome.

No matter how much effort I made writing this book, from various reasons, objective or subjective, I keep the doors open to corrections, additions and novelty and, why not, to reinterpretation.

It's me who will do it or maybe others will do it better than I did.

I wish to gratefully acknowledge the kind assistance of Mrs. Stela Georgescu in typing and correcting the text on the computer and her great effort in arranging the illustrations and the ample bibliography.

I also thank to Dorel Arsene, MD, for his generosity and attention during typing a large part of the text on the computer, and to Mrs. Olga Dumitru, editorial assistant, for her care and accuracy in correcting the entire text and references.

Chapter 18

OCCIPITAL LOBE

Introduction

On the lateral surface of the brain, there are no definite boundaries between the occipital lobes and the parietal and temporal lobes.

The occipital lobe encompasses the most posterior portion of the human cerebral cortex and is primarily responsible for vision. The surface area of the human occipital lobe encompasses approximately 12% of the total surface area of the neocortex of the human brain. Vision begins with the spatial, temporal, and chromatic pattern of light falling onto photoreceptors of the retina and culminates in the perception of the properties of the objects and surfaces within the world around us (Deyoe, 2002). To permit these more cognitive functions, the occipital lobe is heavily interconnected with other lobes of the brain, especially the parietal and temporal lobes, as well as with an array of subcortical structures. Through these connections, the results of visual processing in the occipital lobe enter into and can be influenced by more general processes involved in goal-directed, motivated behavior and "thinking" (Kaas, 1997).

Traditionally, occipital cortex has been subdivided into anatomically distinct regions based on cytoarchitecture. Primary visual cortex is the most distinct region of the occipital lobe. It is also known as striate cortex due to the stria of Gennari, a band of myelinated axons running horizontally in layer 4B which demarcates the extent of striate cortex within and adjacent to the calcarine sulcus.

VISUAL PATHWAYS

The retina arises as an evaginated portion of the brain, the optic pouch, which secondarily is invaginated to form the two layered optic cup. The axons of ganglion cells, at first unmyelinated, are arranged in fine radiating bundles which run parallel to the retinal surface and converge at the optic disk (or optic papilla) to form the optic nerve. This region of the retina contains no photoreceptors and, because it is insensible to light, produces the perceptual phenomenon known as the blind spot. It is the site from which the ophtalmic artery and veins enter (or leave) the eye. The subarachnoid space surrounding the optic nerve is continuous with that of the brain. As a result, increases in intracranial pressure can be detected as papilledema, a swelling of the optic disk.

Optic nerves enter the cranial cavity through the optic foramina and unite to form optic chiasma, beyond which they are continued as the optic tracts. In humans, about 60% of these fibres cross in the chiasma, while the other 40% continue toward the thalamus and midbrain targets on the same side. So, within the chiasma a partial deccussation occurs, the fibres from the nasal halves of the retina crossing to the opposite side, and those from the temporal halves of the retina remaining uncrossed. In binocular vision each visual field, right or left, is projected upon portion of both retinae. Thus the images of objects in the right field of vision are projected on the right nasal and the left temporal half of the retina. In the chiasma the fibres from those two retinal portions are combined to form the left optic tract, which represents the complete right field of vision. By this arrangement the whole right field of vision is projected upon the left hemisphere, and the left visual field upon the right hemisphere. Once past of the chiasma, the ganglion cell axons on each side form the optic tract. Thus, the optic tract, unlike the optic nerve, contains fibres from both eyes. The partial crossing of ganglion cell axons at the optic chiasma allows information from corresponding points on the two retinas to be processed by approximately the same cortical site in each hemisphere.

On each side the optic tract sweeps outward and backward, encircling the hypothalamus and the rostral portion of the crus cerebri (Hubel, 1988).

The ganglion cell axons in the optic tract reach a number of structures in the diencephalon and midbrain. The major target in the diencephalon is the dorsal lateral geniculate nucleus of the thalamus. The lateral geniculate nucleus gives rise to the geniculocalcarine tract which forms the last relay to the visual cortex. Neurons in the lateral geniculate nucleus, like their counterparts in the thalamic relays of other sensory systems, send their axons to the cerebral cortex *via* the internal capsule (Hubel and Wiesel, 1968; Hubel, 1988).

The superior colliculus is concerned with detection of movement with the visual fields and with the coordination of eye and head movements. The pretectal region is concerned with the pupillary light reflex (Fig. 18.1).

Geniculocalcarine tract arises from the lateral geniculate nucleus, passes through the retrolenticular portion of the internal capsule and forms the optic radiations, which end in the striate cortex (also referred to as Brodmann's area 17 or V1), which lies largely along and within the calcarine fissure in the occipital lobe.

The retinogeniculostriate pathway, or primary visual pathway, convey information that is essential for most of what is thought of seeing.

Thus, damage anywhere along this route results in serious visual impairment.

A second major target of the ganglion cell axons is a collection of neurons that lies between the thalamus and the midbrain in a region known as the pretectum. The pretectum is important as the coordinating center for the pupillary light reflex. The initial component of the pupillary light reflex pathway is a bilateral projection from the retina to the pretectum.

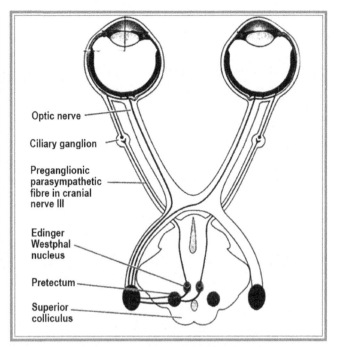

Fig. 18.1. The circuitry responsible for the pupillary light reflex. The pathway includes bilateral projections from the retina to the pretectum and projections from the pretectum to the Edinger-Westphal nucleus. Neurons in the Edinger-Westphal nucleus terminate in the ciliary ganglion, and neurons in the ciliary ganglion innervate the pupillary constrictor muscles. Notice that the afferent axons activate both Edinger-Westphal nuclei *via* the neurons in the pretectum (after Purves et al., 2004).

Pretectal neurons, in turn, project to the Edinger-Westphal nucleus, a small group of nerve cells that lie close to the nucleus of the oculomotor nerve (cranial nerve III) in the midbrain. The Edinger-Westphal nucleus contains the preganglionic parasympathic neurons that send their axons *via* the oculomotor nerve to terminate on neurons in the ciliary ganglion. Neurons in the ciliary ganglion innervate the constrictor muscle in the iris, which decreases the diameter of the pupil when activated. The reduction in the diameter of the pupil occurs when sufficient light falls on the retina.

Under normal condition, the pupils of both eyes respond identically regardless of which eye is stimulated; that is, light in one eye produces constriction of both the stimulated eye (the direct response) and the unstimulated eye (the consensual response). Comparing the response in the two eyes is often helpful in localizing a lesion (Horton, 1992; Hattar et al., 2002).

There are several other important targets of retinal ganglion cell axons. One is suprachiasmatic nucleus of the hypothalamus. The retinohypothalamic pathway is the route by which variation of light levels influences the broad spectrum of visceral functions that are entrained to the day / night cycle. Another target is the superior colliculus, which coordinates head and eye movements to visual (as well as other) targets (Horton, 1992; Hendry and Reid, 2000; Hattar et al., 2002; Purves et al., 2004).

So there is a diversity of ganglion cell types that provide information appropriate to the functions of these different targets. They include not only differences in ganglion cell synaptic connections, but in the locus of the phototransduction event itself. Unlike the majority of ganglion cells, which depend on rods and cones for their sensitivity to light, the ganglion cells that project to the hypothalamus and pretectum express their own light-sensitive photopigment (melanopsin) and are capable of modulating their response to changes in light levels in the absence of signals from rods and cones (Hattar et al., 2002).

Visual field topography

Traditionally, visual field topography has been a primary source of information used to identify and map different visual areas in animals.

In general, there are two types of photoreceptors: cones and rods. Cones are color-selective, less sensitive to dim light than rods, and important for detailed color vision in daylight. Cones are densely packed into fovea, the central part of the retina that we use to look directly at objects to perceive their fine details. Rods contain a different photopigment that is much more sensitive to low levels of light. Rods are important for night vision (dark adaptation). Curiously, there are no rods in the fovea, only cones, and the proportion of rods increases in the periphery. The signals from photoreceptors are processed by a collection of intermediary neurons, bipolar cells, horizontal cells, and amacrine cells, before they reach the ganglion cells, the final processing stage in the retina before signals leave the eye.

The actual cells bodies of ganglion cells are located in the retina, but those cells have long axons that leave the retina at the blind spot and form the optic nerve. Each ganglion cell receives excitatory inputs from a collection of rods and cones – the distillation of information forms a receptive field (Tong and Pearson, 2007). Lateral inhibition (Kuffler, 1953) is important for enhancing the neural representation of edges, regions of an image where the light intensity sharply changes.

As a general rule, information from the left half of the visual world, whether it originates from the left or right eye, is represented in the right half of the brain, and vice versa. Each eye sees a part of visual space that defines its visual field (Fig. 18.2).

A vertical line divides the retina into nasal and temporal division and the horizontal line divides the retina into superior and inferior divisions. Vertical and horizontal lines in visual space intersect at the point of fixation (the point of visual space that falls on the fovea) and define quadrants of the visual field. So, objects in the temporal part of the visual field are seen by the nasal part of the retina, and objects in the superior part of the visual field are seen by the inferior part of the retina.

With both eyes open, the two foveas are normally aligned on a single target in visual space, causing the visual fields of both eyes to overlap extensively. This binocular field of view consists of two symmetrical visual hemifields (left and right). The left binocular hemifield includes the nasal visual field of the right eye and the temporal visual field of the left eye; the right hemifield includes the temporal visual field of the right eye and the nasal visual field of the left eye.

The temporal visual fields are more extensive than the nasal visual fields, reflecting the size of the nasal and temporal retinas respectively. As a result, vision in the periphery of the field of view is strictly monocular, mediated by the most medial portion of the nasal retina (Purves et al., 2004).

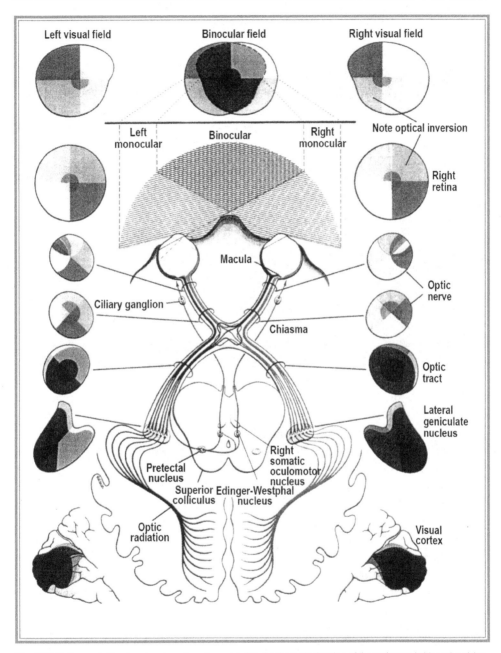

Fig. 18.2. Pathways in the visual system: from the eye to V1. A schematic drawing of the pathways in binocular vision, showing the visual input from left and right visual fields (top of figure) through the optic nerve and optic tract (center of figure), continuing on through the LGN and onto V1 in the cortex (bottom of the figure). (Source: Standring, 2005).

Most of the rest of the field of view can be seen by both eyes; i.e., individual points in visual space lie in the nasal visual field of one eye and the temporal visual field of the other. However, the inferior nasal fields are less extensive than the superior nasal field, and consequently the binocular field of view is smaller in the lower visual field than in the upper.

The topographic arrangement of photoreceptors in the retina is maintained in the central connection. Neurons representing the vertical midline of the visual field are represented in both hemispheres and are functionally linked by interhemispheric, callosal connections. Anyhow, visual space is systematically distorted in the cortical representation.

Ganglion cells that lie in the nasal division of each retina give rise to axons that cross in the chiasma, while those that lie in the temporal retina give rise to axons that remain on the same side. Images of objects in the left visual hemifield fall on the nasal retina of the left eye and the temporal retina of the right eye, and the axons from ganglion cells in these regions of the two retinas project through the right optic tract. Thus, unlike the optic nerve, the optic tract contains the axons of ganglion cells that originate in both eyes and represent the contralateral field of view.

For the primary visual pathway, the map of the contralateral hemifield that is established in the lateral geniculate nucleus is maintained in the projection of the lateral geniculate nucleus to the striate cortex.

Functional neuroimaging (fMRI) has been used to chart the retinotopic organization of visual areas in the human occipital lobe (Zilles and Clarke, 1997). The resulting flat maps show bands of activation corresponding to alternating representations of quadrants of the horizontal and vertical meridian. On the medial wall of the hemisphere, these bands are oriented roughly parallel to the calcarine sulcus (Deyoe and van Essen, 1988; Deyoe, 2002).

From maps of the meridian representations, it is possible to estimate the locations of the borders between different visual areas.

Thus the fovea is represented in the posterior part of the striate cortex, whereas the more peripheral regions of the retina are represented in progressively more anterior parts of the striate cortex. The upper visual field is mapped below the calcarine sulcus, and the lower visual field above it. Like the representation of the hand region in the somatic sensory cortex, the representation of the macula is therefore disproportionately large, occupying most of the caudal pole of the occipital lobe.

Anatomy

The occipital lobes form the posterior pole of the cerebral hemispheres, lying under the occipital bone at the back of the skull. Viewed from the medial surface of the cerebral hemisphere, the occipital lobe is distinguished from the parietal lobe by the parieto-occipital sulcus (Fig. 18.3). No clear landmarks separate the occipital cortex from the temporal or parietal cortex on the lateral surface of the hemisphere, however, because the occipital tissue merges with the other regions. For practical purposes, an imaginary line running laterally from the dorsal tip of the parieto-occipital sulcus to the preoccipital notch is considered the effective boundary separating the occipital lobe from the parietal and temporal lobes.

The lack of clear landmarks makes it difficult to define the extent of the occipital areas precisely and has led to much confusion about the exact boundaries.

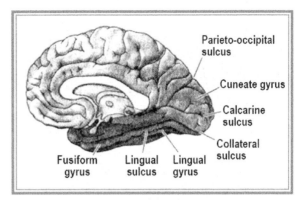

Fig. 18.3. Medical view of the occipital lobe, illustrating the major landmarks (Source: Kolb and Whishaw, 2003).

Within the visual cortex, there are three clear landmarks. The most prominent is the calcarine sulcus, which is flanked above by the cuneus and below by the lingula, and which contains much of the primary cortex. The calcarine fissure divides the upper and lower halves of visual world. On the ventral surface of the hemisphere there are two gyri (lingual and fusiform). The lingual gyrus, separated from the more laterally placed fusiform gyrus by the collateral sulcus, includes part of visual cortical regions V2 and VP, whereas V4 is in the fusiform gyrus.

The fusiform gyrus is then bounded laterally by the occipitotemporal sulcus, although this sulcus tends to be variable and interrupted as it extends posteriorly toward the occipital pole.

The lateral surface of the occipital lobe is especially variable from individual to individual.

Consequently, the lateral occipital gyrus can be irregular and can be split by the lateral occipital sulcus, which has several important variants, sometimes appearing as one, two, or even three small sulci running approximately in the anterior-posterior direction. Most dorsally on the lateral surface there is the transverse occipital sulcus, which often forms the most posterior end of the intraparietal sulcus.

Cytoarchitecture

As for all neocortex, the occipital gray matter is laminated, though the criteria for identifying and naming different layers have varied considerably. The monkey occipital cortex was first divided by Brodmann into three regions (areas 17, 18, and 19), but studies using imaging, physiological, and even anatomical techniques have produced much finer subdivisions.

Although the map is still not complete, the consensus is that the occipital cortex contains at least nine different visual areas (V1, V2, V3, VP, V3a, V4d, V4v, DP, and MT also known as V5) (Tootell and Hadjikhani, 2001) (Fig. 18.4).

The precise locations of the human homologues are still not settled. In a map constructed by Tootell and Hadjikhani there are included all the monkey areas as well as an additional color-sensitive area (V8) (Fig. 18.5).

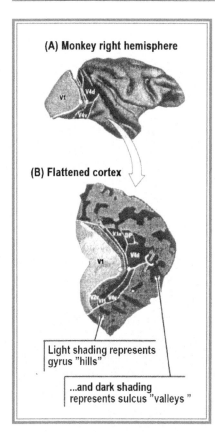

(A) Monkey right hemisphere

(B) Flattened cortex

Light shading represents gyrus "hills"

...and dark shading represents sulcus "valleys"

Fig. 18.4. Topography of the visual cortex of the macaque monkey.
(A) A nearly normal rendition of the lateral surface of the brain in which the sulci are opened slightly. (B) A flattened cortical surface showing both the lateral and medial regions. The shaded areas represent regions that are normally curved up (gyri) or down (sulci). The asterisks refer to the foveal representation in areas B1 and V4. (after Tootell and Hadjikhani, 2001.

Fig. 18.5. Tomography of the human visual cortex. (A) A nearly normal rendition of the lateral surface of the brain in which the sulci are opened slightly. (B) The medial surface in which the sulci are opened slightly. (C) A flattened cortical surface showing both the lateral and medial regions. The shaded areas represent regions that are normally curved up (gyri) or down (sulci). The asterisks refer to the foveal representation in areas V11 and V4. (after Tootell and Hadjikhani, 2001).

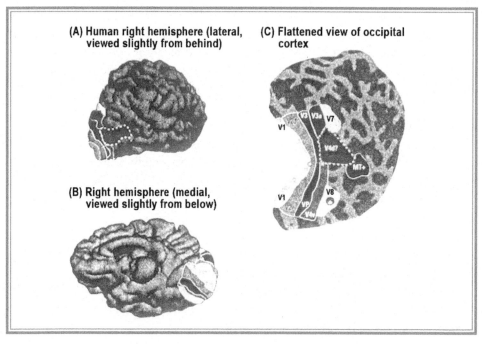

(A) Human right hemisphere (lateral, viewed slightly from behind)

(B) Right hemisphere (medial, viewed slightly from below)

(C) Flattened view of occipital cortex

Some of the areas contain a complete visual field, whereas others have only an upper or lower visual field. This distinction is curious, and Previc (1990) has suggested that the upper and lower fields may have different functions, with the upper more specialized for visual search and recognition and the lower specialized for visuomotor guidance.

Primary visual cortex is the most cytoarchitecturally distinct region of the occipital lobe. It is also known as striate cortex, due to the stria of Gennari, which can be identified even in a cross section of freshly cut tissue (Fig. 18.6).

Fig. 18.6. The visual cortex is highly laminated, as can be seen in a cell body stain (left) or a myelin stain (right) in these sections from a monkey brain. Because of the distinct stripes, the visual cortex is sometimes called the striate cortex (after Kolb and Wishaw, 2003).

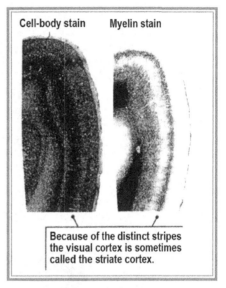

Cell-body stain   Myelin stain

Because of the distinct stripes the visual cortex is sometimes called the striate cortex.

This band of myelinated axons running horizontally in layer 4B demarcates the extent of striate cortex within, and adjacent to, the calcarine sulcus.

Cytoarchitectural differences among visual areas outside the striate cortex (known as extrastriate cortex) tend to be less obvious and more inconsistent, perhaps accounting for significant differences in the accounts of cytoarchitectonic parcellation of occipital cortex by early investigators.

One of the most widely used cytoarchitectonic schemes for subdividing cerebral cortex has been that of Brodmann. According to him, striate cortex is designated area 17 and is immediately surrounded by area 18, which in turn is bounded by area 19. And the portion of Brodmann area 37 may also be included in what is defined here as occipital cortex.

Except for visual areas 17 and 18, Brodmann's areas often correspond poorly with functional distinction identified by more modern techniques such as neuroimaging. This has resulted in diminished use of Brodmann's nomenclature as a basis for describing the functional organization of visual cortex (Fig. 18.7).

Distribution of myelinated fibres within the cortical gray matter has been successful in delineating some functionally defined visual areas. This is certainly the case for the stria of Gennari, which distinguishes the primary visual cortex.

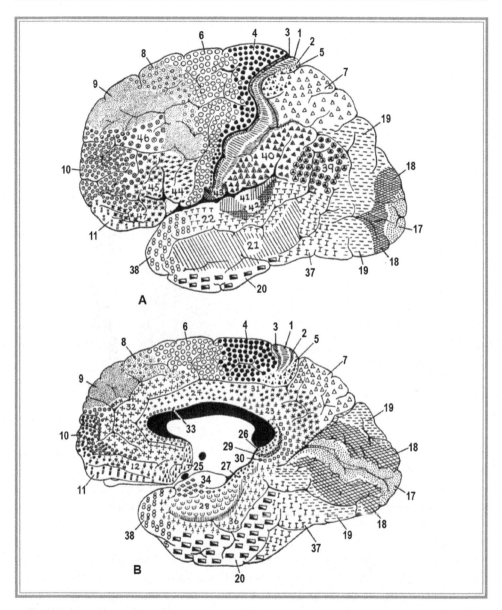

Fig. 18.7. Cytoarchitectural map of human cortex. A, Convex surface; B, medial surface (after Brodmann, 1909).

So, from lateral geniculate nucleus (LGN), neurons send their signals to the primary visual cortex, called V1, because it is the first cortical visual area. The left LGN projects to V1 in the left hemisphere which contains a retinotopic map of the entire right visual field.

The right LGN project to the right V1 which contains a map of the entire left visual field.

Its complex laminar organization is probably the most distinct of all cortical areas. Although we usually say that the cortex has six layers, it is possible to see many more in area V1, partly because layer IV alone features four distinct layers (Kolb and Whishaw, 2003).

Another surprising feature of area V1 is that, although it appears to be anatomically homogeneous, it can be shown to actually be heterogeneous by staining it for the enzyme cytochrome oxidase, which is crucial in making energy available to cells.

Regions of cytochrome-rich areas known as lobes take part in color perception and the interlobes have a role in form and motion perception (Kolb and Whishaw, 2003).

Neurons in V1 are sensitive to a whole host of visual features, not seen in LGN. One of the most important visual features is orientation (Hubel and Wiesel, 1962, 1968). Some V1 neurons respond best to vertical lines, some to 20-degree tilted lined, others to horizontal lines and so forth.

V1 neurons are also sensitive to many other visual features besides orientation (Hubel and Wiesel, 1968). Some neurons respond best to a particular direction of motion, such as upward, leftward or downward motions. Other neurons respond best to particular colors or color differences.

Finally, some neurons respond best to particular binocular disparities (Barlow et al., 1967; Cumming, 2002), which refer to the degree of alignment between images in the two eyes. Small displacements between images in the two eyes are what allows us to perceive stereo-depth when we look at objects with both eyes open.

V1 neurons provide a neural representation of the orientation of visual features that comprise the contours and shapes of the object. From the LGN, V1, V4 to the ventral temporal cortex, you can see that neurons gradually respond to motor complex stimuli from one area to the next (Tong and Pearson, 2007).

So, to summarize, neurons from V1 have small receptive fields that are sensitive to orientation, color, motion or binocular disparity. V1 is functionally heterogeneous.

After visual signals are analyzed in V1, they are sent to higher visual areas for further processing.

Extrastriate visual areas – outside of V1

V1 sends feedforward signals to many higher visual areas including areas such as V2, V3, V4 and motion-sensitive area MT, to name a few (Felleman and Van Essen, 1991).

Area V2 is also heterogeneous when stained with cytochrome oxidase, but instead of lobes, stripes are revealed (Purves et al., 1992). One type, the "thin stripe", takes part in color perception. Two other types, known as thick stripes and pale stripes, have roles in form and motion perception, respectively. The distinction of color function across much of the occipital cortex and beyond (i.e., areas V1, V2, V4, V8) is important because, until recently, the perception of form or movement was believed to be colorblind.

It has now become clear that color vision is integral to analysis of position, depth, motion, and structure of objects (Tanaka et al., 2001). Although the relative amount of color processing certainly varies across occipital regions, with area V4 having color processing as its major function, the processing of color-related information does more than simply allow us to tell red from green. The appreciation of color also enriches our capacity to detect motion, depth, and position.

An example of the advantage of color vision can be seen in the type of photoreceptors in primates.

Sumer and Mollan (2000) found that the color system of primates is optimized for differentiating edible fruits from a background of leaves.

This ability to differentiate is an important advantage when having to select edible fruits from a complex scene and is especially important when the fruits are partly occluded by leaves, which is fairly common. In fact, color provides important information for object recognition in such cases.

According to Zilles and Clarke (1997), dense myelin staining characterizes the middle temporal visual area hMT+, located in the lateral occipital cortex near the confluence of the occipital, temporal, and parietal lobes. In macaque monkeys the third visual area, V3, can also be identified by heavy myelin staining, though it is not clear whether this is also in humans. Human visual areas in lateral cortex appear to be displaced posteriorly toward the occipital pole or onto the medial occipital surface. For example, the hMT+ complex is located posterior to the superior temporal sulcus (STS) in human but it is buried deep within the STS in macaque. Most of the human retinotopic visual areas (V1, V2, V3-VP, V4, V3A) are located entirely or partially on the medial and ventral aspects of the occipital lobe. In macaques, they are located partly or completely on the lateral surface of the brain. This displacement of human visual areas places the foveal representation of the visual field at the occipital pole. Maps of visual field topography provide a good organizational framework for understanding the contributions of different areas to specific visual function such is color or movement perception.

The discovery of circumscribed zones of high cytochrome oxidase activity in striate cortex (puffs, blobs) and extrastriate cortex (V2 "stripes", V4 "patches") triggered the identification and characterization of functionally distinct "modules" within occipital visual areas that had previously been thought to be functionally homogeneous.

So, areas V1 and V2 are functionally heterogeneous and both segregate processing for color, form, and motion. In a sense, areas V1 and V2 appear to serve as little mail-boxes into which different types of information are assembled before being sent on to the more specialized visual areas.

From areas V1 and V2 flow three parallel pathways that convey different attributes of vision. The information derived from the blob area V1 goes to area V4, considered to be a color area. Cells in area V4 are not solely responsive to color, however; some cells respond to both form and color (Farah, 1984; Clarke and Miklossy, 1990; Barbur et al., 1993; Farah, 2000; Goodale, 2000; Kosslyn and Thompson, 2000).

Other information from area V1 (the magnocellular input) also goes to area V2 and then to area V5, which is specialized to detect motion. Finally, an input from area V1 and V2 to area V3 is connected with what Zeki calls "dynamic form" – that is, the shape of objects in motion. Thus, we see that vision begins in the primary cortex (V1), which has multiple functions, and then continues in more specialized zones (Zeki, 1993; Zeki et al., 1999).

It is not surprising to discover that selective lesions up the hierarchy in areas V3, V4, and V5 produce specific deficits in visual processing. People who suffer damage to area V4 are able to see only in shades of gray. Patients not only fail to perceive colors but also fail to recall colors from before their injuries or even to imagine colors. The loss of area V4 results in the loss of color cognition, or the ability to think about color (Meadows, 1974; Sacks and Wasserman, 1987; Tanaka et al., 2001; Tootell and Hadjikhani, 2001).

Similarly, a lesion in area V5 produces an inability to perceive objects in motion. Objects at rest are perceived but, when the objects begin to move, they vanish. In principle, a lesion in area V3 will affect from perception but, because area V4 also processes form, a rather large lesion of both V3 and V4 would be required to eliminate form perception (Zihl et al., 1983; Servas et al., 1993; Ungerleider and Haxby, 1994).

An important constraint of the function of areas V3, V4, and V5 is that all these areas receive major input from area V1. People with lesions in area V1, act as though they are blind, but visual input can still get through to higher levels-partly through small projections of the lateral geniculate nucleus to area V2 partly through projections from the colliculus to the thalamus (the pulvinar) to the cortex. This is the tectopulvinar pathway.

So, projections to the superior colliculus can reach the cortex through relays in the lateral posterior-pulvinar complex of the thalamus. Because this so-called tectopulvinar pathway constitutes the visual system in fish, amphibians and reptiles, we can expect it to be capable of a reasonably sophisticated vision. Because there are two visual pathways to the neocortex, complete destruction of the main pathway, the geniculostriate pathway, does not render a subject completely blind (Poggio, 1968; Kaas, 1987; Livingston and Hubel, 1988).

People with V1 lesions seem not to be aware of visual input and can be shown to have some aspects of vision only by special testing.

Area V1 thus appears to be primary for vision in yet another sense: V1 must function for the brain to make sense out of what the more specialized visual areas are processing. So, people with significant V1 damage are capable of some awareness of visual information, such as motion. Barbur and colleagues (1993) suggested that the integrity of area V3 may allow this conscious awareness, but this suggestion remains a hypothesis.

The functional organization of extrastriate visual areas

Anatomical and electrophysiological studies in monkeys have led to the discovery of multiple areas in the occipital, parietal, and temporal lobes that are involved in processing visual information (Fig. 18.8). Each of these areas contains a map of visual space, and each is largely dependent on the primary visual cortex for its activation (Felleman and Van Essen, 1991; Maunsell, 1992). Neurons in some of these regions are specialized for different aspects of the visual scene.

For example, the middle temporal area (MT) contains neurons that respond selectively to the direction of a moving edge without regard to its color. In contrast, neurons in another cortical area called V4 respond selectively to the color of visual stimulus without regard to its direction of movement.

So, damage to area MT leads to a specific impairment in a monkey's ability to perceive the direction of motion in a stimulus pattern, while other aspects of visual perception remain intact (Zihl et al., 1983; Schiller and Logothetis, 1990; Maunsell, 1992; Zeki, 1993; Chalupa and Werner, 2004).

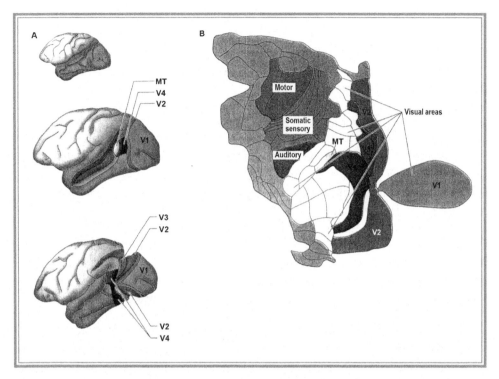

Fig. 18.8. Subdivisions of the extrastriate cortex in the macaque monkey. (A) Each of the subdivisions indicated contains neurons that respond to visual stimulation. Many are buried in sulci, and the overlying cortex must be removed in order to expose them. Some of more extensively studied extrastriate areas are specifically identified (V2, V3, V4 and MT). V1 is the primary visual cortex; MT is the middle temporal area. (B) The arrangement of extrastriate and other areas of neocortex in a flattened view of the monkey neocortex. There are at least 25 areas that are predominantly or exclusively visual in function, plus 7 other areas suspected to play a role in visual processing.
(A after Maunsell and Newson, 1987; B after Felleman and Van Essen, 1991).

Functional MRI studies have indicated a similar arrangement of visual areas within human extrastriate cortex (Sereno et al., 1995). Using retinotopically restricted stimuli it has been possible to localize at least 10 separate representations of the visual field (Fig. 18.9).

One of these areas exhibits a large motion-selective signal, suggesting that it is the homologue of the motion-selective middle temporal area described in monkeys. Another area exhibits color-selective responses, suggesting that it may be similar to V4 in non-human primates.

So, in clinical description, a well-studied patient, who suffered a stroke that damaged the extrastriate region thought to be comparable to area MT in the monkey, was unable to appreciate the motion of objects. The neurologist who treated her noted that she had difficulty in pouring tea into a cup because the fluid seemed to be "frozen". In addition, she could not stop pouring at the right time because she was unable to perceive when the fluid level had risen to the rim. The patient also had trouble following a dialogue because she could not follow the movement of the speaker's mouth. Crossing the street was potentially terrifying because she could not judge the movement of approaching cars.

1422

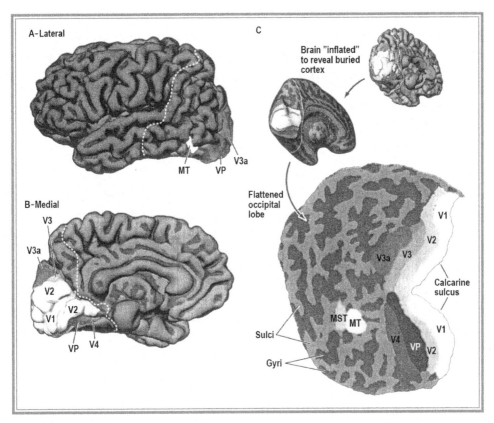

Fig. 18.9. Localization of multiple visual areas in the human brain using fMRI. (A, B) Lateral and medial views (respectively) or the human brain, illustrating the location of primary visual cortex (V1) and additional visual areas V2, V3, VP (ventral posterior area), V4, MT (middle temporal area), and MST (medial superior temporal area). (C) Unfolded and flattened view of retinotopically defined visual areas in the occipital lobe. Dark grey areas correspond to cortical regions that were buried in sulci; light regions correspond to regions that were located on the surface of gyri. Visual areas in humans show a close resemblance to visual areas originally defined in monkeys (after Sereno et al., 1995).

Her ability to perceive other features of the visual scene, such as color and form, was intact (Ungerleider and Mishkin, 1982; Zihl et al., 1983; Sereno et al., 1995; Tootell et al., 1996; Courtney and Ungerleider, 1997; Purves et al., 2004).

Another example of a specific visual deficit as a result of damage to extrastriate cortex is cerebral achromatopsia. These patients lose the ability to see the world in color, although other aspects of vision remain in good working order. The normal colors of a visual scene are described as being replaced by "dirty" shades of gray, much like looking at a poor quality black-and-white movie (Purves et al., 2004).

When achromatopsic individuals are asked to draw objects from memory, they have no difficulty with shapes, but are unable to appropriately color the objects they have represented (Purves et al., 2004).

It is important to distinguish this condition from the color blindness that arises from the congenital absence of one or more cone pigments in the retina. The discovery of the

1423

three human cone types and their different absorption spectra is correctly regarded, therefore, as the basis for human color vision. Nevertheless, how these human cone types and higher-order neurons they contact produce the sensation of color is still unclear.

A fundamental problem has been that, although the relative activities of three cone types can more or less explain the colors perceived in color-matching experiments performed in the laboratory, the perception of color is strongly influenced by the context.

The phenomena of color contrast and color constancy led to a heated, modern debate about how color percepts are generated that now spans several decades. For Land (1986), the answer lay in a series of ratiometric equations that could integrate the spectral returns of different regions over the entire scene. In achromatopsia, the three types of cones are functioning normally; it is damage to specific extrastriate cortical areas that renders the patient unable to use the information supplied by the retina (Purves et al., 2004).

Extrastriate cortical areas are organized into two largely separate systems that eventually feed information into cortical association areas in the temporal and parietal lobes.

One system, called the ventral stream, includes area V4 and leads from the striate cortex into the inferior part of the temporal lobe. This system is responsible for high-resolution form vision and object recognition. Neurons in the ventral stream exhibit properties that are important for object recognition, such as selectivity for shape, color, texture, and faces.

Lesions of the inferotemporal cortex produce profound impairments in the ability to perform recognition tasks but no impairment in spatial tasks.

The dorsal stream, which includes the middle temporal area, leads from striate cortex into the parietal lobe. This system is responsible for spatial aspects if vision such analysis of motion and positional relationships between objects in the visual scene (Purves et al., 2004).

Neurons in the dorsal stream show selectively for direction, and speed of movement.

Lesions of the parietal cortex severely impair an animal's ability to distinguish objects on the basis of their position, while having little effect on its ability to perform object recognition tasks.

These effects are remarkably similar to the syndrome associated with damage to the parietal and temporal lobes in humans.

These discoveries led to the concept that individual cortical visual areas can contain multiple, distinct processing pathways or streams, thereby extending (though not necessarily reiterating) the organizational principle of multiple processing pathway found in the retina and lateral geniculate nucleus.

Connectivity

By the late 1960s, the consensus was that the visual cortex is hierarchically organized, with visual information proceeding from area 17 to areas 18 and 19.

Each visual area was thought to provide some sort of elaboration on the processing of preceding area. This strictly hierarchical view is now considered too simple, and has been replaced by the notion of a distributed hierarchical process, with multiple parallel and interconnecting pathways at each level (Kolb and Whishaw, 2003).

So, the primary visual pathway from the retina to the dorsal lateral geniculate nucleus in the thalamus and on the primary visual cortex is the most important and certainly the most thoroughly studied. Different classes of neurons within this pathway encode the varieties of visual information-luminance, spectral differences, orientation, and motion.

The parallel processing of different categories of visual information continues in cortical pathways that extend beyond primary visual cortex, supplying a variety of visual areas in the occipital, parietal and temporal lobes.

Visual areas in the temporal lobe are primarily involved in object recognition, whereas those in the parietal lobe are concerned with motion. Normal vision depends on the integration of information in all these cortical areas.

So, distinct population of retinal ganglion cells sends their axons to a number of central visual structures that serve different functions. The most important projections are to the pretectum for mediating the pupillary light reflex, to the hypothalamus for the regulation of circadian rhythms, to the superior colliculus for the regulation of eye and head movements, and – most important at all – to the lateral geniculate nucleus for mediating vision and visual perception.

The primary visual pathway (retinogeniculostriate projection) is arranged topographically such that central visual structures contain an organized map of the contralateral visual field.

Visual input

According to Deyoe (2002) visual input from the retina is relayed through the lateral geniculate nucleus (LGN) of the thalamus to terminate in the primary visual cortex (striate, cortex, area 17, V1).

A second major pathway arises from retinal projections that bypass the LGN and project to the superior colliculus. The superior colliculus then projects to the thalamic pulvinar nucleus, which in turn distributes widely to the cortex of the occipital lobe. The layers in the lateral geniculate are distinguished on the basis of cell size. The geniculocortical pathways are subdivided into three main components associated with different neuronal subclasses in the retina and LGN (Maunssell, 1992).

Two ventral layers are composed of large neurons and are referred to as the magnocellular layers, while more dorsal layers are composed of small neurons and are referred to as the parvocellular layers. The axons of the relay cells in the magno- and parvocellular layers of the lateral geniculate nucleus terminate on distinct populations of neurons located in separate strata within layer 4 of striate cortex.

One pathway originates from small P-cells in the retina and is relayed through the parvocellular layers of the LGN to terminate in the layer $4C\beta$ of V1 and more sparsely in layers 4A and 6. A second pathway to striate cortex begins with large M-type retinal ganglion cells and is relayed through the magnocellular layers of the LGN to terminate in layer $4C\alpha$ accompanied by a light projection to layer 6.

The response properties of P and M ganglion cells provide important clues about the contributions of the magno- and parvocellular streams to visual perception.

M ganglion cells have larger receptive fields than P cells, and their axons have faster conduction velocities.

M and P ganglion cells also differ in ways that are not so obviously related to their morphology. M cells respond transiently to the presentation of visual stimuli, while P cells respond in a sustained fashion. Moreover, P ganglion cells can transmit information about color, whereas M cells cannot. P cells convey color information because of their receptive field centers and surroundings are driven by different classes of cones (i.e., cones responding with greatest sensitivity to short-, medium-, or long-wavelength light). For example, some P ganglion cells have centers that receive inputs from long wavelength ("red") sensitive cones and surrounds that receive inputs from medium-wavelength ("green") cones. Others have centers that receive inputs from "green cones" and surrounds from "red cones". As a result, P cells are sensitive to differences in the wavelengths of light striking their receptive field center and surroundings (Ungerleder and Mishkin, 1982; Purves and Lotto, 2003). Although M ganglion cells also receive inputs from cones, there is no difference in the type of cone input to the receptive field center and surroundings; the center and surroundings of each M cell receptive field is driven by all cone types.

A third source of projections to V1 comes from a class of small cells within the koniocellular (K) or intercalar layers of the LGN.

These neurons typically receive input from both the retina and the superior colliculus and terminate in the supragranular layers (above layer 4) of striate cortex. These afferents tend to cluster into "pufflike" regions of layers 2-3 that are also unique for their high levels of metabolic enzyme cytochrome oxidase (co).

Afferents to striate cortex *via* the alternate tectopulvinar pathway terminate most heavily in laminae 1 and upper 2-3 (Horton, 1992; Kaas, 1997; Zilles and Clarke, 1997).

So, neurons contributing to the K-cell pathway reside in the interlaminar zones that separate lateral geniculate layers. These neurons receive inputs from fine-caliber retinal axons and project in a patchy fashion to the superficial layers (layers II and III) of striate cortex. Although the contribution of the K-cell pathway to perception is not understood, it appears that some aspects of color vision, especially information derived from short-wavelength-sensitive cones, may be transmitted *via* the K-cell rather the P-cell pathway (Hubel and Wiesel, 1962; Hubel, 1988; Ungerleider and Mishikin, 1982; Berson, 2003; Chalupa and Werner, 2004).

Neurons of the P, M, and K pathways differ in their visual response properties. Neurons of the parvocellular path have smaller receptive fields, are often color opponents, and are well-suited for conveying information about fine spatial detail and color. Magnocellular neurons tend to have larger receptive fields, prefer low spatial frequencies, and have more transient responses. They tend to have the greatest sensitivity to luminance contrast, especially at low spatial frequencies and low luminance levels. They are optimized for processing rapid temporal changes such as flicker and movement (Fig. 18.10).

The function of K-pathway neurons has appeared to be a major determinant of co-puff cell properties and may play a key role in the modulation of responses evoked by the M and P pathways (Felleman and Van Essen, 1991; Casagrande and Kaas, 1994).

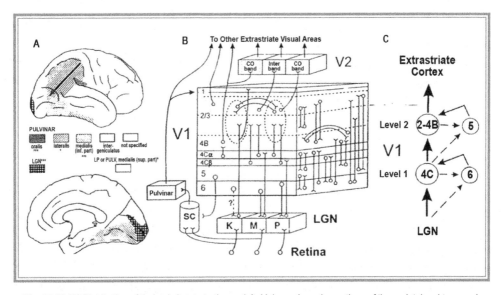

Fig. 18.10 (A) Distribution of thalamic inputs to the occipital lobe and nearby portions of the parietal and temporal lobes. (From Zilles and Clarke, 1997). **(B)** Concurrent input to V1 from K, M, and P retinogeniculate pathways with schematic of intrinsic circuitry and cytochrome oxidase defined puffs (dashed ellipses). V2 receives segregated input from different sets of output neurons in V1 and distributes projections to the different sets of extrastriate visual areas *via* distinct populations of output neurons in different cytochrome oxidase defined compartments. Such circuitry forms the anatomical basis of multiple concurrent processing pathways within and among occipital visual areas (Adapted from Casagrande and Kaas, 1994). **(C)** Functional interpretation of V1 circuitry (Adapted from Callaway, 1989). Abbreviations: LGN, lateral geniculate nucleus; sc, superior colliculus; K, konicellular; M, magnocellular; P, parvocellular.

So, although these three pathways are distinct, their functional capabilities can overlap significantly. It is primarily at the extremes of spatial and temporal frequencies that the M- and P-cell capabilities are most different.

Both M and P pathways may contribute to processing intermediate spatial and temporal frequencies, but P-cell will tend to dominate for high spatial frequencies that are slowly varying. Conversely, magnocellular neurons will respond better than P-cells at low spatial frequencies that are rapidly varying. Chromatically, P-cell color opponency appears to be critical for hue discrimination, but M-cells can respond more strongly to some wavelengths than others, though they are not opponent and their tuning is typically broader than that of P-cells. Under natural viewing conditions, all three inputs to the visual cortex are likely to be concurrently active. Under extreme visual conditions, the specialized capabilities of one or another of the pathways may take over and thereby extend the range of useful sight (Horton, 1992; Callaway, 1998; Deyoe, 2002).

Thus the retinogeniculate pathway is composed of parallel magnocellular and parvocellular streams that convey distinct types of information to the initial stages of cortical processing. Damage anywhere along the primary visual pathway which includes the optic nerve, optic tract, lateral geniculate nucleus, optic radiation, radiation, and striate cortex, results in a loss of vision confined to the predictible region of visual space.

Damage to the magnocellular layers has little effect on visual acuity or color vision, but sharply reduces the ability to perceive rapidly changing stimuli. In contrast, damage to the parvocellular layers has no effect on motion perception, but severely impairs visual acuity and color perception.

Visual information conveyed by the parvocellular stream is particularly important for high spatial resolution vision – the detailed analysis of the shape, size, and color of objects. The magnocellular stream, on the other hand, appears critical for tasks that require high temporal resolution, such as evaluating the location, speed and direction of a rapidly moving object (Zihl et al., 1983; Rodieck, 1998; Purves et al., 2004).

– In sum, primary visual pathway is composed of separate functional streams that convey information from different types of retinal ganglion cells to the initial stages of cortical processing. The magnocellular stream conveys information that is critical for detection of rapidly changing stimuli, the parvocellular stream mediates high acuity vision and appears to share responsibility for color vision with the konicellular stream. Beyond the striate cortex, parcellation of function continues in the ventral and dorsal streams that lead to the extrastriate and association areas in temporal and parietal lobes, respectively. Areas in the inferotemporal cortex are especially important in object recognition, whereas areas in the parietal lobe are critical for understanding the spatial relations between objects in the visual field.

Intrinsic circuitry

The retinal information relayed through the LGN is processed further by the intrinsic circuitry of V1 and then distributed to other cortical areas *via* output neurons in layers 2-3 (Callaway, 1998) (Fig. 18.11). Subcortical projections to the superior colliculus and feedback projection to LGN originate from layers 5 and 6 respectively.

It is through this selective distribution of visual information combined with the characteristics of local processing that different visual areas achieve their functional uniqueness.

Hubel and Wiesel (1962) used microelectrode recording to examine the properties of neurons in more central visual structures. The responses of neurons in the lateral geniculate nucleus were found to be remarkably similar to those in the retina, with a center-surrounded receptive field organization and selectivity for luminance increases or decreases. However, the small spots of light that were so effective at stimulating neurons in the retina and LGN were largely ineffective in the visual cortex. Instead, most cortical neurons in cats and monkeys responded vigorously to light-dark bars or edges, and only if the bars were presented at a particular range of orientations within the cell's receptive field.

The responses of a large number of single cells, Hubel and Wiesel (1962), demonstrated that all edge orientation was roughly equally represented in visual cortex. As a result, a given orientation in a visual scene appears to be "encoded" in the activity of a distinct population of orientation-selective neurons.

Hubel and Wiesel (1962) also found that there are subtly different subtypes within a class of neurons that preferred the same orientation. For example, the receptive field of some cortical cells, which they called simple cells, were composed of spatially separate "on" and "off" response zones, as if the "on" and "off" centers of lateral geniculate cells that supplied these neurons were arrayed in separate parallel bands. Other neurons, referred to as complex cells, exhibited mixed "on" and "off" responses throughout their receptive fields as if they received their inputs from a number of simple cells. Further analysis uncovered cortical neurons sensitive to the length of the bar of light, decreasing their rate of response when the bar exceeded a certain length. Still other cells responded selectively to the direction in which an edge moved across their receptive field. Anyhow, there is little doubt that the specificity of the receptive field properties of neurons in the striate cortex (and beyond) play an important role in determining the basic attributes of visual scenes (Purves et al., 2004).

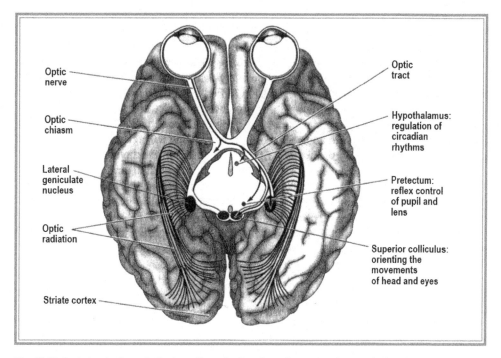

Fig. 18.11. Central projections of retinal ganglion cells. Ganglion cell axons terminate in the lateral geniculate nucleus of the thalamus, the superior colliculus, the pretectum, and the hypothalamus. For clarity, only the crossing axons of the right eye are shown (view is looking up at the inferior surface of the brain) (after Purves et al., 2004).

Another feature is the binocularity. Most cortical neurons have binocular receptive field, and these fields are almost identical, having the same size, shape, preferred orientation, and roughly the same position in the visual field of each eye.

Bringing together the inputs from the two eyes at the level of the striate cortex provides a basis for stereopsis, the special sensation of depth that arises from viewing nearby objects with two eyes instead of one. Because the two eyes look at the world from slightly different angles, objects that lie in front of or behind the plane of fixation project to noncorresponding points on the two retinas. For a small disturbance on either side of the plane of fixation, where the disparity between the two views of the world remains modest, a single image is perceived; the disparity between the two eye views of objects nearer or farther than the point of fixation is interpreted as depth (Purves et al., 2004).

An important advance in studies of stereopsis was made in 1959 when Julesz (1971, 1995) discovered an ingenious way of showing that stereoscopy depends on matching information seen by the two eyes without any prior recognition of what object(s) such matching might generate.

Although the neurophysiological basis of stereopsis is not understood, some neurons in the striate cortex and in other visual cortical areas have receptive field properties that make them good candidates for extracting information about binocular disparity.

Unlike many binocular cells whose monocular receptive fields sample the same region of visual space, these neurons have monocular fields that are slightly displaced (or perhaps differ in their internal organization) so that the cell is maximally activated by stimuli that fall on noncorresponding parts of the retinas (Purves et al., 2004).

Some of these neurons (so-called far cells) discharge to disparities beyond the plane of fixation, while others (near cells) respond to disparities in front of the plane of fixation. The pattern of activity in these different classes of neurons seems likely to contribute to the sensation of stereoscopic depth (Julesz, 1995; Tootell et al., 1996).

So, the intrinsic processing of V1 can be divided into two major levels. Input from LGN terminates at the first level in the different subdivisions of layer 4C. Information is then distributed primarily to level 2 output neurons within layers 2-3, and 4B. The latter output signals are modified by neurons in layers 5 and 6 that combine information about the inputs and outputs of each processing level and feed it back onto neurons at the same level (Zilles and Clarke, 1997; Kaas, 1997).

The laminar organization of V1 circuitry is complemented by horizontal connections that tend to connect functionally similar zones distributed within specific laminae.

In layers 2-3, long horizontal projections preferentially interconnect puff-like zones containing cells that have similar visual response properties and that are rich in the metabolic enzyme cytochrome oxidase.

Likewise, interpuff zones tend to be interconnected most strongly with other interpuff zones. In V2, a similar pattern of specific horizontal connections link co-defined compartments termed the thick-, thin-, and interstripe zones (Kaas, 1997; Callaway, 1998).

Together, the laminar specificity of vertical intrinsic connections and the functional specificity of horizontal connections provide an anatomical substrate for creating different subsets of output neurons whose visual response properties reflect different combinations of the P, M, and K afferent pathways, as well as modulatory effects of cortical feedback pathways and other subcortical inputs (Felleman and Van Essen, 1991; Zilles and Clarke, 1997; Kaas, 1997; Callaway, 1998).

Output neurons in layer 4B of V1 are dominated by M-pathway characteristics, as are the responses of the extrastriate visual areas, such as V2 thick stripes and area MT, to which the 4B cells project.

In contrast, output neurons in the interpuff regions of V1 tend to be strongly biased by P-cell characteristics, which are subsequently imparted to downstream visual areas such as V2 (thin- and interstripe compartments), VP, and V4. Output neurons in co-puff subdivisions tend to exhibit characteristics that appear to reflect a mixture of influences.

As a result, later processing stages, such as V4, can also be shown to exhibit a mixture of influences.

Overall, then the intrinsic circuitry of V1 acts to process, combine, and redistribute the visual information available in the different afferent pathways, thereby creating a new set of output signals that reflects the afferent inputs, but that also encodes more complex visual properties or features. Intrinsic circuitry within subsequent cortical processing stages, though less well-studied, presumably functions in a similar manner (Callaway, 1998; Deyoe, 2002).

Corticocortical connectivity

The output neurons of layers 2-3 and 4B of V1 selectively distribute different types of visual information to subsequent processing stage in extrastriate visual cortex. Each extrastriate visual area itself has unique feedforward and feedback connections within and, often, outside the occipital lobe. These patterns of selective connectivity are a primary determinant of the functional specificity of each visual area. Finally, interhemispheric projections through the corpus callosum connect the left and right halves of each visual area into a functionally integrated whole (Kaas, 1997; Callaway, 1998; Deyoe, 2002).

In monkey, connections among cortical visual areas tend to follow a consistent pattern of laminar distribution that differentiates forward, backward, and lateral types of connectivity (Felleman and Van Essen, 1991).

Generally, forward connections arise from neurons in layers 2-3 of the lower area and distribute to layer 4, tapering off into the lower reaches of layer 3 in the higher visual area. In some visual areas, however, forward projections can also originate in subgranular layers (below layer 4), though the terminal distribution remains targeted at layer 4 of the recipient area (Felleman and Van Essen, 1991; Callaway, 1998; Deyoe, 2002).

In contrast, backward-type projections tend to originate in layer 6 of the higher area and distribute outside the layer of the lower area, though some feedback projections can have a bilaminar origin. Finally, some visual areas have interconnections, whose terminal fields engage nearly all laminae. This distribution pattern is thought to characterize lateral connections between visual areas at approximately the same processing level. On the basis of these patterns of connectivity, it is possible to arrange the various occipital visual areas into a processing hierarchy (Felleman and Van Essen, 1991).

The extent to which this plan applies to human visual cortex is not known, though the overall scheme is likely to be similar (Deyoe and Van Essen, 1988).

This connectional hierarchy incorporates several important organizational features. First, it is generally consistent with the concept that successively more complex visual response properties are represented at successive processing stages, though a detailed comparison of the response properties of efferent neurons at one stage with the properties of recipient neurons at the next stage are generally lacking. Another key aspect of this cortico-cortical network is that nearly every forward connection is matched by a corresponding backward connection, thereby establishing reciprocity between visual areas.

Alternate connectivity schemes based on the strength of response correlation among visual areas rather than anatomical connectivity have stressed this reciprocity and suggest that a less hierarchical, more dynamic, processing network may also provide a useful model of occipital connectivity. A third important principle is that multiple, parallel pathways exist within, and between, each processing level (Felleman and Van Essen, 1991).

The arrangement of multiple parallel pathways within the cortex thereby provides a basis for concurrent processing of different aspects of the incoming visual information. Thus, the M, P, and K pathways that provide concurrent processing within the retina and LGN are further modified in V1 to yield a new set of signals.

These are then passed on to subsequent stages of processing *via* distinct sets of corticocortical output neurons. This same process is then reiterated at each successive processing stage (Felleman and Van Essen, 1991; Deyoe, 2002).

Not long ago, it seemed that these intracortical pathways were simply a continuation of the geniculostriate pathways – that is, the magnocellular pathway provided input to the dorsal stream and the parvocellular pathway provided input to the ventral stream. More recent work has indicated that the temporal pathway has clearly access to the information conveyed by both the magno- and parvocellular stream; and the parietal pathway, while dominated by inputs from the magnocellular stream, receives inputs from the parvocellular streams. Thus, interaction and cooperation between the magno- and parvocellular stream appear to be the rule in complex visual perception.

Patterns of organization within the sensory cortices: Brain modules

Observations over the last 40 years have made it clear that there is an iterated substructure within the sensory cortical maps. This substructure takes the form of units called modules, each involving hundreds or thousands of nerve cells in repeating patterns (Purves et al., 2004).

The observation that the somatosensory cortex comprises elementary units of vertically linked cells was first noted in the 1920s by Lorente de No (1949) based on his studies in the rat.

Mountcastle (1957, 1988) found that vertical microelectrode penetrations in the primary somatosensory cortex of the monkeys encountered cells that responded to the same sort of mechanical stimulus presented at the same location on the body surface. Soon after Mountcastle's pioneering work, Hubel and Wiesel (1977) discovered a similar arrangement in the cat primary visual cortex. These and other observations (Woolsey and Van der Loos, 1970; Hubel, 1988; Purves et al., 1992) led Mountcastle (1988) to the general view that "the elementary pattern of organization of the cerebral cortex is a vertically oriented column or cylinder of cells capable of input-output functions of considerable complexity". Since these discoveries, the view that modular circuits represent a fundamental feature of mammallian cerebral cortex has gained wide acceptance, and many such entities have now been described in various cortical regions (Figures 18.12 and 18.13).

Fig. 18.12. Examples of iterated, modular substructures in the mammallian brain. (A) Ocular dominance columns in layer IV in the primary visual cortex (V1) of a rhesus monkey. (B) Repeating units called "blobs" in layers II and III in V1 of the squirrel monkey. (C) Stripes in layers II and III in V2 of squirrel monkey. (D) Barrels in layer IV in primary somatic sensory cortex of a rat. (E) Glomeruli in the olfactory bulb of a mouse. (F) Iterated units called "barreloids" in the thalamus of a rat. These and other examples indicate that modular organization is commonplace in the brain. These units are of the order of one hundred to several hundred microns across. (From Purves et al., 1992).

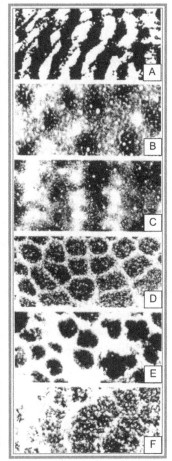

Fig. 18.13. Columnar organization of orientation selectivity in the monkey striate cortex. Vertical electrode penetrations encounter neurons with the same preferred orientations, whereas oblique penetrations show a systematic change in orientation across the cortical surface. The circles denote the lack of orientation-selective cells in layer IV. (after Purves et al., 2004).

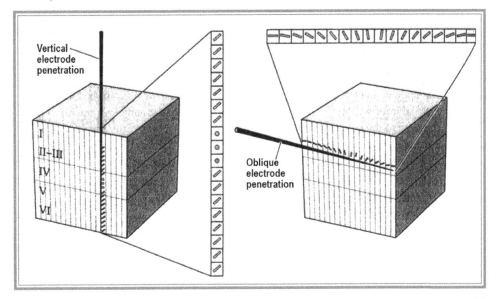

This patterned circuit has led to conclude that modules are a fundamental feature of the cerebral cortex, essential for perception, cognition, and perhaps even consciousness.

Although modular circuits of a given class are readily seen in the brains of some species, they have not been found in the same brain regions of other, sometimes closely related, animals. Second, not all regions of the mammillian cortex are organized in a modular fashion. And third, no clear function of such modules has been discerned (Purves et al., 2004).

The columnar organization of the striate cortex

In general, the responses of neurons are qualitatively similar at any one point in primary visual cortex, but tend to shift smoothly across its surface. With respect to orientation, all the neurons encountered in an electrode penetration perpendicular to the surface at a particular point will very likely have the same orientation preference, formatting a "column" of cells with similar response properties (Weliky et al., 1996). Adjacent columns usually have slightly different orientation preference; the sequence of orientation preferences encountered along a tangential electrode penetration gradually shifts as the electrode advances (Obermayer and Blasdel, 1993; Purves et al., 2004).

Thus, orientation preference is mapped in the cortex, much like receptive field location (Blasdel and Salma, 1986).

Unlike the map of visual space, however, the map of orientation preference is iterated many times, such that same orientation preference is repeated at approximately 1 mm intervals across the striate cortex.

This iteration presumably ensures that there are neurons for each region of visual space that represent the full range of orientation values (Bonhoefer and Grinvald, 1993, 1996). The orderly progression of orientation preferences accommodated within the orderly map of visual space by the fact that the mapping is relatively coarse.

Each small region of visual space is represented by a set of neurons whose receptive fields cover the full range of orientation preferences, the set being distributed over several millimeters of the cortical surface (Bonhoeffer and Grinvald, 1996; Weliky et al., 1996; Purves et al., 2004).

The availability of optical imaging techniques has made it possible to visualize how response properties, such as the selectivity for edge orientation or ocular dominance, are mapped across the cortical surface. These methods generally rely on intrinsic signals (changes in the amount of light reflected from the cortical surface) that correlate with levels of neural activity. Such signals are thought to arise at least in part from local changes in the ratio of oxyhemoglobin and deoxyhemoglobin that accompany such activity, more active areas having a higher deoxyhemoglobin / oxyhemoglobin ratio.

This change can be detected when the cortical surface is illuminated with red light (605-700 nm). Under these conditions, active cortical regions absorb more light than the less active ones. With the use of sensitive video camera, and averaging over the number of trials (the changes are small, 1 or 2 parts per thousand) it is possible to visualize these differences and use them to map cortical patterns of activity (Bonhoeffer and Grinvald,

1993; Obermeyer and Blasdel, 1993). This approach has now been applied to both striate and extrastriate areas in both experimental animals and human patients undergoing neurosurgery (Purves et al., 2004). The results emphasize that maps of stimulus features are general principle of cortical organization.

This powerful technique can also be used to determine how maps for different stimulus properties are arranged relative to one another, and to detect additional maps such as that for direction of motion. A comparison of ocular dominance hands and orientation preference maps shows that pinwheel centers are generally located in the center of ocular dominance bands, and that the iso-orientation contours that emanate from the pinwheel centers run orthogonal to the border of ocular dominance bands (Bonhoeffer and Grinvald, 1993; Obermeyer and Blasdel, 1993).

These systematic relationships between the functional maps that coexist within primary visual cortex are thought to ensure that all combinations of stimulus features (orientation, direction, ocular dominance, and spatial frequency) are analyzed for all regions of visual space (Bonhoeffer and Grinvald, 1993; Obermeyer and Blasdel, 1993).

Although most neurons in the striate cortex respond to stimulation of both eyes, the relative strength of the inputs from the two eyes varies from neuron to neuron. At the extremes of this continuum are neurons that respond almost exclusively to the left or right eye; in the middle are those that respond equally well to both eyes. As in the case of orientation preference, vertical electrode penetrations tend to encounter neurons with similar ocular preference (or ocular dominance), whereas tangential penetrations show gradual shifts in ocular dominance (Tootell et al., 1996; Hubel and Wiesel, 1977; Tootell et al., 1996; Chalupa and Werner, 2004; Purves et al., 2004). These shifts in ocular dominance result from the ocular segregation of the inputs from lateral geniculate nucleus within cortical layer IV (Horton, 1992).

In short, the striate cortex is composed of repeating units, or modules, that contain all the neuronal machinery necessary to analyze a small region of visual space for variety of different stimulus attributes.

A number of other cortical regions show a similar columnar arrangement of their processing circuitry.

Compared to retinal ganglion cells, neurons at higher levels of the visual pathway become increasingly selective in their stimulus requirements. Thus, most neurons in the striate cortex respond to light-dark edges only if they are presented at a certain orientation; some are selective for the length of the edge, and others to movement of the edge in a specific direction. Indeed, a point in visual space is related to a set of cortical neurons, each of which is specialized for processing a limited set of the attributes in the visual stimulus. The neural circuitry in the striate cortex also brings together information from the two eyes; most cortical neurons (other than those in layer IV, which are segregated into eye-specific columns) have binocular responses. Binocular convergence is presumably essential for the detection of binocular disparity, an important component of depth perception (Purves et al., 2004).

Functional subsystem

The incoming visual information is relayed from the retina through the lateral geniculate nucleus to V1 and then to V2 and other extrastriate visual areas.

So, V1 (the striate cortex) is the primary vision area: it receives the largest input from the lateral geniculate nucleus of the thalamus and it projects to all other occipital regions. V1 is the first processing level in the hierarchy.

V2 also projects to all other occipital regions. V2 is the second level.

After V2, three distinct parallel pathways emerge on route to the parietal cortex, superior temporal sulcus, and inferior temporal cortex, for further processing.

As we shall see in more detail shortly, the parietal pathway, or dorsal stream, has a role in the visual guidance of movement, and the inferior temporal pathway, or ventral stream, is concerned with object perception (including color).

The middle pathway along the superior temporal sulcus is probably important in visuospatial functions.

At hierarchical levels beyond V1 and V2, part of the visual information goes to areas V3 and VP (Horton, 1992).

Motion perception

Human hMTS+ respond selectively to moving vs. stationary stimuli, but also responds to other aspects of motion stimuli in ways that appear to parallel reported single-unit response properties or perceptual effects. Motion produces a significant change in activation within hMT+, yet it can result in little or no change in activation V1-V2 (Deyoe, 2002).

Though retinal image motion often indicates the movement of objects (or self), motion cues can also be used to identify the boundaries and 3-dimensional shape of objects rather than their trajectories.

In summary, the middle-temporal area, or what is commonly called area MT, is important for motion perception. Almost all of the neurons in area MT are direction-selective, meaning that they respond selectively to a certain range of motion directions and do not respond to directions beyond that range (Zeki, 1974; Albright, 1984). Moreover, some of these neurons respond well to the pattern of motion (Albright, 1992), meaning that these neurons can integrate many different motion directions and calculate what the overall direction of an object might be. The activity in this region seems to be closely related to motion perception and, when activity in this region is disrupted, motion perception may be severely impaired (Tong and Pearson, 2007).

Color

The most studies have identified several distinct foci within human visual areas VP and V4 that are activated somewhat more strongly by chromatic than by archromatic stimuli. Anyhow, greater selectivity and task specificity are found anterior to V4v. Such selectivity has been shown to be associated with visual area V8 and, in some tasks, with a more anterior site. V8 is retinotopically distinct from V4v and contains a representation of both superior and inferior visual fields.

Color-selective activation sites in dorsal occipital cortex have also been observed on occasion, but their location and identity remain poorly defined.

The presence of occipitotemporal color-related sites is consistent with human lesion studies in which damage to ventral cortex results in diminished or absent color discrimination (achromatopsia) (Zeki, 1990). Often, color perception losses in both upper and lower visual fields, even though the lesion appears to be confined to ventral cortex.

In contrast, area V8, which is located within the lesion-sensitive zone, does have both upper and lower field representations, thereby making it a prime candidate for the achromatopsia site (Zeki, 1990). Moreover, V8 is located adjacent to the fusiform face area (FFA). This juxtaposition of V8 and FFA is likely to account for the fact that prosopagnosia (inability to recognize face) is commonly associated with cerebral achromatopsia.

In humans, cerebral achromatopsia does not arise from lesions of V4v but from more anterior lesions encompassing V8 and / or additional neighboring areas. This does not necessarily imply that V8 or any single visual area is solely responsible for color vision or for all color-related deficits. In fact, moving stimuli consisting of pure chromatic contrast can readily activate human hMT+.

So, to summarize, area V4 is known to be especially important for the perception of color (Zeki, 1997) and some neurons in this area respond well to more complex features or combination of features (Pasupathy and Connor, 2002). For example, some V4 neurons are sensitive to curvature of two lines that meet at a specific angle. These neurons might signal the presence of a curving contour or of a corner (Tong and Pearson, 2007).

Area V4 sends many outputs to higher visual areas in the ventral visual pathway, which is important for object recognition (Ungerleider and Mishkin, 1982). The anterior part of ventral visual pathway consists of the ventral temporal cortex, which is especially important for object recognition.

Form

There is general agreement that a major portion of the form processing system is located in the ventral occipitotemporal cortex.

Passive viewing of luminance-based contour and edges readily activates retinotopic visual areas of the medial and ventral occipital cortex in humans. The size of a detectable increment in the contrast of a plaid grating was quite precisely tracked by a proportional increment in fMRI response of visual area V1, V2d, V3 and V4A. In area hMT+, the fMRI response tends to saturate above a few percent contrast, consistent with the high contrast sensitivity of MT neurons studied in animals (Kaas, 1997).

Single-cell recording in animals has shown that neurons in V2, but less in V1, are capable of responding selectively to these contours, thereby suggesting a hierarchical processing mechanism. Neuroimaging studies with human subjects have shown that some types of illusory contours may preferentially activate later processing stages including V3A, V4v, V7, V8 and LO (lateral occipital visual complex).

The most selective responses to motion-defined contours and shapes have been associated with a region termed the kinetic-occipital area (KO).

It is located approximately 1.5 cm posterior to hMT+ in the lateral occipital cortex.

Cue invariance

In humans, several neuroimaging studies have tested for cue-invariant responses to contours, edges, or outline figures defined by luminance, color, texture, binocular disparity, or motion. In the most comprehensive study, similar responses were observed for luminance-, texture-, and motion-defined figures in lateral occipital cortex posterior to hMT+ (labeled LO) and in, or near, area V3A. The cue-invariant representation of contour information in LO and V3A may represent an important stage of abstraction in influence of object attributes from the available retinal information (Deyoe, 2002).

Figure-ground segmentation

It has been proposed that a swath of cortex located posterior to area hMT+ forms a complex specialized for the segmentation and processing of object information. This area, labeled LO, is more strongly activated by discrete objects than by gratings, textures, or motion fields (Deyoe, 2002).

In summary, lateral occipital (LO) cortex seems to have a general role in object recognition and responds strongly to a variety of shapes and objects (Malach et al., 1995). LO prefers intact shapes and objects more than scrambled visual features.

This region seems to represent the particular shapes of objects.

Presumably, different neurons in this region respond best to different kinds of objects. A method to test object selectivity is to measure neural adaptation to a particular shape. This is exactly what LO does, even when the repeated object is presented in a new location or in a different format so that retinotopic visual areas (V1-V4) will not adapt to the image (Grill-Spector et al., 1999; Kourtzi and Kanwisher, 2001).

Parahippocampal place area (PPA) is another strongly category-selective region that responds best to houses, landmarks, indoor and outdoor scenes (Epstein and Konwisher, 1998).

In comparison, this brain area responds more weakly to other types of stimuli such as faces, bodies or inanimate objects. Because this region responds to very different stimuli than the fusiform face area, many studies have taken advantage of the different response properties of the FFA and PPA to study the neural correlates of visual awareness (Tong and Pearson, 2007).

Complex forms

Regions of cortex in the collateral sulcus and adjacent lingual gyrus that is similar to retinotopically defined V4 and / or VP, the fusiform gyrus or adjacent inferior temporal gyrus, sometimes extending into area LO, encompass a swath of cortex that extends from the occipital lobe into ventral temporal cortex. This swath not functionally homogeneous is perhaps most consistently apparent for the analysis and recognition of face. The posterior extent of this region is lateral to the area activated during color processing (V8) or during the presentation of "scrambled" faces and has been termed the fusiform face area (FFA).

Face stimuli and face discrimination have been studied extensively. In the human studies it has been shown that the fusiform gyrus from the occipital junction forward to midtemporal lobe is activated by tasks requiring face recognition.

This region responds more to human, animal, and cartoon faces than to a variety of non-face stimuli, including hands, bodies, eyes shown alone, back views of heads, flowers, buildings and inanimate objects (Kanwisher et al., 1997; Mc Carthy et al., 1997; Tong et al., 2000; Schwarzlose et al., 2005).

In a recent study, Tsao et al. (2006) recorded the activity of single neurons in this face area and discovered that 97 per cent of the neurons in this region responded more to face than to other kinds of objects.

This region seems to be important for the conscious perception of face.

Lesions that cause prosopagnosia tend to have common involvement of the fusiform gyrus within the general vicinity of the FFA (Fig. 18.4).

In summary, single unit recordings in monkeys have revealed that many neurons in the ventral temporal cortex respond best to contour, simple shapes, or complex objects. Same neurons in this region are highly selective and respond to only a particular kind of object, such as a hand, a face shown from a particular viewpoint, a particular animal, a familiar toy or an object that the monkey has learned to recognize and so forth (Desimone et al., 1984; Gross, 1992; Logothetis et al., 1995; Tanaka, 1996).

Human neuroimaging studies have revealed many brain areas involved in processing objects. These object-sensitive areas, which lie just anterior to early visual areas V1-V4, respond more strongly to coherent shapes and objects, as compared to scrambled, meaningless stimuli.

The lateral occipital complex lies on the lateral surface of the occipital lobe, just posterior to area MT. Because this region is strongly involved in object recognition, Tong and Pearson (2007) consider it as part of the ventral pathway.

The fusiform face area lies on the fusiform gyrus, on the ventral surface of the temporal lobe. The parahippocampal place area lies on the parahippocampal gyrus, which lies medial to the fusiform gyrus on the ventral surface of the temporal lobe.

Written words and dyslexia

Because this function is most highly developed in humans, it may distinguish us from other primates. Some neuroimaging studies have implicated ventral occipitotemporal cortex near, but distinct from the FFA, in the analysis of visual word form, though other studies have obtained different results.

Specifically, dyslexics appear to have an impaired function of magnocellular-dominated pathways extending into dorsal occipital cortex, especially through hMT+ to the parietal cortex (Kaas, 1997).

Depth and the analysis of space

The analysis of space involves the assignment of distances of objects and surfaces relative to the self and each other, the representation of spatial maps for navigation, the extraction of locations and orientations of objects relative to the limbs for purposes of manipulation, and, finally, the computation of object positions relative to the center of gaze or relative to the current focus of attention.

Visual information allows us to direct our movements to objects in space and to assign meaning to objects. But spatial location is not a unitary characteristic. Objects have location relative to an individual (egocentric space) and relative to one another (allocentric space).

Egocentric visual space is central to the control of your actions toward objects. It therefore seems likely that visual space is coded in neural systems related to vision for action. In contrast, allocentric properties of objects are necessary for you to construct a memory of spatial location (Kolb and Whishaw, 2003).

The available evidence indicates that the cortical analysis of space heavily involves parietal and medial temporal lobe structures that receive direct or indirect projection from occipital lobe visual areas. Under passive viewing, the 3-dimensional stimuli evoked stronger fMRI activation in hMT+ and in several other foci, which included LO, V3A, and several parietal foci that are likely to receive projections from hMT+ or V3A (Zilles and Clarke, 1997).

Visual areas involved in the extraction of spatial information may be involved in the analysis of eye movements. This is supported by the observation that parietal visual areas such as VIP and LIP in macaques contain cells that are active during different types of eye movements and may be capable of compensating for such movements.

Other aspects of spatial processing such as the representation of mental maps of space appear to involve visual areas in the parietal, frontal, and medial temporal cortices outside the occipital lobe.

Given that there are a number of functionally distinct areas in macaque parietal cortex (e.g., VIP, LIP, MIP, PRR), it is likely that a similar multiplicity related, in part, to spatial processing will be described for human parietal cortex in the near future.

The ventral and dorsal pathways

The distinction between the ventral and the dorsal streams can be seen clearly in a series of patients studied by Milner and Goodale (1995). They first described D.F., a patient who was blind but who nevertheless shaped her hand appropriately when asked to reach for objects. Her dorsal stream was intact, as revealed by the fact that she could "unconsciously" see location, size, and shape.

On the other hand, Milner and Goodale noted that patients with dorsal-stream damage consciously reported seeing objects but could not reach accurately or shape the hand appropriately when reaching. Milner and Goodale proposed that the dorsal stream should be thought of as a set of systems for the one-line visual control of action. Their argument is based on three main lines of evidence.

1) The predominant characteristic of the neurons in posterior parietal regions is that they are active during a combination of visual stimulation and associated behavior. For example, cells may be active only when a monkey reaches out to a particular object. Looking at an object in the absence of movement does not activate the neurons. Thus, these "visual" neurons are unique in that they are active only when the brain acts on visual information.

2) These posterior parietal neurons can therefore be characterized as an interface between analysis of the visual world and motor action taken on it. The demands of action have important implications for what type of information must be sent to the parietal cortex – information such as object shape, movement, and location. Each of these visual features is likely to be coded separately, and at least three distinct pathways within the dorsal stream run from area V1 to the parietal cortex. One pathway goes from area V1 directly to area V5 to parietal cortex, a second goes from area V1 to areas V5 and V3a and then to parietal regions, and a third goes from area V1 to area V2 to the parietal cortex. These three pathways must certainly be functionally dissociable.

3) Most of the visual impairment associated with lesions to the parietal cortex can be characterized as visuomotor or orientational (Jakobson et al., 1991; Goodale et al., 1991; Felleman and van Essen, 1991; Goodale, 1993; Kosslyn and Thompson, 2000).

The Milner-Goodale model is an important theoretical advance in understanding how our visual brain is organized (Fig. 18.14).

Fig. 18.14. A summary of the visual processing hierarchy. The dorsal stream, which takes part in visual action, guides movements such as the hand postures for grasping a mug or pen, as illustrated. The ventral stream, which takes part in object recognition, identifies object such as mugs and pens in our visual world. The dorsal and ventral stream exchange information through polysensory neurons in the superior temporal sulcus stream, as shown by doubleheaded arrows. (after Goodale, 1993).

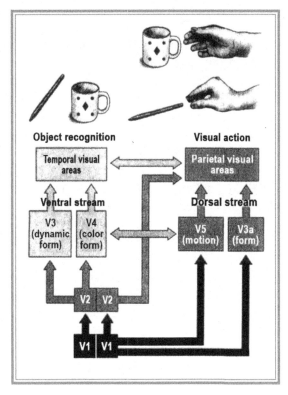

So, the two distinct visual streams have evolved to use visual information in two fundamentally different ways: the dorsal stream for guiding movements and the ventral for identifying objects.

Anyhow, according to Kolb and Whishaw (2003), the third stream of visual processing, which originates from structures associated with both the parietal and the temporal pathways and flow to a region of the temporal lobe is buried in the superior temporal sulcus. The superior temporal sulcus is characterized by polysensory neurons-neurons that are responsive to both visual and auditory or both visual and somatosensory input. The interaction of the parietal and temporal streams in the superior temporal sulcus is probably due to the interaction between the dorsal and the ventral -the "action" and "recognition"-streams (Kolb and Whishaw, 2003).

Brain regions associated with specific visual pathways were identified by measuring the regional blood flow (Ungerleider and Haxby, 1994; Haxby et al., 1999, 2000). In their studies subjects were given two tasks. In the first, the subjects indicated which of two faces was identical with a sample face. In the second, the subjects were asked to identify which of two stimuli had a dot (or square) in the same location as in a sample. The results showed activation of the temporal regions for the facial stimuli and activation of the posterior parietal region for the location task. Note, in addition, the activation of frontal areas for the spatial task supporting the idea that the frontal lobe plays a role in certain aspects of visual processing. Anyhow, in that time subjects have to make eye movements, which activate regions in the dorsal stream; so, whether the spatial or the movement components activate the parietal region is not clear. A similar dissociation was identified among the processes that detect motion, color, and shape (Campbell et al., 1986; Kingdom et al., 2001; Kolb and Whishaw, 2003). Detection of motion activates regions in the vicinity of area V5, whereas detection of shape activates regions along the superior temporal sulcus and the ventral region of the temporal lobe. The perception of color is associated with activation of the region of the lingual gyrus, which is the location of area V4. One study also found activation of a lateral occipital region, which is difficult to interpret in the light of lesion studies.

In sum, studies of regional blood flow in normal subjects show results consistent with the general notion of two separate visual streams, one to the parietal lobe and the other to the temporal lobe (Kolb and Whishaw, 2003).

The ventral pathway leading from V1 to the temporal lobe that is important for representing "what" object are and a dorsal pathway leading from V1 to the parietal lobe that is important for representing "where" objects are located. This important organizational principle of the visual system was proposed by Ungerleider and Mishkin (1982).

In the dorsal pathway, signals from V1 travel to dorsal extrastriate areas, such as areas MT and V3A, which then send major projections to many regions of the parietal lobe. The dorsal pathway is important for representing the locations of objects, so that the vision system can guide actions towards those objects (Goodale and Humphrey, 1998). This type of vision requires detailed information about the precise location, size, and orientation of the object.

Areas MT and V3A are important for processing visual motion and stereo-depth.

In the ventral pathway, many signals from V1 travel to ventral extrastriate areas V2, V3 and V4 and onward to many areas of the temporal lobe. The ventral or "what" pathway is important for processing information about the color, shape, and identity of visual objects, processing which emphasizes the stable, invariant properties of objects. The parietal and temporal lobes send projections to some common regions in the prefrontal cortex, where information from each pathway can also be reunited (Tong and Pearson, 2007).

Visual consciousness

In the brain there are a lot of areas responsible for consciousness. These areas work together to achieve this remarkable feat. Primary visual cortex seems to be important for our ability consciously to perceive any visual feature, while higher visual areas may have a more specialized role in perceiving certain visual features or objects (Tong, 2003).

Different cortical visual areas and neurons involved in processing a specific kind of visual stimuli (color, orientation, motion, faces, objects, etc.), together with other cortical areas and subcortical structures (thalamus, hypothalamus, reticular formation, etc.) seems to play different roles in our conscious visual experience.

According to one theory of visual consciousness, called *hierarchical theory* (Crick and Koch, 1995; Rees et al., 2002), higher visual areas respond to more complex stimuli, such as entire objects, and can integrate information about many visual features, which are processed in early visual areas. *The interactive* theory of visual consciousness emphasizes a different idea. It turns out that the signals entering the brain do not simply travel up the visual hierarchy: higher visual areas send feedback signals back down to early visual areas, especially to area V1 (Bullier, 2001). There are as many feedback projections as feedforward projections in the visual system, neurons projecting from higher visual areas to lower visual areas.

According to the interactive theory, once a stimulus is presented, feedforward signals travel up the visual hierarchy, activating many neurons in its path, but this feedforward activity is not enough for consciousness. Instead, high-level areas must send feedback signals back to lower-level areas where the feedforward signals come from, so that neural activity returns full circle, forming a neural circuit (Pollen, 1999; Lamme and Roclfsema, 2000).

This combination of feedforward - feedback signals is important for awareness, because higher areas need to check the signals in nearly areas and confirm if they are getting the right message, or perhaps to link neural representation of an object to the specific features that make up the object (Tong and Pearson, 2007).

Unconscious perception

According to Tong and Pearson (2007) the term unconscious perception refers to situations when subjects report not seeing a given stimulus, but their behavior or brain activity suggests that specific information about the unperceived stimulus was indeed processed by the brain.

Neurons may fire in a stimulus-specific way at many levels of the brain, but this activity may not be strong enough, last long enough, or involve enough neurons or brain areas to lead to awareness. One of the best examples of this comes from neural recordings in animals under anesthesia; visual neurons in many brain areas still show strong stimulus-selective responses (Tong and Pearson, 2007). If you become conscious of a particular stimulus, then neurons in your brain that represent that pattern will become highly active.

Anyhow, without enough activity in the right brain areas, awareness may simply fail: the result is unconscious perception. When two different stimuli are flashed briefly enough in quick succession, the visual system can no longer separate the two stimuli. Instead, what people perceive is a mix, or a fused blend of the two images.

For example, if we were to expose you to a red square, then quickly follow it with a green square, what you might experience is a combination of the two – a yellow square (Tong and Pearson, 2007). This method can be used to present invisible patterns, such as a face or a house, by flashing red contours on a green background to one eye and the opposite colors to the other eye.

When subjects were presented with such images in the fMRI scanner, the fusiform face area responded more strongly to faces and the parahippocampal place area responded more to house, even though subjects were no longer aware of the images (Moutoussis and Zeki, 2002). This is an example of unconscious perception. The activity in ventral temporal parts of the brain could differentiate, to some degree, whether a face or house was presented, even though the subject could not verbally report a difference.

Area MT, a brain area specialized for processing motion, also responds to unperceived motion. When moving stimulus is presented far out in the periphery of the visual field and is crowded by other stimuli, area MT still responds to motion, even when subjects are not aware of the motion (Moutoussis and Zeki, 2006). In this experiment, the motion stimulus was flanked on two sides by flickering stimuli, making the visual space so busy and cluttered that subjects could not see the motion in the display. Although MT responded somewhat to the perceived motion stimulus, it responded much more strongly when the surrounding flickering stimuli were removed and motion stimulus was clearly perceived.

In other studies, researchers used binocular rivalry to render pictures of fearful faces invisible.

The expression of the faces carried emotional content, although the subjects were never aware of seeing the faces. The amygdala that normally responds to emotional stimuli also responded to the invisible fearful faces (Pasley et al., 2004).

It is clear that many brain areas may continue to show stimuli-specific activity despite the fact that we are unaware of that stimulus.

In most of these studies, greater activity was found when subjects were aware of a stimulus than when they were not, suggesting that a minimum level of activity may be needed to make the difference between no awareness and awareness. A low level of neural activity below a specific threshold might not be adequate to result in being aware of a stimulus (Tong and Pearson, 2007).

In sum, Tong and Pearson (2007) can conclude that at least two things are needed for visual awareness: (1) activity in the right neurons or brain areas; and (2) activity that exceeds a critical threshold.

Visual attention

Visual attention refers to the ability to prepare for, select, and maintain awareness of specific locations, objects, or attributes of the visual scene (or an imagined scene) (Deyoe, 2002).

The center of gaze typically follows the focus of attention, but the observer can intentionally dissociate the two, thereby demonstrating that the neural systems controlling eye movements and attention are at least partially distinct (Deyoe, 2002). Some visual attributes are:

– enhance the detection of subtle changes in brightness, color, or virtually any other attribute;

– require focused attention to be perceived correctly. In a crowded visual environment directed attention may be required if different attributes of the same object are to be correctly associated. Certain behaviors can be performed with little, if any, focused attention, whereas others are highly sensitive to the allocation of attention. Automatic processes direct behavior that occurs without intention, involuntarily, without conscious awareness, and without producing interference with ongoing activities. Automatic processing may be an innate property of the way in which sensory information is processed or it can be produced by extended training (Logan, 1992, Bargh and Ferguson, 2000).

Operations that are not automatic have been referred to by various terms, including controlled, effortful, attentive, and conscious. Conscious operations differ fundamentally from automatic processing in that they require focused attention. A person stopping at a red light is an example of bottom-up processing, whereas a person actively searching for a street at which to turn is an example of top-down processing (Treisman, 1986).

Bottom-up processing is data driven; that is, it relies almost exclusively on the stimulus information being presented in the environment. In contrast, top-down processing is conceptually driven. It relies on the use of information already in memory, including whatever expectation might exist regarding the task at hand. So, automatic and conscious processing can reasonably be presumed to require at least some different cortical circuits (Logan, 1992; Naatanen, 1992; Neibur, 2002).

Treisman (1986) and Treisman and Gormican (1988) concluded that, although practice can speed up feature processing, it remains dependent on specific automatic neural associations between features and a serial-processing pathway. Feature processing appears to be innate to the visual system.

Posner and Raichle (1993) suggest that, in a sense, the attentional process provides the "glue" that integrates features into a unitary object. When features have been put together, the object can be perceived and held in memory as a unit. A clear prediction from Treisman's theory is that neurons in the visual areas outside area V1 and probably outside area V2 should respond differentially, depending on whether attention is focused on the corresponding receptive field. Treisman (1986) presumes that features are the properties that cells in the visual system are coded to detect. But features may perhaps be biologically significant stimuli, as illustrated in an experiment by Eastwood and colleagues (2001). The task was to identify the odd face, which could be a happy face in a sea of sad ones or vice versa. Before you try to do so, turn your book upside down.

Subjects were faster at detecting sad faces, whereas they were upside down or right side up. Furthermore, when Eastwood and colleagues redid the experiment with abstract targets that signified either a happy or sad state, subjects still found the sad-related feature faster.

Given that the features should be equally conspicuous in the happy and sad conditions, it follows that there is something biologically more important to detecting sad (negative) than happy (positive) stimuli.

It appears that negative stimuli (potentially dangerous or threatening features as well as sad ones) are attended to very efficiently and demand attention more than to targets for positive features.

From an evolutionary perspective, favoring the nervous system that attends to stimuli that can make a difference to an animal's survival makes sense. The evolution of biological targets is likely more important to survival than are the simplest targets detected by cells in area V1.

How and where attention exerts its effects over the processing of incoming visual information are becoming clearer. Ample evidence from animals and humans now shows that attention can modulate the responses of neurons in occipital visual cortex.

Moran and Desimone (1985) trained a monkey to hold a bar while it gazed at a fixation point on a screen. A sample stimulus (for instance, a vertical blue bar) appeared briefly at one location in the receptive field, followed about 500 ms later by two stimuli: one at the same location and another in a separate one. The key point is that both targets were in the cell's receptive field, but only one target was in the correct location. When the test stimulus was identical with the sample and in the same location, the animal was rewarded if it released the bar immediately. In this way, the same visual stimulus could be presented to different regions of the neurons' receptive field, but the importance of the information varied with its location.

– As the animal performed the task, the researchers recorded the firing of cells in the area V4. Cells in area V4 are color and form sensitive; so, different neurons responded to different conjunctions of features. Thus, a given cell might respond to one stimulus (for example, a horizontal green bar) and not to another (for example, a vertical red bar). These stimuli were presented either in the correct location or in an incorrect location for predicting reward.

So, when effective stimulus was presented in the correct location, the cell was highly active. When the same stimulus was presented in an incorrect location, however, the cell was not responsive. It appears that, when attention is focused on a place in the visual world, the cell responds only to stimuli appropriate to that place.

Moran and Desimone (1985) considered the possibility that visual area activated earlier (V1) or later (TE) in visual processing might also show attentional effects. Presumably the features detected in area V1 were too pimple to direct attention, whereas those in area TE could.

So, the cells showing constraints in spatial attention were in the areas V4 and TE, both parts of the object-recognition stream. Neurons in this system are coding spatial location.

Moran and Desimone's monkeys did not make a movement in space. If they did, we would predict that cells in the posterior parietal cortex would be significant to attentional demands.

In fact, Mountcastle (1995) reported just such results. These cells are responding not to the features of the stimuli but rather to the movements needed to get to them. Thus, there appear to be two types of visual attention, one related to the selection of stimuli and the other to the selection and direction of movements.

Kahneman (1973) noted that perceptual system does not always work at peak efficiency. He proposed that the capacity to perform mental activity is limited and that this limited capacity must be allocated among concurrent activities. Thus, for Kahneman, one aspect of attention is the amount of effort that is directed toward a particular task.

When you attempt a difficult maneuver with a car, such as parking in a tight spot, you turn down your car radio.

Spitzer and colleagues (1988) wandered if cells in area V4 might vary their firing characteristics in accord with the amount of effort to solve a particular visual problem.

Spitzer and colleagues (1988) reasoned that it should be easy for cell to discriminate between a stimulus within its preferred orientation or color and a stimulus outside this orientation of color. Animals' performance confirmed that the finer discrimination was more difficult: 93% of their responses were correct under the easy conditions as compared with 73% under the difficult conditions.

The change in response characteristics of the area V4 cells is intriguing. First, under the difficult conditions, the cells increased their firing rate by an average of about 20%. Second, the tuning characteristics of the cells changed.

The more difficult task appears to have required increased attention to the differences between the stimuli, as manifested in a change in the stimulus selectivity of neurons in area V4.

It is not known how this attentional effect can alter the cell's activity. The result of studies using monkeys have led to the idea that the critical region may be the pulvinar, which is a thalamic nucleus that projects to secondary visual areas in the tectopulvinar system.

Petersen and his colleagues (1987) found that neurons in the pulvinar respond more vigorously to stimuli that are targets of behavior than they do to the same stimuli when they are not targets of behavior. That is, when a visual stimulus is present but has no meaning for the animal, the cells have a low firing rate. When the same stimulus now signifies a reward, the cells become more active.

Because the pulvinar complex projects to the posterior parietal cortex, temporal cortex, and prefrontal cortex, it may play same role in directing Treisman's "spotlight" to different parts of space.

Petersen and his colleagues tested this prediction by finding that disrupting the pulvinar does disrupt spatial attention. The pulvinar receives visual inputs from the colliculus, which is known to play a role in orienting to visual information; so it may be a collicular-pulvinar spotlight that is at work.

PET measurements showed that the selective-attention task activated specific visual regions, the region varying with the feature detected (Corbetta et al., 1991, 1993). Thus, attention to color activated a region probably corresponding to area V4, whereas attention to shape activated regions corresponding to areas V3 and TE. The selective task also activated the insula, the posterior thalamus (probably, pulvinar), the superior colliculus, and the orbital frontal cortex (Corbetta et al., 1991, 1993).

Taken together, the results of the Corbetta studies show that different coortical areas are activated in different attentional tasks:

The parietal cortex is activated for attention to location; the occipital-temporal cortex is activated for attention to features such as color and form.

The anterior cingulate and prefrontal areas show activation during both visual tasks. Thus, attention appears to generally require the activation of anterior cingulate and some prefrontal areas in addition to the activation of specific sensory areas related to a particular sensory modality, such as vision or touch.

So, tactile stimulation activated areas S1 and S2, but in addition, during the attentional task, there was activation in the posterior parietal cortex, like in Brodmann's area 7. Thus, distinct regions in the posterior parietal cortex appear to have roles in attention to different types of sensory inputs (Burton et al., 1999).

CLINICAL EFFECTS AND SYMPTOMS

Visual field defects

Brain lesions studies are important for understanding what brain areas may be necessary for certain kind of visual awareness – awareness of color, motion, faces, objects, or the capacity to be aware of seeing anything at all! (Tong and Pearson, 2007).

Brain lesions may be investigated in humans who have suffered from unfortunate injury to certain parts of the brain, which may result from strokes, tumors, trauma, or neurodegenerative disease.

Different visual deficits can result from neural damage at different levels of the visual processing hierarchy.

Because a spatial relationship in the retinas is maintained in central visual structures, a careful analysis of the visual fields can often indicate the site of neurological damage. Relatively large visual field deficits are called anopsias and smaller ones are called scotomas.

Damage to the retina or one of the optic nerves before it reaches the chiasma results in a loss of vision that is limited to the eye of origin.

The main causes of unilateral and bilateral optic neuropathy are: demyelinative, ischemic, parainfectious, toxins and drugs, deficiency states, heredofamilial and developmental, compressive and infiltrative.

Observable changes in the optic disc are, therefore, of particular importance. They may reflect the presence of raised intracranial pressure (papilledema or "choked disc"), infarction of the optic nerve head (disc edema), congenital defects of the optic nerves (optic pits or colobomas), hypoplasia and atrophy of the optic nerves, and glaucoma.

Lesions of the chiasma, optic tract and geniculocalcarine pathway cause bitemporal hemianopsia, homonymous hemianopsia or superior homonymous quadrantanopsia (contralateral temporal and ipsilateral nasal quadrants) (Meyer's loop).

Parietal lobe lesions are said to affect more the inferior quadrants of the visual field than the superior ones, but this is difficult to document; with a lesion of the right parietal lobe, the patient ignores the left half of space, and with a left parietal lesion, the patient is often aphasic.

Damage in the region of the optic chiasma results in specific types of deficits that involve the visual field of both eyes. For example, damage to the middle portion of the optic chiasma can affect the fibres that are crossing from the nasal retina of each eye, leaving the uncrossed fibres from the temporal retinas intact. The resulting loss of vision is confined to the temporal visual field of each eye and is known as bitemporal hemianopsia. It is also called heteronomous hemianopsia to emphasize that the parts of the visual field that are lost in each eye do not overlap. Individuals with this condition are able to see in both left and right visual fields, provided both eyes are open (Fig. 18.15). Damage to structures that are central to the optic chiasma, including the optic tract, lateral geniculate nucleus, optic radiation, and visual cortex, results in deficits that are limited to the contralateral visual hemifield.

Because such damage affects the corresponding parts of the visual field in each eye, there is a complete loss of vision in the affected region of the binocular visual field, and the deficit is referred to as a homonymous hemianopsia.

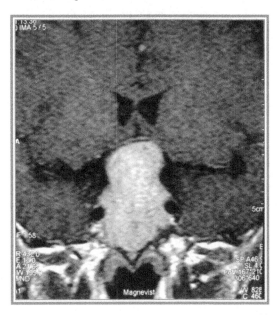

Fig. 18.15. A 56-years-old female patient harboring a very large nonfunctioning macroadenoma with suprasellar extension and bitemporal hemianopsia.

Damage along the optic radiation in its course from the lateral geniculate nucleus to the striate cortex is rarely complete. Some of the optic radiation axons run out into the temporal lobe on their route to the striate cortex, a branch called Meyer's loop. Meyer's loop carries information from the superior portion of the contralateral visual field. More medial parts of the optic radiation, which pass under the cortex of the parietal lobe, carry information from the interior portion of the contralateral visual field. So, superior fibres that leave the lateral geniculate body go straight back to the primary visual cortex; inferior fibres loop anteriorly around the superior temporal horn of the lateral ventricle (Meyer's loop). Because these fibres are approximately 5 cm from the top of the temporal lobe, they are sometimes damaged during temporal lobectomy, can thus result in a superior homonymous quadrantanopsia. Damage to the optic radiation underlying the parietal cortex results in an inferior homonymous quadrantanopsia.

Macular vision is represented most posteriorly at the occipital tips. Each fovea appears to project in both occipital lobes. Injury to central visual structures can lead to a phenomenon called macular sparing. Macular sparing is commonly found with damage to the cortex, but can be a feature of damage anywhere along the length of the visual pathway.

The nonoverlapping part of the most peripheral temporal field (monocular temporal crescent) represents unpaired crossed axons from the nasal retina, which project to the most anteromedial part of the visual cortex. The primary visual cortex has interconnections with numerous visual association areas (Zeki, 1993).

Visual agnosia

The disorder of vision and higher visual functions are common in many patients with neurological disease. The visual system is the most widely researched and best understood higher order sensory system in the brain.

Object agnosia is a rare condition first described by Lissauer in 1890. It consists of a failure to name and indicate the use of a seen object by spoken or written words or by gesture. The patient cannot even tell the generic class of the seen object. Visual acuity is intact, the mind is clear, and the patient is not aphasic – conditions requisite for the diagnosis of agnosia. If the object is palpated, it is recognized at once, and it can also be identified by smell or sound if it has an odor or makes noise. Moving the object or placing it in its customary surroundings facilitates recognition. Lissauer conceived the visual object recognition as consisting of two distinct processes – the construction of a perceptual representation from vision (apperception) and the mapping of this perceptual representation onto stored percepts or engrams of the object's functions and associations. Lissauer proposed that impairment of either of these processes could give rise to a defect in visual object recognition.

Teuber was credited in 1968 with the classic definition of agnosia – that is, a normal percept stripped of its meaning. In the setting of visual agnosia, such a definition implies normal or near normal sensory perception in the context of impaired recognition of the object being perceived. Most patients with visual agnosia can be shown to have abnormality of perception.

The traditional way to classify visual-object agnosia is to distinguish two broad forms: associative agnosia and apperceptive agnosia (Lissauer, 1888).

Associative agnosia

Associative agnosia corresponds to a "pure" visual agnosia, as reflected in Teuber's definition, and means the ability to recognize an object despite any apparent perception of the object. Thus, the associative agnostic can copy a drawing rather accurately, indicating a coherent percept, but he cannot identify it.

Failure of object recognition is a defect in memory, that affects not only past knowledge about the object, but also the acquisition of new knowledge. Associative agnosias are more likely with damage to region in the ventral stream that are farther up the processing hierarchy, such as the anterior temporal lobe. So, associative agnosia usually results from damage to the ventral temporal cortex.

Apperceptive agnosia

Apperceptive visual agnosia refers to an abnormality of visual recognition in which perceptual features are so prominent as to dominate the clinical picture. Basic visual functions (acuity, color, motion) are preserved. The fundamental deficit is an inability to develop a percept of the structure of an object or objects. In the simplest case, patients are simply unable to recognize, copy, or match simple shapes.

Many patients have another unusual symptom, too-often referred to as simultan-agnosia. In this case patients can perceive the basic shape of an object, but they are unable to perceive more than one object at a time. Such patients often act as though they were blind, possibly because they are simply overwhelmed by the task at hand. Such patients can still recognize objects by using other senses such as touch, hearing or smell, so the loss of function is strictly visual.

Apperceptive agnosia does not result from a restricted lesion but usually follows gross bilateral damage to the lateral parts of the occipital lobes including regions sending outputs to the ventral stream. Such injuries are probably most commonly associated with carbon monoxide poisoning, which appears to produce neuronal death in "watershed" region – that is, regions lying in the border areas between territories of a different arterial system (Kolb and Whishaw, 2003).

In the course of assessing patients with possible agnosia, it is important to distinguish between defects in naming and defects in recognition. This is a distinction that is commonly either blurred or completely unappreciated in the scientific and clinical literature on agnosia. The key is to understand that an object can be recognized without being named but cannot be named without being recognized. Thus, if a patient is asked to identify an object and fails to produce its name, it is important to probe the patient regarding features of the object to establish that a true recognition defect exists.

Visual agnosia does not appear to result from damage to the dorsal stream. The most affected region is the tissue at the occipitotemporal border, which is part of the ventral visual pathway.

James et al. (2003) propose that the dorsal system is not only responsible for processing "where" objects are, but also "how" action can be performed toward a particular object, such as pointing at or reaching for that object. Apparently, visual processing in the dorsal system is not accessible to consciousness – the patient cannot report the orientation of the slot – yet the dorsal system can guide the right action. Complementary studies of patients with optic ataxia have revealed the opposite pattern of visual deficits, indicating a double dissociation between conscious visual perception and visually guided action. Optic ataxia typically results from damage to the parietal lobe, which is part of the dorsal pathway. These patients can perceive visual orientations and recognize objects well, but have great difficulty in performing visually guided actions.

Simultanagnosia

Wolpert (1924) originally described a patient who demonstrated a "spelling dyslexia" (an inability to read all but the shortest words, spelled out letter by letter) and a failure to perceive simultaneously all the elements of a scene and to properly interpret the scene. In the framework of gestalt psychology, the patient could recognize the parts but not the whole. A cognitive defect of synthesis of the visual impressions was thought to be the basis of this condition, which Wolpert called simultanagnosia. Some of the patients with this disorder have a right homonymous hemianopsia; in others, the visual field is full. This is part of the Balint syndrome, the other components of which are faulty visual scanning (ocular apraxia) and visual reaching (optic ataxia), suggesting that a fault in ocular scanning might underlie all the defects.

Through tachistoscopic testing, Kinsbourne and Warrington (1963) have noted that reducing the time of stimulus exposure permits single objects to be perceived in an instant, but not two objects. Rizzo and Robin (1990) have proposed that the primary defect is in sustained attention to incoming visual-spatial information. Nielsen (1946) has attributed this disorder to a lesion of the inferolateral part of the dominant occipital lobe (area 18). In a patient who presented with an isolated "spelling dyslexia" and simultanagnosia, Kinsbourne and Warrington (1963) found a localized lesion within the inferior part of the left occipital lobe. In other instance, the lesions have been bilateral in the superior part of the occipital association cortices.

Prosopagnosia

The earliest mention of the symptom was made by Quaglino, an Italian ophthalmologist, who, in 1867, reported a patient suffering from left hemianopsia, achromatopsia, and inability to recognize familiar faces – problems caused by a cerebrovascular accident.

The symptom had to await Bodamer's report in 1947 to be identified as a distinct form of agnosia, deserving a distinctive name (prosopagnosia, from the Greek word prosopon, meaning "face").

Since the 1940's, more than a hundred case reports (Farah, 1990) have been published, and some patients have been extensively and repeatedly investigated.

The clinical picture. Prosopagnosia refers to an impairment in familiar face recognition. Patients with facial agnosia cannot recognize any previously known faces, including their own as seen in a mirror or photograph. They can recognize people by face information, however, such as a birthmark, moustache or characteristic hairdo, by voice, gait, context or other nonface cues.

With a few exceptions, they can discriminate its gender, race, and approximate age, although finer age estimation may be impaired (De Renzi et al., 1989). Face recognition disorders do not extend to the identification of emotional expressions, which is preserved in the great majority of prosopagnosics, while it may be impaired in patients who do not have problems in recognizing familiar faces (Kurucz and Feldmar, 1979), providing evidence that discrete neural structures subserve the two abilities. It has been shown that patients with prosopagnosia demonstrate nonconscious recognition of familiar faces.

Patients with prosopagnosia, particularly those of the associative type, often have normal judgments of facial emotional expressions.

That is, despite the inability to identify the face, judgments related to facial emotional expression (e.g., happy, sad, angry, and surprised) are similar to those of controls.

The opposite dissociation has been described. In these studies, it was demonstrated that patients with bilateral damage to amygdala were unable to judge emotional facial expressions accurately, despite normal recognition of identity (Adolphs et al., 1994, 1995, 1998). Patients with bilateral amygdala damage were significantly impaired in judging faces that looked "unapproachable" or "untrustworthy". These findings were interpreted to support the proposition that the amygdala was involved in social judgment as well as judgment of emotion based on facial features (Jones and Tranel, 2001, 2002). The findings indicate the complex, complimentory and reciprocal relationship between multiple areas of the brain, in the processing of different aspects of face information (e.g., identity, emotion, and social valence) (Jones and Tranel, 2002). In patients with proso-pagnosia caused by acquired brain damage (e.g., by stroke, tumor, or other lesion), there may be some visual field defect, usually a superior quadrantanopsia of one or both visual fields. Such patients have otherwise normal neurologic and neuropsychological exams and do not evidence aphasia, amnesia, dementia, or disorders of executive functions. Visual acuity and visual perception may be normal or near normal in associative prosopagnosia, although many cases with clear visual perceptual defects have been described (and probably correspond to an apperceptive type).

It was demonstrated that patients with acquired prosopagnosia show that the recognition defect often extends to objects other than faces. Anyhow, there are some remarkable exceptions that have been reported. Patients with prosopagnosia are still able to recognize objects well, but have great difficulty in recognizing or telling apart faces (Bodamer, 1947; Meadows, 1974).

Studies have revealed a few patients who can discriminate between subtle differences in objects but can no longer distinguish between faces (McNeil and Warrington, 1993). Another patient could no longer recognize upright faces accurately and was actually better at recognizing upside-down faces, which is just the opposite of normal subject performance (Farah et al., 1995).

A study of a very unusual object agnosic patient, who was very impaired at recognizing objects could recognize upright faces just as well as normal subjects (Moscovitch et al., 1997). Remarkably, if the face were turned upside-down, the patient became severely impaired, performing six times worse than normal participants under these conditions. Apparently the patient has an intact system for processing upright faces, but the system responsible for processing objects and upside-down faces is badly damaged (Valentine, 1988). Taken together, evidence from that patient and prosopagnostic patients provide evidence of a double dissociation between the visual processing of upright faces as compared to objects and upside-down faces (Tong and Pearson, 2007). Prosopagnosics may not accept the fact that they cannot recognize their own faces, probably because they know who must be in the mirror and thus see themselves. According to Damasio and colleagues, most facial agnosics can tell human from nonhuman faces and can recognize facial expression normally (Damasio et al., 1982; 1989).

Scientists have also described a third form of prosopagnosia termed "developmental prosopagnosia" (De Haan and Campbell, 1991; Kracke, 1994; De Haan, 1999; Jones and Tranel, 2001). Developmental prosopagnosia refers to a selective face recognition defect that begins in childhood and is not associated with any identifiable structural lesion. In general, such cases have shown significant apperceptive features, although one reported case was believed to be an essentially associative prosopagnosia. Similar to cases of acquired prosopagnosia, such patients recognize individuals by gait, voice, or other nonface features. In one case there were features of a broader visual object agnosia. In those cases in which neuroimaging has been completed, no structural brain abnormalities have been identified. Functional imaging has not been done in such cases. These patients appear to manifest the face recognition disability over many years. Although first identified in childhood, in at least one case the disorder persisted into adulthood.

Similar to cases of acquired prosopagnosia, in at least one case nonconscious electrodermal recognition of familiar faces was demonstrated.

Prosopagnosia can result from bilateral damage around the regions of the lateral occipital cortex, inferior temporal cortex and the fusiform gyrus (Meadows, 1974; Bouvier and Engel, 2006). In some cases, unilateral damage to the right hemisphere may lead to this impairment. Because lesions are usually quite large and might damage fibre tracts leading to a critical brain region, it is difficult to identify a precise site. Nonetheless, the brain lesion sites associated with prosopagnosia appear to encompass the fusiform face area and extend much more posteriorly (Tong and Pearson, 2007).

All postmortem studies on facial agnosias have found bilateral damage, and the results of imaging studies in living patients confirm the bilateral nature of the injury in most patients, with the damage centered in the region below the calcarine fissure at the temporal junction. These results imply that the process of facial recognition is probably bilateral, but asymmetrical (Kolb et al., 1983; Boussaud et al., 1990; Hancock et al., 2000).

Visual object agnosia

The term visual object agnosia is reserved for patients who have difficulty with identification of entities at basic object level. Thus, visual object agnosia refers to a visual recognition defect at the level of nonunique objects rather than at the level of specific members of a category (Damasio et al., 2000). For example, a patient with visual agnosia may not know that a violin is a violin, that a dog is a dog, or that a car is a car (Jones and Tranel, 2002). Memory is normal, and there is defect in judgment, basic verbal intellectual skills, or language.

Associated conditions often include defects in color recognition and naming and defects in reading. Lesions associated with visual object agnosia are typically more extensive than those in case of prosopagnosia, including occipitotemporal cortex bilaterally, extending dorsally into visual association cortex, and almost always involving underlying white matter. There is evidence that the left hemisphere plays a more critical role than the right in the development of visual object agnosia (Jones and Tranel, 2002).

Disorder of reading

The study of alexia dates at least to the contributions of Déjérine, who in 1891 and 1892 described two patients with quite different patterns of reading impairment.

Déjérine's first patient (Déjérine, 1891) developed an impairment in reading and writing subsequent to an infarction involving the left parietal lobe. Déjérine termed this disorder "alexia with agraphia" and attributed the disturbance to a disruption of the "optical image for words", which he thought to be supported by the left angular gyrus. Déjérine concluded that reading and writing required the activation of these "optical images" and that the loss of the images resulted in an inability to recognize or write familiar words.

Déjérine's second patient (Déjérine, 1892) was quite different. This patient was unable to read aloud or for comprehension but could write, a disorder that Déjérine designated "alexia without agraphia" (also known as agnosic alexia and pure alexia). The patient had a right homonymous hemianopsia from a left occipital lesion, which included the fibres carrying visual information from the right to the left hemisphere. Déjérine explained alexia without agraphia in terms of a "disconnection" between visual information confined to the right hemisphere and the left angular gyrus, which he assumed to be critical for the recognition of words.

The study of acquired dyslexia was revitalized by Marshall and Newcombe (1973). These investigators described a patient (GR) who read approximately 50 percent of concrete nouns but was severely impaired in the reading of abstract nouns and all other parts of speech. The most striking aspect of GR's performance, however, was his tendency to produce errors that appeared to be semantically related to the target word (e.g., speak read as "talk"). Marshall and Newcombe (1973) designated this disorder "deep dyslexia". These investigators also described two patients whose primary deficit appeared to be an inability to derive the pronunciation of irregularly spelled words, such as "yacht". This disorder was designated "surface dyslexia".

Pure alexia refers to the inability to read with preserved ability to write. These patients are not aphasic, nor is there a defect in memory, orientation, basic intellectual skills, or verbal arithmetic skills. The neurologic exam is normal apart from a typical finding of a right homonymous hemianopsia.

An inability to read has often been seen as the complementary symptom to facial-recognition deficits.

Alexia is most likely to result from damage to the left fusiform and lingual areas. Either hemisphere can read letters, but only the left hemisphere appears able to combine the letters to form lexical representations (that is, words). The lesion typically abuts the splenium. Thus, visual information is regarded only by the right occipital lobe, and such information is blocked from passing to the left hemisphere by virtue of the retrosplenial lesion. This information thus cannot be decoded into lexically meaningful words by association areas in the left parietal cortex, specifically surrounding the left angular gyrus (Jones and Tranel, 2002). In the instance, when a patient is asked to trace letters with his or her hand, there is no such disconnection between sensorimotor cortex on the left and the left angular gyrus. The key in this case is that the visual system is bypassed (Jones and Tranel, 2002).

Alexia can be conceived as a form of object agnosia in which there is an inability to construct perceptual wholes from parts or to be a form of associative agnosia, in which case word memory (the lexical store) is either damaged or inaccessible (Farah, 1990; 1998; Behrmann et al., 1992).

In evaluating patients with pure alexia, it is useful to ask them to copy printed material, to write a sentence by dictation, and to write a sentence spontaneously. However, such patients will have difficulty in copying sentences, given their inability to read. If the examiner asks the patient to trace letters with the patient's finger, the patient may be able to discern the meaning of the written word (Jones and Tranel, 2002).

Disorder of color processing

Normal color vision depends on the integrity of cone cells, which are most numerous in the macular region. When activated, they convey information to special columns of cells in the striate cortex. Three different cone pigments with optimal sensitivities to blue, green, and orange-yellow wavelengths are said to characterize these cells; presumably each cone possesses only one of these pigments. Transmission to higher centers for the perception of color is believed to be effected by neurons and axons that encode at least two pairs of complementary colors. In the optic nerve and tracts, the fibres for color are of small caliber and are preferentially sensitive to noxious agents and pressure. The geniculostriate fibres for color are separate from but course along with fibres that convey information about form and brightness; hence there may be a homonymous color hemianopsia (hemiachromatopsia). The visual fields for blue-yellow are smaller than those for white light, and the red and green fields are smaller than those for blue-yellow.

Assessment of color imagery depends primarily on the self-report on the patient. Patients may complain that they cannot "remember" the colors that various objects should have (this complaint may also indicate color agnosia).

The patients may note that, following a brain lesion, they no longer dream in color. Interestingly, it has been suggested that recall of most personal memories depends on color and other visual imagery (Ogden, 1993).

Achromatopsia

Diseases may affect color vision by abolishing it completely (achromatopsia) or partially by quantitatively reducing one or more of the three attributes of color – brightness, hue and saturation. Or, only one of the complementary pairs of color may be lost, usually red-green. The disorder may be congenital and hereditary or acquired. The commonest form, and the one to which the term color blindness is usually applied, is a male sex-linked inability to see red and green while normal visual acuity is retained.

Patients with achromatopsia complain that colors appear to be black and white, washed out, gray or dirty. Such patients may also demonstrate some color desaturation and dyschromatopsia rather than complete lack of color.

Lesions associated with achromatopsia are characteristically found in the infracalcarine medial occipital lobe, typically involving the lingual and fusiform gyri. When the lesion is unilateral, the color defect is in the contralateral visual space. When the lesion is bilateral, the color defect subsumes the entire visual field. There may well be visual field cuts, typically involving superior quadrants.

Damasio (1985) has drawn attention to a group of acquired deficits of color perception with preservation of form vision, the result of focal damage (usually, infarction) of the visual association cortex and subjacent white matter. Color vision may be lost in a quadrant, half of the visual field, or the entire field. The latter, or full-field achromatopsia, is the result of bilateral occipitotemporal lesions involving the fusiform and lingual gyri, a localization that accounts for its frequent association with visual agnosia (especially, prosopagnosia), and some degree of visual field defect. A lesion restricted to the inferior part of the right occipitotemporal region, sparing both the optic radiation and striate cortex, causes the purest form of achromatopsia (left hemiachromatopsia). With a similar left-sided lesion, alexia may be associated with the right hemiachromatopsia.

In addition to the losses of perception of form, movement, and color, lesions of the visual system may also give rise to a variety of positive sensory visual experiences. The simplest of these are called phosphenes, i.e., flashes of light and colored spots in the absence of luminous stimuli. Mechanical pressure on the normal eyeball may induce them at the retinal level, as every child discovers.

In patients with migraine, ischemia of nerve cells in the occipital lobe gives rise to the bright zigzag lines of a fortification spectrum.

Formed or complex visual hallucinations are observed in a variety of conditions, notably in the withdrawal state following chronic intoxication with alcohol and other sedative-hypnotic drugs, in Alzheimer disease, and in disease of the occipitoparietal or occipitotemporal regions or the diencephalon ("peduncular hallucinosis"). In color blindness a genetic abnormality of cone pigments is postulated, but the defect cannot be seen by inspecting the retina. A failure of the cones to develop or a degeneration of cones may cause a loss of color vision, but in the latter condition visual acuity is often diminished, a central scotoma may be present, and, although the macula appears to be normal ophthalmoscopically, fluorescein angiography shows the pigment epithelium to be defective. Congenital color visions are usually protan (red) or detan (green), leaving yellow-blue color vision intact; acquired lesions may affect all colors.

Lesion of the optic nerves usually affects red-green more than blue-yellow; the opposite is true of retinal lesions. An exception is a dominantly inherited optic atrophy, in which the scotoma mapped by a large blue target is larger than that for red.

Color anomia

The term color anomia refers to an inability to name colors in the context of normal performances on tests of matching color or of color generation. This disorder is usually associated with pure alexia and right homonymous hemianopsia.

Color naming can be affected independently of color perception, imagery, and recognition (Geschwind and Fusillo, 1966; Damasio et al., 1979; Rizzo and Damasio, 1989; Rizzo et al., 1993).

Color anomia is relatively rare, and, in fact, naming of color is often relatively spared in patients who have severe naming defects for other classes of stimuli. Goodglass and coworkers (1986) found that color naming was very infrequently impaired in various aphasic patients and was, in fact, one of the categories that tended to stand out as being especially intact – a finding consistent with an older case study (Yamadori and Albert, 1973). Such patients are able to match same-color chips and associate colors with objects. When shown a specific color, such patients are unable to name it with appropriate verbal tag. This defect seems to be exacerbated when less contextual information is available.

Given the site of the lesion in color anomia, there is some suggestion that this may represent a disconnection syndrome. That is, in the left visual field (ipsilateral to the lesion) color perception is normal, but perception is limited to primary visual cortex in the right hemisphere only. This elementary perceptual information is blocked by a retrosplenial lesion in the mesial left occipital lobe, thereby rendering such information unavailable to the left hemisphere (Jones and Tranel, 2002).

Color agnosia

Following the Teuber (1968) definition of agnosia as a "normal percept stripped of its meaning", color agnosia refers to the loss of the ability to retrieve color knowledge pertinent to a given stimulus that is not caused by deficient color perception. So, color agnosia is a rare condition defined as an inability to retrieve color information in the context of normal perception and language. Color agnosia is often associated with visual object agnosia and may be associated with category-related recognition defects, particularly for living entities as opposed to artifactual entities. The defect should also be distinguished from color anomia and from color imagery impairment. In the latter condition, the patient cannot bring into mind's eye a particular color, but the patient still knows what the color is and can give verbal or nonverbal testimony to that knowledge – for instance, by performing normally on tasks requiring matching of color or names with objects. A patient with color agnosia, by contrast, has lost the "knowing" of colors and will not perform such tasks normally (Tranel, 1997). For example, a patient with color agnosia will be unable to remember the color of common entities (e.g., "what color is a banana?") and will be unable to provide a list of objects that come in various colors (e.g., "name things that are red") (Jones and Tranel, 2002). Some authors have argued that especially in cases in which the defect is "two-ways" – i.e., when the patient cannot name colors from color stimuli and cannot point the colors given the color names – the designation of agnosia is accurate. Color agnosia is rare. Only a few well-studied cases have been reported (Kinsbourne and Warrington, 1964; Farah et al., 1988; Schnider et al., 1992; Luzzatti and Davidoff, 1994, etc.). Based on a handful of well-studied patients, the neuroanatomical correlates of color agnosia include the occipital-temporal region either unilaterally on the left or bilaterally.

Functional imaging studies suggest that areas associated with color knowledge are probably anterior and lateral to areas associated with color perception.

Visual neglect

Neglect can be defined as "the failure to report, respond, or orient to novel or meaningful stimuli, presented to the side opposite a brain lesion, when this failure cannot be attributed to either sensory or motor defects". In the visual modality, the most common form of neglect is hemispatial neglect. The essential feature of spatial neglect is that the patient ignores objects in the visual hemifield contralateral to the lesion, in the absence of a visual field cut.

Such neglect is commonly associated with right hemisphere lesions resulting in left hemispatial visual neglect.

Right hemispatial visual neglect, though rare, can be seen during the acute period in some cases of left hemisphere lesions. The typical lesion is in the occipital-temporal-parietal border zone (Jones and Tranel, 2002).

So, damage to the dorsal pathway can lead to optic ataxia (impairments in visual guided actions) or visual neglect. Damage to the ventral temporal cortex can lead to impairments in visual perception, object recognition or face recognition. Patients with brain injuries in the ventral and dorsal pathways reveal a dissociation between the conscious perception of basic shapes and orientations and the ability to perform visually guided actions.

The finding of neglect is often not restricted to the visual modality and may be demonstrated in both sensorimotor and auditory systems concurrently with visual neglect.

One of the ways to evaluate hemispatial visual neglect in affected patients is to perform a double simultaneous stimulation task, in which the examiner introduces a visual stimulus to the left visual field, to the right visual field, and then to both fields simultaneously. The most clear evidence of neglect from this procedure is that the patient will identify each stimulus individually, but when presented simultaneously the patient will identify only the stimulus presented ipsilateral to the lesion.

Furthermore, methods of detecting hemispatial neglect include drawing tasks, line bisection-tasks, or line cancellation tasks (Jones and Tranel, 2002).

So, material in one visual field – usually the left – can be seen but remain unnoticed unless the patient's attention is drawn to it (Chaves and Caplan, 2001). This form of visual inattention, also known as unilateral sensory or spatial neglect, typically occurs when there is right parietal lobe involvement as well as occipital lobe damage. Right occipital lesions are less likely to give rise to inattention. The so-called "visual inattention" associated with occipital lobe damage is similar to simultaneous agnosia in that the patient spontaneously perceives only one thing at a time. It differs from simultaneous agnosia in that the patient will see more than one object if others are pointed out: this is not the case in a true simultaneous agnosia.

In addition to demonstrating neglect in other modalities (sensorimotor and auditory), associated signs observed in neuropsychological testing of patients with neglect include constructional dyspraxia, anosodiaphoria, and anosognosia.

Other visuospatial anomalies

Occasionally, patients with an attention hemianopsia may displace an image to the nonaffected half of the field of vision (visual allesthesia), or visual image may persist for minutes to hours, or it may reappear episodically, after the exciting stimulus has been removed (palinopsia or paliopsia); the later disorder also occurs in defective but not blind homonymous fields of vision. *Polyopia* (polyopsia), the perception of double or multiple images when a single stimulus (object) is presented, is said to be associated predominantly with right occipital lesions and can occur with either eye. Usually there is one primary and a number of secondary images, and their relationships may be constant or changing.

Bender and Krieger (1951), who described several such patients, attributed the polyopia to unstable fixation. *Oscillopsia*, or illusory movement of the environment, occurs mainly with lesions of the labyrinthine-vestibular apparatus and is described with disorder of ocular movement.

Other visuospatial anomalies associated with occipital lesions include *astereopsis* (loss of stereoscopic vision), *metamorphopsias* (visual distortions), *optic allesthesia* (misplacement of percepts in space), and *palinopsia* (persevered visual percept) (Damasio, 1988; Benson, 1989; Zihl, 1989; Barton and Caplan, 2001; Dănăilă and Golu, 2006). These are very rare conditions but of theoretical interest as they may provide clues to cortical organization and function. Lesions associated with these conditions tend to involve the parietal cortex as well.

Cortical blindness and Anton's syndrome

With bilateral lesions of the occipital lobe (destruction of area 17 of both hemispheres), there is a loss of sight and a loss of reflex closure of the eyelids to a bright light or threat. The degree of blindness may be equivalent to that which follows enucleation of the eyes or severance of the optic nerves. The pupillary light reflexes are preserved, since they depend upon visual fibres that terminate in the midbrain, short of the geniculate bodies. Usually no changes are detectable in the retinas, though van Buren (1963) has described slight optic atrophy in monkeys long after occipital ablation. The eyes are still able to move through a full range, but optokinetic nystagmus cannot be elicited. Visual imagination and visual imagery in dreams are preserved. With very rare exceptions, no cortical potential can be evoked in the occipital lobes by light flashes or pattern changes (visual evoked response), and the alpha rhythm is lost in the EEG. There may also be visual hallucinations of either elementary or complex types. The usual cause of cortical blindness is occlusion of the posterior cerebral arteries (embolic or thrombotic). The infarction may also involve the medial temporal regions and thalami with a resulting Korsakoff amnesic defect and a variety of other neurologic deficits referable to the high midbrain and diencephalon. Hypoxic-ischemic encephalopathy, Schilder disease and other leukodystrophies, Creutzfeldt-Jakob disease, progressive multifocal leukoence-phalopathy, and bilateral gliomas are other causes of cortical blindness.

A commonly associated phenomenon with cortical blindness is ***Anton's syndrome***, in which the patient with cortical blindness denies all visual difficulties. Anton's syndrome is considered a special form of anosognosia and is frequently seen only in the acute epoch (within 2 or 3 months following the event).

The main characteristic is denial of blindness by a patient who obviously cannot see. The patient acts as though he could see, and when attempting to walk, he collides with objects, even to the point of injury. He may offer excuses for his difficulties: "I lost my glasses", "The light is dim", etc., or there may be only an indifference to the loss of sight.

The lesion in cases of negation of blindness extend beyond the striate cortex to involve the visual association areas.

Cortical blindness and Anton's syndrome may also result from subcortical lesions to optic radiations. Pupillary responses are preserved, but visual evoked potential cannot be demonstrated (Jones and Tranel, 2002).

Bilateral lesions of primary visual cortex result in cortical blindness, a condition commonly caused by bilateral infarction of the posterior cerebral arteries.

Rarely, the opposite condition may arise: a patient can see small objects but claims to be blind. This individual walks about avoiding obstacles, picks up crumbs or pills from the table, and catches a small ball thrown from a distance. Damasio et al. (1980) suggests that this might be a type of visual disorientation but with sufficient residual visual information to guide the hand, and that the lesion will be in the visual association areas superior to the calcarine cortex.

Topographical disorientation

The term topographical disorientation refers to an acquired inability to navigate the environment in daily life (Tranel et al., 1997; Barrash, 1998; Damasio et al., 2000).

The most striking manifestation of spatial memory deficit is topographic disorientation – namely, the inability to find one's way in a familiar environment and to learn new paths, in the absence of global amnesia, severe mental deterioration, or disorders of visual perception and exploration. Förster (1890) and Meyer (1900) must be credited with having provided the first exhaustive description of its features. With restitution of function or in milder cases from the beginning, navigation is impaired only in environments that the patient has first experienced since the onset of disease (Habib and Sirigu, 1987).

Two broad types of topographical disorientation can be discerned. The first may be termed anterograde topographical disorientation, which involves a defect in new learning. Patients with this disorder will complain that they become lost in new places, cannot learn new routes, or cannot retrace their path in real life. Associated clinical findings may include left hemispatial neglect, left visual field cuts, and constructional dyspraxia. The site of lesion associated with the disorder is the medial occipitotemporal area, particularly on the right and including the posterior parahippocampal gyrus and lingual gyrus. Anterograde topographical agnosia has been described in cases of right parietal dysfunction, and of left mesial occipitotemporal dysfunction but in these cases the clinical phenomenon appears to be more transient and less severe.

Retrograde topographical disorientation refers to the inability to recognize previously well-known spatial / topographical routes. The patient with retrograde topographical disorientation will be unable to recognize either previously known visual scene (e.g., rooms in their home and the street on which they lived) or landmarks (e.g., their house and the local grocery). Patients with retrograde topographical disorientation are unable to describe in verbal terms from memory familiar scenes or routes. The lesion most commonly associated with this disorder is in the mesial occipitotemporal cortices of the right hemisphere, thus disconnecting primary visual cortex from higher order association cortices (Jones and Tranel, 2002).

It is apparent that the basic deficit underlying the patient's difficulty is the inability to retrieve and abstract map of the route, which specifies the spatial relationships defining the position of a place with respect to other places and the subject and to transform them in guidelines for walking.

Landmark recognition and spatial map construction are the main mental operations that assist navigation through familiar surroundings and their discrete disruption underlies two forms of route-finding disability, topographic agnosia and topographic amnesia (Paterson and Zangwill, 1945). The failure to identify a specific building might result from perceptual impairment that prevents the appreciation of the small distinctive features identifying an exemplar of a category whose elements are similar or from the inability to match the perceived building with its representation stored in memory. Prosopagnosia is a frequent, but not necessarily concomitant, topographic agnosia. Landis and coworkers (1986) found prosopagnosia in only 7 of 16 patients suffering from what they called "environmental agnosia".

Failure to recognize familiar environments is by no means a constant feature of patients with topographic disorientation. De Renzi and Scotti (1969) who were unable to identify famous building did not improve in taking his bearing when their names were provided by the examiner because he could not remember their position with respect to other sites of the city. The amnestic nature of this form of topographic disorientation is confirmed by the patient's failure to give a verbal description of the route, to trace it on a road map, and to draw a map of a familiar place.

The dissociation between topographic amnesia and topographic agnosia is exemplified by patient 5 of Aimard et al. (1981) who was unable to find a room in his apartment but, when he eventually opened its door, immediately recognized it. Of course, agnosic and amnesic disorders can coexist in the same patient, as both are dependent on right hemispheric damage.

The study of the anatomic correlates of topographic disorientation has pointed out the crucial role played by the posterior regions of the brain, especially of the right hemisphere. In some cases damage is bilateral (Förster, 1890; Wildbrand, 1892; Dunn, 1895; Peters, 1896; Meyer, 1900), but in others it is confined to the right side, where the areas more frequently involved are the parietal lobe (Paterson and Zangwill, 1945; Hécaen et al., 1956; Assal, 1969; Aimard et al., 1981; Newcombe and Ratcliff, 1990) and the medial occipitotemporal cortex (Gloning, 1965; Whitty and Newcombe, 1973; Hécaen et al., 1980; Aimard et al., 1981; Landis et al., 1986; Habib and Sirigu, 1987). The most frequent etiology is an infarction in the territory of the right posterior cerebral artery, which supplies blood to the medial surface of the occipital and temporal lobe. Habib and Sirigu (1987) argued that the crucial lesion is located in the right parahippocampal gyrus (posterior to the uncus and anterior to the subsplenial region), but it is difficult to reconcile this assumption with the lack of topographic disorientation found in patients submitted to right temporal ablation, although they showed psychometric signs of spatial learning impairment (Milner, 1965; Milner, 1971; Smith and Milner, 1981).

In the animal, parietal area 7, corresponding to the inferior parietal lobule in humans, has strong connections with the posterior parahippocampal gyrus, but the evidence that its damage results in route-finding impairment is meager and based only on the report that monkeys are hesitant and slow in finding their way to the cage after bilateral (Ettlinger and Wegener, 1958; Bates and Ettlinger, 1960) and also unilateral ablation (Sugishita et al., 1978) of areas 5 and 7.

Episodes of topographic disorientation are frequently seen in the advanced stages of degenerative dementia of Alzheimer type.

Eleven cases have been reported (Moretti et al., 1983; Stracciari, 1992; Stracciari et al., 1994). During the attack which lasted from 5 to 40 min, the patients were perfectly aware of what was happening to them and retained the ability to recognize places, shops, streets, and so on, but they could not find their way out. None of them showed signs of mental deterioration, or of verbal and spatial dysmnesia when the episode was over. This reflects a transient dysfunction of unknown origin of the right occipitotemporal region.

Defects in constructional skills

Constructional ability can be defined as the ability to manipulate materials to form an intended final construction (Jones and Tranel, 2002).

Copying drawings is a task that enjoys particular popularity in clinical practice because it is easy to administer at the bedside and is the simplest way to bring out constructional apraxia. This ability is well known to most practitioners, examples of tests of constructional ability are the Draw a Clock test, the block design subtest from the Wechsler Adult Intelligence Test, and the intersecting pentagons from the Mini Mental State Examination. The test of constructional ability presumes that the patient has adequate visual acuity to see the test and that motor skills are adequate to complete the test.

The mechanisms whereby a patient manifests defects in constructional abilities may be determined by examination of the process of construction or by examination of the final product.

The symptoms known by the neurologists for more than seventy years (Kleist, 1934) consist in the inability to assemble the elements of a bidimensional or tridimensional whole, respecting their orientations and spatial relationship. For example, visual neglect may be determined by a drawing task in which the item to be drawn (or copied) is placed far to the side of the page (usually the right side, indicating left hemispatial visual neglect). Hemispatial neglect may also be shown in a case in which one side of the object is distorted or missing. Finally, in the absence of neglect, there may be a lack of appreciation of visual spatial relationships apparent in the production of a drawing by the patient, in which elements of the object to be constructed are present but are distorted in their spatial relationship to one another (Jones and Tranel, 2002).

Kleist (1934) viewed constructional apraxia as a left parietal deficit, due to the disruption of a center (tentatively localized in the left angular gyrus) that would represent the interface between the analysis of visuospatial information and the planning of hand movements. On this assumption, the deficit would be attributable to neither a perceptual nor an executive impairment but to the stage where movement programs, which are organized by the left hemisphere, must be monitored by spatial analysis. This hypothesis was abandoned when it was shown that constructional apraxia is by no means limited to left parietal damage and is indeed as frequent or even more frequent following right brain damage.

The evidence that constructional apraxia reflects the disruption of different abilities, depending on the damage side, is most suggestive but has not been unequivocally demonstrated. Although an executive impairment remains a possible component of the defective performance of left brain-damaged patients, visuospatial disorders are likely to be influential in both hemispheric groups. Parietal damage is a frequent anatomic correlate of constructional apraxia after damage to either hemisphere, although the association is closer in right brain-damage patients than in left brain-damage patients (Ajuriaguerra et al., 1960).

Reproduction of a structured model is a sequential task that requires a certain degree of planning and is, therefore, liable to be sensitive to the functioning of frontal structures (Luria and Tsvetkova, 1964; Benton, 1968).

Supportive of the idea that different mechanisms underlie parietal and frontal constructional apraxia is the finding that the disorder is associated with poor performance on a line bisection task in right brain-damaged patients having damage to the parietooccipital cortex but not in those with frontal, subcortical damage (Pillon, 1981; Marshall et al., 1994).

In conclusion, the site of lesion associated with defects in constructional skills is typically the right occipital cortices and adjacent visual association cortex. There may be a greater perceptual component to the defect with more ventral lesions and a greater defect of spatial relationship with more dorsal lesions. In some cases, constructional disabilities can be observed in left-sided lesions in these same sites, but such patients often have a fluent aphasia, a lesser or more transient constructional defect, and the defect is more likely to show a lack of appreciation of spatial relationships and preserved visuoperception (Jones and Tranel, 2002). Since the introduction of imaging techniques in clinical practice, it has been increasingly recognized that subcortical structures contribute to cognitive functions, and disorder of language, praxis, lateralized attention, and so on, have been reported following damage to basal nuclei.

Visual illusions (metamorphopsias)

According to Adams and colleagues (1997), these may present as distortions of form, size, movement, or color; also visual images may fail to arouse visual memories and their associated effect, resulting in a sense of strangeness or inexplicable familiarity, as it occurs in the "dreamy state" of temporal lobe epilepsy.

Visual illusions take the form of objects seeming too small (*microppsia*) or too large (*megalopsia or macropsia*) or that appear to be moving toward or away from the patient. In other cases, objects may appear elongated, swollen, or run together or the vertical and horizontal orientation of the image may shift (*metamorphopsia*). Inverted vision, irradiation of contour, disappearance of color (*achromatopsia*), illusional coloring (*erythropsia), polyopia* (one object appearing as two or more objects), *monocular diplopia* (vertical, concentric, especially triplopia), illusions of movement of stationary objects, too rapid displacement of moving objects or imperception of movement are other form of illusory visual experience. Also, there may be a loss of stereoscopic vision, perseveration or periodic reappearance of visual images long after the cessation of the visual stimulus (*palinopsia or paliopsia*), or a false orientation of objects in space (*optic allesthesia)* (Hécaen, 1962).

Illusions of these types have been reported with lesions of the occipital, occipitoparietal, or occipitotemporal regions, and the right hemisphere appears to be involved more often than the left one. Illusions of movement occur more frequently with posterior temporal lesions, polyopia (polyopsia) more frequently with occipital lesions (although it may occur in hysteria), and palinopsia with both parietal and occipital lesions.

Visual field defects are present in many of the cases.

Hoff and Potzl (1935) have insisted that an element of vestibular disorder underlies the metamorphopsias of parieto-occipital lesions (the vestibular and proprioceptive systems are represented in the right parietal lobe and lesions there are responsible for misperceptions of movement and spatial relations). The illusion of tilting of the environment or upside-down vision occurs more often with lesions of the vestibular nuclei than with those of the occipital-parietal cortex.

Pharmacological agents like atropine, lysergic acid, and mescaline cause many of the afore-mentioned illusory phenomena.

Visual hallucinations

A hallucination is a perception in the absence of an adequate peripheral stimulus; it must be distinguished from an illusion, which is a misinterpretation of a perception. Illusions occur in normal people, especially when they are tired, inattentive, or in states of high expectation.

Visual hallucinations are less frequent in schizophrenia than auditory ones, but when they are present, they often occur in association with other hallucinations. Visual hallucinations of small animals are noted in delirium, especially delirium tremens, and fornication, the sensation that animals are crawling under the skin or over the body, have been associated with cocaine psychosis.

Traditionally it has been taught that the lesions responsible for visual hallucinations, if identifiable, are usually situated in the occipital lobe or posterior part of the temporal lobe, and that elementary hallucinations have their origin in the occipital cortex, and complex ones, in the temporal cortex. However, the complexity of visual hallucinations has only limited diagnostic value; in some cases, formed hallucinations are localizing with lesions of the occipital lobe and unformed ones with lesions of the temporal lobe (Weinberger and Grant, 1941).

Also, as emphasized by these authors, lesions that give rise to visual hallucinations, simple or elaborate, need not be confined to central nervous structures but may be caused by lesions at every level of the neuro-optic apparatus (retina, optic nerve, chiasma, etc.).

So, visual hallucinations caused by a neurological disease are attributable to lesions anywhere in the visual system from the retina (macular degeneration, cataracts, enucleations), optic nerve and tract, midbrain, geniculocalcarine radiation (multiple sclerosis, ischemia, compression, stroke, tumors), to the occipital or temporal cortex (stroke, tumors, seizures). They sometimes reflect sensory deprivation.

Other visual hallucinations appear in migraine, narcolepsy, Alzheimer's disease, diffuse Lewy body disease, Parkinson's disease with dopaminergic treatment, drug intoxication or withdrawal, metabolic encephalopathies (delirium), schizophrenia, and depression or mania (mood congruent). The clinical setting for the occurrence of visual hallucinations varies. The simplest black and white moving scintillations are part of migraine. Others, some colored, can occur as a seizure aura. Often they are associated with a homonymous hemianopia, as indicated earlier. Frequently they occur as part of a confusional state or delirium. In the "peduncular hallucinosis" of Lhermitte (1971), the hallucinations are purely visual, appear natural in form and color, sometimes in pastels, move about as in an animated cartoon, and are usually considered to be unreal, abnormal phenomena (preserved insight). Similar phenomena may occur as part of hypnagogic hallucinations in the narcolepsy-cataplexy syndrome.

In their material, McKee and associates (1990) emphasize that so-called peduncular hallucinosis has been associated mainly with high mesencephalic lesions and, more particularly in one case, with lesions of the pars reticulata of the substantia nigra. The hallucinations in this disorder are purely visual; if hallucinations are polymodal, the lesion is always in the occipitotemporal parts of the cerebrum.

Visual hallucinations may be elementary or complex, and both types have sensory as well as cognitive aspects.

Elementary (or unformed) hallucinations include flashes of light, colors, luminous points, stars, multiple lights (like candles), and geometric forms (circles, squares, and hexagons). They may be stationary or moving (zigzag, oscillations, vibrations, or pulsations). They are much the same as the effects that Foerster and Penfield (1930) obtained by stimulating the calcarine cortex in a conscious person. Complex, or formed, hallucinations include objects, persons or animals. They are indicative of lesions in the visual association areas or their connections with the temporal lobe. They may be of natural size, lilliputian, or grossly enlarged.

With hemianopsia, they may appear in the defective field or move from the intact field toward the hemianopsic one. The patient may realize that the hallucinations are false experiences or may be convinced of their reality. Patient's response is usually in accord with the nature of the hallucination or he may react with fear to a threatening vision.

A special syndrome of ophthalmopathic hallucinations occurs in the blind person. The visual images may be of elementary or complex type, usually of people or animals, and are polychromic (vivid colors). The hallucinations may occupy all of the visual field, the field of one eye, or corresponding blind fields in the patient with homonymous hemianopia (hemianopsia). Moving the eyes or closing the affected eye has variable effects, sometimes abolishing the hallucinations. A similar phenomenon in the elderly (with preserved vision) has been called the "syndrome of Bonnet", following the report by this author of visual hallucinations occurring in a "sane" person. The topic of senile hallucinations has been extensively reviewed by Gold and Robin (1989).

The hallucinatory phenomena of delirium are nonlocalizable, but sometimes the evidence points to an origin in the temporal lobe. In ophthalmopathic hallucinations, there is visual loss from retinal, optic nerve or tract, or occipital lobe lesions, and, with the latter locations, a slight impairment of mental function as well.

Visual imagery

Visual mental imagery refers to the evocation of visual images in the "mind's eye" in the absence of sensation through the retina.

Early studies demonstrated that patients with various types of deficits in higher order visual functions (e.g., achromatopsia and spatial neglect) tended to show similar deficits in mental imagery. For example, when asked to imagine walking down a familiar street, a patient with left hemispatial visual neglect would describe only the buildings on the right side of the street. When asked to imagine turning around and walking the other direction up the street, the same patient would describe buildings on the other side of the street that had previously been neglected (Heilman et al., 1993; Farah, 2001; Tranel, 2001).

Similarly, patients with deficits in color perception due to cerebral lesions have been shown to have deficits in imaging colors of objects (Temple, 1992; Farah, 2001). So, visual perceptual deficits in patients can often be demonstrated in some way by similar deficits in visual imagery.

Visualization is crucial in problem-solving tasks such as mental arithmetic, map reading, and mechanical reasoning.

Behrmann and colleagues (1992) described a patient, CK. The curious thing about CK is that, although he cannot recognize objects, he can imagine them and can draw them in considerable detail from memory. This ability implies some dissociation between the neural system dealing with object perception and that dealing with the generation of images. Kolb and Whishaw (2003) conclude that neural structures mediating the perception and visualization of objects are unlikely to be completely independent, but it is clear that a deficit in object perception cannot be due simply to a loss of mental representations (that is, memory) of objects.

Farah (1984, 1990) and Kosslyn and Thompson (2000) proposed that mental rotation of objects probably entails both hemispheres, with some degree of right-hemisphere superiority.

Nonetheless, it does seem likely that mental rotation implicates structures related to the dorsal stream. We can imagine that, before a brain could visualize rotating an object, it would first have to have actually rotated it manually. This requires the activation of at least part of the motor cortex – the region needed to actually do it. Farah (1984, 1990) concluded that, although the data designed to identify the natural events underlying the generation of a mental image are noisy, a reasonably consistent answer is emerging from the results of imaging studies.

D'Esposito and colleagues (1997) addressed this question in an fMRI study by asking subjects to generate mental images from memory, cued by an aurally presented word such as "tree". The subjects kept their eyes closed throughout the experiment so that any neural activation could be attributed to imagery rather than to direct activation of the visual pathways. The results show that visualizing concrete words increases activation in the left posterior temporo-occipital region corresponding to the fusiform gyrus (area 37). There was no activation in area V1, the fMRI data are consistent to those of other imaging studies, as well as to a case history of a patient with a left-occipital lobectomy (including area 37) who had hemianopia in both real and imagined stimuli. The pronounced asymmetry is consistent with Farah's hypothesis that, in most people, the left hemisphere is specialized for image generation.

Mental imagery appears to be a top-down activation of a subset of the brain's visual areas. In other words, at least some cortical areas are used both for perception and for visualization.

These common areas carry the same representational functions for both purposes, carrying information specifically about color, shape, spatial location, and so on. There is evidence for a distinct mechanism for image generation as well, one separates from the processes needed for perception. Farah notes that the evidence, although mixed, points to a region in the left temporo-occipital region as the key location for this mechanism.

Anyhow, the neural underpinnings of deficits in visual imagery have been located primarily in visual association cortex (areas 8 and 19) and more anterior association cortices. However, data from functional MRI studies suggest that primary visual cortex (area 17) may be more actively involved in mental imagery than there had previously been suspected.

Summary
Lesions in the primary visual area

A unilateral lesion in the primary visual area (Brodmann's area 17) results in blindness of the contralateral visual field, referred to as a contralateral homonymous hemianopsia. If distruction of the primary visual cortex is the result of a vascular lesion, macular sparing may occurs, that is, central vision is unaffected.

It is believed that this due to the presence of collateral anastomotic channels between the middle and posterior cerebral arteries.

A bilateral lesion in the primary visual area results in complete blindness, also referred to as cortical blindness.

The usual cause of cortical blindness occlusion of the posterior cerebral arteries (embolic and thrombotic). A transitory form of cortical blindness may occur with head injury, migraine, or the antiphospholipid antibody syndrome of lupus erythematous, and as a consequence of intravascular dye injection and administration of a number of drugs such as interferon-alpha or cyclosporine.

Lesions in the association with visual areas

A lesion in the association with visual areas (Brodmann's areas 18 and 19) (usually, bilaterally) results in visual agnosia. Since the visual pathways and primary visual cortex are intact, the individual is able to "see" an object or person. However, although he may be locking at a familiar object or person, he is unable to identify them, or describe the function of it.

Selective disorders of form discrimination (including depth perception and the integration of features into a whole) as well as disorders affecting the surface properties of objects (such as their texture or color) have been documented.

An individual with visual agnosia may recognize an object one day but not the next. Also, he may recognize certain familiar objects but not others. Interestingly, an object may be identified by other senses, such as touch.

Dyslexia is a type of visual agnosia. Four patterns of dyslexia have been recognized: letter-by-letter, deep, phonological, and surface dyslexia.

Letter-by-letter dyslexia is equivalent to pure alexia without agraphia. Deep dyslexia is a severe reading disorder in which patients recognize and read aloud only familiar words, especially concrete, imageable nouns and verbs. Phenological dyslexia is similar to deep dyslexia, with poor reading of nonwords, but single nouns and verbs are read in a nearly normal fashion and semantic errors are rare. The fourth type, surface dyslexia, involves spared ability to read laboriously by grapheme-phoneme conversion but inability to recognize words at a glance.

Individuals with dyslexia are unable to read and write words, although they can see and recognize letters.

REFERENCES

Adams RD, Victor M, Ropper AH, Neurologic disorders caused by lesions in particular parts of the cerebrum. In: RD Adams et al. (eds.). *Principles of Neurology*. Sixth Edition, chap 22; New York, St Louis, San Francisco, etc., McGraw-Hill, 435-471, 1997.

Adolphs R, Tranel D, Damasio H, Damasio AR, Impaired recognition of emotion in facial expressions following bilateral damage to the human amygdala. Nature 372; 669-672, 1994.

Adolphs R, Tranel D, Damasio H, Damasio AR, Fear and the human amygdala. J Neurosci 15; 5879-5891, 1995.

Adolphs R, Tranel D, Damasio AR, The human amygdala in social judgment. Nature 393; 470-474, 1998

Aimard G, Vighetto A, Confavreux C, Devic M, La désorientation spatiale. Rev Neurol 137; 97-111, 1981.

Ajuriaguerra J, Hecaen H, Angelergues R, Les apraxies: Variétés cliniques et latéralisation lésionnelle. Rev Neurol 102; 566-594, 1960.

Albright TD, Direction and orientation selectivity of neurons in visual area MT of macaque. J. Neurophysiol 52; 1106-1130, 1984.

Albright TD, Form-cue invariant motion processing in primate visual cortex. Science 255; 11141-1143, 1992.

Assal G, Régression des troubles de la reconnaissance des physionomies et de la mémoire topographique chez un malade opéré d'un hématome intracérébral pariétotemporal droite. Rev Neurol 121; 184-185, 1969.

Barbur JL, Watson JDG, Franckowiak RSJ, Zeki S, Conscious visual perception without V1. Brain 116; 1293-1302, 1993.

Bargh JA, Ferguson MJ, Beyond behaviorism: On the automaticity of higher mental processes. Psychological Bulletin 126; 925-945, 2000.

Barlow HB, Blakemore C, Pettigrew JD, The neural mechanism of binocular depth discrimination. J. Physiol 193; 327-342, 1967.

Bates JAV, Ettlinger G, Posterior biparietal ablation in the monkey. Arch Neurol 3; 177-192, 1960.

Barrash J, A historical review of topographical disorientation and its neuroanatomical correlates. J Clin Exp Neuropsychol 20; 807-827, 1998.

Barton JJ, Caplan LR, Cerebral visual dysfunction. In: J Bogousslavsky and LR Caplan (eds). *Stroke Syndromes*. (2nd ed) Cambridge, UK: Cambridge University Press, 2001.

Behrmann M, Winocur G, Moscovitch M, Dissociation between mental imagery and object recognition in a brain-damaged patient. Nature 359; 636-637, 1992.

Bender MB, Krieger HP, Visual function in perimetric blind field. Arch Neurol Psychiatry 65; 72, 1951.

Benson DF, Disorders of visual gnosis. In: JW Brown (ed), *Neuropsychology of Visual Perception*. New York: IRBN Press, 1989.

Benton AL, Differential behavioral effects in frontal lobe disease. Neuropsychologia 6; 53-60, 1968.

Berson DM, Strange vision: ganglion cells as circadian photoreceptors. Trends Neurosci 26; 314-320, 2003.

Blardel GG, Salama G, Voltage-sensitive dyes reveal a modular organization in monkey striate cortex. Nature 321; 579-585, 1986.

Bonhoffer T, Grinvald A, Optical imaging based on intrinsic signals: The methodology. In: A Tage (ed), *Brain Mapping: The Methods.* New York: Academic Press, 1996.

Bonhoffer T, Grinvald A, The layout of iso-orientation domains in area 18 of the cat visual cortex: Optical imaging reveals a pinwheel-like organization. J Neurosci 13; 4157-4180, 1993.

Bodamer J, Die Prosopagnosie. Arch Psychiatr Nervenkrank 179; 6-53, 1947.

Boussaud D, Ungerleider GL, Desimone R, Pathways for motion analysis: Cortical connections of the medial superior temporal and fundus of the superior temporal visual areas in the macaque. Journal of Comparative Neurology 296; 462-495, 1990.

Bouvier SE, Engel SA, Behavioral deficits and cortical damage loci in cerebral achromatopsia. Cereb Cortex 16; 183-191, 2006.

Bullier J, Feedback connections and conscious vision. Trend Cogn. Sci. 5; 369-370, 2001.

Burton H, Abend NS, MacLeod A-MK, et al., Tactile attention tasks enhance activation in somatosensory regions of parietal cortex: A positron emission tomography study. Cerebral Cortex 9; 662-674, 1999.

Callaway EM, Local circuits in primary visual cortex of the macaque monkey. Ann Rev Neurosci 21; 47-74, 1998.

Campbell R, Landis T, Regard M, Face recognition and lip reading: A neurological dissociation. Brain 108; 509-521, 1986.

Casagrande VA, Kaas JH, The afferent, intrinsic, and efferent connections of primary visual cortex in primates. In: A Peters and K Rockland (eds), *Cerebral Cortex,* Vol. 10, Plenum Press, New York; 201-259, 1994.

Chaves CJ, Caplan LR, Posterior cerebral artery. In: J Bogousslavsky and LR Caplan (eds). *Stroke Syndromes.* Cambridge, UK: Cambridge University Press, 2001.

Clarke S, Miklossy J, Occipital cortex in man. Organization of callosal connections, related myelo- and cytoarchitecture, and putative boundaries of functional visual areas. Journal of Comparative Neurology 298; 188-214, 1990.

Corbetta M, Mierzin FM, Dobmeyer S, et al., Selective and divided attention during visual discrimination of shape, color, and speed: Functional anatomy by positron emission tomography. Journal of Neuroscience 11; 2383-2402, 1991.

Corbetta M, Mierzin FM, Shulman GL, Petersen SE, A PET study of visuospatial attention. Journal of Neuroscience 13; 1202-1226, 1993.

Courtney SM, Ungerleider LG, What fMRI has taught us about human vision. Curr Op Neurobiol 7; 554-561, 1997.

Chalupa LM, Werner JS (eds), The Visual Neuroscience. Cambridge, MA: MIT Press, 2004.

Crick E, Koch C, Are we aware of neural activity in primary visual cortex? Nature 375; 121-123, 1995.

Cumming BC, An unexpected specialization for horizontal disparity in primate primary visual cortex. Nature 418; 633-636, 2002.

Damasio AR, Disorder of complex visual processing: Agnosia, achromatopsia, Balint's syndrome and related difficulties of orientation and construction. In: Mesulam MM (ed), *Principles of Behavioral Neurology.* Philadelphia, Davis; 259-288, 1985.

Damasio AR, Regional diagnosis of cerebral disorders. In: JB Wyngaarden and LH Smith, Jr (eds), *Textbook of Medicine* (18th ed). Philadelphia: Saunders, 1988.

Damasio AR, McKee J, Damasio H, Determinants of performance in color anomia. Brain Land 7; 74-85, 1979.

Damasio A, Yamada T, Damasio H, et al., Central achromatopsia: Behavioral, anatomic, and psychologic aspects. Neurology 30; 1064, 1980.

Damasio AR, Damasio H, Van Hoesen GW, Prosopagnosia: Anatomical basis and behavioral mechanisms. Neurology 32; 331-341, 1982.

Damasio AR, Tranel D, Damasio H, Disorders of visual recognition. In: F Boller and J Grafman (eds), *Handbook of Neuropsychology,* Vol. 2, Amsterdam, Elsevier, 1989.

Damasio AR, Tranel D, Rizzo M, Disorders of complex visual processing. In: MM Mesulam (ed), *Principles of Behavioral and Cognitive Neurology.* Oxford Univ Press, New York, 332-372, 2000.

Dănăilă L, Golu M, *Tratat de Neuropsihologie,* Vol 2, Editura Medicală Bucureşti; 261-319, 2006.

De Haan EHF, A familial factor in the development of face recognition deficits. J Clin Exp Neuropsychol 21; 312-315, 1999.

De Haan EHF, Campbell R, A fifteen year follow-up of a case of developmental prosopagnosia. Cortex 27; 489-509, 1991.

De Renzi E, Scotti G, The influence of spatial disorders in impairing tactual discrimination of shapes. Cortex 5; 53-62, 1969.

De Renzi E, Bonacini MG, Faglioni P, Right posterior patients are poor assessing the age of a face. Neuropsychologia 27; 839-848, 1989.

Déjérine J, Sur un cas de cécité verbale avec agraphie, suivi d'autopsie. CK Séances Soc Biol 3; 197-201, 1891.

Déjérine J, Contribution à l'étude anatomo-pathologique et clinique des différents variétés de cécité verbale. CR Séances Soc Biol 4; 61-90, 1892.

Desimone R, Albright TD, Gross CG, Bruce C, Stimulus-selective properties of inferior temporal neurons in the macaque. J. Neurosci 4; 2051-2062, 1984.

Deyoe EA, Occipital lobe. In: VS Ramachandran (ed.), *Encyclopedia of the Human Brain,* Vol. 3, Academic Press, Amsterdam, Boston, London, etc.; 677-7115, 2002.

Deyoe EA, van Essen DC, Concurrent processing streams in monkey visual cortex. Trends Neurosci 11; 219-226, 1988.

Dunn D, Double hemiplegia with double hemianopsia and loss of a geographical center. Trans Coll Phys Philadelphia 17; 45-55, 1895.

D'Esposito M, Detre JA, Aguirre GK, et al., A functional MRI study of mental image generation. Neuropsychologia 35; 725-730, 1997.

Ettlinger G, Wegener J, Somaesthetic alternation, discrimination and orientation after frontal, and parietal lesions in the monkey. Q J Exp Psychol 10; 177-186, 1958.

Eastwood JD, Smilek D, Merikle PM, Differential attentional guidance by unattended faces expressing positive and negative emotion. Perception and Psychophysics 63; 1004-1013, 2001.

Epstein R, Konwisher N, Representation of perceived object shape by the human lateral occipital complex. Science 293, 1506-1509, 1998.

Farah MJ, The neurological basis of mental imagery. A componential analysis. Cognition 18; 245-272, 1984.

Farah M, Visual agnosia: Disorders of object recognition and what they tell us about normal vision. Cambridge, MA: MIT Press, 1990.

Farah MJ, The neuropsychology of mental imagery. In: F Boller and J Grafman (eds.), *Handbook of Neuropsychology.* Vol. 2, Amsterdam, Elsevier, 1990.

Farah MJ What is "special" about face perception? Psychological Review 105; 482-498, 1998.

Farah MJ, The neural basis of mental imagery. In: MS Gazzaniga (ed.), *The New Cognitive Neurosciences.* 2nd ed. Cambridge MA: MIT Press; 965-974, 2000.

Farah MJ, The neuropsychology of mental imagery. In: F Boller and J Grafman (eds), *Handbook of Neuropsychology.* 2nd ed. Vol 4, Elsevier, Amsterdam; 239-248, 2001.

Farah MJ, Levine DN, Calvanio R, A case study of mental imagery deficit. Brain Cog 8; 147-164, 1988.

Farah MJ, Tanaka JW, Drain HM, What causes the face inversion effect? J Psychol Hum Percept Perform 21; 628-634, 1995.

Felleman DJ, Van Essen DC, Distributed hierarchical processing in the primate cerebral cortex. Cerebral Cortex 1; 1-47, 1991.

Förster R, Ueber Rindenblindheit. Albrecht v. Graefe Arch Ophtalmol 38; 94-108, 1890.

Foerster O, Penfield W, The structural basis of traumatic epilepsy and results of radical operation. Brain 53; 99-119, 1930.

Geschwind N, Fusillo M, Color naming defectes in association with alexia. Arch Neurol. 15; 137-146, 1966.

Gloning K, Die Cerebralen Bedingten Stoerungen de Raumlichen Sehens und des Raumerlebens. Vienna, Maudrig, 1965.

Gold K, Robin PV, Isolated visual hallucinations and the Charles Bonnet syndrome: A review of the literature and presentations of six cases. Comp Psychiatry 30; 90, 1989.

Goodale MA, Visual pathways supporting perception and action in the primate cerebral cortex. Current Opinion in Neurobiology 3; 578-585, 1993.

Goodale MA, Perception and action in the human visual system. In: MS Gazzaniga (ed), *The New Cognitive Neurosciences.* 2nd ed. Cambridge MA: MIT Press; 365-377, 2000.

Goodale MA, Humphrey GK, The objects of action and perception. Cognition 67; 181-207, 1998.

Goodale MA, Millner DA, Jakobson LS, Carey JDP, A neurological dissociation between perceiving objects and grasping them. Nature 349; 154-156, 1991.

Goodglass H, Wingfield A, Hyde MR, Theukrauf JC, Category specific dissociations in naming and recognition by aphasic patients. Cortex 22; 87-102, 1986.

Grill-Spector K, Kushner T, Edelman S, et al., Differential processing of objects under various viewing conditions in the human lateral occipital complex. Neuron 24; 187-203, 1999.

Gross CG, Representation of visual stimuli in inferior temporal cortex. Philos Trans R Soc Lond B Biol Sci 335, 3-10, 1992.

Habib A, Sirigu A, Pure topographical disorientation: A definition and anatomical basis. Cortex 23; 73-85, 1987.

Hancock PJB, Bruce V, Burton M, Recognition of unfamiliar faces. Trends in cognitive Science 4; 330-337, 2000.

Hattar S, Liao HW, Takao M, et al., Melanopsin-containing retinal ganglion cells: Architecture, projections, and intrinsic photosensitivity. Science 295; 1065-1070, 2002.

Haxby JV, Ungerleider LG, Clark VP, et al., The effect of face inversion on activity in human neural systems for face and object perception. Neuron 22; 189-199, 1999.

Haxby JV, Hoffman EA, Gobbini MI, The distributed human neural system for face perception. Trends in Cognitive Science 4; 223-233, 2000.

Hécaen H, Penfield W, Bertrand C, Malno R, The syndrome of apractognosia due to lesions of the minor cerebral hemisphere. Arch Neurol Psychiatry 75; 400-434, 1956.

Hécaen H, Clinical symptomatology in right and left hemispheric lesions. In: VB Mountcastle (ed) *Interhemispheric Relations and Cerebral Dominance.* Baltimore, Johns Hopkins. Ch. 10; 215-263, 1962.

Hécaen H, Tzortzis C, Randot P, Loss of topographical memory with learning deficits. Cortex 16; 525-542, 1980.

Heilman KM, Watson RT, Valenstein E, Neglect and related disorders. In: KM Heilman and E Valenstein (eds), *Clinical Neuropsychology.* 3rd ed. Oxford Univ Press, New York; 279-336, 1993.

Hendry SH, Reid RC, The koniocellular pathway in primate vision. Anu Rev Neurosci 23; 127-153, 2000.

Hoff H, Potzl O, Zür diagnostischen Bedeutung der Polyopie bei Tumoren des Okzipithalhirns. Z Gesante Neurol Psychiatr 152; 433, 1935.

Horton JC, The central visual pathways. In: WM Hart (ed.), *Alder's Physiology of the Eye.* St Louis: Mosby Yearbook, 1992.

Hubel DH, *Eye, Brain and Vision.* New York: Scientific American Library, 1988.

Hubel DH, Wiesel TN, Receptive fields, binocular interaction and functional architecture in the cat's visual cortex. J Physiol (Lond) 160; 106-154, 1962.

Hubel DH, Wiesel TN, Receptive fields and functional architecture of monkey striate cortex. J Physiol (Lond) 195; 215-243, 1968.

Hubel DH, Wiesel TN, Functional architecture of macaque monkey visual cortex. Proc R Soc (Lond) 198; 1-59, 1977.

Jakobson LS, Archibald YM, Carey DP, Goodale MA, A kinematic analysis of reaching and grasping movements in a patient recovering from optic ataxia. Neuropsychologia 2; 803-809, 1991.

Jones R, Tranel D, Severe "associative" developmental prosopagnosia in a child with superior intellect. J Clin Exp Neuropsychol 23; 265-273, 2001.

Jones RD, Tranel D, Visual disorder. In: VS Ramachandran (ed), *Encyclopedia of the Human Brain,* Vol 4. Amsterdam, Boston, London etc., Academic Press; 775-789, 2002.

Julesz B, Foundations of Cyclopean Perception. Chicago: The University of Chicago Press, 1971.

Julesz, B, Dialogues on Perception. Cambridge, MA: MIT Press, 1995.

James TW, Culham J, Humphrey GK, et al., Ventral occipital lesions impair object recognition but not object-directed grasping. An fMRI study. Brain 126; 2463-2475, 2003.

Kaas JH, The organization and evolution of neocortex. In: SP Wise (ed), Ed. *Higher Brain Function.* New York: Wiley, 1987.

Kaas J, The organization of visual cortex in primates: Problems, conclusions, and the use of comparative studies in understanding the human brain. In: K Rockland (ed), *Cerebral Cortex,* Vol. 12, Plenum Press, New York, 1997.

Kahneman D, Attention and Effort. Englewood Cliffs, NJ: Prentice-Hall, 1973.

Kanwisher N, Mc Dermott J, Chun MM, The fusiform face area: a module in human extrastriate cortex specialized for face perception. J. Neurosci. 17, 4302-4311, 1997.

Kingdom F, Li H-CO, Mac Aulay EJ, The role of chromatic contrast and luminance polarity in stereoscopic segmentation. Vision Research 41; 375-383, 2001.

Kinsbourne M, Warrington EK, The localizing significance of limited simultaneous visual form perception. Brain 86; 697, 1963.

Kinsbourne M, Warrington EK, Observations on color agnosia. J Neurol Neurosurg Psychiatry 27; 296-299, 1964.

Kleist K, *Gehirnpathologie.* Leipzig, Barth, 1934.

Kolb B, Whishaw JQ, The occipitals lobes. In: B Kolb and JQ Whishaw (eds), *Fundamentals of Human Neuropsychology* Fifth Edition, Worth Publishers, New York; 318-344, 2003.

Kolb B, Milner B, Taylor L, Perception of faces by patients with localized cortical excisions. Canadian Journal of Psychology 37; 8-18, 1983.

Kosslyn SM, Thompson WL, Shared mechanisms in visual imagery and visual perception: Insight from cognitive neuroscience. In: MS Gazzaniga (ed.), *The New Cognitive Neurosciences.* 2nd ed. Cambridge MA: MIT Press; 975-986, 2000.

Kourtzi Z, Kanwisher N, Representation of perceived object shape by the human lateral occipital complex. Science 293, 1506-1509, 2001.

Kracke J, Developmental prosopagnosia in Asperger syndrome: Presentation and discussion of an individual case. Dev Med Child Neurol 36; 873-886, 1994.

Kuffler SW, Discharge patterns and functional organization of mammallian retina. J Neurophysiol 16; 37-68, 1953.

Kurucz J, Feldmar G, Prosopo-affective agnosia as a symptom of cerebral organic disease. J Am Geriatric Soc 23; 225-230, 1979.

Lamme VA, Roclfsema PR, The distinct models of vision offered by feedforward and recurrent processing. Trends Neurosci 23, 571-579, 2000.

Land E, Recent advances in Retinex theory. Vis Res 26; 7-21, 1986.

Landis T, Cummings JL, Benson DF, Palmer EP, Loss of topographical familiarity. An environmental agnosia. Arch Neurol. 43; 132-136, 1986.

Lhermitte F, Chain F, Escourolle, et al., Etude des troubles perceptifs auditifs dans les lésions temporales bilatérales. Revue Neurol. (Paris) 124; 329-351, 1971.

Lissauer H, A case of visual agnosia with a contribution to theory. Cognitive Neuropsychology 5; 157-192, 1888.

Lissauer H, Ein Fall von Seelenblindheit nebst eine Beitrag zur Theorie des selben. Arch für Psychiatrie und Nervenkrankheiten 21; 222-270, 1890.

Livingston M, Hubel D, Segregation of form, color, movement and depth: Anatomy, physiology, and perception. Science 240; 740-749, 1988.

Luria AR, Tsvetkova LS, The programming of constructive activity in local brain injuries. Neuropsychologia 2; 95-108, 1964.

Logan GD, Attention and preattention in theories of automaticity. American Journal of Psychology 105; 317-340, 1992.

Logothetis NK, Paulus J, Poggio T, Shape representation in the inferior temporal cortex of monkeys. Curr Biol 5, 552-563, 1995.

Lorente de No R, The structure of the cerebral cortex. Physiology of the Nervous System, 3rd ed. New York: Oxford University Press, 1949.

Luzzatti C, Davidoff J, Impaired retrieval of object-color knowledge with preserved color naming. Neuropsychologia 32; 933-950, 1994.

Marshall JC, Newcombe F, Patterns of paralexia : A psycholinguistic approach. H Psycholing Res 2; 175-199, 1973.

Marshall RS, Lazar RM, Bindcr JR, ct al., Intrahemispheric localization of drawing dysfunction. Neuropsychologia 32; 493-501, 1994.

Maunsell JHK, Functional visual streams. Curr Opin Neurobiol 2; 506-510, 1992.

Mc Carthy G, Puce A, Gore JC, Allison T, Face-specific processing in human fusiform gyrus. J. Cogn Neurosci 9, 605-610, 1997.

McKee AC, Levine D, Kowall NW, Richardson EP, Peduncular hallucinations associated with isolated infarction of the substantia nigra pars reticulata. Ann Neurol 27; 500, 1990.

McNeil JE, Warrington EK, Prosopagnosia: a face-specific disorder. Q J Exp Psychol 46; 1-10, 1993.

Meadows JC, The anatomical basis of prosopagnosia. J Neurol Neurosurg Psychiatr 37; 489-501, 1974.

Meadows JC, Disturbed perception of color associated with localized cerebral lesions. Brain 97; 615-632, 1974.

Meyer O, Ein- und doppelseitige homonyme Hemianopsie mit Orientierungstoerungen. Monatschr Psychiatr Neurol 8; 440-456, 1900.

Milner B, Visually-guided maze learning in man: Effects of bilateral hippocampal, bilateral frontal and unilateral cerebral lesions. Neuropsychologia 3; 317-338, 1965.

Milner B, Interhemispheric differences in the localization of psychological processes in man. Brit Med Bull 27; 272-277, 1971.

Milner AD, Goodale MA, The Visual Brain in Action. Oxford: Oxford University Press, 1995.

Moran J, Desimone R, Selective attention gates visual processing in the extrastriate cortex. Science 229; 782-784, 1985.

Moretti G, Cafarra P, Parma M, Transient topographical amnesia. Ital J Neurol Sci 3; 361, 1983.

Moscovitch M, Winocur G, Behrmann M, What is special about face recognition? Nineteen experiments on a person with visual object agnosia and dyslexia but normal face recognition. J Cogn Neurosci 9; 555-604, 1997.

Mountcastle VB, Modality and topographic properties of single neurons of cat's somatic sensory cortex. J Neurophysiol 20; 408-434, 1957.

Mountcastle VB, Perceptual Neuroscience: The Cerebral Cortex. Cambridge: Harvard University Press, 1988.

Mountcastle VB, The parietal system and some higher brain functions. Cerebral Cortex 5; 377-390, 1995.

Moutoussis K, Zeki S, The relationship between cortical activation and perception investigated with invisible stimuli. Proc Natl Acad Sci USA 99; 9527-9532, 2002.

Moutoussis K, Zeki S, Seeing invisible motion: a human fMRI study. Curr Biol 16; 574-579, 2006.

Naatanen T, Attention and Brain Function. Hillsdale NJ, Lawrence Erlbaum, 1992.

Newcombe F, Ratcliff G, Disorders of visuospatial analysis. In: F Boller, J Grafman (eds): *Handbook of Neuropsychology*. Amsterdam, Elsevier, vol 2; 333-356, 1990.

Niebur E, Hsiao SS, Johnson KO, Synchrony: A neuron mechanism for attentional selection?, Current Opinion in Neurobiology 12; 190-194, 2002.

Nielsen JM, *Agnosia, Apraxia, Aphasia: Their Value in Cerebral Localization*, 2nd ed, New York, Hoeber, 1946

Obermayer K, Blasdel GG, Geometry of orientation and ocular dominance columns in monkey striate cortex. J Neurosci 13; 4114-4129, 1993.

Ogden JA, Visual object agnosia, prosopagnosia, achromatopsia, loss of visual imagery, and autobiographical amnesia following recovery from cortical blindness. Case MH. Neuropsychologia 31; 571-58, 1993.

Paterson A, Zangwill OL, A case of topographical disorientation associated with a unilateral cerebral lesion. Brain 68; 188-221, 1945.

Pasley BN, Mayes LC, Schultz RT, Subcortical discrimination of unperceived objects during binocular rivalry. Neuron 42; 163-172, 2004.

Pasupathy A, Connor CE, Population coding of shape in area V4. Nat Neurosci 5; 1332-1338, 2002.

Peters A, Ueber die Beziehungenzwieschen Orientierungsstoerungen und ein- und doppelseitiger Hemianopsie. Arch Augenheilk 32; 175-187, 1896.

Petersen SE, Robinson DL, Morris JD, Contributions of the pulvinar to visual spatial orientation. Neuropsychologia 25; 97-106, 1987.

Pillon B, Troubles visuoconstructifs et methodes de compensation: Resultats de 85 patients atteints de lésions cerebrales. Neuropsychologia 19; 375-383, 1981.

Posner MI, Raichle ME, *Images of Mind*. New York: Scientific American Library, 1993.

Poggio GF, Central neural mechanisms in vision. In: VB Mountcastle (ed), *Medical Physiology*. St Louis: Mosby, 1968.

Pollen DA, On the neural correlates of visual perception. Cereb. Cortex 9; 4-19, 1999.

Previc FH, Functional specialization in the lower and upper visual fields in humans: Its ecological origins and neurophysiological implications. Behavioral and Brain Science 13; 519-575, 1990.

Purves D, Lotto RB, *Why We See What We Do: An Empirical Theory of Vision*, Chapter 3 and 4. Sunderland MA: Sinauer Associates; 41-87, 2003.

Purves D, Riddle DR, La Mantia AS, Iterated patterns of brain circuitry (or how the brain gets its spots). Trends in Neuroscience 15; 362-368, 1992.

Purves D, Augustine GJ, Fitzpatrick D, et al., Central visual pathways. In: D Purves, Augustine GJ, Fitzpatrick D et al., (eds), *Neuroscience*. Third Edition. Chapter 11, Sinauer Associates Inc Publishers. Sunderland, Massachusetts, USA; 259-282, 2004.

Quaglino A, Emiplegia sinistra con amaurosi – Guarigione. Perdita totale della percezione dei colori e della memoria della configurazione degli oggetti. Annotazione alla medecima di GB Borelli. Giorn Oftalmol Ital 10; 106-117, 1867.

Rees G, Kreiman G, Koch C, Natural correlates of consciousness in human, Nat Rev Neurosci in human, Nat Rev Neurosci 3, 261-270, 2002.

Rizzo M, Damasio AR, Acquired central achromatopsia, In: JJ Kulikowski, CM Dickinson, KK Murray (eds), *Seeing Contour and Color*, England: Pergamon Press; 758-763, 1989.

Rizzo M, Robin DA, Simultanagnosia: A defect of sustained attention yields insights on visual information processing. Neurology 40; 447, 1990.

Rizzo M, Smith V, Pokorny J, Damasio AR, Color perception profiles in central achromatopsia. Neurology 43; 995-1001, 1993.

Rodieck RW, *The First Step in Seeing*. Sunderland, MA: Sinauer Associates, 1998.

Sacks O, Wasserman R, The case of the colorblind painter. New York: Review of Books 34, 25-33, 1987.

Schiller PH, Logothetis NK, The color-opponent and broad-band channels of the primate visual system. Trends Neurosci 13; 392-398, 1990.

Schnider A, Landis T, Regard M, Benson DF, Dissociation of color from object in amnesia. Arch Neurol 49; 82-985, 1992.

Schwarzlose RF, Baker CJ, Kanwisher N, Separate face and body selectivity on the fusiform gyrus. J. Neurosci. 25, 11055-11059, 2005.

Sereno MI, Sale AM, Reppas JB, Kwong KK, Belieweau JW, Brody TJ, Rosen BR, Tootell RB, Borders of multiple visual areas in humans revealed by functional magnetic resonance imaging. Science 268; 889-893, 1995.

Servas P, Goodale MA, Humphrey GK, The drawing of objects by a visual form agnosic: Contribution of surface properties and memorial representations. Neuropsychologia 31; 251-259, 1993.

Smith ML, Milner B, The role of the right hippocampus in the recall of spatial location. Neuropsychologia 19; 781-793, 1981.

Spitzer H, Desimone R, Moran J, Increased attention enhances both behavioral and neuronal performance. Science 240; 338-340, 1988.

Stracciari A, Transient topographical amnesia. Ital J Neurol Sci 13; 593-596, 1992.

Stracciari A, Lorusso S, Pazzaglia P, Transient topographical amnesia. J Neurol Neurosurg Psychiatry 57; 1423-1425, 1994.

Sugishita M, Ettlinger G, Ridley RM, Disturbance of cage-finding in the monkey. Cortex 14; 431-438, 1978.

Sumer P, Mollon JD, Catarrhine photopigments are optimized for detecting targets against a foliage background. Journal of Experimental Biology 203; 1963-1986, 2000.

Tanaka J, Weiskopf D, Williams P, The role of color in high-level vision. Trends in Cognitive Sciences 5; 211-215, 2001.

Tanaka K, Inferotemporal cortex and object vision. Annu Rev Neurosci 19, 109-139, 1996.

Temple CM, Developmental memory impairment: Faces and patterns. In: R Campbell (ed), *Mental Lives: Case Studies in Cognition*. Blackwell, Oxford; 199-215, 1992.

Teuber HL, Alteration of perception and memory in man. In: L Weiskrantz (ed.). *Analysis of Behavioral Change*. New York: Harper and Row; 269-375, 1968.

Tong F, Primary visual cortex and visual awareness. Nat Rev. Neurosci 4; 219-229, 2003.

Tong F, Nakayama K, Moscovitch M, et al., Response properties of the human fusiform face area. Cogn Neuropsychol 17; 257-279, 2000.

Tong F, Pearson J, Vision. In: BJ Baars and NM Gace (eds). *Cognition, Brain, and Consciousness. Introduction to Cognitive Neuroscience*. Chapter 6. Amsterdam-Boston-Heidelberg etc. Academic Press is an imprint of Elsevier; 149-181, 2007.

Tootell RBH, Hadjikhani N, Where is "dorsal V4" in human visual cortex? Retinotopic topographic and functional evidence. Cerebral Cortex 11; 298-311, 2001.

Tootell RB, Dale AM, Sereno MI, Malach R, New images from human visual cortex. Trends Neurosci 19; 481-48, 1996.

Tsao DY, Freiwold WA, Tootell RB, Livingstone MS, A cortical region consisting entirely of face-selective cells. Science 311; 670-674, 2006.

Tranel D, Disorders of color processing (perception, imagery, recognition, and naming). In: TE Feinberg and JM Farah (eds), *Behavioral Neurology and Neuropsychology*. New York, St Louis, San Francisco etc., McGraw-Hill, Health Profession Division; 257-265, 1997.

Tranel D, Central color processing and its disorders. In: F Boller and J Grafman (eds), *Handbook of Neuropsychology*. 2nd ed., Vol. 4, Elsevier, Amsterdam; 1-14, 2001.

Tranel D, Damasio H, Damasio AR, A neural basis for the retrieval of conceptual knowledge. Neuropsychologia 35; 1319-1324, 1997.

Treisman A, Features and objects in visual processing. Scientific American 254; 14-124, 1986.

Treisman A, Gormican S, Feature analysis in early vision. Psychological Review 95; 15-30, 1988.

Ungerleder JG, Mishkin M, Two cortical visual systems. In: DJ Ingle, MA Goodale and RJ Mansfield (eds). *Analysis of Visual Behavior*. Cambridge MA: MIT Press; 549-586, 1982.

Ungerleider LG, Haxby JV, "What" and "where" in the human brain, Current Opinion in Neurobiology 4; 15-165, 1994.

Valentine T, Upside-down faces: A review of the effects of inversion upon face recognition, British Journal of Psychology 79; 471-491, 1988.

Van Buren JM, Trans-synaptic retrograde degeneration in the visual system of primates. J Neurol Neurosurg Psychiatry 26; 402, 1963.

Weinberger LM, Grant FC, Visual hallucinations and their neuro-optical correlates, Arch Ophthalmol 23; 166, 1941.

Weliky M, Bosking WH, Fitzpatrick D, A systematic map of direction preference in primary visual cortex. Nature 379; 725-728, 1996.

Whitty CWM, Newcombe F, Oldfield's study of visual and topographical disturbances in a right occipito-parietal lesion after 30 years duration. Neuropsychologia 11; 471-475, 1973.

Wildbrand H, Ein Fall von Seelenblindheit und hemianopsie mit Sections-Befund. Dtsch Z Nervenheilk 2; 361-387, 1892.

Wolpert J, Die Simultanagnosie-Storung der Gesamtauffassung. Z Gesamte Neurol Psychiatr 93; 397, 1924.

Woolsey TA, Van de Loos H, The structural organization of layer IV in the somatosensory region (SI) of mouse cerebral cortex. The description of a cortical field composed of discrete cytoarchitectonic units. Brain Res 17; 205-242, 1970.

Yamadori A, Albert ML, Word category aphasia. Cortex 9; 83-89, 1973.

Zeki SM, Functional organization of a visual area in the posterior bank of the superior temporal sulcus of the rhesus monkey. J Psychol 236; 549-573, 1974.

Zeki S, A century of cerebral achromatopsia. Brain 113; 1721-1777, 1990.

Zeki S, *A Vision of the Brain*. Oxford: Blackwell Scientific Publications, 1993.

Zeki SM, Dynamism of PET Image: Studies of visual function. In: RSJ Franckowiak, KJ Frith, et al., (eds), *Human brain function*. San Diego: Academic Press, 1997.

Zeki S, Aglioti S, McKeefry D, Berlucchi G, The neurological basis of conscious color perception in a blind patient. Proceedings of the National Academy of Science of the United States of America 96; 14124-14129, 1999.

Zihl J, Von Cramon D, Mai N, Selective disturbance of movement vision after bilateral brain damage. Brain 106; 313-340, 1983.

Zihl J, Cerebral disturbances of elementary visual functions. In: JW Brown (ed.). *Neuropsychology of visual perception*. New York: IRBN Press, 1989.

Zilles K, Clarke S, Architecture, connectivity, and transmitter receptors of human extrastriate visual cortex: Comparison with nonhuman primates. In: K Rockland (ed.), *Cerebral Cortex*, Vol. 12, Plenum Press, New York, 1997.

Chapter 19

WHITE MATTER
OF CEREBRAL HEMISPHERE

The central nervous system (CNS) is composed of white and gray matter.

White matter consists mostly of nerve cell axons, whereas gray matter consists mostly of nerve cell bodies.

Gray matter is arranged into nuclei or cortex. The cerebral cortex consists of 50-100 billion nerve cell bodies arranged into a three to six layered sheet that laminates the brain surface.

All information entering (afferent fibres) or leaving the cerebral cortex (efferent fibres) or connecting one part of the cortex with another must pass through the subcortical white matter. Thus, the cerebral cortex receives the following **afferent** (input) fibres: corticocortical (association and commissural) excitatory fibres (which release glutamate or aspartate) from ipsilateral and contralateral areas, thalamocortical excitatory fibres from thalamus nuclei, cholinergic excitatory fibres from the basal forebrain nuclei, noradrenergic inhibitory fibres from the brain stem locus ceruleus, and serotonergic inhibitory fibres from the brain stem raphe nuclei (Patestas and Gartner, 2008). Cortical **efferent** fibres arise from the output neurons of the cerebral cortex: the pyramidal and fusiform cells. Their myelinated axons course deep, pass into the subcortical white matter, and then are distributed to widespread regions of the CNS.

The central core white matter of the cerebral hemispheres is composed of myelinated nerve fibres of varied sizes and their supporting neuroglia. These nerve fibres which make up the white matter of the cerebral hemispheres are either **association** fibres which link different cortical areas in the same hemisphere; **commissural** fibres, which link corresponding cortical areas in the two hemispheres; or **projection** fibres, which connect the cerebral cortex with the corpus striatum, diencephalon, brain stem and the spinal cord.

Association fibres

The association fibres interconnect various areas of the cortex within the same hemisphere. Association fibres also known as arcuate fibres are axons of small pyramidal cells and fusiform neurons primarily from cortical layers II and III. Association fibres that connect various cortical areas make up most of subcortical white matter. These fibres gather to form fasciculi that connect different lobes, but like a two-way highway, fibres merge into and exit these fasciculi all along their course. These arcuate fibres restricted to a single hemisphere are subdivided into two major categories, short and long fibres (Fig. 19.1).

The short arcuate fibres connect adjacent gyri (U-shaped fibres). These fibres leave the cortex of one gyrus, enter the underlying white matter, and then loop around the pit of a sulcus and project into the cortex of an adjacent gyrus. Thus, many pass subcortically between adjacent gyri, some merely pass from one wall of sulcus to the other, and most of them are confined to cortical gray matter.

The long arcuate fibres which connect distant nonadjacent gyri, and different lobes of the same hemisphere consist of the following fibre tracts; the uncinate fasciculus, cingulum, superior longitudinal fasciculus, inferior longitudinal fasciculus, and the superior and inferior fronto-occipital fasciculus.

The fibres follow a sharply curved course across the stem of the lateral sulcus, near the anteroinferior part of the insula.

The uncinate fasciculus which extends from the anterior temporal to motor speech (Broca's) area and orbital gyri, forms fronto-temporal interconnections.

The cingulum which extends from medial cortex below the rostrum to parahippocampal gyrus and parts of the temporal lobe is located internal to the cingulate gyrus continuing into the parahippocampal gyrus. The cingulum is a prominent association bundle in the cingulate gyrus. This bundle of long and short association fibres carries impulses to and from the parahippocampal gyrus.

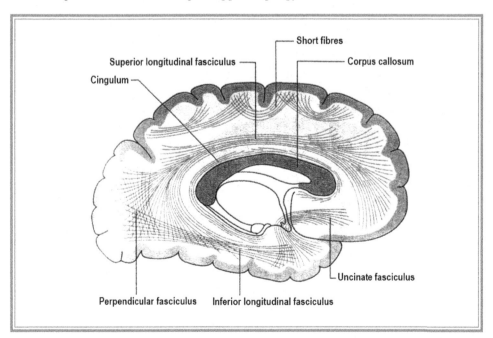

Fig. 19.1. The organization of the principal association fibres projected upon a sagittal section of the left cerebral hemisphere. (after Crossman, 2008).

The superior longitudinal fasciculus extends from anterior frontal lobe to occipital, parietal, and temporal lobes and is located in the core of the hemisphere. It is the largest of long association fasciculi. It starts in the anterior frontal region and arches back, above the insular area contributing fibres to the occipital cortex (areas 18 and 19). It curves down and forwards, behind the insular area, to spread out in the temporal lobe.

The superior longitudinal fasciculus contains a group of fibres, the arcuate fasciculus that forms a distinct arch posterior to the insula. This fasciculus links Broca's area (the frontal lobe motor area for speech) with Wernicke's area (the temporal lobe area for language comprehension).

The superior fronto-occipital fasciculus (subcalosal bundle) interconnects the frontal lobe with the occipital lobe.

The fronto-occipital fasciculus starts at the frontal pole. It passes back deep to the superior longitudinal fasciculus, separated from it by the projection fibres in the corona radiata. It lies lateral to the caudate nucleus near the central part of the lateral ventricle. Posteriorly, it fans out into the occipital and temporal lobes, lateral to the posterior and inferior horns of the lateral ventricle (Crossman, 2008).

The inferior longitudinal fasciculus extends from posterior region of the parietal and temporal lobes to anterior region of occipital lobe. Its fibres, probably derived mostly from areas 18 and 19, sweep forward, separated from the posterior horn of the lateral ventricle by the optic radiation and tapetal commissural fibres, and are distributed throughout the temporal lobe (Crossman, 2008).

The inferior fronto-occipital fasciculus, which like their superior counterpart also interconnects the frontal and occipital lobes, radiates in the frontal lobe, passes through the temporal lobe inferior to the insula, to also radiate in the occipital lobe. Some of its fibres curve around on the deep aspect of the lateral sulcus, interconnecting the frontal and temporal lobes, as a result of their hook-like path are referred to as the uncinate fasciculus (Patestas and Gartner, 2008).

The external capsule is insinuated between the claustrum and putamen, and the extreme capsule is located between the claustrum and the insular cortex (Haines and Mihailoff, 2006).

Projection fibres

Projection fibres include ascending fibres from lower centers to the neocortex, such as projections from the thalamus, and descending fibres from the neocortex to the brain stem and spinal cord.

Projection fibres are restricted to a single hemisphere and connect the cerebral cortex with lower levels, namely the corpus striatum, diencephalon, brain stem, and spinal cord. The majority of these fibres are axons of pyramidal cells and fusiform neurons.

These fibres are component part of the internal capsule, which is subdivided into the anterior limb (Fig. 19.2), genu (Fig. 19.3), posterior limb (Fig. 19.4), restrolentiform, and sublentiform regions. The projection fibres may be subdivided into corticopetal and corticofugal fibres.

Fig. 19.2. A coronal section of the rostral part of the human cerebral hemispheres at the level of the anterior limb of the internal capsule where it separates the caudate nucleus from the putamen (after Augustine, 2008).

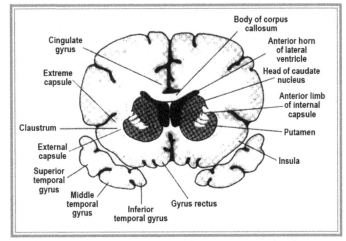

Fig. 19.3. A coronal section of the human cerebral hemispheres at the level of genu of the internal capsule (after Augustine, 2008).

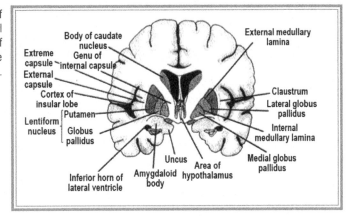

Fig. 19.4. A coronal section of the human cerebral hemispheres at the level of the posterior limb of the internal capsule. The cortical origin and partial course of the projection fibres that form the internal capsule are illustrated including fibres of the corona radiata (after Augustine, 2008).

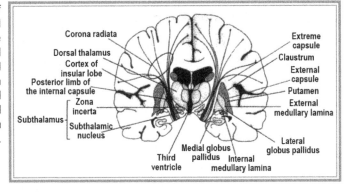

Corticopetal fibres are afferent fibres that bring information from the thalamus to the cerebral cortex. They consist of thalamocortical fibres.

Thus corticopetal fibres include: (1) thalamocortical fibres arising from the VPL, VPM, ventral lateral (VL), and ventral anterior (VA) nuclei of the thalamus relaying sensory information such as touch, pressure, conscious proprioception, two-point tactile

1483

sensation, as well as pain and temperature sensation from the body and head to the sensory cortex; (2) the MGN (medial geniculate nuclei) of the thalamus relaying auditory information *via* the auditory radiation to the auditory cortex; and (3) the LGN (lateral geniculate nuclei) of the thalamus relaying visual information *via* the optic radiation to the visual cortex. Although these afferent fibres terminate in layers I-IV of the cerebral cortex, most terminate in layers IV. The cholinergic and serotonergic afferents of the cerebral cortex function in the control of the sleep and arousal.

Corticofugal fibres are efferent fibres that transmit information from the cerebral cortex to lower centers of the brain and spinal cord.

These fibres consist of axons arising from large pyramidal cells that course in the corona radiata and internal capsule to terminate in the basal ganglia, the brain stem, and the spinal cord.

Corticofugal fibres consist of the corticothalamic, corticoreticular, corticorubral, corticotegmental, corticopontine, corticobulbar and corticospinal tracts.

Commissural fibres

The commissural fibres ensure the anatomical and functional connections of the two cerebral hemispheres. Therefore, it is possible to coordinate their integrative-reflex actions.

Commissural fibres arise in one cerebral hemisphere and cross the midline to terminate in the corresponding cortical area of the contralateral hemisphere. These fibres provide an avenue of communication between corresponding cortical areas of the two hemispheres which is essential in the integration of information in the two sides of the brain. Commissural fibres consist of the myelinated axons of medium-sized pyramidal neurons residing in various layers of the cerebral cortex. Cortical commissural fibres emerge mainly from the pyramidal cells residing in the cortical superficial layers and the external granular (layer II) and external pyramidal (layer III) layers.

In the adult brain there are four major hemispheric commissures: the anterior commissure, the posterior commissures that bridge the temporal lobes, the hippocampal commissure (commissure of the fornix) connecting hippocampal formation of two hemispheres, and the corpus callosum.

Anterior commissure

The anterior commissure is a compact bundle of myelinated nerve fibres located caudal to the rostrum of the corpus callosum but rostral to the main part of the fornix. Here it is embedded in the lamina terminalis where it is part of the anterior wall of the third ventricle (Fig. 19.5).

In sagittal suction it is oval. Its long (vertical) diameter is approximately 1.5 mm. Laterally it splits into anterior and posterior bundles. The smaller anterior bundle curves forwards on each side to the anterior perforated substance and olfactory tract. The posterior bundle curves posterolaterally on each side in a deep grove on the anteroinferior aspect of the lentiform complex, and subsequently fans out into the anterior part of the

Fig. 19.5. A coronal section of the human cerebral hemispheres, at the level of the anterior commissure. Some commissural fibres that form the corpus callosum and the anterior commissure are illustrated (after Augustine, 2008).

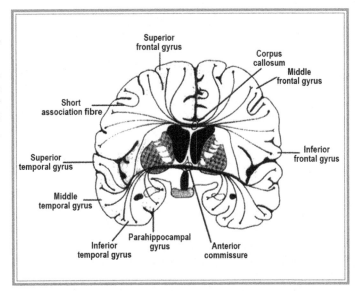

temporal lobe, including the parahippocampal gyrus (Crossman, 2008). It connects the right and left amygdala, the olfactory bulb and anterior olfactory nucleus, the anterior perforated substance, olfactory tubercle and diagonal band of Broca; the prepyriform cortex; the entorhinal area and adjacent parts of the parahippocampal gyrus; part of the amygdoid complex (especially the nucleus of the lateral olfactory stria); the bed nucleus of the stria terminalis and the nucleus accumbens; the anterior regions of the middle and inferior temporal gyri.

Thus, anterior commissure is a relatively small one in the basal forebrain lying above the optic chiasma and anterior to the main columns of the fornix that connects homologous areas of the middle and inferior temporal gyri, including parts of the olfactory cortices (Mendoza, 2011).

Posterior commissure

The posterior commissure which is of unknown constitution in man is a small fasciculus that crosses the midline at the base of the pineal gland and just posterior (dorsal) to the cerebral aqueduct.

Various small nuclei are associated with it. Among these are the interstitial nuclei of the posterior commissure, the nucleus of Darkschewitscz in the periaqueductal grey matter, and the interstitial nucleus of Cajal near the upper end of the oculomotor complex, closely linked with the medial longitudinal fasciculus. Fibres from all these nuclei and the fasciculus cross in the posterior commissure. It also contains fibres from thalamic and pretectal nuclei and the superior colliculi, together with fibres that connect the tectal and habenular nuclei. The destinations and functions of many of these fibres are obscure (Crossman, 2008).

Thus, the posterior commissure connects the right and left pretectal region and related cells group of the mesencephalon.

The habenular commissure which is a small fascicle running along the upper aspect of the posterior commissure, interconnected the habenular nuclei. However, the pretectal area and pretectal nuclei are parts of the epithalamus, that are three fibre bundles: the posterior commissure, habenular commissure, and the habenulo-interpeduncular tract.

Hippocampal commissure

The hippocampal commissure (commissure of the fornix) is formed by fibres that originate in the hippocampal formation and cross the midline as a thin layer inferior to the splenium of the corpus callosum. Thus, this commissure joins the right and left hippocampi to one another.

Corpus callosum

The corpus callosum is the most massive commissure in the entire nervous system. It is the largest axonal tract of the adult brain that provides symmetrical connections between the two hemispheres. It provides a bridge for the passing of information from one cerebral hemisphere to the other by 200-300 million myelinated and unmyelinated axons (Dupree, 2011).

Although the corpus callosum is the largest white matter tract of the brain, it is not essential for life.

The corpus callosum begins development around the 11th week of gestation and continues through adolescence. Initially, the corpus callosum is composed of astrocytic processes which serve as conduits for growing axons extending to the contralateral hemisphere (Paul et al., 2007).

Corpus callosum is composed of four parts: the rostrum, the genu, the body (also known as the trunk), and the splenium. Each portion of the corpus callosum is responsible for connecting symmetrical regions of the two hemispheres, with the rostrum and genu connecting portions of the prefrontal and premotor cortices, the body interconnecting the premotor, motor, supplementary motor, and the posterior parietal cortices, while the splenium connects portions of the temporal, occipital, and parietal lobes.

Internal capsule and corona radiata

Projection fibres are organized into a large, compact bundle called the internal capsule, which has intimate structural associations with the diencephalon and basal ganglia. In an axial plane through the hemisphere, the internal capsule appears as a prominent "V"-shaped structure with the "V" pointing mediatelly (Fig. 19.6).

Thus, the internal capsule is a massive, fan-shaped collection of fibres (white matter) that connect the thalamus to the cerebral cortex, and another which descends to the lower portion of the brain stem and the spinal cord.

Fibres which reciprocally connect the thalamus and the cortex constitute the **thalamic radiation**. These thalamocortical and corticothalamic fibres form a continuous fan that emerges along the whole lateral extent of the caudate nucleus. Fibre bundles radiating forward, backward, upward, and downward form large portions of various parts of the internal capsule.

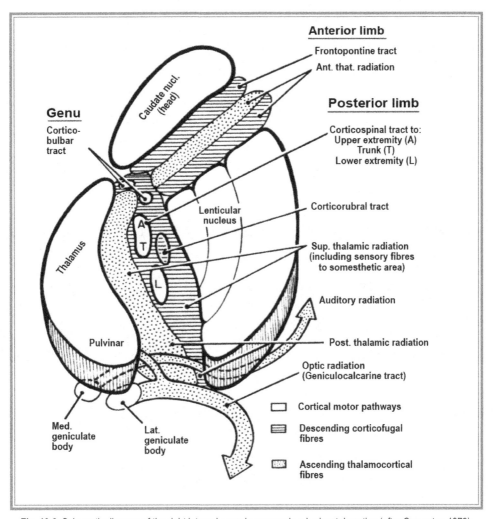

Fig. 19.6. Schematic diagram of the right internal capsule as seen in a horizontal section (after Carpenter, 1979).

Although the radiations connect with practically all parts of the cortex, the richness of connections varies considerably for specific cortical areas. Most abundant are the projections of the frontal granular cortex, the precentral and postcentral gyri, the calcarine area and the gyrus of Heschl. The posterior parietal region and adjacent portions of the temporal lobe also have rich thalamic connections, but relatively scanty radiations go to other cortical areas (Walker, 1938).

The thalamic radiation are grouped into four subradiations designated as the thalamic peduncles.

The anterior or frontal peduncle connects the frontal lobe with the medial and anterior thalamic nuclei.

The superior or centroparietal peduncle connects the Rolandic area and adjacent portion of the frontal and parietal lobes with the ventral tier thalamic nuclei. The fibres, carrying general sensory impulses from the body and head, form part of this radiation and terminate in the postcentral gyrus.

The posterior or occipital peduncle connects the occipital and posterior parietal convolutions with the caudal portions of the thalamus. It included the optic radiations (geniculocalcarine) from the lateral geniculate body to the calcarine cortex (striate area).

The inferior or temporal peduncle is small and includes the scanty connections of the thalamus with the temporal lobe and the insula. Includes in this are the auditory radiations (geniculotemporal) from the medial geniculate body to the transverse temporal gyrus of Heschl (Carpenter, 1979).

Thalamocortical and corticofugal fibres within the internal capsule occupy a comparatively small, compact area.

The cerebral hemisphere is connected with the brain stem and spinal cord by the extensive projection system of the internal capsule. Thus, descending motor fibres arising from the motor cortex destined for the brain stem and the spinal cord also descend in the internal capsule.

Fibres of the internal capsule flare out into the hemisphere as they pass distal to the caudate and putamen. This abrupt divergence of internal capsule fibres forms the **corona radiata** ("radiating crown"), which contains converging corticofugal fibres, as well as diverging corticopetal fibres (Haines, 2006). Thus, fibres arise from the whole extent of the cortex, enter the while substance of the hemisphere and appear as a radiating mass of fibres, the **corona radiata,** which converges toward the brain stem (Fig. 19.7). On reaching the latter they form a broad compact fibre band, the internal capsule, flanked medially by the thalamus and caudate nucleus and the lateral by the lenticular nucleus.

Thus, the internal capsule is composed of all the fibres, afferent and efferent, which go to, come from, the cerebral cortex. A large part of the capsule is obviously composed of the thalamic radiation described above. The rest is composed mainly of corticofugal fibre systems (efferent cortical fibres) which descend to the lower portion of the brain stem and the spinal cord.

In an axial plane through the hemisphere the internal capsule can be divided into an anterior limb, a genu (L "knee") and a posterior limb. The two limbs converge toward the genu, the angle between the anterior and posterior limb.

The anterior limb is interposed between the head of the caudate nucleus and the lenticular nucleus. This anterior limb contains the anterior thalamic radiation (thalamocortical / corticothalamic fibres) or peduncle, and the prefrontal corticopontine tract.

These frontopontine fibres, which arise from the cortex in the frontal lobe, synapse with cells of the pontine nuclei. Axons of these cells enter the opposite cerebellar hemisphere through the middle cerebellar peduncle. Anterior thalamic radiations interconnect the medial and anterior thalamic nuclei and limbic structures with the frontal cortex.

The genu, located at the intersection of the anterior and posterior limbs, is situated approximately at the level of the interventricular foramen. The genu abuts the third ventricle medially and the globus pallidus forms its lateral border. The genu of internal capsule contains corticonuclear (corticobulbar) fibres that arise in the frontal cortex just rostral to precentral sulcus (area 4), form the precentral gyrus (primary motor cortex) and terminate mostly in the contralateral motor nuclei of cranial nerves. Anterior fibres of the superior thalamic radiation, between the thalamus and cortex, also extend into the genu.

Lesions of these fibres give rise to motor deficits of cranial nerves, most notably deficits related to the facial and hypoglossal nerves (Haines, 2006).

The posterior limb of the internal capsule is larger, more complex and includes the corticospinal tract. The fibres concerned with the upper limb are anterior. More posterior regions contain fibres representing the trunk and lower limbs.

Other descending axons include frontopontine fibres, particularly from areas 4 and 6 and corticorubral fibres, which connect the frontal lobe to the red nucleus. Most of the posterior limb also contains fibres of the superior thalamic radiation (the somaesthetic radiation) ascending to the postcentral gyrus (Crossman, 2008).

This posterior limb is divided into a **thalamolenticular part** (which lies between the lenticular nucleus and the dorsal thalamus), a **sublenticular part** (fibres passing ventral to the lenticular nucleus) and a **retrolenticular part** (fibres extend caudally for a short distance behind the lenticular nucleus). In this caudal region a number of fibres passing beneath the lenticular nucleus to reach the temporal lobe collectively form the **sublenticular portion** of internal capsule.

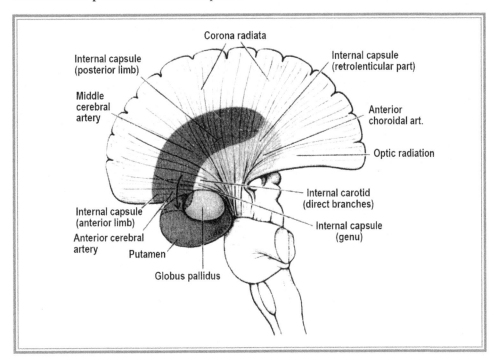

Fig. 19.7. Diagram of the blood supply of the internal capsule and corpus striatum. The putamen and globus pallidus are shown rotated ventrally away from their normal position adjacent to the internal capsule. Regions supplied by branches of the middle and anterior cerebral arteries are shown in black and portions of the internal capsule and corpus striatum supplied by the anterior choroidal artery. Direct branches of the internal carotid artery supply the genu of internal capsule (Alexander, 1942).

However, contemporary terminology and common usage refer to the "thalamo-lenticular part" as the posterior limb, and the "sublenticular part" as the sublenticular limb. By this scheme the internal capsule consists of five parts: an anterior limb, genu, posterior limb, sublenticular limb, and retrolenticular limb (Haines, 2006).

Thus, the posterior limb of the internal capsule contains: (1) corticospinal fibres, (2) frontopontine fibres, (3) the superior thalamic radiation, and (4) a relatively smaller number of corticotectal, corticorubral and corticoreticular fibres. Corticospinal fibres are organized in a specific manner so that those closest to the genu are concerned with cervical portions of the body, while succeeding, more caudal regions are related to the upper extremity, trunk and lower extremity, respectively.

Fibres of superior thalamic radiation, located caudal to the corticospinal fibres, project impulses concerned with general somatic sense to the postcentral gyrus (Carpenter, 1979).

The retrolenticular portion of the posterior limb contains the posterior thalamic radiations and the optic radiation and interconnections between the occipital and parietal lobes and caudal parts of the thalamus, especially the pulvinar. These include the optic radiation, parietal and occipital corticopontine fibres and fibres from the occipital cortex, to the superior colliculi and pretectal region.

Visual input from the lateral geniculate body to the occipital cortex is conveyed *via* geniculocalcarine radiation (optic radiations) through the retrolenticular limb. Optic radiations form a distinct lamina of fibres immediately lateral to the tapetum as they course caudally into the occipital lobe. It sweeps backwards, intimately related to the superolateral aspect of the inferior horn and the lateral aspect of the posterior horn of the lateral ventricle, from which it is separated by the tapetum.

The sublenticular part of the internal capsule contains temporopontine and some parietopontine fibres, the auditory radiation from the medial geniculate body to the superior temporal and transverse temporal gyri (areas 41 and 42), and a few fibres that connect the thalamus with the temporal lobe and insula. Fibres of the auditory radiation sweep anterolaterally below and behind the lentiform complex to reach the cortex.

Thus, geniculotemporal radiation (auditory radiations) convey auditory information from the medial geniculate nucleus to the transverse temporal gyri through the sublenticular limbs.

Vascular supply. The anterior limb of the internal capsule is supplied by the anterior cerebral artery, and anterior choroidal artery.

The posterior limb is supplied by penetrating branches of the middle cerebral artery (De Piero, 2011) (Fig. 19.8).

Function. Descending fibres of the corticobulbar and corticospinal tracts travel through the internal capsule. Corticobulbar fibres, controlling facial musculature, larynx, and tongue, are located in the genu. Posterior to the genu there are corticospinal tracts controlling arm, followed by leg. The most posterior part of the internal capsule contains ascending axons of the spinothalamic tract, carrying sensory input from the body to the thalamus.

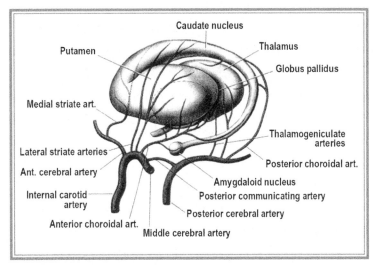

Fig. 19.8. Diagrammatic representation of the arterial supply of the corpus striatum and thalamus (modified from Aitken, 1909).

The anterior limb of the internal capsule contains axons to and from frontal association cortex (Martin, 2003; Fix, 2008; De Piero, 2011).

Pathology. The posterior limb of the internal capsule is a frequent site for lacunar strokes. The most common syndrome is that of pure motor hemiplegia. The lenticulostriate arteries, penetrating branches of the middle cerebral artery, are frequently damaged by hypertension, diabetes, and aging, and can be occluded, causing strokes.

Less commonly small aneurysms (Charcot-Bouchard aneurysms) may develop, and cause intracerebral hemorrhage, sometimes referred to as intraparenchymal hemorrhage (De Piero, 2011).

Thrombosis or hemorrhage of the anterior choroidal, striate or capsular branches of the middle cerebral arteries are responsible for most injuries to the internal capsule.

Vascular lesions in the posterior limb of the internal capsule may result in contralateral hemianesthesia of the head, trunk, and limbs due to injury of thalamocortical fibres en route to the sensory cortex. There is also a contralateral hemiplegia due to injury of the corticospinal tract (Aitken, 1909; Alexander, 1942).

If the genu of the internal capsule is involved in the injury, corticobulbar fibres are also destroyed. Lesions in the posterior third of the posterior limb may include the optic and auditory radiations.

In such instances there may be a contralateral triad consisting of hemianesthesia, hemianopsia and hemihypoacusia. More extensive vascular lesions may include the thalamus or corpus striatum, so that affective changes and symptoms due to injury of the basal ganglia may be added to those characteristic of injury to the internal capsule (Alexander, 1942; Dănăilă and Păiş, 1988, 2004). Thus, lesions in this area produce more widespread disability than lesions in any other region of the nervous system.

Lesions in cerebral white matter sever connections between lower and higher centers or between cortical areas. White matter lesions are found in many dementing disorders and appear to be specifically associated with attentional impairments (Junkué et al., 1990; Filley, 2001).

REFERENCES

Aitken HF, A report on the circulation of the lobar ganglia: made to Dr. James B. Ayer. Boston Med Surg J Suppl 160; 25, 1909.

Alexander L, The vascular supply of the striopallidum. A Res Nerv & Ment Dis Proc 21; 77-132, 1942.

Augustine JR, *Human Neuroanatomy*. An Introduction. Academic Press, Amsterdam, Boston, Heidelberg etc.; 316-318, 2008.

Carpenter MB, *Human Neuroanatomy*. Seventh Edition. The Williams and Wilkins Company, Baltimore; 162-165, 1979.

Crossman AR, Basal ganglia. In: S Standring (ed.), *Gray's Anatomy*. Fortieth Edition. Churchill Livingstone, Elsevier; 354-359, 2008.

Dănăilă L, Păiş V, *Ateroscleroza cerebrală din sistemul carotidian*, Ed. Ştiintifică şi Enciclopedică, Bucureşti, 1988.

Dănăilă L, Păiş V, *Ateroscleroza cerebrală ischemică*. Editura: Editura Medicala, Bucureşti, 2004.

De Piero TJ, Internal Capsule. In: JS Kreutzer, J De Luca, B Caplan (eds) *Encyclopedia of Clinical Neuropsychology*. Vol. 2, Springer, New York, Dordrecht, Heidelberg, London; 1343, 2011.

Dupree J, Corpus Callosum. In: JS Kreutzer, J De Luca, B Caplan (eds.), *Encyclopedia of Clinical Neuropsychology*. Vol. 1, Springer , New York, Dordrecht, Heidelberg, London; 709, 2011.

Filley CM, *The Behavioural Neurology of White Matter*. Oxford: Oxford University Press, 2001.

Fix JD, *Neuroanatomy* (3rd ed.), Baltimore, MD: Lippincott, Williams and Wilkins, 2008.

Haines DE, *Fundamental neuroscience for basic and clinical applications*. 3rd ed, Philadelphia, PA: Churchill Livingstone, Elsevier; 2006.

Haines DE, Mihailoff GA, The telencephalon. In: DE Haines (ed.), Fundamental neuroscience for basic and clinical applications. Philadelphia. Churchill-Livingstone-Elsevir; 244-259, 2006.

Junqué, C, Pujol, J, Vendrell P, et al., Leuko-araiosis on magnetic resonance imaging and speed of mental processing. Arch Neurol 47; 151-156, 1990.

Mendoza JE, Anterior Commissure. In: JS Kreutzer, J De Luca, B Caplan (eds) *Encyclopedia of Clinical Neuropsychology*. Vol. 1, Springer, New York, Dordrecht, Heidelberg, London; 187, 2011.

Martin J, *Neuroanatomy: Text and atlas* (3rd ed). New York, Mc Graw-Hill, 2003.

Patestas AM, Gartner LP, *A Textbook of Neuroanatomy*. Blackwell Publishing, USA, 2009.

Paul LK, Brown WS, Adolphs R, et al., Agenesis of the corpus callosum: genetic, developmental and functional aspects of connectivity. Nature Review Neuroscience 8; 287-299, 2007.

Walker AE, The thalamus of chimpanzee. IV. Thalamic projection of the cerebral cortex. J Anat 73; 37-93, 1938.

Chapter 20

CORPUS CALLOSUM

Anatomy of the corpus callosum

The midline longitudinal cerebral fissure, occupied in life by the falx cerebri, incompletely separates the two cerebral hemispheres from one another.

The link between the hemispheres is provided by the corpus callosum. This large arch of white matter constitutes the floor of the cerebral fissure.

The corpus callosum is the largest fibre tract in the brain, and it contains over 200 million axons originating from layers 2 and 3 of both hemispheres (Aboitiz et al., 1992).

The corpus callosum (from the Latin callus, meaning "hard body") is the largest structure on the medial surface of each hemisphere.

This enormous bundle of myelinated fibres forms an anatomical and functional connection between the right and left hemispheres.

The corpus callosum links mainly corresponding areas of the neocortex of the two cerebral hemispheres. It, however, also contains commissural fibres that arise in certain cortical areas of one cerebral hemisphere and cross to the opposite side to terminate in noncorresponding areas of the contralateral hemispheres.

This is true for fibres arising in the primary visual cortex of one cerebral hemisphere that cross to the opposite side to terminate in the visual association cortex of the contralateral hemisphere.

Similarly, parts of the motor and somesthetic cortical areas where the hand is represented, do not receive commissural fibres from the corresponding motor and sensory cortical areas of the contralateral hemisphere.

However, the somesthetic association areas receive commissural fibres that connect the two cerebral hemispheres, thus each hemisphere samples information available to the contralateral hemisphere.

While the left and right hemispheres have some different functions, the corpus callosum has the same 200 million fibres, constantly trafficking back and forth, which serves to integrate information from both sides.

The corpus callosum has fibres that project between the hemispheres in an orderly way, with regions in the anterior portion connecting similar brain areas in the frontal lobes and regions in the posterior portion connecting similar brain areas in the occipital lobe.

A variety of individual differences in callosal size and pattern are suggested to exist. For example, Witelson (1986) reported that the corpus callosum is larger in left-handers than in right-handers and in the women than in the man.

Thus, the size and the shape of the corpus callosum vary greatly from individual to individual, and there are sex differences in the shape of the callosum. The splenium is more bulbous shaped in women and has a greater maximum width but it is more tubular shaped in men. There are age related changes in the corpus callosum during childhood and adulthood. In some cases, the corpus callosum is lacking, a condition termed agenesis of the corpus callosum.

The corpus callosum originates from the area of the lamina terminalis as a structure initially composed of astrocytic processes. Axons from developing neurons in each hemisphere traverse this glial structure across to the contralateral side. As this takes place the corpus callosum enlarges in a caudal direction to form the prominent structure found in adults.

The corpus callosum is located superior to the diencephalon and forms the roof of much of the lateral ventricles, and the floor of the longitudinal fissure.

Its antero-posterior length is of 96 mm in men and 98 in women when measured through by projecting the farthest anterior and posterior points on a horizontal line (Velut et al., 1998). The anterior end is located 4 cm away from the frontal pole, and the posterior end is found at 6 cm from the occipital pole. However, the corpus callosum is organised with a great deal of regularity (Brodal, 1981; Colonier, 1986; Witelson, 1995; Clarke et al., 1998)

This huge bundle of commissural fibres, the corpus callosum, consists, from rostral to caudal, of five segments: the anteriormost region, the **rostrum**, the curved **genu**, the relatively flattened **body** (also called the trunk) forming the roof of the lateral ventricle, the **isthmus**, and its posteriormost region, the **splenium** (Fig. 20.1).

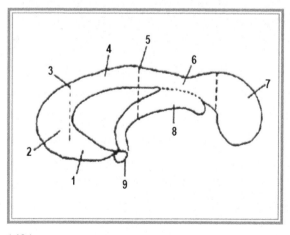

Fig. 20.1. The aspect of corpus callosum on a sagital section: 1. Rostrum; 2. The genu of the corpus callosum; 3. The line that separates the genu from the body (trunk); 4. Trunk (body) of the corpus callosum; 5. The line that unites the point located 5 cm anterior from the central sulcus with the superior margin of intraventricular foramen; 6. The isthmus of corpus callosum; 7. Splenium; 8. Fornix; 9. Anterior commisure.

The rostrum represents the most anterior part and it forms a curve downwards. It continues towards the posterior with a lamina of white matter of various widths. This horizontal lamina descends in a beak-like shape that reaches the superior margin of the white anterior commissure.

The peaked posterior extremity of the rostrum is located between the subcallous area downward and the septum pellucidum upwards. Consequently, the posterior elongation of this white lamina separated, from the subcallous area by the posterior paraolfactory sulcus, locates itself above the paraterminal gyrus which covers the septal nuclei (Velut et al., 1998).

The genu of the corpus callosum which presents a significant anterior convexity is situated anterior to the rostrum. Thus, the anterior extent of the corpus callosum, known as the genu, bends inferiorly and turns posteriorly where it forms a slender connection, the rostrum, with the anterior commissure.

Inferior to the genu and rostrum is the subcallosal area – a collective term including the subcallosal gyrus and, inferior to it, the septal area. The term, **rhinencephalon** (Greek, nose brain) refers to cerebral structures related to olfaction, particularly in lower animals. In humans, this area of the brain consists of many structures on the medial and inferior surfaces of each cerebral hemisphere.

One, the anterior perforated substance, is posterior to the olfactory trigone and best visualised on the inferior surface of the brain.

Another, the **subcallosal area**, is on the medial surface of each cerebral hemisphere inferior to the genu and rostrum of the corpus callosum. It includes a dorsally located subcallosal gyrus and a ventrally located septal area. As the cingulate gyrus turns into the subcallosal area, it is continued with the subcallosal gyrus that is inferior to the rostrum of the corpus callosum.

The virtual separation of the genu from the rostrum and body consists of a vertical line that crosses through the most posterior area of the genu. The genu is located between the septum pellucidum, which is inserted in a posterior medial line and the gyrus cinguli which is located anteriorly.

The insertion of the septum pellucidum is frequently doubled (in 83% of cases according to Winkler et al., 1997) resulting in a double septum and septal cavity (Fig. 20.2).

The septum pellucidum is bilaminar with a potential space between its layers (cavum septi pellucidi) that is normally absent at birth but may remain open as a median cleft. There is an enormous variability in the reported incidence of cavum septi pellucidi (from 2% to 71.5%).

Enlargement of the cavum, though rare in healthy individuals, has been reported in patients with schizophrenia (Augustine, 2008).

Many of the fibres passing through the rostrum and genu arch rostrally to interconnect the anterior cortical areas of the frontal lobes; these form the **minor** (or **frontal) forceps**.

The body (trunk) of the corpus callosum is continued behind the genu and consists of most of the commissural fibres that interconnect the remaining frontal lobe, parietal lobe, and part of the temporal lobe. Thus, midcallosal areas contain a mixture of fibres coming from both anterior and posterior regions.

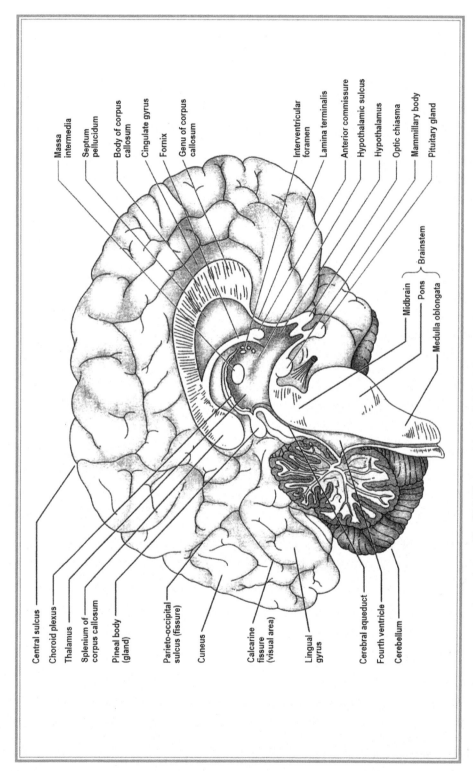

Central sulcus

Choroid plexus

Thalamus

Splenium of corpus callosum

Pineal body (gland)

Parieto-occipital sulcus (fissure)

Cuneus

Calcarine fissure (visual area)

Lingual gyrus

Cerebral aqueduct

Fourth ventricle

Cerebellum

Massa intermedia

Septum pellucidum

Body of corpus callosum

Cingulate gyrus

Fornix

Genu of corpus callosum

Interventricular foramen

Lamina terminalis

Anterior commissure

Hypothalamic sulcus

Hypothalamus

Optic chiasma

Mammillary body

Pituitary gland

Midbrain

Pons

Medulla oblongata

Brainstem

Fig. 20.2. Diagram of the medial view of a sagital section of the brain.

1496

Either rectangular or upwards in a convex shape, its larger axis is horizontal or a little ascending in an antero-posterior direction.

According to Winkler et al. (1997), the average width of the corpus callosum is 6.12 mm but ranges between 4 and 8 mm.

The body is located between the cingular gyrus (from which it is separated by the callous sulcus), which is located upwards, and the septum pellucidum, downwards. Thus, throughout its entire length, the convex facet of the corpus callosum is separated from the cingular gyrus by a deep callous sulcus.

Thus, dorsal to, and following the contours of the corpus callosum, is the cingulate gyrus that then passes behind the splenium, narrows into the cingulate isthmus, before becoming continuous with the parahippocampal gyrus. Separating the cingulate gyrus from the corpus callosum is the sulcus of the corpus callosum. The cingulate gyrus is continued rostrally with the subcallosal gyrus (the dorsal part of the subcallosal area).

On the superior aspect of the body there are two bundles of fibres which form the medial and lateral longitudinal striae.

The former is better identified. It passes on each side of the median line and is adherent to the surface of the corpus callosum.

The lateral longitudinal striae is more difficult to identify because it is located deeper in the callosum sulcus and is marked through a small shape located between the inferior facet of the cingular gyrus and the superior facet of the corpus callosum.

Between these two striae, the plane surface of the corpus callosum is covered with a grey matter lamina called **indusium griseum**. Anteriorly it passes around the knee and rostrum in order to reach the paraterminal gyrus. Inferiorly it continues with Broca's diagonal band and then with the anterior perforated substance and the periamygdaloid area. Posteriorly it leaves the surface of the splenium of the corpus callosum. It elongates through the **subsplenial gyrus** and then the **fasciolar gyrus** into the hyppocampal region between the **fimbria** upwards and the **dentate gyrus** downwards. The origin and structure of the medial and lateral longitudinal striae are uncertain (Duvernoy, 1998). They are considered to be aberrant fibres of the fornix (the medullar stria blends with the fasciola cinerea, a posterior extension of the dentate gyrus and the lateral stria blends with the fasciolar gyrus).

The isthmus of corpus callosum is located in the posterior area of the body. Anteriorly it is thinner than the body, and posteriorly it is larger, thus its name. According to Witelson (1989) the anterior limit is given by the vertical line that passes through the junction between the anterior 2/3 and the posterior 1/3 of the corpus callosum. The posterior limit is given by another vertical line located between the anterior 4/5 and the posterior 1/5 of the corpus callosum. According to Velut et al. (1998) the inferior limit corresponds to the adhesion point of the fornix, and the posterior limit is given by the vertical line that passes through the anterior facet of the splenium.

The most important particularity of the isthmus is represented by its adhesion to the superior facet of the fornix body. This adhesion of the corpus callosum to the fornix creates the risk of sectioning the interhyppocampal commissure of the fornix while performing a low posterior callosotomy.

For Winkler et al. (1997) the distance between the M line (the line that unites the point located 5 cm anterior from the central sulcus with the superior margin of the interventricular foramen) and the most anterior point of the adhesion of the corpus callosum to the fornix varies between 10 and 40 mm (the average is 23.79 mm). One must also take notice of the fact that the antero-posterior length of this adhesion is highly variable. Its maximum is greater than 10 mm.

Finally, Winkler et al. (1997) highlights the fact that the separation of the corpus callosum from the fornix is very easy in 77% of cases and difficult or impossible in the remaining cases. These variations highlight the importance on an MRI scan before every callosotomy.

The splenium is the region located in the most posterior area of the corpus callosum, and closes the "callous C". The fibres interconnecting the occipital lobes, loop through the splenium of the corpus callosum forming the major (or occipital) forceps. Fibres from the visual cortex at the posterior pole of the cerebrum occupy the posterior end portion of the callosum.

The tapetum, which is located in the lateral wall of the atrium and posterior horn of the lateral ventricle, is also composed of fibre bundles that cross in the splenium and separate the ventricle from the optic radiation.

Thus, the posterior extent of the corpus callosum, known as the splenium, is bullous in shape. This portion of the corpus callosum consists of commissural fibres interconnecting the posterior parietal, posterior temporal and occipital cortices. Lesions in this area are associated with the well-known neurobehavioral disconnection syndrome of alexia without agraphia.

Contrary to the rest of the corpus callosum that is hidden between the two hemispheres, the splenium emerges in the ambient cistern or the superior cerebellar lake surrounded in its posterior region by the falco-tentorial junction. The splenium forms a thicker area which is the superior limit of this cistern through its inferior convexity.

The anterior limit is given by the medial pineal body and the lateral pulvinar, and downwards and forwards there is the mesencephalic tectum. Downwards, the cistern is limited by the culmen of the vermis, and in its posterior area it is limited by the free margin of the cerebellar tentorium, which curves upwards and internally in order to bond with the free margin of the cerebral falx. This falco-tentorial junction forms the original triangle of the right sinus. At this level the width of the cingular gyrus, which moulds on the posterior region of the splenium, decreases and forms the **isthmus**. This isthmus forms away from the median line and is continued interiorly by the parahippocampal gyrus.

The subsplenial gyrus, which is between the isthmus and the splenium, is continued with the fasciolar gyrus. Above and ahead of the splenial formation, there is the body of the fornix which contains in its posterior area the interhyppocampal fibres of its commissure. It is called the psalterium. In the lateral area, each lateral margin of this body is continued by the fornix cross which becomes the fimbria that roles around the pulvinar area.

Then, the fimbria emerges above the fasciolar gyrus and away from the splenium, which remains above these structures.

In sum, in humans, the different regions of the corpus callosum described on the medial sagittal section are: the rostrum, the genu, the body or the trunk, the isthmus and the splenium.

Callosal fibres radiating to the frontal lobe (radiations of the corpus callosum) form the genu from the frontal forceps; those radiating from the splenium in the occipital lobe form the occipital forceps. Attached to the inferior border of the corpus callosum is the thin septum pellucidum – a transparent, membranous partition that separates the right and left cerebral ventricles and forms their medial wall.

The callous fibres

The nervous fibres of the corpus callosum radiate into the white matter of each hemisphere. Afterwards they disperse into the cerebral cortex. The dissection of the posterior extremity of the rostrum does not allow the identification of some commissural fibres, but the white median tissue unites in the posterior with the anterior commissure (Velut et al., 1998).

In the lateral region, the fibres of the rostrum blend with the lateral fibres of the anterior commissure. These are located in the posterior area and make a loose curve with the concavity towards the posterior. The fibres located in the most posterior region of the rostrum pass in the anterior region below the putamen. Internally there is the accumbens nucleus which continues the head of the caudate nucleus in its inferior and lateral area (Nieuwenhuys and Meek, 1990).

The fibres of the genu draw a perfect horseshoe shape with an anterior concavity – an assembly named the **minor forceps**. The inferior fibres of this forceps appear above the gyrus rectus. These are fibres coming from the ventral and median regions of the prefrontal cortex, which cross through the rostrum and the ventral area of the genu of the corpus callosum (Pandya and Seltzer, 1986; Habib and Pelletier, 1994).

The fibres which come from the prefrontal dorso-lateral cortex are located in the dorsal area of the genu of the corpus callosum. The fibres of the genu are arched by the cingular fibres and have a sagittal direction. These are located below the cortex of the gyrus holding the same name. These cingular fibres are connected in their posterior area with the septal nuclei. The fibres of the corpus callosum are arched by the cingular fibres (Fig. 20.3).

Laterally, the callous fibres spread in the white substance, forming a curve with its concavity located in its superior area. The more they are located towards the dorsal area of the corpus callosum, the larger the concavity.

They cross the fibres of the corona radiata in the core of this white matter and form, according to Klingler (1956), an arched line, which Velut et al. (1998) did not find. Nevertheless, the callous fibres and those of the corona radiata are oriented so that they crisscross in an oblique angle. This makes it difficult to identify them. The fibres of the corona radiata condense in the lower internal capsule. The angle in which the callous fibres and those of the corona radiata connect is located immediately above the body of the caudate nucleus, and below the subependymal layer it forms the lateral margin of the body of the lateral ventricle (Velut et al., 1998).

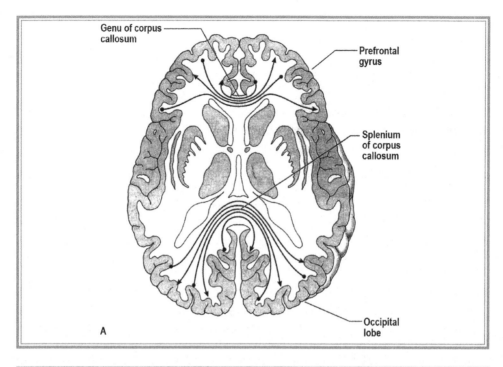

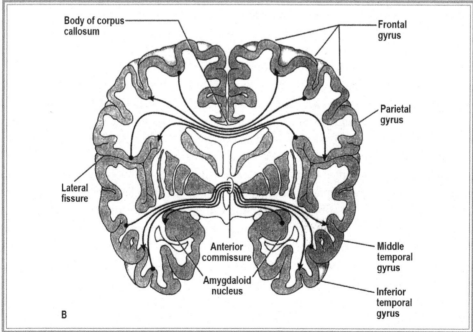

Fig. 20.3. (A) Horizontal schematic representation of the brain showing the fibre connections of the genu and splenium of the corpus callosum. (B) Coronal schematic representation of the brain showing the fibres of the anterior comissure and the body of the corpus callosum. (Modified from Young PA and Young PH, 1997. Basic Clinical Neuroanatomy. Williams and Wilkins, Baltimore).

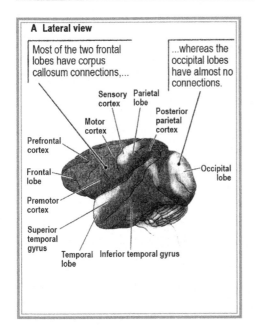

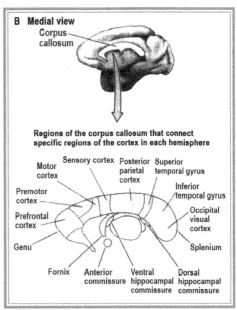

Fig. 20.4. Patterns of commissural connections. (A) The areas shaded show regions of the cortex of a rhesus monkey that receive projection from the contralateral hemisphere through the corpus callosum.
(B) Regions of the corpus callosum showing zones through which a radioactive label was transported after injections into specific locations in the cortex (after Pandya and Seltzer, 1986).

The fibres of the anterior half of the callous body connect to the premotor dorsolateral cortex and the median supplementary motor area. The middle area of the body connects to the motor area M1, the insula and the anterior cingulate cortex (Pandya and Seltzer, 1986; Habib and Pelletier, 1994).

More towards its posterior region, the callous areas connect to the somatosensory areas S1 and S2. The posterior area of the body connects to the associative parietal cortex, and more towards the posterior it connects to the superior temporal areas (including the hearing area), the insula and the posterior cingulum. The areas M1, S1 and S2 related to the foot and hand are not connected. Thus, the motor and sensory areas for distal parts of the limbs (mainly the hands and feet) lack connections. It could be argued that, because their essential function is to work independently of one another, connections are not necessary. Among the areas that do receive interhemispheric connections, the density of projections is not homogeneous (Fig. 20.4 A) (Pandya and Seltzer, 1986).

Areas of the cortex that represent the midline of the body – such as the central meridian of the visual fields, auditory fields, and trunk of the body on the somatosensory and motor cortex – have the densest connections. The functional utility of this arrangement is that movements of the body or actions in central space require interhemispheric cooperation.

Thus, the corpus callosum bonds together the representations of the midpoints of the body and space that are divided by the longitudinal fissure. The corpus callosum connects identical points in the contralateral hemisphere. One group of projections goes to areas to which the homotopic areas on the contralateral side project. Another group of projections has a diffuse terminal distribution. The pattern of connections between the hemisphere in the rhesus monkey is illustrated in figure 20.4B (Pandya and Seltzer, 1986). Thus the fibres passing through the body of the corpus callosum are proceeding from front to back, from the premotor, motor, somatosensory, and posterior parietal cortex.

Many studies proved that the transfer of somato-sensitive information needs to integrate the trunk of the corpus callosum (Diamond et al., 1977; Bogen, 1987). In particular, the fibres that pass through the posterior area of the trunk are crucial to finishing the tasks that need the crisscross location of a tactile stimulus. Geffen et al. (1985) showed that if the trunk of the corpus callosum is the regular path for the sensitive information, the splenium can maintain up to 50% of this function.

The fibres of the splenium form a posterior concavity that is larger than the one of the genu which is called the **major forceps** (Young and Young, 1997).

Outside and at a distance from the median line, the splenium is arched by the isthmus of the cingulate gyrus. The fibres from the superior area of the splenium connect to the inferior temporal cortex and the parahippocampal gyrus. In its anterior area (and the superior one) the fibres connect to the superior parietal lobules and the juxtastriate region (Pandya and Seltzer, 1986; Habib and Pelletier, 1994) (Fig. 20.5).

The dissection of the fibres located in the splenium really demonstrates that the inferior fibres that are located in the splenial area go towards the striate regions and form **the major forceps.** Areas 17 are not connected. The more these fibres are located in the posterior region of the splenium, the closer they are to the median line of the occipital lobe. So, fibres in the posterior part, or splenium, are from the superior temporal, inferior temporal, and visual cortex (Pandya and Seltzer, 1986).

The superior splenial fibres go towards the occipito-temporal and temporal regions (Velut et al., 1998). This location of the special fibres forms the **tapetum.**

Initially, the fibres are located on the roof of the ventricular atrium. Afterwards they form into a fan like shape from back to front, and spread in an anterior direction below the lateral ependymal area of the atrium and the inferior horn of the lateral ventricle. Thus, the tapetum is located between this ependyma and the optic radiations.

In order to reveal the optic radiations at the level of the roof of the inferior horn in the lateral ventricle it is necessary to perform the ablation of the fibres located in the tapetum. Finally, the fibres located mostly towards the anterior area of the anterior tapetum are next to the tail of the caudate nucleus, which is located above the stria terminalis. Thus, according to Pandya and Seltzer (1986), most of the primary visual cortex (area V1) is devoid of interhemispheric connections, except for that part representing the midline of the visual world, the visual meridian. The lack of such connections has been explained in functional terms: this cortex represents the visual world topographically, and there is no need for one half of the representation to be connected to one other.

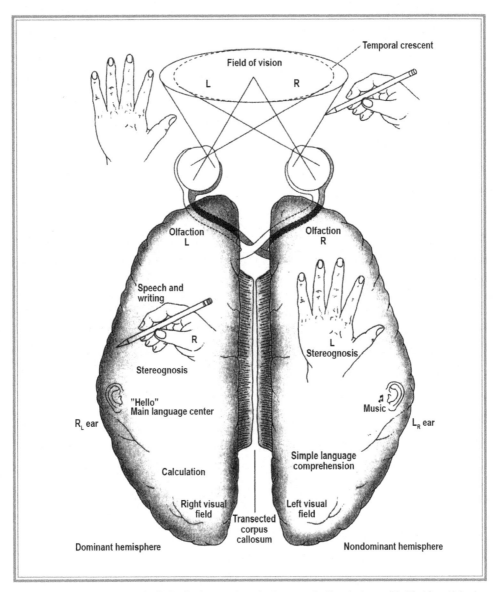

Fig. 20.5. Functions associated with the dominant and nondominant cerebral hemispheres. (Modified from Noback, CR et al. (1996), The Human Nervous System, 5ᵗʰ edn. Williams and Willkins, Baltimore).

Klingler's method allows the dissection of fibres in each of these areas and the establishment of their connections to the corona radiata and the optic radiations.

Finally each segment of the corpus callosum takes part in forming the walls of the lateral ventricle.

Despite the size and the large number of commissural fibres, the information regarding the functional role of the corpus callosum is limited. In humans the total number of fibres is approximately 200 million. However, there is detailed data missing regarding the callous connections of many regions. The first investigations have been done in the visual area. The somatic and sensitive areas are connected to the contralateral ones, but the **right and left areas related to** the hand and foot lack commissural callous connections (Powell, 1981).

It is not well defined if there are callous connections between the visual cortex and the two hemispheres. They exist only to represent the vertical meridian (or visual area) of the retina. It can be claimed that the connected cortical areas are in relation with a medium retinal region which is very narrow and from which the ganglion cells send axons that spread and send collaterals in the optic tract on both sides. The commissural bonds are specific because they gather together cortical columnar units in a bilateral function.

The function of the corpus callosum

The description of this structure was made by Galen in the second century BC, but the hypothesis of its involvement in the functional connection of the two hemispheres dates from 1543 and belongs to Vesalius. However, in 1739 the corpus callosum was considered by La Peyronie to be the centre of the soul (Brion and Jedynak, 1975).

During the seventeenth century Schmidt (1676) called attention to the rather striking phenomenon of loss of reading ability with preservation of the capacity to write as a sequel to stroke. Many descriptions of the condition which was by then called "pure word blindness" and which was often attributed on theoretical grounds to the destruction or dysfunction of a "reading centre" in the angular gyrus appeared during the 1870's and 1880's (Benton, 2000). No clinicopathologic correlations were made, however, until 1892, when Déjérine published his famous post-mortem study of a case of pure alexia following a stroke. His patient, an educated man and an accomplished musician, suddenly lost the ability to read musical scores as well as conventional written material. He had a right visual field defect – in all probability a hemiachromatopsia, not a hemianopsia (Damasio, 1983). The autopsy study disclosed infarctions in the territory of the left posterior cerebral artery, specifically, the medial occipital area and the splenium of the corpus callosum. Déjérine inferred that the lesions had the effect of preventing the transmission of visual information to the language centres of the left hemisphere, thus making reading impossible while leaving the interpretation of nonverbal visual stimuli intact. Déjérine claimed that the lesion of the splenium led to a disconnection of the speech areas located in the left hemisphere, from the intact cortical areas in the right hemisphere, therefore the impossibility of the patient to decode the verbal visual stimuli (Brion and Jedynak, 1975).

His concept of pure word blindness as a disconnection symptom, and not as a result of destruction of a "reading centre", was validated by later investigators. This theory was later confirmed by Trescher and Ford (1937), Maspes (1948), Geschwind (1965).

Thus, most of our knowledge related to the callous function comes from studying adult subjects which suffered spontaneous or surgical lesions of the corpus callosum.

Although the corpus callosum is the largest of the interhemispheric commissures, relatively little has been known of its functions until recently. According to Carpenter (1979), the first convincing evidence regarding its function was the demonstration of its importance in interhemispheric transfer of visual discrimination learning in cats with a longitudinal section of the optic chiasma (Fig. 20.6) (Meyers, 1956).

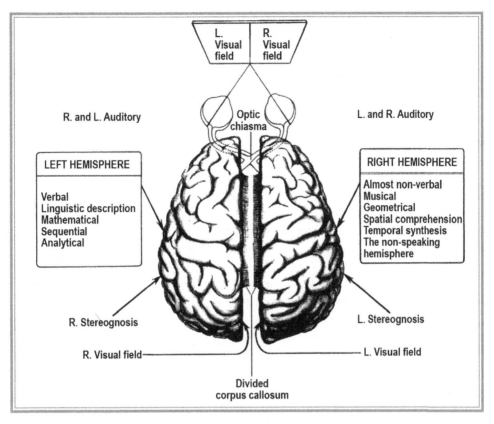

Fig. 20.6. A top view of the two hemispheres. Schematic drawing of the two halves of the cerebral cortex, showing some major functions of the right and left hemispheres. Note the massive bridge of the corpus callosum connecting the two sides. The eyes on top focus on converging lines in order to enable stereoscopic depth perception. (Standring, 2005).

Following the section of the optic chiasma and corpus callosum, cats trained with one eye masked were unable to remember simple visual discriminations learned with the first eye.

The untrained eye could be trained to make reverse-type discrimination without interfering with the patterned discrimination learned on the opposite side. This functional independence of the surgically separated cerebral hemispheres with respect to learning, memory and other gnostic activities has been the stimulus for considerable investigations (Mountcastle, 1962).

Thus, interhemispheric connections function to allow each hemisphere to work as a coordinated unit.

Callosal disconnections of either inter- or intrahemispheric connections can produce a variety of neurological syndromes including apraxia, aphasia, agnosia, alexia, and unilateral agraphia.

The most systematic investigation of hemispheric specialisation and hemispheric integration in cases of callosal disconnection has been carried out with patients who have undergone callosotomy in order to control their intractable epilepsy.

These so-called split-brain patients are the focus of most studies.

Akelaitis (1941, 1944) failed to discover cognitive sequelae of the surgery using standard neuropsychological procedures.

It was the Bogen group that recognised the importance of providing a nonverbal means of response to demonstrate the presence of two independent cognitive systems within the same subject (Bogen and Gazzaniga, 1965; Sperry et al., 1969).

Initial studies confirmed the neurologists' assertion that the left hemisphere was dominant for language whereas the right could neither name nor describe objects presented to it visually or tactually, although it could perform certain visuospatial tasks.

The left hemisphere is dominant for conceptual similarities, for detail and for a gestalt synthesizer. The right hemisphere perceives forms but is lacking a phonological analyser.

However, interactive processes between hemispheres in the normal undivided brain may further modulate such strategic differences, in some cases reducing them, in others enhancing them.

Moreover, even in the divided brain, undivided subcortical processes may provide a surprising degree of interhemispheric cross-talk.

However, the corpus callosum plays an important role in the interhemispheric transfer of learned discrimination, sensory experience and memory.

Further – refined experiments continue to develop our understanding of perceptual cognitive, mnemonic, and linguistic processes and their integration into coherent thought and behavior (Baynes and Gazzaniga, 1997).

The clinic of the corpus callosum

The clinical effects of disconnection were first seriously considered by Wernicke in 1874 and were very much a part of early neurology. He predicted the existence of an aphasic syndrome (conduction aphasia) that would result from severing fibre connections between the anterior and posterior speech zones. Later, in 1892 Déjérine was the first to demonstrate a distinctive behavioral deficit resulting from the pathology of the corpus callosum.

The first real description of a callous syndrome had been made by Raymond in 1893 (Lassonde et al., 1996).

In a series of papers published in about 1900, Liepmann (1900, 1905) and Liepmann and Maas (1907) most clearly demonstrated the importance of severed connections as an underlying factor in the effects of cerebral damage. Liepmann wrote extensively on the principle of disconnection, particularly about the idea that same apraxias might result from disconnection. He reasoned that, if a patient were given a verbal command to use the left hand in a particular way, only the verbal left hemisphere would understand the command. To move the left hand, a signal would then have to travel from the left hemisphere through the corpus callosum to the right hemispheric region that controls movement of the left hand.

By interrupting the part of the corpus callosum that carries the command from the left hemisphere to the right, one disconnects the right hemisphere's motor region from the command. Thus, although the subject would comprehend the command, the left hand would be unable to obey it. Necessarily then, callosal interruption would result in an inability to follow verbal commands with the left hand although there would be no loss of comprehension (as expected from a left hemisphere lesion) and there would be no weakness or incoordination of the left hand (as expected from a right hemisphere lesion). We now recognise the notion that spatial or pictorial instructions understood by the right hemisphere may require a callosally mediated interhemispheric communication for correct left hand execution.

In humans, the highlighting of many callous related symptoms was done in patients with tumors, degenerative disease, partial vascular lesions and agenesis of the corpus callosum.

The study of epileptic patients, where the ablation of a commissure (anterior, posterior, hippocampal) or a callosotomy (sectioning of corpus callosum) had been performed as therapy, allowed the description of the main components of the callous disconnection syndrome.

One should keep in mind that callosal lesions, surgical as well as naturally occurring, are often accompanied by damage to or pressure upon neighbouring structures, resulting in several distinct types of signs: (a) signs of hemisphere disconnection, (b) neighbourhood signs, and (c) nonlocalising signs such as meningismus or signs of increased intracranial pressure. Here, attention is given mainly to signs of the first type.

Thus, the earliest clinical report of a surgical division of commissural pathways to prevent the spread of an epileptic attack was made by Van Wagenen and Herren in 1940, coincident with Erickson's report of the experimental observations in primates of seizure spread *via* the corpus callosum (Erickson, 1940). Van Wagenen and Herren (1940) were inspired to perform the surgery on patients with severe intractable epilepsy after observing that one of their epileptic patients experienced considerable relief after developing a tumor in his corpus callosum. Epileptic seizures are caused by abnormal electrical discharges that reverberate across the brain from one hemisphere to the other. Severing all or part of the corpus callosum can reduce seizure activity by 60-70% in 80% of the patients. Van Wagenen and his colleagues feared that one of the side effects of the surgery would be that it might produce a split personality, or a dual consciousness.

However, after 20 of the surgeries were conducted in the 1940's, researchers like Akelaitis never found psychological side effects (Akelaitis, 1941, 1945). The surgery did not appear to create two minds, each with its own personality and consciousness, fighting over the control of the body. The absence of a dual consciousness continued to be observed when the surgery was revived by Bogen, in the early 1960's, and Sperry.

In 1965, Bogen advocated this approach as a surgical treatment for epilepsy, and further reports appeared in the 1970's (Luessenhop, 1970; Wilson et al., 1975). However, despite the phenomenal academic interest generated by the function of the corpus callosum and lateralised hemispheric function in humans, this therapeutic approach did not arouse much clinical interest until several reports appeared in the mid-1980's. The procedure was medically beneficial, leaving some patients virtually seizure-free afterwards, with minimal effects on their everyday behavior.

However, more extensive, psychological testing by Sperry, Gazzaniga and Bogen (1969) soon demonstrated a unique behavioral syndrome that has been a source of new insights into the nature of cerebral asymmetry.

Although the callosotomy is not as dangerous as it was in the 1940's, given the advent of microsurgery technique, it is still a treatment of last resort. And the procedure is even rarer now, since pharmacological treatments have greatly improved, as well as presurgical techniques to localise the origin of seizure (Gazzaniga and Miller, 2009). But the callosotomy surgery offers a lot of hope to patients with no other treatment options, and in the 1940's those other options were much fewer.

This right-to-left aspect of callosal function was not part of Liepmann's original callosal concept although, in retrospect, it seems a natural corollary. Liepmann himself considered the left hemisphere to be the organiser of complex (particularly learned) motor behavior. Whether and in what way the left hemisphere is dominant for skilled movements generally (and not just those linguistically related) are currently matters of active controversy (Kimura and Archibald, 1974; Zaidel and Sperry, 1977; Haaland and Delaney, 1981; Jason, 1983; Hampson and Kimura, 1984; Bogen, 1987).

Liepmann's deduction, although brilliant, was ignored by a number of neurologists. The earliest systematic studies of the effects of commissural sections in humans are those of Akelaitis (1943). Very few behavioral deficits were observed, such as in jocular despair.

Lashley (1950) declared that the corpus callosum served only to keep the hemispheres from sagging. Testing procedures at the time were far from subtle, but more importantly we now know that, rather far from the anterior commissure, enough of the splenium may have been spared to permit transfer of some visual information.

An important series of papers by Myers (1956) and Sperry (1974, 1976, etc.), revived interest in the effects of disconnecting neocortical regions.

Their work confirmed others' earlier observations that the animals were virtually indistinguishable from their surgically intact counterparts and indeed appeared normal under most testing and training conditions.

Unlike those of earlier studies, however, the results of their studies revealed that, under special training procedures, the animals could be shown to have severe deficits. Thus, if the sensory information were allowed to separate access to each hemisphere, each could be shown to have its own independent perceptual, learning, and memory processes (Mishkin, 1979). The corpus callosum does indeed serve important functions. This conclusion has been confirmed in subsequent studies on the effects of surgical disconnection of the human cerebral hemispheres as a treatment of intractable epilepsy (Kolb and Whishaw, 2003).

The examination of the callous disconnection syndrome also depends on the age at which the callosotomy is performed. According to Ptito and Lepore (1983), a callosotomy that had been performed on an animal before the end of myelinisation of the corpus callosum allows at least a partial interhemispheric visual transfer. It is well known that the myelination of fibres is one of the last events in the maturation of the neural system.

Mitchel (1987) found that human infants younger than about 1 year are like split-brain patients in that they are unable to transfer information about objects obtained by touch.

Rudy and Stadler-Morris (1987) found that rats trained on spatial-navigation tasks learned the task with one hemisphere at 22 days of age but could not learn it with the other.

By the time they were 25 days old, they did display interocular equivalence. The researchers suggest that the 22-day-old rat behaves like a split-brain animal. After the end of myelinisation no transfer can be performed. In cats, the period of myelinisation in callous fibres begins around the age of 28 days (Elberger, 1982), and in humans it extends until the end of the tenth year of existence (Yakovlev and Lecours, 1967).

Due to this reason, a callosotomy performed before the age of 10 should remain almost asymptomatic.

Transfer tests in children with a callosotomy performed before the age of ten, revealed minor or no deficit (Geoffroy et al., 1983, 1986; Lassonde et al., 1986). The reaction time, much longer than in normal persons, confirms the limits of the compensation mechanisms in these subjects (Sauerwein and Lassonde, 1983; Lassonde et al., 1991, 1996).

A commissurotomy performed between age ten and fifteen leads to not very severe signs of callous disconnection (ideomotor apraxia, unilateral anomia, etc.), similar to the ones in adults. It is possible that this mildness is based on certain forms of plasticity that determines a cerebral reorganisation. Its quality and efficacy depends on how early the lesion was produced (Lassonde et al., 1996).

Related to different aspects of the interhemispheric disconnection syndrome in children, youth and adults, Ramackers and Nijokiktjien (1991) released theirs concept of development.

Young children may be considered subjects with a physiological split-brain. In the first decade, the transfer capacity of tactile information is limited, but it increases with age (Quinn and Geffen, 1986).

The fact that the physiological disconnection syndrome disappeared is an ontogenetic phenomenon (Galin et al., 1977) that corresponds to a degree of myelinisation (Ptito and Lepore, 1983).

Thus, some authors stress about the hypothesis of a dysfunction in the corpus callosum in some dyslexic subjects (Ramackers and Nijokiktjien, 1991). This phenomenon of plasticity in subjects with no corpus callosum or subjects, who underwent an early callosotomy, was related to the critical period of development that coincides with synaptic hyperproduction (Hommet and Billard, 1998).

However, the precise relation between the callous malformation and the interhemispheric dysfunction is suspected but not yet proved in the development pathology.

We performed callosotomies (Fig. 20.7) for intractable seizures in four patients. They were 17, 19, 25 and 27 year-old. After surgery we obtained remission of 8-43 months and a decrease in the number and severity of the epileptic seizures. The routine

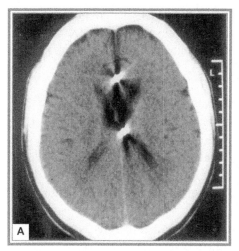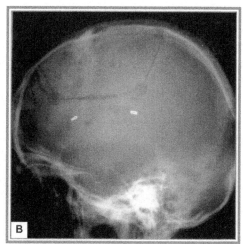

Fig. 20.7. Postoperative CT-scan shows a partial disconnection (A + B) in a patient with contractable seizures. Control clips have been fixed in order to see the location and extension of the colostomy. The postoperative results were very good.

neurological examination did not record any significant change in walking, orthostatism, cutaneous and myotatic reflexes, cranial nerves, sight, hearing and smell. The extraocular movements of the face, tongue, mandible and those of each limb were normal. However, the coordination of the hands was affected if a task that needed both hands was performed without seeing.

When studied under more stringent experiment condition where sensory input was limited to one hemisphere, the consequences of callosal disconnection readily became apparent. Thus, when deprived of visual feedback, the commissurotomised participant was unable to name an object held in the left hand because the left (naming) hemisphere no longer had access to information in the right hemisphere. For the same reason, when deprived of visual input, one hand was unable to select an object held by the other. While the left hand was unable to write an intelligible sentence, it may surpass the efforts of the right in copying a complex geometric design. If emotionally charged images are restricted to the left visual field, a split-brain patient may evidence an appropriate affective response; however, because the speaking left hemisphere is disconnected from the hemisphere that saw the image, he or she may be unable to explain their reaction.

On rare occasions, patients have been dismayed that one hand (usually the left) might be carrying out some activity of which the left (speaking hemisphere) is unaware or find that one hand is working in a counter-productive fashion to the other (e.g., one hand pulling pants up and the other pushing them down) (Mendoza, 2011).

However, according to Kolb and Whishaw (2003), for dualists who hold that the brain has a separate corresponding mental representation (the mind), these are compelling reasons to consider that a split-brain person possesses two brains and two minds. For materialists, who hold that behavior is explained as a function of the nervous system, without recourse to mind, the philosophical implications are not so weighty. But for everyone, there is a challenge to understand how persons with separated hemispheres function in a seemingly integrated way (Kolb and Whishaw, 2003).

Further on, we will describe the disconnection syndrome in direct relation with the disruption of communication between the motor and sensorial areas. Because of the crossing of these tracts, each hemisphere controls the contralateral half of the body. The operational efficacy of the two hemispheres is based on the transfer of information that takes place between them and on their bilateral integration (Jeeves, 1990).

Specificity of callosal fibres

It has long been noted that separating up to two-thirds of the anterior callosum leads to little if any changes in ability (Risse et al., 1989). The symptoms of callous disconnection may vary depending on the location of the lesion. Thus, located lesions allowed determining these commisural areas that play a primary role in producing each of the elements of the callous disconnection syndrome. Commissurotomies and callosotomies disrupt the interhemispheric transfer of many types of information. However, both cerebral hemispheres are believed to make significant contributions to most routine daily functions, including language-based activities being carried out primarily by the left hemisphere and the right hemisphere apparently being more important for certain perceptual and emotional functions.

If the anterior split continues far enough, a disruption of the ability to transfer sensory and position information from hand to hand will be observed. In contrast, the section of the splenium disrupts the transfer of visual information between the hemispheres, which isolates lateralised visual input. After a posterior section, although explicit identification and naming of left visual field stimuli is not possible, some transfer of higher-order information may occur (Sidtis et al., 1981).

In cases with inadvertent surgical sparing, very specific transfer of information has been found (Gazzaniga et al., 1989). Occasionally, strokes yield partial callosal lesions as well; one such patient with damage to the body of the corpus callosum demonstrates left-hand tactile anomia and agraphia (Baynes and Gazzaniga, 1997).

The disconnection syndrome

Most of our knowledge related to the function of the corpus callousum comes from studying adult subjects who suffered spontaneous or surgical lesions of the corpus callosum.

Classically, the syndrome of interhemispheric disconnection or the callous syndrome consists of a series of symptoms of variable complexity in which one can include transfer defects of elementary sensorial information that is symmetrically organised in the two hemispheres.

One might also include dysfunctions of elaborate cognitive functions (speech, praxias) in which one hemisphere is more or less exclusively specialised, and even psychic symptoms with a dissociative character.

Thus, the complete section of the corpus callosum, which has come to be used increasingly as a treatment for medically intractable epilepsy (Reeves, 1985) is regularly followed by a wide variety of neurological and neuropsychological deficits. The deficits that are most apparent immediately after operation make up the acute disconnection syndrome (Wilson et al., 1977). Those deficits that persist make up the stabilised syndrome of hemisphere disconnection (Sperry et al., 1969; Bogen, 1978; 1985 a, b).

A partial section of the corpus callosum may produce a fraction of the full syndrome, depending upon the part of the corpus callosum that has been cut as well as the amount and nature of any associated extracallosal damage.

In general, most of the disconnection deficits, both acute and chronic, are not present as long as the splenium is spared (Apuzzo et al., 1982; Gordon et al., 1971; Dănăilă and Golu, 2002). But certain partial sections do entail a few inevitable deficits, as well as some common complications, whose recognition is important for the surgeon utilising transcallosal approaches.

Sperry, Gazzaniga and others have extensively studied the effects of hemispheric disconnection on behaviours related to both motor and sensory systems.

The patients with divided brain (split-brain) operated by Akelaitis (1943 and 1944) and Bogen and Vogel (1962) for epileptic seizures, have been examined by Sperry et al. (1969) and Sperry (1986). Thus, with the exception of several transitory postoperatory phenomena observed just in some of the patients (mutism, left hemiapraxia, etc.), the respective patients did not seen to stand out in any way compared to the ones who did not undergo surgery. However, when these patients went through adequate psychological tests, they showed some particular signs and symptoms.

Afterwards, they have been grouped under the name "callous disconnection syndrome" (Bogen and Vogel, 1962; Bogen and Gazzaniga, 1965; Gazzaniga, 1970; Hécaen and Assal, 1973; LeDoux and Gazzaniga, 1978; Bogen, 1985; Sperry, 1986).

The signs of callous disconnection are based upon the principle of a specialised left hemisphere involved in the verbal behavior and a right hemisphere involved in spatial and visual-perceptive abilities.

The communication between the two hemispheres is based upon the registration of sensorial or motor information coming from the callous commissure in each of them. Or, in some cases, it is based upon the bilateral transport of information.

Thus, signs of disconnection may be observed when the callous commissure is sectioned, and the motor or sensorial information is limited to a single hemisphere (Lassonde et al., 1996).

There are four conditions in which the hemispheres become completely or partial separated.

First, in humans, the interhemispheric fibres are sometimes cut as a therapy for intractable epilepsy.

Second, people are born with congenitally reduced or completely missing interhemispheric connections.

Third, in animals, disconnections are performed to trace functional systems, to model human conditions and to answer basic questions about interhemispheric development.

Four, a stroke involving the anterior and / or posterior cerebral artery.

The effects of complete disconnection

Epileptic seizures may begin in a restricted region of one hemisphere (most often the temporal lobes) and then spread through the fibres of the corpus callosum or anterior commissure to the homologous location in the opposite hemisphere.

In some cases the medication is of little value, and the seizures may actually become life threatening because they recur often, sometimes several times in an hour.

To relieve this seizure condition, the corpus callosum and anterior commissure can be surgically sectioned. In these patients we can obtain substantial relief from their epilepsy and often show marked improvements in personal well being, competence, and intelligence.

As a result of the surgery, each hemisphere retains fibres that allow it to see only the opposite side of the visual world. Likewise, each hemisphere predominantly receives information from the opposite side of the body and controls movements on the opposite side of the body. The surgery also isolates speech in those persons with lateralised speech.

About a year or so is required for recovery from the surgical trauma. Within 2 years, the typical patient is able to return to school or work.

Specific tests, however, can show differences between the functioning of split-brain patients and that of people with normal cerebral connections. In the split-brain, each hemisphere can be shown to have its own sensations, percepts, thoughts, and memories that are not accessible to the other hemisphere (Purves et al., 1988).

Thus, after hemisphere disconnection in the human, unilateral tactile anomia, left hemialexia, and unilateral apraxia are typical. That is a right-hander with complete cerebral commissurotomy cannot name aloud objects correctly manipulated (hence, recognised) with the left hand, cannot read aloud written material presented solely to the left half-field of vision, and cannot execute with the left hand actions verbally named or described by the examiner, although these actions are readily imitated when demonstrated.

The apraxia usually recedes within a few months, whereas the hemialexia and unilateral anomia can persist for years (Bogen, 1987).

Finally, the subjects with total callosotomy still have the possibility to transfer a piece of this information probably through extracallous interhemispheric tracts (or through ipsilateral projections of tactile information) (Habib, 1998). The absence of direct callous connections between primary sensitive areas of the distal extremity of the limbs makes one suppose that the transfer of sensitive information is performed through associative areas rich in callous connections, therefore after processing the signal to some extend (Cusik and Kaas, 1986).

The effects of partial disconnection

According to Kolb and Whishaw (2003), surgeons have experimented with partial surgical disconnection of the hemispheres, hoping to attain the same clinical relief from seizures but with fewer neuropsychological side effects.

Thus, partial disconnection, in which the posterior part of the corpus callosum is left intact, appears to combine markedly milder effects than those of a complete commissurotomy and the same therapeutic benefits.

Sperry (1974) and Sperry et al. (1979) have found that patients with partial disconnection are significantly better at motor tasks such as those needed to use the Etch-a-Sketch.

The results of research on monkeys with partial commissurotomies suggest that the posterior part of the corpus callosum (splenium) subserves visual transfer, whereas the region just in front of the splenium affects somatosensory transfer (Pandya and Seltzer, 1986).

Acute disconnection syndrome

During the first few days after a complete cerebral commissurotomy, the patients commonly respond reasonably well, to simple commands, with their right limbs. But they are easily confused by three- or even two-part commands, each part of which is obviously understood. The patients often lie quietly and may seem mildly "akinetic", although cooperating when stimulated (Bogen, 1987).

There is sometimes an "imperviousness" resembling the one often seen with naturally occurring genu lesions (Alpers and Grant, 1931; Bogen, 1978, 1987). The patients are often mute even when willing to write short (usually one-word) answers.

The left-side apraxia to verbal command is usually severe and can be mistaken for hemiplegia. Similarly, a disregard for the left half-field of vision can be mistaken for a hemianopsia.

Left side weakness in the first week or so due to retraction edema in the right hemisphere sometimes confounds the picture. There may be competitive movements between the left and right hands. Moreover, some patients have focal motor seizures, manifested by clonic contractions on alternating sides of the body and without loss of consciousness, occasionally followed by transient unresponsiveness of whichever limbs were involved.

The patients commonly have bilateral Babinski signs as well as bilateral absent superficial abdominal reflexes (Bogen, 1987).

Well-coordinated but repetitive reaching, groping, and grasping with the left hand sometimes resembles a grasp reflex. The left arm hypotonia, the responses bilaterally to plantar stimulation, and the mutism were regularly observed.

One of Bogen's patient's condition worsened at the end of the first week associated with an alkalotic hyponatremia present on days 5 to 7. When the hyponatremia was corrected the patient rapidly improved with respect to alertness and left side coordination. But some degree of mutism persisted for another month. The duration of mutism seems to be related to the extent of extracallosal damage (Bogen, 1987). There was also, as in every one of Bogen's 12 right-handers tested after complete commissurotomy, a persistent anomia in the left hand.

A positive Babinski sign can be found not only contralateral to the retracted hemisphere but also, for at least a day or two, on the ipsilateral side. The best explanation for this ipsilateral Babinski sign is probably that the diaschistic shock effect on the unexposed hemisphere after an extensive callosal section is sufficient to depress for a few days the corticofugal inhibition of the primitive extensor response (Bogen, 1974;

Van Gijn, 1977). In any event, the Babinski signs rapidly subside bilaterally and are not present over a long term (Botez and Bogen, 1976).

As the severity of the acute disconnection syndrome subsides in a week or so, a phenomenon variously called "intermanual conflict" or "the alien hand" appears (Bogen, 1987). Almost all complete commissurotomy patients manifest some degree of intermanual conflict during the early postoperative period.

Intermanual conflict was observed after commissurotomy by Wilson et al. (1977) and by Akelaitis (1944-1945), who called it "diagnostic dyspraxia".

While doing the block design test unimanually with his right hand, his left hand came up from beneath the table and was reaching for the blocks when he slapped it with his right hand and said, "That will keep it quiet for a while". Examples of intermanual conflict have been reported in detail by Rayport et al. (1983) and Ferguson (1985). In rare instances, the intermanual conflict may reappear even years later.

One of Bogen's patients remained seizure-free for 8 years and then had a status epilepticus a few months after her family physician discontinued her anticonvulsant medication (Bogen, 1985). Her seizures were readily controlled when her medication was reinstituted. Her left-handed anomia was still readily demonstrable 21 years postoperatively. This persistence of unilateral tactile anomia was also true of all their other patients (Bogen et al., 1981).

Chronic disconnection syndrome

According to Bogen (1987), within a few months after surgery, the symptoms of acute hemisphere disconnection become compensated to a remarkable degree. In personality and social situations the patient appears much as before.

When input is lateralised, each hemisphere seems to have its own learning processes and its own separate memories.

Split-brain patients soon accept the idea that they have capacities of which they are not conscious such as left-hand retrieval of objects not nameable. They may quickly rationalise such acts, sometimes in a transparently erroneous way (Gazzaniga and LeDoux, 1978). But even many years after operation the patients will occasionally be quite surprised when some well-coordinated or obviously well-informed act has just been carried out by the left hand. This is particularly common under conditions of continuously lateralised input (Zaidel, 1983).

In sum, split-brain is a condition resulting from surgical lesioning of all or a substantial portion of the corpus callosum, thus interrupting the normal flow of information between the two hemispheres of the brain (Mendoza, 2011).

Geschwind and Kaplan (1962) discovered that their patient produced lucid writing with the right hand (left hemisphere, but "aphasic" writing with the left hand (right hemisphere). They also reported anomia for objects placed in the left hand but not the right.

By the middle of the 20th century, Sperry and his associate noted that if both the corpus callosum and the optic chiasma were lesioned in animals (thus, restricting visual information from each eye to the ipsilateral hemisphere), dramatically different results were obtained. Not only could the animal not carry out a discrimination task previously learned by one eye (cerebral hemisphere) when only the opposite eye was left uncovered, but each eye (cerebral hemisphere) could learn conflicting tasks, depending on which eye was used.

In other classic series in the 1960s, Gazzaniga, Boegen and Sperry clearly demonstrated the effects of split-brain preparations in human subjects (Mendoza, 2011).

Following commisurotomy, behavioral deficits were not always obvious. This is probably due to the extensive cross-cueing that normally takes place, especially through vision where the right hand sees what the left one is doing and vice-versa.

Although in cases of naturally occurring callosal lesion in humans, or even more surprisingly in cases of callosal agenesis, there is typically a failure to evidence the signs of a disconnection syndrome (Mendoza, 2011).

The psychological examination emphasised discrete elements of unilateral agraphia on the left side, unilateral constructive apraxia on the right side, tactile anomia of the left hand, disorder in naming objects presented in the left visual area and amnestic elements.

In addition to providing insights into how the two hemispheres normally interact and their respective strengths, studies of split-brain patients have raised some intriguing questions about the presumed unitary nature of consciousness.

The transfer of sensorial information

Visual effects

The organisation of the tract in the visual system directs the information coming from each hemi-field towards the opposite hemisphere. As far as the transfer of visual information is concerned, the data pleads for its location to be at the level of the enlarged splenial area, a region dedicated for the passage of interoccipital fibres.

In the visual system, connections in each hemisphere run from area V1 to area V2 and to area V3, V4 and V5 in the same hemisphere (Mishkin, 1979). Connections from V3, V4 and V5 cross the corpus callosum to the analogous area on the opposite side, and also connect with area TE on the same side (Fig. 20.8). Area TE connects to the anterior temporal cortex and the amygdala on the same side and connects, through the anterior commissure, to these structures on the opposite side.

By using different tasks, Mishkin (1979) has demonstrated that bilateral lesions in area V1, V2 or TE result in an impaired or abolished ability to solve visual-discrimination problems in monkeys.

Because unilateral lesions do not have such an effect, what seems to be necessary is one intact trio of areas V1, V2 and TE. There is, however, one constraint: the remaining cortical regions must be connected to. Thus, as illustrated in figure 20.8 B, a lesion in area V1 on the right and in area TE on the left does not disturb performance, because an intact system still functions.

If the connection between the hemispheres is severed, the neocortical areas are still intact but are not connected, and the result is failure of the visual-discrimination ability (Fig. 20.8 C). Clearly, the neocortical regions do not function properly if they are not connected to one another.

Fig. 20.8. Disconnection effects in the visual system of monkeys.
(A) The visual system is intact.
(B) After lesioning (dark gray areas), the left visual cortex still has access to the visual association cortex of the right hemisphere, and so vision is still possible.
(C) The intact components of the visual system are disconnected (jagged line) after lesioning, producing major visual deficits. (After Mishkin, 1979).

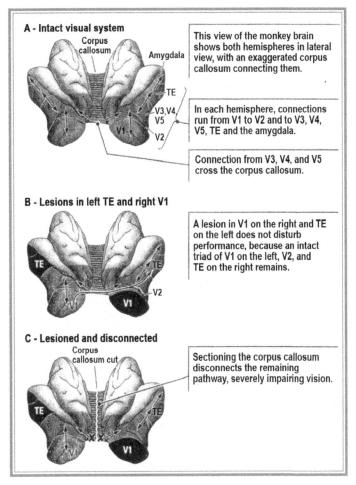

A - Intact visual system
Corpus callosum
Amygdala
TE
V3,V4, V5
V1
V2

This view of the monkey brain shows both hemispheres in lateral view, with an exaggerated corpus callosum connecting them.

In each hemisphere, connections run from V1 to V2 and to V3, V4, V5, TE and the amygdala.

Connection from V3, V4, and V5 cross the corpus callosum.

B - Lesions in left TE and right V1
TE
TE
V2
V1

A lesion in V1 on the right and TE on the left does not disturb performance, because an intact triad of V1 on the left, V2, and TE on the right remains.

C - Lesioned and disconnected
Corpus callosum cut
TE
TE
V1

Sectioning the corpus callosum disconnects the remaining pathway, severely impairing vision.

Mishkin (1979) studied area TE, thinking of it as the final step in the neocortical visual system. He later studied the problem of how visual stimuli might gain what he calls "motivational" or "emotional" significance. Monkeys with bilateral temporal lobotomies including the amygdala attach no significance to visual stimuli. That is, they will repeatedly eat nasty-tasting objects or place inedible objects in the mouth.

In 1965, Geschwind proposed that this symptom represents a disconnection of the amygdala from the visual system. Area TE connects with the amygdala on the same side and the amygdala on the opposite side through the anterior commissure.

The result of Mishkin (1979) and Nakamura and Mishkin (1980) point to an important role of the nonvisual cortex in visual perception and demonstrate the importance of studying the connections to a functional system as well as its areas. If an animal cannot move in response to visual information, it appears to be essentially blind, even though the visual system may be processing the sensory input.

We can speculate at this point that it is an extreme example of a disconnection syndrome because the brain is disconnected from both its inputs and outputs. It seems likely that, although the brain could still function, it would be unconscious in the absence of inputs or outputs (Kolb and Whishaw, 2003).

In human beings, visual material can be presented selectively to a single hemisphere by having the patient fix his gaze on a projection screen onto which pictures of objects or symbols are projected to the right, left or both visual half-fields using exposure times of 0.1 second or less (Bogen, 1987).

In short, the visual system is crossed, so information flashed to one visual field travels selectively to the contralateral hemisphere. By using this fact, researchers have demonstrated left- and right-visual-field superiority for different types of input.

For example, verbal material is perceived more accurately when presented to the right visual field, presumably because the input travels to the left, linguistic hemisphere.

On the other hand visuospatial input (such as a map) produces a left-visual-field superiority, because the right hemisphere appears to have a more important role in analysing spatial information (Kolb and Whishaw, 2003).

However, words presented to the left visual field, and hence right hemisphere, are sometimes perceived, not as accurately or consistently as when they are presented to the right visual field. These relative effects occur because either hemisphere potentially has access to input to the opposite hemisphere through the corpus callosum, which connects the visual areas. Thus, the visual-field superiority observed in normal subjects is relative (Myers, 1956; Sperry, 1974; Nakamura and Mishkin, 1980; Lepore et al., 1986; Lassonde 1986; Lassonde et al., 1986; Fantie and Kolb, 1989).

A commissurotomy patient no longer has such access, because the connection is severed. Given that speech is usually housed in the left hemisphere of right-handed patients, visual information presented to the left visual field will be disconnected from verbal associations because the input goes to the right, nonlinguistic hemisphere.

Similarly, complex visual material presented to the right visual field will be inadequately processed, because it will not have access to the visuospatial abilities of the right hemisphere. It follows that, if material is appropriately presented, it will be possible to demonstrate aphasia, agnosia, alexia, and acopia (the inability to copy a geometric design) in a patient who ordinarily exhibits none of these symptoms, as Kolb and Whishaw (2003) demonstrated.

If verbal material is presented to the left visual field, the commissurotomy patient will be unable to read it or to answer questions about it verbally, because the input is disconnected from the speech zones of the left hemisphere.

Presentation of some verbal material to the right visual field presents no difficulties, because the visual input projects to the verbal left hemisphere (Downer, 1961; Geschwind, 1965; Gazzaniga, 1970; Schrift et al., 1986; Fabri et al., 2001; Kolb and Whishaw, 2003).

Similarly, if an object is presented to the left visual field, the patient will be unable to name it and thus will appear agnosic and aphasic. If presented to the right visual field, this same object will be correctly named, because the left visual cortex perceives the object and has access to the speech zones. Thus, we can see that the split-brain patient is aphasic, alexic, and agnosic if verbal material or an object requiring a verbal response is presented visually to the right hemisphere, but this person appears normal if material is presented to the left hemisphere (Downer, 1961; Geschwind, 1965; Gazzaniga, 1970; Schrift et al., 1986; Fabri et al., 2001; Kolb and Whishaw, 2003).

A further deficit can be seen if the patients are asked to copy a complex visual figure. Because the right hemisphere controls the left hand, we might predict that the left hand will be able to copy the figure but right hand being deprived of the expertise of the right hemisphere, will be severely impaired. This result is indeed the case: the left hand draws the figure well, whereas the right hand cannot and is, thus, acopic (Kolb and Whishaw, 2003).

The complete splenial sections are exceptional. There are only few documented observations of spontaneous lesions that led to splenial destruction with no previous lesions (Damasio et al., 1980; Degas et al., 1987; Habib et al., 1990). The typical behavior of subjects with callous disconnection, in the case of a short tachistoscopic projection of a stimulus representing an image, a letter, a word etc., in the lateral region of this visual area refers only to reporting a light or a "flash" in the left side. The same stimulus presented on the right side leads to its immediate recognising. In case of subjects with cerebral division, a simultaneous bilateral projection of stimuli in each visual hemifield shows that it is difficult to distinguish them and that the images cannot overlap. Each hemisphere responds independently to its respective stimulus (Lassonde et al., 1996). In the case of chimerical figures (faces of people, shapes etc.), formed by two unpaired halves, each of the elements in a compound pair was projected in a single hemisphere. Under these conditions, if a verbal answer is required, the subject communicates only the stimulus directed towards the left hemisphere. When he is asked to point with the left hand, the subject indicates the stimulus analysed by the right hemisphere (Levy et al., 1972).

With the help of this test it is possible to confirm the difference between specific functions for each hemisphere. So, the stimuli presented in the right hemifield which is controlled by the left hemisphere can be read and described verbally. The right hemisphere could not name, neither verbally, nor in writing, the visual material presented in the left hemifield.

With the left hand the subject can indicate with no difficulty, in a collection of things, the object that is presented to him as an image or verbally.

The failure of the right hand is due to the fact that the left hemisphere, on which it depends, is not informed about the stimulation exerted exclusively upon its homologue (LeDoux and Gazzaniga, 1978).

Thereinafter, it was proved that patients with callosotomy, too, have a superior visuospatial function of their hemisphere, while their left hemisphere uses electively visual imagery that consists of letters.

The use of tactile information in order to form representations of abstract shapes is better developed at the level of the parietal lobe in the right hemisphere. The analysis of information from unfamiliar **facial figures**, too, belongs to the right hemisphere, while the left hemisphere is more able to generate voluntary expressions. However the facial mimic, which is part of a spontaneous emotion, is the result of both hemispheres. Consequently, the right hemisphere has proved its superiority in analysing perceptual and spatial performances, while the left hemisphere is essential for finding solutions to complex visual problems, speech, tasks that involve deductions, generalisation, and intelligent behaviours.

In the case of a callosotomy, visual and tactile perceptions remain isolated in each hemisphere. Even though the subjects are able to report independently the visual material that was received and saved in one of the two hemispheres, they cannot compare the two hemifields because the perception remains isolated in each hemisphere (Baynes and Gazzaniga, 1997).

These facts correspond to the concept of a specialised left hemisphere for treating significant information.

Besides the infraconscious treatment of information received in the right hemisphere, it has proved that subjects with callosotomy are able to transfer messages related to movement, light, and location of targets in the lateral area of the visual field, between the two hemispheres (Habib, 1998). Sergent (1990) proved that "split-brain" subjects are capable of a certain level of conscious treatment, in particular a semantic one of some stimuli (numbers, facial expressions) that are addressed to the right hemisphere. It is supposed that the subcortical commissures are responsible for the transfer of this information. The fact was proved in rats but they were considered to be accessories or inexistent in primates (Berlucchi, 1990). Consequently, the subcortical commissures, in particular the anterior commissure, are able to maintain a part of the visual information transfer that is depending on the splenium.

The loss of the ability to transfer information from the left hemisphere to the right hemisphere and vice-versa seems to have no impact on their overall psychological state.

In sum, although individuals seem normal following callosotomy, postoperative studies have revealed some interesting findings. Thus, when patients were asked to read words that were presented in their right visual field, they were able to see and to read the words. However, when words were presented in their left visual field, they could not read them as they were not even aware that the words were there. One explanation is as follows: visual information from the right visual field is relayed to the left cerebral hemisphere (*via* the visual pathway, which was not affected when the corpus callosum was sectioned), which is the dominant hemisphere in the processing of language in most individuals.

Thus the patients were able to see and read the words. In contrast, visual input from the left visual field is relayed to the right cerebral hemisphere (again, *via* the visual pathway, which was not affected when the corpus callosum was sectioned), the nondominant hemisphere for language.

As a result of the bisection of the corpus callosum, the visual input relayed to the right cerebral hemisphere has no way of also reaching the left hemisphere containing the language area.

Consequently, patients could not see or read the words, as if they had a left homonymous hemianopsia. These individuals are not blind.

When they were asked to select with their hand an object that corresponds to the object that was presented in their left visual field, they selected the matching object. This showed that the visual system is functioning properly, and that it is the language function that is not.

Although the above studies support the finding that the left cerebral hemisphere is the "dominant" hemisphere in the processing of language, other studies indicate that the right hemisphere may also be involved to some extent in language comprehension (Patestas and Gartner, 2008).

Language

The most striking observation regarding split-brain subjects is the presence of complex generative language in only one hemisphere. Nonetheless, the series of patients operated on by Bogen demonstrated a well-developed right hemispheric lexicon in the majority of patients examined, although that lexicon appeared to be limited to simple auditory and visual comprehension and some written output (Gazzaniga et al., 1962; Sperry et al., 1969; Levy et al., 1971).

Assessing the scientific significance of the data obtained after the examination of the four left-handed patients with face localised in the right hemisphere, we may state that:

a. they confirm other studies of this kind which pointed out the poorer lateralisation of the speech structure in left-handed patients as compared with right-handed ones (Gazzaniga, 1983).

b. they demonstrated the role of the right hemisphere in the integration and production of speech in left-handed patients. It extends its competence in performing impressive speech. On the other hand it begins to directly control the articulating apparatus and, implicitly, to participate in the production of expressive speech;

c. correlated with the data supplied by the analysis of right-handed patients with lesions in the right hemisphere, they show that the linguistic dominance of the left hemisphere does not completely eliminate but only limits the participation of the right hemisphere in the production of verbal behavior (Dănăilă and Golu, 1987).

The Wilson-Roberts series, demonstrated much less frequent right hemispheric participation in even rudimentary language processing. By 1983, of the 28 completed callosotomies, only 3 patients had a documented right hemispheric lexicon (Gazzaniga, 1983). Moreover, there was considerable variation in the quality and sophistication of the language available to the right hemisphere (Sidtis et al., 1981).

The visual and auditory lexicons of the right hemisphere appear to be similar, albeit somewhat smaller than the corresponding left hemispheric lexicons (Gazzaniga et al., 1984).

Both hemispheres can make a variety of semantic judgments, recognising categorical, functional and associative relations. The ability to discriminate words from nonword letter strings is limited but possible, which suggest that the visual word form is represented in the right hemisphere of the patients (Reuter-Lorenz and Baynes, 1992).

Phonologic information is difficult for the right hemisphere to manipulate, although it may possess limited phonologic competence and be able to produce speech. Sidtis et al. (1981) assessed discrimination of phonemes (such as "ba" versus "pa") in two callosotomy patients. The right hemisphere of one patient was able to discriminate but not identify phoneme contrasts and was also able to identify rhyming words. However, this patient was able to produce some verbal responses to left visual field stimuli within a year of her completed surgery (Gazzaniga et al., 1984).

The other patient remained mute until more than 10 years after the surgery; he has now gained rudimentary control of speech within the right hemisphere (Baynes et al., 1995).

Although he remained unable to make accurate judgments that require moving from letter to sound, he was able to integrate visual and auditory phonologic information within his right hemisphere (Baynes et al., 1994, 1995). This remarkable development has implications for the limits of functional plasticity and for the role of the right hemisphere in long-term recovery from aphasia (Baynes and Gazzaniga, 1997).

The linguistic prowess of the right hemisphere does not appear to extend to the use of grammatical rules for comprehension or the production of sentences.

In a left-handed patient with right hemispheric language dominance, comprehension of grammatical relations appears to be possible only for the right hemisphere (Lutsep et al., 1995).

Right hemispheric reading proceeds more slowly than the left hemispheric reading and may use a different mode of processing as has been reported for some deep dyslexic patients (Reuter-Lorenz and Baynes, 1992).

Likewise, a right hemispheric lexicon with a more diffuse or associative organisation than that of the left hemisphere has been suggested as the source of certain reading errors in deep dyslexic (Coltheart, 1980; Schweinger et al., 1989) and pure alexic patients (Coslett and Saffran, 1989).

The language profile seen in callosotomy patients is more consistent with the profile reported by Coslett and Saffran (1989) for the preserved reading of their pure alexic patient than with that reported for deep dyslexic patients (Baynes and Gazzaniga, 1997).

Thus, auditory comprehension of words by the disconnected right hemisphere is suggested by the subject's ability to retrieve with the left hand various objects if they are named aloud by the examiner. Visual comprehension of printed words by the right hemisphere is often present: after a printed word is flashed to the left visual half-field, the subject is often able to retrieve with the left hand the designated item from among an array of hidden objects. Control by the left hemisphere is excluded in these tests because incorrect verbal descriptions given immediately after a correct response by the left hand show that only the right hemisphere knew the answer.

While the disconnected right hemisphere's receptive vocabulary can increase considerably over the years, single word comprehension is rarely accompanied by speech. The most extreme cases of right hemisphere language ability in right-handed (and left hemisphere-speaking) split-brain subjects include two patients with right hemisphere speech, both with an intact anterior commissure (Sidtis et al., 1981; McKeever et al., 1982). Right hemisphere language in the split-brain subject has other limitations, with the syntactic ability being rudimentary at best. Whereas phonetic and syntactic analysis seems to specialise heavily in the left hemisphere, there is a rich lexical structure in the right hemisphere (Zaidel, 1978).

However, after a commissurotomy, each hemisphere can be tested separately, demonstrating in a positive way those things that each hemisphere can do better than the other, rather than inferring from its loss of function what a hemisphere is able to do if injured.

Representative reviews are included in the references (Bogen and Bogen, 1969; Levy, 1974; Nebes, 1974; Sperry, 1974; Zaidel, 1983; Bradshaw and Nettleton, 1983; Trevarthen, 1984).

Right-handers can write legibly, albeit not fluently, with the left hand. This ability is commonly lost with callosal lesions, especially those that cause unilateral apraxia. An inability to write to dictation is common with left hemisphere lesions, almost always affecting both hands. The left hand may be dysgraphic if affected by a right hemispheric lesion, such as a frontal lesion causing forced grasping (Bogen, 1978).

That the left dysgraphia after callosal sectioning is not simply attributable to an incoordination or paresis can be established if one can demonstrate other abilities in the left hand requiring as much control as would be required for writing. The left hand may spontaneously doodle or it may copy various designs or diagrams. It is not so much the presence of a deficit but rather the contrast between certain deficits and certain retained abilities that is most informative (Bogen, 1987).

Simple or even complex geometric figures previously made with the patient's own right hand can often be copied by a left hand that cannot write or even copy writing (Bogen and Gazzaniga, 1965; Bogen, 1969; Kumar, 1977; Zaidel and Sperry, 1977).

Postcallosotomy mutism

After a complete section of the cerebral commissures, there was in almost every case a postoperative period of mutism, of varying duration, during which speech was absent or extremely sparse, although comprehension and writing were retained.

In these cases, there was little if any paraphasia: when the ability to talk returned there was no nominal amnesia; in some cases there was a definite lack of bodily spontaneity and motor initiative for a time, but only partially correlated in duration with the loss of speech.

As the mutism subsided, there was a stage of partial recovery that usually included hoarseness or whispering, but without paraphasia, anomia, or novel semantic or syntactic errors, except for 1 right-hander (corpus callosum was operated from the left) (Bogen, 1987).

However, postcommissurotomy deficits depend mainly upon the nature and amount of preexisting extracallosal damage (Sperry et al., 1969; Gordon et al., 1971; Bogen, 1976).

Postcommissurotomy mutism was originally considered a simple neighbourhood sign, a partial akinetic mutism from the retraction affecting the anterior end of the third ventricle (Cairns, 1952; Ross and Stewart, 1981). In contrast to the cases of complete commissurotomy in other patients all of the same structures (including the massa intermedia and the anterior commissure) were severed, except the splenium, and there was no immediate postoperative mutism (Gordon et al., 1971).

Such cases are evidence not only against a third ventricle origin for mutism, but also against a right supplementary cortex origin. On the other hand, Ross et al. (1984) reported mutism after anterior callosal sections but not after posterior callosal sections.

After a complete callosotomy in two stages, Rayport et al. (1985) observed in three of eight cases a marked decrease in spontaneous speech unaccompanied by paraphasia or a comprehension deficit or inability to sing. The authors suggested that, in these most affected cases, mixed hand dominance may have been an important consideration.

Of particular importance was the absence of any language or speech problems after the first stage of callosotomy (rostrum, genu, and most of the trunk). The mutism appeared only after the second stage of the callosotomy (the splenium and remainder of the trunk).

This result does not totally eliminate the retraction on the supplementary motor cortex as a partial contributory cause.

Rayport et al. (1985) have suggested that mutism could result from an interhemispheric conflict. But they emphasize more the aspect of mixed dominance, which might indicate a greater role than usual of the corpus callosum in the production of speech.

A diaschisis secondary to differentiation of speech areas accounts for deficits in terms of left hemisphere dysfunctions even when the left hemisphere in unmolested.

So, the diaschisis of the left hemisphere (from a complete section) must affect the speech "centres" or "circuits" more than it affects writing "centres" or "circuits". This implies, in turn, that the writing function is more robust or resistant in some sense than that for speech, in spite of having developed later in both phylogeny and ontogenesis (Bogen, 1978).

A more speculative possibility is that speech usually requires interhemispheric integration in order to control the larynx and other midline structures in the following sense: One can suppose that left hemisphere speech ordinarily includes a corollary discharge (Sperry, 1950) to the other hemisphere.

When the commissures are completely severed a downstream interhemispheric conflict occurs at the level of the motor nuclei for the larynx, which results in dysphonia (Bogen, 1987).

Those concerned with the normal physiology of speech will be more interested in the temporary (several weeks to months) mutism after splenial sections (either as part of a total callosotomy or as a second stage) than the long-lasting mutism (many months to years) of those whose anomalous laterality is associated with long-standing cortical lesions. But for the surgeon using a transcallosal approach to the third ventricle, neither of these is apt to be as important as transient mutism (several days to weeks) after the section of callosal segments (such as the trunk) well anterior to the splenium (Bogen, 1987).

However, the lack of speech could be considered a mutism of the type often associated with akinesia of either cingulate or subfrontal origin. Ross et al. (1984) think of the postcommissurotomy state as a sort of "forme fruste" of akinetic mutism, in which mutism is much more evident than is akinesia.

The occurrence of mutism in callosotomy cases without entry into the third ventricle could be explained as the result of a subfrontal retraction while sectioning the rostrum.

Arguing against this is the paucity of postoperative mutism in four of Ross et al. (1984) patients whose splenium was spared but who underwent a section of both the rostrum and the anterior commissure under direct vision. Thus, transitory mutism (for a few days or months) immediately after surgery (commissurotomy) is classic but not completely explained.

For Bogen (1987), keeping an intact splenium of the corpus callosum was sufficient in order to avoid such a disorder.

In case of sectioning the intermediary area between the genu and the trunk of the corpus callosum, the transitory mutism would be due to the inclusion of interhemispheric fibres from the cingular area 24, which are associated, to the elemental mechanisms of speech (Ross et al., 1984). According to Reeves (1991), an anterior callosotomy produces a speech disorder which evokes an "adynamic" aphasia of variable gravity (from a simple bradyarthria to complete mutism). The reasons for this type of disorder still remain unknown but there probably are multiple ones: preparatory associated lesions, the phenomenon called diaschisis of the hemisphere that dominates speech, a functional imbalance between the two hemispheres in relation to the brutal disruption of an assembly of cortical and cortico-subcortical connections.

Reeves (1991) shows that these disorders are associated with a certain number of symptoms which evoke a dysfunction of the medial regions in the non-dominant frontal cortex.

They manifest through a deficit of the inferior left limb and grasping of the left hand which indicates a lesion of the right SMA.

In such situations the author invokes a surgical injury of the right internal frontal region.

Long-term dysphasic disorders after a callosotomy are very rare and debatable. After a complete callosotomy, Fergusson et al. (1985) and Spencer et al. (1988) reported multiple cases of an important and long-term lack of variability in spontaneous speech, with no disorders in understanding or repetition. The respective authors suggest that such a disorder occurs mainly in patients whose speech depends on the interhemispheric interaction and very large bilateral representations. This is why before every commissurotomy there is a mandatory test with amobarbital. We can probably be reassured with respect to the risk of severe postoperative mutism by a favorable response to carotid amobarbital testing. This test can give ambiguous results, but it can be used to exclude critical dependence upon the commissures. That is, if the patient continues to speak intelligibly when the hemisphere minor for speech is narcotised, then the disconnection of this minor hemisphere will probably not deprive the patient of an essential resource with respect to speech production.

Except these particular cases, the callous disconnection is considered to be an intervention that does not affect speech.

However, in "split-brain" cases, there are some very subtle disorders of speech as for instance an influence on very elaborate or pragmatic speech. Zaidel (1990) shows that the most obvious pragmatic deficits appear in subjects whose right hemisphere has a rather important role in speech development. One of Zaidel's (1990) "split-brain" subjects used subtlety of speech and clinch in a pertinent manner. They were formally correct from a lexical and semantic point of view. In normal subjects, they are dependent on the right hemisphere, and are disturbed by its lesions (Hannequin et al., 1987).

Zaidel (1990) affirms that the respective functions are sensible to transcallous inhibition.

Corpus callosum and reading

In patients with verbal capacities controlled by the right hemisphere there is more conceptual and semantic information in that hemisphere compared to syntactic and phonologic information.

However, the ability of discrimination of words from a row of letters is limited, which proves that the visual shape of words is represented in the right hemisphere (Eviator and Zaidel, 1991; Reuter-Lorentz and Baynes, 1992; Baynes and Gazzaniga, 1997). The left hemisphere is dominant not only for speech but also for the possibility of deduction, interpreting of behavior and emotions and giving a rational meaning for events we are confronted with.

The interhemispheric mechanism involved in reading can be approximated due to a tachistoscopic method.

If a visual-linguistic stimulus (letter or word) is projected for a short period of time in a visual field, the stimulus at first reaches only the contralateral hemisphere. In subjects with an intact corpus callosum, the letter or words that are projected on the left side are perceived in the right hemisphere, and are immediately recognised by the left hemispheric circuits that are responsible for decoding the visual-linguistic information and transformed in oral language.

On the contrary, in "split-brain" subjects the information remains stored in the right hemisphere that has a variable decoding capacity according to individual and decoding material. However, it cannot achieve a complete processing of information. Consequently, its capacity of expressive formulation is considered to be quasi-nil and leads to an incapacity of the individual to name the respective oral stimulus (Habib, 1998).

This left hemialexia that is characteristic to the callous disconnection syndrome is thoroughly documented in literature. Sidtis et al. (1981) discuss the case of a patient with commissurotomy in the posterior half of the corpus callosum. When significant stimuli have been projected in his right hemisphere he could not name, but could describe them, a phenomenon called "bout de langue". This fact suggested that a lesion of the posterior area of the corpus callosum is responsible of the absence of perceptive characteristic transfers of the stimulus, while the anterior area is intact and capable of transferring whichever level of significant representation. On the other hand, Sergent (1987) interprets this phenomenon to be a result of an extracallous transfer through the profound subcortical structures of the brain stem.

One of the first neurologic syndromes related to an interhemispheric disconnection is the syndrome of pure alexia (Déjérine, 1892). People suffering from alexia following a lesion of the left occipital region, lesion which is frequently vascular, are incapable of understanding or reading words.

However, after a period of total alexia they can decipher the words by splitting them into syllables ("letter by letter dyslexia"). Messages coming from the right hemisphere (the only one receiving information due to a right homonymous hemianopsia) are interrupted by a lesion of the splenial fibres at the level they enter the left hemisphere, consequently to an occipital lesion, spread the forward and into depth.

Therefore, the absence of interhemispheric transfer leads to some speech disorder directly related to the dominance of the left hemisphere.

In right-handed "split-brain" patients, the deficits manifest through left tactile anomia, left lateral homonymous pseudohemianopsia, left ideomotor apraxia to verbal orders and agraphia of the left hand.

The linguistic potential of the right hemisphere in a patient with cerebral division, seems to be limited to verbal, heard or read understanding but only for certain categories of words, and his capacity of expressing himself is extremely limited, but not quite inexistent (Bogen, 1985).

The analysis of subjects with callous lesions consists of a privileged pattern for understanding the role of the right hemisphere in reading (Michel et al., 1996).

Corpus callosum and the visual-spatial aptitudes

A unilateral constructive apraxia was reported for patients with callosotomy (Bogen and Gazzaniga, 1965). A drawing made with the left hand is inaccurate but the three dimensional characteristics are conserved because of the fact that the right hemisphere is dominant in treating spatial data necessary for building three-dimensional shapes.

On the other hand, the drawing made with the right hand, although it has correct graphics, it lacks several of the spatial attributes, particularly the three-dimensional ones, making it difficult to identify it. Consequently, the right hand is apraxic because of the isolated left hemisphere that is not completely adapted for visuospatial tasks.

The location of the callous lesion that is responsible for the right constructive apraxia is not precisely known. Degas et al. (1987) and Habib (1998) assume that right hemisphere information that is necessary for the hemisphere borrow the fibres in the junction between the splenium and the trunk of the corpus callosum in order to allow the right hand to perform visual-constructive tasks.

The lesions located before this region are not accompanied by a constructive apraxia (Kazuis and Sawanda, 1993), and keeping the splenium does not involve it happening.

Somesthesis

The somatosensory system is completely crossed. Thus, an object placed in the left hand can be named because the tactile information projects to the right hemisphere, crosses to the left, and subsequently has access to the speech zones. Similarly, if a subject is blindfolded and the right hand is moulded to form a particular shape, the left hand is able to copy the shape. The tactile information goes from the right hand to the left hemisphere and then across the corpus callosum to the right hemisphere, and the left hand forms the same shape (Kolb and Whishaw, 2003).

The lack of interhemispheric transfer after hemisphere disconnection can be demonstrated with respect to somesthesis (including touch, pressure, and proprioception) in a variety of ways. The somatosensory functions of the left and right parts of the body become independent.

Consequently, unseen objects in the right hand are handled, named, and described in a normal fashion but the subjects with total callosotomy cannot do so if the object is placed in the left hand, because the sensory input is disconnected from the left (speech) hemisphere.

Thus, the most useful single sign of hemisphere disconnection is unilateral tactile anomia: this is an inability to name or describe an object when it is left by one hand whereas it is readily named (or well described if the name is unknown) when it is placed into the other hand or when it is presented either to vision or to audition.

This unilateral tactile anomia was present in every patient with complete commissurotomy studied by Gazzaniga and LeDoux (1978), McKeever et al. (1981) and Bogen (1978), despite sparing the anterior commissure. Although there are many signs of brain bisection, one of the most convincing ways to demonstrate hemisphere disconnection is to ask the patient to feel with one hand then name various small, common objects such as a button, coin, safety pin, paper clip, pencil stub, a rubber band or key. Vision must be excluded (Bogen, 1987).

The patient with a hemisphere disconnection is generally unable to name or describe an object in the left hand although he readily names objects in the right hand. Sometimes the patient will give a vague description of the object although unable to name it, but there is a contrast with the ability to name the object readily when it is placed into the right hand.

The most certain proof that the object has been identified is for the subject to retrieve it correctly from a collection of similar objects.

However, astereognosis can be reasonably excluded.

Specific posture impressed on one (unseen) hand by the examiner cannot be mimicked in the opposite hand. A convenient way to test for lack of interhemispheric transfer of proprioceptive information is as follows: the patient extends both hands beneath the opaque screen (or vision is otherwise excluded) and the examiner impresses a particular posture on one hand. For example, one can put the tip of the thumb against the tip of the little finger and have the other three fingers fully extended and separated. The split-brain patient cannot mimic with the other hand a posture being held by the first hand.

This procedure should be repeated with various postures and in both directions. After complete commissurotomy there is a partial loss of the ability to name exact points stimulated on the left side of the body.

This defect is least apparent, if at all, on the face and it is most apparent on the distal parts, especially the finger tip. This deficit is not dependent upon language; it can be shown in a nonverbal (picture identification) fashion, in which case the deficit is present in both directions (right-to-left and vice versa) (Bogen, 1987).

According to Bogen (1987), an easy way to demonstrate cross localisation of the defect is to have the subject's hand extended, palms up (with vision excluded). One touches the tip of one of the four fingers with the point of a pencil, asking the patient to then touch the same point with the tip of the thumb of the same hand. Repeating this manoeuvre many times produces a numerical score, about 100% in normal people, for either hand. In the absence of a parietal lesion, identification of any of the four finger tips by putting the thumb tip upon the particular finger can be done at nearly 100% level by the split-brain patient.

One then changes the task so that the finger tip is to be indicated, not by touching it with the thumb of the same hand, but by touching the corresponding finger tip of the other hand with the thumb of that (other) hand. Sometimes the procedure should be demonstrated with the patient's hand in full vision until the patient understands what is required. This cross localisation cannot be done by the split-brain patient at much better than chance level (25%), whereas most normal adults do better than 90%.

An incompetence to cross localize or cross match has been found in young children (Galin et al., 1979) possibly because their commissures are not yet fully functioning (Yakovlev and Lecours, 1967).

Nociceptive and thermal information is transmitted from the extra lemniscal spinothalamic system through partially bilateral paths, which are not significantly damaged by the disconnection following the callosotomy. Nevertheless, the hemispheric disconnection might be highlighted as far as the fine tactile actions are concerned, as well as in cases that need an active exploration (stereognosia, the recognition of physical characteristics of stimuli, localizing of tactile areas) (Lassonde et al., 1996).

A right handed patient with a split-brain cannot, without seeing a familiar object (spoon, fork, pencil, key, etc.) that he can touch with the left hand, but after numerous manipulations he can give hints about the nociceptive character of the tip of the scissors, the thermal aspect (cold metal), weight, and other attributes that help him identify the object. The use of these hints, called "cross-cueing" or crisscross naming, is highly common in patients with callosotomy, who try, consciously or not, to compensate their deficits (Lassonde et al., 1996).

Gazzaniga et al. (1962), Brion and Jedinak (1975) and McKeever et al. (1981) described the details of anomia, but it is important to mark the fact that a left unilateral anomia cannot be related to astereognosia, because the patient must choose a series of stimuli that he perceives with the left hand.

Neither is it aphasia because he correctly names these objects with the right hand (Barbizet and Duizabo, 1985). Consequently, a left tactile anomia is due to the fact that the sensitive information that allows the recognition of an object reaches the right hemisphere but cannot reach the speech area of the left hemisphere. A left visual anomia is due to the fact that visual information coming from the left temporal visual area reaches the right occipital region, but cannot reach the speech area located in the left hemisphere.

Finally, the patient with a divided brain cannot perform tasks that include intermanual comparison. Without seeing, he cannot reproduce with one arm or hand the specific postures of the opposite limb.

According to Bentin et al. (1984) and Gaffen et al. (1985), one of the most sensitive tests for evaluating the callous disconnection is that of crisscross tactile localisation. It consists of applying light pressure upon the extremity of the finger, outside the visual area of the patient. With the help of the thumb of the same hand, the patient indicates without difficulty which of the fingers had been stimulated. If the tests are performed separately with the fingers from the opposite hand the patient will be constantly wrong.

Audition

The auditory system is more complex than the other sensory system because it has both crossed and uncrossed connections.

A naturally occurring lesion near the callosal trunk can result in the suppression of one ear when tested dichotically. Hence, one might accept similar changes after a section of the callosal trunk. However, several authors showed the place of the callosal transfer of audible information.

Springer and Gazzaniga (1975) were the first to report a left dichotic extinction in a case of a parietal callosotomy in which the splenium had been preserved. Musier and Reeves (1986) noticed that complete callosotomies lead to an alteration of performance of the left ear when undergoing dichotic tests. This fact explains the disruption of transfer for verbal information that was initially received from the left ear / right hemisphere.

On the other hand, the two ears have a deficit in tests of pattern recognition for sound frequency. This suggests that the test needs both hemispheres (Habib, 1998).

However, the performance of subjects with an anterior callosotomy are very variable, therefore the conclusion that pertinent fibres for audible information transfer are located in the posterior half of the commissurotomy. This fact had been confirmed in some cases with spontaneous parietal lesions of the corpus callosum (Damasio et al., 1980; Degas et al., 1987; Habib et al., 1990).

According to Damasio et al. (1980) and Degas et al. (1987), the splenial lesion had been accompanied by an alteration of the dichotic hearing test. This fact suggests that the passage of pertinent intertemporal fibres for audible transfer is located in the splenium.

Alexander and Warren (1988) came to the conclusion that the interhemispheric passage of audible information is located near the somatosensorial information from the posterior area of the trunk, i.e., the isthmus. Damasio and Damasio (1979), Poncet et al. (1987) point out that in order to finish the extinction of the left ear it is necessary for the callous fibres to be touched in general in the interior of the left hemisphere and not at the level of the corpus callosum itself.

This "paradoxical extinction" of the left ear accompanied by a moderate aphasia became the classic sign of a lesion of the profound white matter in the left hemisphere, similar to the sensitive differentiation or ideomotor apraxia to which it is associated (Poncet et al., 1987).

Therefore, the audible attributes are bilateral, but each sound stimulus is analysed by both hemispheres due to the interhemispheric transfer through the corpus callosum. Because the contralateral tracts are more important due to the number of fibres they contain, they are dominant over the information directed through the ipsilateral tracts. Nevertheless, the patient with a split-brain can report with no difficulty the verbal or nonverbal stimuli that are present in one ear only.

However, the verbal stimuli perceived by the right ear are analysed mainly by the left temporal region (linguistic). Due to the fact that the right hemisphere is responsible for musicality, the musical material is analysed with less difficulty in the left ear, from where it is massively directed towards the right temporal area. However, after a cerebral commissurotomy, the patient readily identifies single words (and other sounds) if they are presented to one ear at a time.

But if different words are presented to the two ears simultaneously ("dichotic listening"), only the words presented to the right ear will be reliably reported (Milner et al., 1968; Sparks and Geschwind, 1968; Efron et al., 1977). Therefore, words played into the left ear can travel directly to the hemisphere or can go to the right hemisphere and then to the left through the corpus callosum. However, the direct access does not appear to exist when the hemispheres are disconnected.

This large advantage of the right ear is usually considered the result of two concurrent circumstances: (a) the ipsilateral pathway (from the left ear to the left hemisphere) is suppressed by the presence of simultaneous but differing inputs, as it is in intact individuals during dichotic listening (Kimura, 1967; Teng, 1981). (b) the contralateral pathway from the left ear to the right hemisphere has now been severed and conveys information that ordinarily reaches the left (speaking) hemisphere by the callosal pathway. Although left ear words are rarely reported, their perception by the right hemisphere is occasionally evidenced by appropriate actions of the left ear (Gordon, 1973).

Contralateral ear suppression commonly appears after hemispherectomy or the creation of another large hemispheric lesion. Because there is usually suppressed by left hemisphere lesions, the suppression of the left ear by a left hemisphere lesion has been called "paradoxical ipsilateral extinction". Further observations have led to the conclusion that, whether the lesion is in the left or the right hemisphere, or if it is close to the midline, the suppression of left ear stimuli is probably attributable to an interruption of interhemispheric pathways (Sparks et al., 1970; Michel and Peronnet, 1975; Damasio and Damasio, 1979).

In any case, the auditory effects are unlikely to be of clinical importance, although one can anticipate certain patients in whom slight auditory alterations might be quite important.

Olfaction

The olfactory tract is not essentially crisscrossed. The interhemispheric communication between the cortical areas responsible for the olfactory analysis is ensured rather through the anterior commissure, than thorough the corpus callosum.

According to Bouchet and Cuilleret (1983), areas 23 and 24 of the anterior and posterior region of the cingular circumvolution could be responsible for olfaction. Their interhemispheric communication fibres transit, at least in monkeys, through the dorsal facet of the corpus callosum.

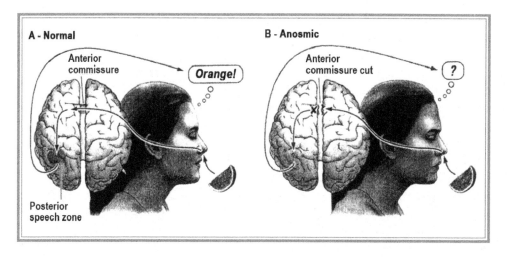

Fig. 20.9. Anosmia. (A) In the normal condition, olfactory input to the right nostril transvers directly back into the right hemisphere and crosses the anterior commissure, thus gaining access to the left (speech) hemisphere. (B) Anosmia results from section of the anterior commissure. (The jagged line indicates the lesion.) When the pathway is severed., the information is blocked, and the left hemisphere has no way of knowing what odor the right hemisphere perceived. (after Kolb and Whishaw, 2003).

In humans no such fact could be confirmed. Therefore, there are no symptoms of disconnection shown for this sensorial attribute, other than patients whose commissurotomy included the anterior commissure (Risse et al., 1978). These patients could not perceive smell presented in the right nostril with their right hemisphere to which it was transmitted. Right anosmia does not hinder the left hand to find the object that produces the sensation in a collection of stimuli (Gazzaniga et al., 1975). However, if smell perceived by the right nostril is unpleasant, the subject may be disgusted, but cannot verbally express the feeling (Gordon and Sperry, 1968).

A patient whose anterior commissure is severed cannot name odour presented to the right nostril because the speaking left hemisphere is disconnected from the information. The right hemisphere has the information but has no control of speech (Fig. 20.9) (Kolb and Whishaw, 2003).

Thus, unlike all the other senses the olfactory system is not crossed. Input from the left nostril goes straight back to the left hemisphere, and input from the right nostril goes to the right hemisphere. Fibres travelling through the anterior commissure join the olfactory regions in each hemisphere, just as fibres travelling thorough the corpus callosum join the motor cortex of each hemisphere (Kolb and Whishaw, 2003).

The transfer of motor information

Movement

Observations by Akelaitis (1943) about the first patients with surgical callosotomies show an extraordinary discretion of the neuropsychological changes induced by callous sections.

The most obvious change consists of the impossibility to perform two simultaneous actions with each hand (Gazzaniga et al., 1967).

In fact, the most certain functional correlation in matter of the topographic anatomy of the corpus callosum refers to the existence of important difficulties in bimanual coordination consequent to sectioning the anterior half of the callous commissure.

Zaidel and Sperry (1977) observed that in 5-10 years after surgery an important quantitative and qualitative alteration of bimanual coordination still persists during tasks that involve either a rapid alternative movement of both hands, or a complex bimanual coordination.

Kreuter et al. (1972) also demonstrated that during the synchronised or alternant bimanual tapping test, the "split-brain" subjects cannot perform the task unless they significantly slow down the rhythm of motor act.

Preilowski (1990), who studied the role of commissural fibres in bimanual coordinated movements, believes one needs an unharmed anterior area of the corpus callosum in order to complete these actions.

The information coming from a hemisphere needs to be transferred to the contralateral hemisphere as an interhemispheric exchange of "motor corollary discharges". This role normally belongs to the premotor frontal cortex or more specifically to the supplementary motor area (SMA) or the medial premotor system (Goldberg, 1985).

Through the genu of the corpus callosum, in the anterior area of the body, the SMA is richly connected to the contralateral SMA as well as to the primary motor area. The connections between the two motor and premotor systems of the corpus callosum are crucial for performing coordinate actions with the two superior limbs.

However, a total callous section alters the synchronisation of the two hands more severely than an anterior section. This fact suggests the partially compensatory role of regions located more posterior which transmit proprioceptive information through the presplenial region (Ellenberg and Sperry, 1979).

If a hand performs rapid alternative movements of pronation-supination one can notice, particularly in children, the natural tendency of performing mirror movements with the other hand (Njiokiktjien et al., 1986) when the subject is involved in a bimanual activity. This tendency is found in subjects with callous agenesis, but is more severe. Dennis (1976) supposes that this tendency of performing mirror gestures generally means the callous transfer systems are immature.

Here, the corpus callosum has an inhibitory action that suppresses mirror involuntary movements which disturb the coordinated bimanual movements.

For Dennis (1976), these inhibitory systems borrow the posterior region of the corpus callosum. The callous connections may also play an important role in some motor activities such as moving a hand during learning a particular motor action (Habib, 1998).

Therefore, patients with callosotomy present many disorders of interhemispheric disconnections when a monomanual answer is expected. Thus, in right-handed patients, writing with the left hand results in a unilateral left agraphia which is characterised by drawing illegible letters of the alphabet, paragraphia, and the impossibility of copying words if not written in printed form.

These symptoms presented by the left hand (in right-handed patients) are consequent to the fact that the right hemisphere is essentially aphasic, while writing with the right hand (which depends on the left hemisphere) is normal. In the preoperatory phase a unilateral left ideomotric apraxia appears, but only for verbal orders (Lassonde et al., 1996).

However, according to Kolb and Whishaw (2003), because the motor system is largely crossed, we might predict that the disconnection of the hemispheres will induce a form of apraxia and agraphia, because the left hand would not receive instructions from the left hemisphere. These disabilities would not be seen in the right hand because it has access to the speech hemisphere.

So, if a patient was asked to use the right hand to copy a geometric design, it might be impaired (**acopia**) because it is disconnected from the right hemisphere, which ordinarily has a preferred role in rendering.

Preilowski (1975) and later Zaidel and Sperry (1977) stated that the severity of the deficit declines significantly with the passage of time after surgery, possibly because the left hemisphere's ipsilateral control of movements is being used.

A second situation that might produce severe motor deficits in commissurotomy patients is one in which the two arms must be used in cooperation.

Thus, patients were severely impaired at alternating tapping movements of the index finger.

A high degree of manual cooperation is required to trace a diagonal line smoothly. If the hemispheres have been disconnected, the cooperation is severely retarded, because the left and right motor systems cannot gain information about what the opposite side is doing, except indirectly by the patient's watching them.

Dramatic illustrations of conflict between hands abound (Kolb and Whishaw, 2003).

It is of interest to note that while inhibiting these episodes of intermanual conflict were able to use their left hands in a purposeful and cooperative manner when "not thinking of what they were doing (Preilowski, 1975).

Praxic and graphometric activities

When there is a major disconnection between the two hemispheres, the language-linked dominant hemisphere agent that maintains its primary control over the contralateral dominant limb effectively loses its direct and linked control over the separate "agent" based in the nondominant hemisphere (and, thus, the nondominant limb), which had been previously responsive and "obedient" to the dominant agent. The possibility of purposeful action in the nondominant limb occurring outside the realm of influence of the dominant agent thus can occur (Goldberg and Goodwin, 2011).

Disturbing some general activities that reach only the left hemi-body following surgical or spontaneous disconnection represents the most obvious test for specific praxic functions in the left hemisphere. The locations of two lesions are capable of inducing it. One affects the genu of the corpus callosum, probably through the disconnection of fibres that interconnect the premotor areas (Geschwind and Kaplan, 1962) and another located in the posterior, at the level of the callous isthmus, engrams through the disconnection of the left hemispheric motor (Heilman, 1979).

Therefore, one can distinguish two types of callous agraphies of the left hand: one related to the disruption of premotor fibres from the anterior area of the corpus callosum, characterised not only by affecting the handwriting but also the capacity of typewriting or the use of letters on a mobile phone with the left hand.

The other one is related to the presplenial lesion which disconnects the left angular gyrus and affects only handwriting.

Thus, the left hemisphere, which lacks the spatial support of the right hemisphere, becomes apraxo-agnosic. The drawing or copying of a drawing which had been well executed with the right hand before surgery becomes unrecognisable after operation. The left hand may however reproduce the drawing. In this case, Bogen and Gazzaniga (1965) speak about a constructive apraxia, and Preilowski (1975) and Zaidel and Sperry (1977) speak about a dysfunction of the ability of bimanual motor coordination. The situation becomes more dramatic when a task must be performed without seeing.

According to Watson and Heilman (1983), at the level of the left hemisphere, in right handed people, there are two types of programs or engrams: a verbal-motor one, that controls the linguistic nature of the written message, and another one named video-kinaesthetic, that controls the graphic aspects that allow a spatial-temporal structure.

Finally, Sugishita et al. (1980) and Gersh and Damasio (1981) insist upon the dissociated character of callous apraxia and agraphia. Degas et al. (1987) consider that a lesion of the splenium, and of the posterior fourth of the body of the corpus callosum, provoked agraphia without left apraxia.

Kazuis and Sawada (1993) had a patient with a lesion located in the posterior half of the body of the corpus callosum leaving the juxta-splenial area of the isthmus intact. They observed this patient showed left apraxia without agraphia.

These data show that the interhemispheric fibres that allow the transfer of graphic information from the left to the right hemisphere are located in the posterior area of the body of the corpus callosum and those that control the gestures of the left hand are located in its anterior region.

Thus, if a lesion of the corpus callosum disconnects the left hand from the left hemisphere, that hand is unable to respond to verbal commands and is considered apraxic.

Suppose, however, that the right hand is unable to respond to verbal commands. Geschwind (1965) speculated that this deficit results from a lesion in the left hemisphere that disconnects its motor cortex (which controls the right hand) from the speech zone (Fig. 20.10). Thus, the right hand cannot respond to verbal commands and is considered apraxic.

Although Geschwind's model can explain bilateral apraxia in some patients, it must be emphasized that disconnection is not the only cause of apraxia. Because the posterior cortex has direct access to the subcortical neural mechanisms of arm and body movements, parietal input need not go through the motor cortex, except for the control of finger movements. Further, patients with sections of the corpus callosum are initially apraxic but show substantial recovery despite a disconnection of the motor cortex of the left and right hemisphere.

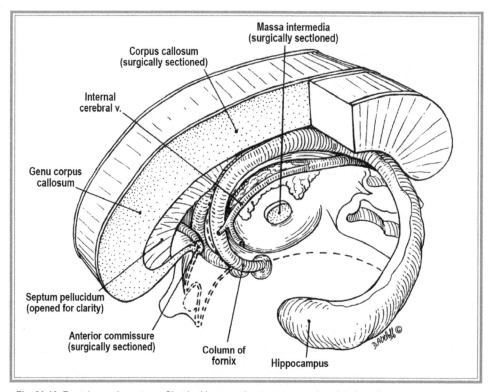

Fig. 20.10. Frontal commissurotomy: Sketched here are the structures sectioned during a frontal commissurotomy. This includes most of the corpus callosum (sparing the splenium), the ventral hippocampal commissure (between the fornices), and the anterior commissure (after Bogen, 1987).

A diagnosed apraxia is a rare manifestation, but a more spectacular one of this intercortical disconnection (Brion and Jedynak, 1975; Poncet, 1983; Bogen, 1985). The cited example is of a female patient who was struggling to button her shirt with the right hand, while she was doing the opposite with the left one.

This complex, variable behavior showed that what appears to be the effect of the callous lesion is due to a self and contradictory activity of the right hemisphere that is freed by the control of the left hemisphere which is normally dominant.

Tanaka et al. (1996) compared through MRI the callous lesions of three patients suffering from this syndrome and noticed that the diagnosed dyspraxia appears after a lesion that specifically affects the most posterior area of the callous body, which passes through a region of fibres that unite the left and right superior parietal areas.

Authors came to the conclusion that a diagnosed apraxia is due to the disconnection between the superior left parietal lobe, which is dominant for voluntary control of movement, and the right hemisphere, which controls the movements of the left hand. Even though it is tempting, this hypothesis has not yet been confirmed (Habib, 1998). Consequently, a diagnosed apraxia is a complex behavior in which the left hand or even the assembly of the left hemi-body performs elaborate actions which come against the free will of the patient.

Agnosia and alexia

Geschwind (1965) theorized that agnosia and alexia can disconnect the posterior speech area from the visual association cortex. Both symptoms can be produced by a lesion that disconnects the visual association region on the left from the speech zone or by a lesion that disconnects the right visual association cortex from the speech zone by damaging the corpus callosum. Thus, the patient, although able to talk, is unable to identify words or objects, because the visual information is disconnected from the posterior speech zone in the left hemisphere (Kolb and Whishaw, 2003).

Transfer of complex asymmetrically organized information

What best differentiates the human brain from that of other mammals is mainly its asymmetrical way of functioning. Diverse functions known as cognitive functions mainly depend on either one or the other hemisphere. A lesion of the corpus callosum may disrupt the access of a certain function of the so called "minor" hemisphere to the contralateral hemisphere which is able to better or even exclusively treat the given information.

Unilateral apraxia

In 1907, Liepmann and Maas described a patient with a right hemiparesis from a lesion of the pons. The patient also had a lesion of the corpus callosum. This patient was unable to correctly pantomime to command with his left arm. Because he had a right hemiparesis, his right hand could not be tested.

Since the work of Broca, it has been known that right-handers' left hemisphere is dominant for language. Liepmann and Maas could have attributed their patient's inability to pantomime to a disconnection between language and motor areas so that the left hemisphere that mediates comprehension of verbal commands could not influence the right hemisphere's motor areas that are responsible for controlling the left hand.

However, this patient also could not initiate gestures or correctly use actual tools or objects, therefore, a language-motor disconnection could not account for these findings. Liepmann and Maas posited that the left hemisphere of right-handers contains movement formulas and that the callosal lesion in this patient disconnected these movement formulas from the right hemisphere's motor areas.

Geschwind and Kaplan in 1962, Geschwind in 1965, and Gazzaniga et al. (1967) also found that their patients with callosal disconnection could not correctly pantomime to command with the left hand. Unlike the patient reported by Liepmann and Maas, however, their patients could imitate and correctly use actual tools and objects with the left hand. The preserved ability to imitate and use actual tools and objects suggests that the inability to gesture to command in these patients with callosal lesions was induced by a language-motor disconnection rather than a movement formula-motor disconnection.

In addition, a disconnection between the movement formula and motor areas should produce spatial and temporal errors, but many of the errors made by Liepmann and Maas' patient appeared to be content errors. In 1983, Watson and Heilman described a patient with an infarction limited to the body of the corpus callosum. Their patient had no weakness in her right hand and performed all tasks flawlessly with her right hand. With her left hand, however, she could not correctly pantomime to command, imitate, or use actual tools. Immediately after her cerebral infarction she made some content errors, but later on, she made primarily spatial and temporal errors.

Her performance indicated that not only language but also movement representations were stored in her left hemisphere and that her callosal lesion disconnected these movement formulas from the right hemisphere.

Thus, left limb dispraxia can be attributed to the simultaneous presence of two deficits: poor comprehension by the right hemisphere (which has good control over the left hand) and poor ipsilateral control by the left hemisphere (which understands the commands).

Failure to correctly position a limb, to move the limb correctly in space, and to properly orient the limb is called **ideomotor apraxia**. Apraxia has been subclassified into ideational apraxia, and limb-kinetic apraxia (Liepmann, 1900).

Ideational apraxia is a loss of the conception of a gesture or skilled movement. In this form, the patient does not seem to know what to do, and the motor activity is not facilitated by the use of actual objects.

Ideomotor apraxia affects the implementation of movement, producing spatial and timing errors. The patient seems to know what to do but cannot carry movement out properly.

Limb-kinetic apraxia refers to clumsiness, awkwardness of a limb in the performance of a skilled act that cannot be accounted for by paresis, ataxia, or sensory loss. This apraxia manifested by the inability to make finely graded, precise limb movements.

Apraxia may be differentiated by the body elements involved in the impaired movement, using the term limb apraxia, oral or buccofacial apraxia, trunk or axial apraxia.

The terms dressing apraxia and **constructional apraxia** are sometimes used to describe certain symptoms of unilateral extinction or neglect (amorphosynthesis) that characterize partial lobe lesions.

These patients also make temporal errors and may fail to correctly imitate movements, but some patients imitate worse than they gesture in response to command.

In right-handed individuals, ideomotor apraxia is almost always associated with left hemisphere lesions, but in left-handers, ideomotor apraxia is usually associated with right hemisphere lesions. Ideomotor apraxia is associated with lesions in a variety of structures, including the corpus callosum, the inferior parietal lobe, and the premotor areas.

Ideomotor apraxia has also been reported with subcortical lesions that involve the basal ganglia and white matter.

Alien hand syndrome. Symptoms: anarchic hand, callosal apraxia, diagnostic dyspraxia, Dr. Strangelove syndrome, intermanual conflict, magnetic apraxia, wayward hand.

Alien hand syndrome is a relatively rare manifestation of damage to specific brain regions involved in voluntary movement (Goldberg and Goodwin, 2011). The core observation is the patient's report that one of his / her hand is displaying purposeful, coordinated, and goal-directed behavior over which the patient feels he / she has no voluntary control. The hand seems to possess the capability of acting autonomously, independent of their conscious voluntary control.

The patient fails to recognize the action of one of his hands as his own. The hand, effectively, appears to manifest a "will of its own" (Goldberg and Goodwin, 2011).

This definition excludes disordered, non-purposeful, and dyskinetic movements associated with other involuntary movement disorders.

Three forms of alien hand syndrome have been described: frontal, callosal, and posterior.

The frontal form is associated with damage to the medial surface of the cerebral hemisphere in the frontal region. The frontal variant involves the medial aspect of the premotor cortex anterior to the primary motor cortex including the supplementary motor area and anterior cingulate cortex. Generally, these alien behaviours appear in the hand contralateral to the damaged hemisphere regardless of hemispheric dominance.

The posterior or "sensory" form appears most often with a parietal or parieto-occipital focus of circumscribed damage (Pack et al., 2002). As in the frontal variant, the alien behavior appears in the hand contralateral to the damaged hemisphere. The movement of the affected alien limb is typically less organized and often has an ataxic instability particularly with visually guided reaching. The limb may also show pro-prioceptive sensory impairments with hypaesthesia, so that the kinaesthetic impairment limits the monitoring of limb position. Visual field deficits as well as hemi-inattention may be seen on the same side as the alien hand (Goldberg and Goodwin, 2011).

Alien hand behavior has also been reported in association with a subcortical thalamic infarction.

The fMRI study of cortical activation patterns associated with alien and non-alien movement has demonstrated that alien movement is in fact characterized by the isolated activation of the primary motor cortex in concert with the activation of interhemispheric premotor regions (Assal et al., 2007).

The callosal form is seen with an isolated lesion of the corpus callosum.

The voluntary motor systems of the two hemispheres are isolated from each other due to lost interhemispheric communication following callosotomy.

In the "callosal" variant of alien hand syndrome, the appearance of "intermanual conflict" or "self-oppositional" behaviours is the predominant feature (Goldberg and Goodwin, 2011). In the callosal variant, the problematic alien hand is consistently the nondominant hand, while the dominant hand is the identified "good", controlled hand. The patient may express frustration and bewilderment at the conflicting and disruptive behavior of the alien hand whose motivations remain inaccessible to consciousness (Goldberg and Goodwin, 2011).

There may be an attentional component that modulates the appearance of these episodes of self-oppositional behavior since intermanual conflict is observed more frequently when the patient is fatigued, stressed, or is engaged in effortful multitasking activity.

Occasionally, the two hands are observed to be engaged in two different and entirely unrelated activities as if being guided by completely separate and independent intentions (Goldberg and Goodwin, 2011).

The callosal and frontal variants are often seen in combination with a corresponding overlap of observed behavior. However, a clear differentiation between an apparent intermanual conflict due to attempts to restrain alien behaviours associated with the frontal variant, and a true intermanual conflict, in which the two hands are directed towards an independently contradictory purpose, may be difficult to make (Biran and Chatterjee, 2004).

The patient may become fearful that they will be held accountable for consequences of an action of the alien hand over which they do not feel control (Giovannetti et al., 2005).

The patient may display "auto-criticism" complaining that the alien hand is not doing what it has been "told to do" and is therefore characterized as disobedient, wayward, or "evil". Given the predicament created, the patients may develop depersonalization and dissociate themselves from the unintended actions of the hand (Biran and Chatterjee, 2004; Giovannetti et al., 2005; Assal et al., 2007; Sumner and Husain, 2008; Goldberg and Goodwin, 2011).

In alien hand syndrome, different regions of the brain are able to command purposeful limb movements, without generating conscious feeling or self-control over these movements. This process, impaired in alien hand syndrome, normally produces the conscious sensation that movement is being internally initiated and produced by an active self (Frith et al., 2000; Scepkowski and Cronin-Golomb, 2003; Sumner and Husain, 2008).

However, an evaluation of callosal apraxia and impairment of interhemispheric transfer of information should be included. There is no definitive treatment for the alien syndrome but a number of different rehabilitative approaches have been described.

Corpus callosum and memory

Changes in mnemonic capacity after callosotomy are due to lesions of the discrete processing capacities in the isolated hemispheres.

Loss of general memory capacity as measured by standardised tests has been reported for same patients (Zaidel and Sperry, 1974; Zaidel, 1990). Clark and Geffen (1989) suggested that discrepancies in memory function reported after callosotomy might be due to the involvement of the hippocampal commissure.

Phelps et al. (1991) observed a decrease in verbal and visual recall following a posterior callosal section, which may damage the hippocampal commissure, but preserved or even improved memory after an anterior callosal section. Recognition memory was relatively intact in both groups.

The left hemisphere appears to make greater use of general knowledge schemas to explain perceptions and experiences and to use them to "interpret" events, than does the right hemisphere, and this predilection has an impact on the accuracy of memory (Gazzaniga, 1985; Phelps and Gazzaniga, 1992). A left hemisphere "interpreter" constructs theories to assimilate perceived information into a comprehensible whole. By doing so, however, the elaborative processing involved has a deleterious effect on the accuracy of perceptual recognition.

This result extended to include verbal material (Metcalfe et al., 1995).

However, this predilection has an important role in memory accuracy (Baynes and Gazzaniga, 1997). Thus, the left hemisphere interprets the theoretical constructions by assimilating information in a comprehensible whole with the help of verbal material.

Corpus callosum and attention

The cerebral substrate of attention mechanisms as well as that of other cognitive functions is now considered to be overlapping an assembly of interconnected neurons that are organized in a distributive network. Part of it is functionally lateralized in the right hemisphere of the human brain (Mesulam, 1990). Several authors proved that the corpus callosum does not possess a primary role in the distribution of attention resources in the two hemispheres; therefore it acts as a regulator that is capable to distribute cognitive energy to each hemisphere according to the existence of each situation and task.

According to Levy (1974), the regulation of the awakening function and its distribution between hemispheres depends on the reciprocal inhibition from the level of the brain stem and the reciprocal facilitation in the corpus callosum.

In "split-brain" subjects, there were reports about certain attention disorders both during general awakening (Diamond et al., 1977) and during the distribution of attention in the outside space of the body (Ellenberg and Sperry, 1979).

In Kinsbourne's model, the regulation of attention involves the existence of an interaction between the controlled activity of one hemisphere by mesencephalic structures and the reciprocal inhibiting or facilitating relation achieved through the corpus callosum (Kinsbourne, 1970 and 1973). Each hemisphere controls the attention from the contralateral perceptive area and the activity balance between hemispheres appears to be a result of the interaction between the activity of the mesencephalic systems and the inhibition / facilitation game with the callous fibres (Habib, 1998).

According to this model, the most competent hemisphere in a certain task increases its level of activity in a specific manner, while the opposite hemisphere decreases it. Therefore, the role played by the corpus callosum is essential in ensuring the modulation of equilibrium depending not only on the cognitive attributes of the task, but also on non-specific factors such as motivation, the difficulty of the task or a voluntary attention path. A particular case is the one of two competing tasks. In this situation, the capacity of the receptor hemisphere for one task can be rather active than inhibited, which depends on the attributes of the competing task (Kinsbourne, 1973). This reveals the attention control through hemisphere interaction.

In subjects with a commissurotomy, the observed symptoms are interpreted by Kinsbourne not as an interruption of a path that allows passage of information, but as the inactive hemisphere being incapable of ensuring the treatment of information that it is less specialized for.

A similar explanation is given by Mayer et al. (1988) in a subject with a spontaneous callous lesion who presented an extinction of the left hand in the task of dichaptic palpation. However, with the help of sight the authors managed to attract the patient's attention to the left hand.

Concerning this tactile-kinaesthetic model, scientists came to the conclusion that attracting attention towards the tactile recognition of the left hand by changing the procedure suggests the special role played by the corpus callosum in the attention mechanisms.

Corpus callosum and the emotional function

Amongst the cerebral functions that are asymmetrically organized, the emotional functions are, without doubt, the ones with a very uncertain anatomical substrate. Neuropsychologists admit that the right hemisphere is specialized in the treatment of emotional information, both at a perceptive level and at an expressive level. In case of a lesion of the right hemisphere, revealing emotional control disorders (anosodiaphoria, anosognosia, hemiasomatognosia, affective indifference) and disorders of the prosody of speech, represent two more valid examples.

On an intact brain it is difficult to measure the importance of the corpus callosum in the support mechanisms of these functions. In patients with commissurotomy, Sperry et al. (1979) presented emotional stimuli to the right hemisphere of "split-brain" subjects. They noticed that the "affective aura", meaning the poorly defined feeling of an affective event immediately goes to the left hemisphere, through subcallous connections that unite the limbic structures, the place where the emotional experience is probably built. The only role in this field presently given to the corpus callosum is that of allowing an individual who has an affective stimulus with characteristics best analysed by the right hemisphere, to give a cognitive judgment and a verbal meaning to the stimulus.

Hoppe and Bogen (1977) and then Ten Houten et al. (1986) suggested applying the concept of alexithymia (characterizing some difficulties in verbalizing emotions presented to psychosomatic patients) to subjects with commissurotomy. The degree of ease or difficulty the subject encounters in the verbal test of expressing emotion as well as expressing the richness or purpose of his fantastic world are highly discriminative between normal subjects and "split-brain" subjects. This fact suggests how a high degree of alexithymia appears after a callous section and the important role of the corpus callosum in the respective transfer of information.

The interhemispheric transfer of elaborate behavior

In this model of connectivity for premotor systems, Goldberg (1985) suggests that each of the two median premotor systems (SMA and the neighbouring cortex), have, among other functions, the role of volitional control of movements in the opposite hemibody.

In lesions of the median facet of the frontal lobe, which also simultaneously involve the SMA and the callous fibres, the author often observed an unusual behavior of the hemi-body that is opposite to the lesion, in which the superior limb has the tendency of performing movements without voluntary control of the subject.

Thus, most often appear movements of attraction to a certain visual target with the purpose of grabbing the objects that are close. Goldberg associates this behavior to an excessive addiction of the motor cortex to the environment, because the motor cortex is freed of the premotor median cortical control and left under the influence of only the lateral system (its role is to control movements oriented as a response to stimuli from the environment).

Goldberg calls this "foreign hand sign" behavior, which is often misinterpreted.

This is why Poncet et al. (1987) replaces the term with "stubborn hand". This symptom must be differentiated from the motor behavior observed after a callous lesion, which is called apraxia.

In practice, it is important to make a difference between the stubborn hand sign and the apraxia. The first is related to a double lesion, both median frontal and callous, which affects the hand opposite to the harmed frontal lobe, and the latter appears only after a callous lesion that affects exclusively the superior left limb (Habib, 1998).

The median fusion

The median fusion is the process that ensures the continuity of the proprio- and exteroceptive space, beyond the median line (Lassonde et al., 1996). Thus, the stimuli of a hemi-body or a hemi-visual field stimulate the neurons in one hemisphere, and after passing through the median line they also stimulate the ones in the opposite hemisphere, without recording any discontinuity, because the second hemisphere had already been prepared to receive this information through the corpus callosum (Guillemot et al., 1987, 1988). Most callous connections of the motor and sensitive cortical regions from the anterior area of the corpus callosum are designed, from a functional point of view, for the median line of the corpus (the trunk) and to a smaller extend they are designed for the proximal regions of the limbs (Manzoni et al., 1980; McKenna et al., 1981; Pandya and Seltzer, 1986; Innocenti, 1986; Lepore et al., 1986; Guillemot et al., 1988).

Exploring the somato-sensorial sensitivity thresholds through the discrimination test for two points, shows that the thresholds are indeed higher for the axial corporal region (trunk) both in subjects with no corpus callosum and in those with callosotomy. In the case of visual testing, the receptor fields of the callous neurons are found near the vertical meridian, which they reach and sometimes cross (Berlucchi, 1972, 1983; Lepore et al., 1983).

Subjects with no corpus callosum are incapable of evaluating the distance between stimuli if they must use the parallax movement index in their central vision (Rivest et al., 1996). It even seems that cells from the primary additive cortex that are tight to the corpus callosum functionally correspond to the omnidirectional cells involved in the analysis of sound in the central area of the hearing field or in the perception of sounds presented in front of the subject (Imig et al., 1986).

In tests of indicating the location of fixed sound and in those that simulate movement, the results showed an inferior performance of subjects with no corpus callosum compared to the witnesses, both for sounds transmitted for the pericentral region and for sounds transmitted for the lateral region. These data do not seem to support the hypothesis of a privileged relation of the corpus callosum with the median line (Poirier et al., 1993). Consequently, the entire pathology of the callous system should affect the median fusion process because it is certain that the corpus callosum participates in the making of this median fusion.

However, participation is more important for the systems that are certainly contra-lateralized (visual, and lemniscal somatosensorial (Lepore et al., 1994; Lassonde et al., 1996).

Interhemispheric transfer time

The interhemispheric transfer time, which is tributary to the integrity of the callous commissure, is prolonged (30 – 87 milliseconds) (Sergent and Myers, 1985; Di Stefano et al., 1992), in people with commissurotomy compared to normal subjects (2 milliseconds) (Berlucchi et al., 1977; Berlucchi, 1990).

A longer reaction period of 12.7 to 50.5 milliseconds had also been noticed with the help of simple tests of video-motor reaction in persons with no corpus callosum (Milner and Lines, 1982; Rugg et al., 1984).

Syndromes after callosotomy

Frontal commissurotomy

By "frontal commissurotomy", Gordon et al. (1971) refer to a section of the anterior two-thirds of the corpus callosum together with the anterior commissurotomy. A section of the anterior commissure was done under direct vision and the third ventricle was entered between the two fornices so the section also included the ventral hippocampal commissure (Fig. 20.10). The same operation was used on a few occasions by Wilson et al. (1977).

Because these patients had retraction within the third ventricle to allow section of the anterior commissure under direct vision, mutism in cases with more extensive sections was not likely of third ventricular origin (Bogen, 1987). All of these patients had retraction of the medial aspect of the right frontal lobe, comparable with that in the complete cases: therefore the retraction on the supplementary motor cortex does not seem to be a sufficient explanation for mutism after callosotomy (Bogen, 1987).

In the long term, Preilowski (1972) could show some deficits of motor coordination in two patients with frontal commissurotomy. But exhaustive testing for usual disconnection deficits has shown that, with retention of splenium, such deficits should not be expected (Gordon et al., 1971; Gazzaniga et al., 1975; Greenblatt et al., 1980; Bogen et al., 1981).

The patient of Geschwind and Kaplan (1962) that presented on operated left frontal glioma and an accidental lesion of the anterior cerebral artery, was writing normally with the right hand according to dictation, but had an aphasic behavior of the left hand. This patient could not recognize the objects he was holding with the left hand, although he could do it with the same hand put in front of a group of objects. The authors imagined a lesion of the corpus callosum (confirmed by autopsy) that did not affect the splenium, but led to an interruption of the callous tract between the motor centres in the right hemisphere which controls the left hand and the speech areas located near the left hemisphere.

Gersh and Damasio (1981) reported cases of people with apraxia but no agraphia of the left hand that followed the sectioning of the anterior region of the trunk in the corpus callosum. The authors came to the conclusion that praxic impulses use fronto-frontal tracts, thus the apraxia, but no agraphia of the left hand, appear when the section affects exclusively the anterior area of the trunk in the corpus callosum.

Risse et al. (1989) noticed that the sectioning of the two-thirds located in the anterior area of the corpus callosum leads to small or no changes. Here an example (Fig. 20.11).

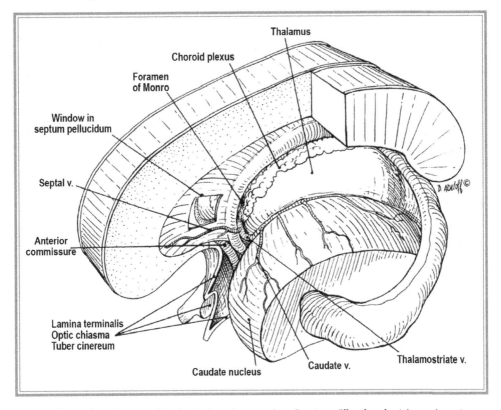

Fig. 20.11. Anterior callosotomy. This sketch shows how anterior callosotomy differs from frontal commissurotomy. There are two principal differences: the anterior commissure is spared, and third ventricle is not entered by separating the fornices (after Bogen, 1987).

In the case of a larger anterior section there appears a disruption of the ability to transfer sensorial and position information from one hand to the other. On the contrary, a section of the splenium disrupts the transfer of visual information between hemispheres and isolates the lateral visual inputs.

Thus, a section of the corpus callosum that spares the splenium (as well as the anterior commissure) but is otherwise complete can be readily accomplished *via* an exposure anterior to the rolandic bridging vein (Bogen, 1987). This procedure which avoids entry into the third ventricle has come to be the most popular version of commissural section for epilepsy or tumors. After this operation one does not observe most of the acute disconnection syndrome. This smoother postoperative course is not surprising because the acute disconnection syndrome does not usually occur after frontal commissurotomy, which is essentially the same procedure plus a section of the anterior commissure and massa intermedia.

Absence of significant mutism with callosotomy sparing the splenium has been reported by Rayport et al. (1985) and Bogen (1987).

Ross et al. (1984) reported transient (1- to 10- day) mutism with this procedure. This difference could depend upon the amount of retraction particularly if there has been a retraction of the left hemisphere below the falx as well as the usual right hemisphere retraction. Even a lesser callosal section may be followed by mutism when it is associated with a concurrent thalamic lesion (Bogen, 1987).

Midcallosal section

A midcallosal section is an incision through the trunk sparing not only the splenium but also most of the genu. Such an incision affords ready access to the foramina of Monro with practically no obligatory physiological cost as presently assessable (Gordon et al., 1971; Ozgur et al., 1977; Shucart and Stein, 1978; Winston et al., 1979; Long and Leibrock, 1980; Antunes et al., 1980; Apuzzo et al., 1982). I operated on 115 cases of tumors of the third ventricle. The clinical picture was dominated by the signs of intracranial hypertension. Neuropsychological signs (40%) were sometimes under-estimated, revealing the disease in only 17% of cases. Ophthalmologic signs and endocrine disorders have been found in 32% of these cases. In planning the surgical approach, we took into account the localization and size of the tumors: transcallosal approach for the third ventricle, primary tumors (58,2%) (Figures 20.12, 20.13, 20.14, 20.15).

Microsurgery has been used in all cases – Laser with CO_2 and Nd: YAG was used in 12 (10,4%) cases.

The somesthetic nontransfer has not been detected in most cases of midcallosal section. But if the task is made more difficult, so that normal individuals commonly make mistakes, some deficits (as compared with normal subjects) have been elicited.

Splenial section

In the case of a section of the posterior half of the trunk, the agraphia of the left hand with no associated apraxia is due to the fact that the graphic impulses transit over the posterior area, through parietal tracts.

The visual interhemispheric transfer is done especially through the splenium. A lesion at this level leads to alexia without agraphia (Figures 20.16, 20.17, 20.18, 20.19, 20.20, 20.21).

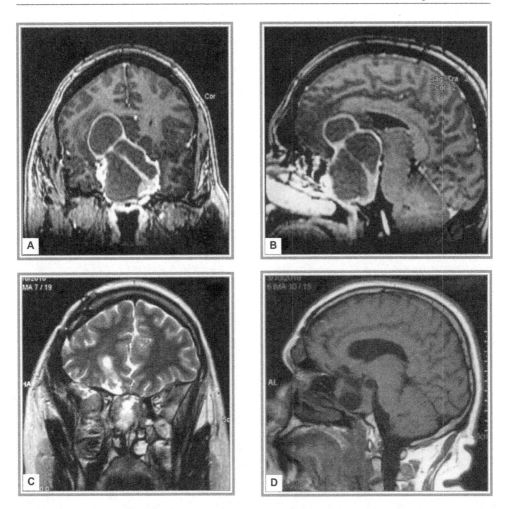

Fig. 20.12. (A and B) Preoperative coronal and sagittal T1-weighted gadolinium-enhanced MRI demonstrating details of an anterior giant cystic craniopharyngioma with sellar enlargement, and suprasellar component and cystic extension into the third ventricle. (C and D) images were obtained after almost complete removal of tumor with very good results. Excision was accomplished through a midline anterior transcallosal and interfornicial corridor.

Thus, whereas more anterior section of the corpus callosum entails minimal long term physiological cost, a section of the splenium commonly causes a left hemialexia (Trescher and Ford, 1937; Maspes, 1948; Wechsler, 1972; Iwata et al., 1974; Damasio et al., 1980). This inability to read in the left visual half-field may be accompanied by a so called colour anomia, an inability to give the names of colours presented to the patient's view although the colours can be matched and the patient can give (speak or write) the colour names of objects, for example "yellow" when asked the colour of a banana (Geschwind and Fusillo, 1966).

When the hemialexia and associated deficits are more severe they can be mistaken for a left homonymous hemianopsia.

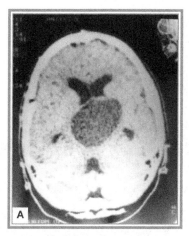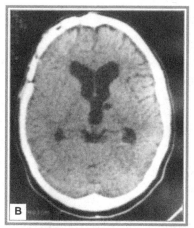

Fig. 20.13. (A) A contrast enhanced axial CT-scan of a 32-year-old man with a large third ventricle tumor (craniopharyngioma). (B) Axial CT-scan, 6 months, postoperatively, confirming total removal of the tumor with excellent results. Excision was accomplished through a midline anterior transcallosal corridor.

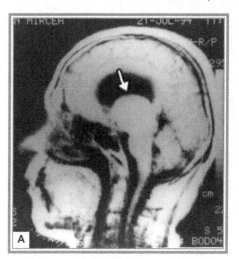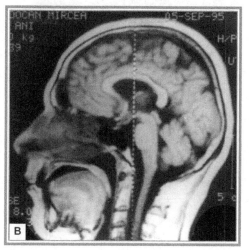

Fig. 20.14. (A) Sagittal MRI demonstrating details of a big third ventricular tumor (dermoid cyst) who was excized transcallosal with very good results. (B) Sagittal MRI after complete removal of the tumor.

In a review (Sugishita et al., 1985), hemialexia is considered of two types: an inability to match written words with objects and an inability to read aloud written words or letters. Both of these are said to be mimicked by the condition of visual hemineglect.

The splenial disconnection can be quite crippling for almost any literate person when the callosal lesion is combined with left occipital lesions or indeed any lesion causing a right hemianopsia.

Such individuals typically have alexia without agraphia: that is, they can write but are unable to read, even what they have just written correctly to dictation. This remarkable dissociation of reading from writing has been known for nearly a century (Déjérine, 1892; Benson, 1985).

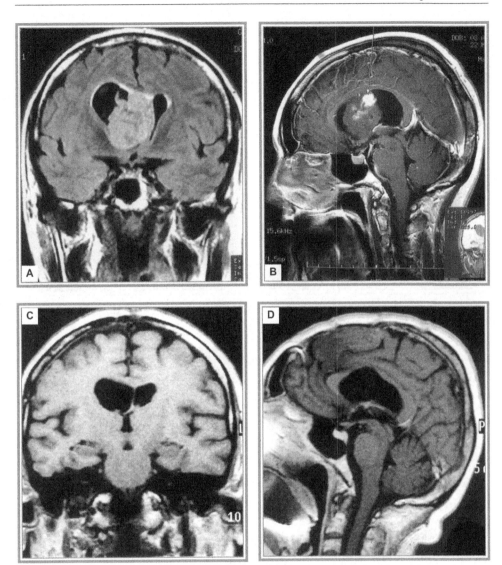

Fig. 20.15. (A and B) Preoperative coronal and sagittal T1-weighted gadolinium-enhanced MRI demonstrating of an anterior third ventricle tumor (astrocytoma). (C and D). Images were obtained after complete removal of the tumor with excellent results. Excision was accomplished through a midline transcallosal approach.

In splenial lesions the right occipital cortex is disconnected from the left hemisphere. Thus, the left hemisphere retains competence to write to dictation but no longer has access to information arriving in the right occipital lobe from the left visual half-field.

Generally, alexia is a cortical disorder of reception in which there is a loss of the ability to comprehend written material manifested as an impairment of reading. Those afflicted with alexia have at one time the ability to read but no longer comprehend written material.

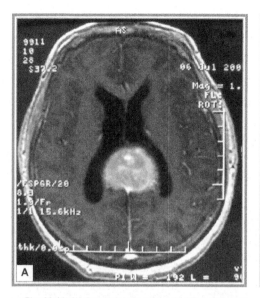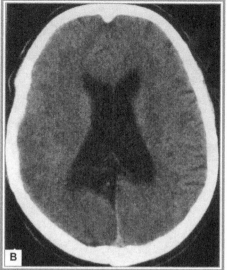

Fig. 20.16. (A) Contrast enhanced axial CT-scan in a 39-year-old woman shows a large, well-delimitated pineal region tumor (meningioma). (B) Postoperative CT-scan after total removal of the tumor.

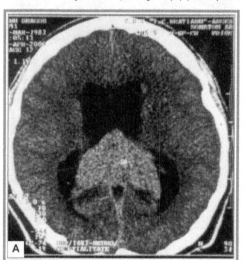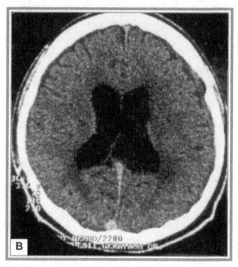

Fig. 20.17. (A) CT-scan showing a large pineal region tumor with involvement of the third and lateral ventricle. (B) Postoperative CT-scan after the excision of that pineal region tumor (germinoma).

Hemialexia is the loss of reading ability in the nondominant visual field as the result of a surgical section of the corpus callosum.

Alexia without agraphia (visual verbal agnosia) is a syndrome, in which a literate person loses the ability to read aloud, to understand written script, and, often, to name colours, i.e., to match a seen colour to its spoken name – visual verbal colour anomia. Such a person can no longer name or point on command to words, although he is sometimes able to read letters or numbers (Adams et al., 1997).

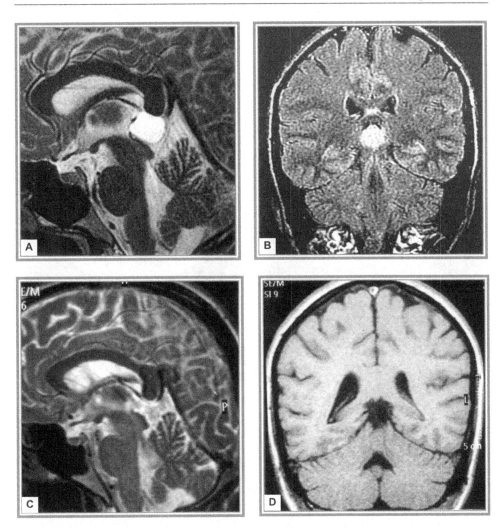

Fig. 20.18. (A and B) Sagittal and coronal T1-weight gadolinium-enhanced MRI, demonstrating a medium-sized pineocytoma. (C and D) Postoperative MRI after total removal of the tumor.

Understanding spoken language, repetition of what is heard, writing spontaneously and to dictation, and conversation are all intact. The ability to copy words is impaired but is better preserved than reading, and the patient may even be able to spell a word or to identify a word by having it spelled to him or by reading one letter at a time (letter-by-letter reading). In some cases, the patient manages to read simple letters but not join them together (**asyllabia**).

The most striking feature of the syndrome is the retained capacity to write fluently, after which the patient cannot read what has been written (alexia without agraphia).

When the patient with alexia or dyslexia also has difficulty in auditory comprehension and in repeating spoken words, the syndrome corresponds to Wernicke's aphasia (Adams et al., 1997).

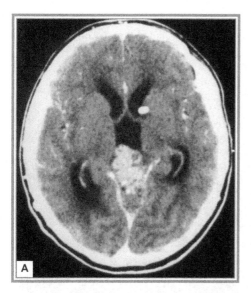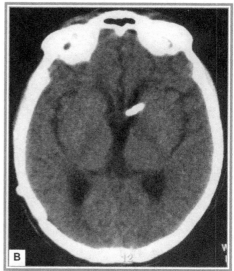

Fig. 20.19. (A) Contrast enhanced axial CT-scan shows a large germinoma of the pineal region with involvement of the third ventricle. (B) Postoperative CT-scan (five month after operation) shows total removal of the tumor.

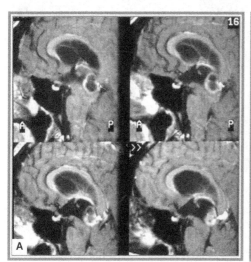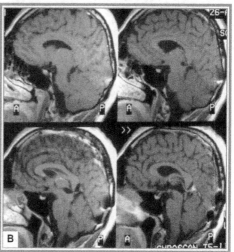

Fig. 20.20. (A) Sagittal T1-weight gadolinium-enhanced MRI in a 31-year-old male patient, shows a pineal tumor. (B) Postoperative MRI after removal of a germinoma. The tumor was removed by the infratentorial supracerebellar approach.

Autopsies of such cases have usually demonstrated a lesion that destroys the left visual cortex, and underlining white matter, particularly the geniculocalcarine tract, as well as the connection of the right visual cortex with the intact language areas of the dominant hemisphere.

In the case originally described by Déjérine (1892), the disconnection occurred in the posterior part (splenium) of the corpus callosum, wherein lie the connection between the visual association areas of the two hemispheres.

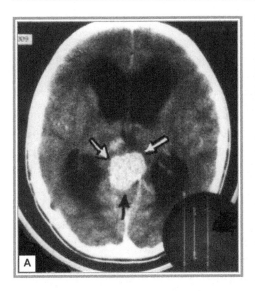 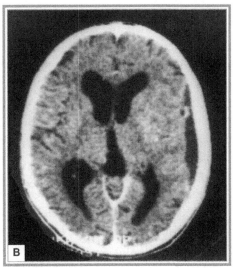

Fig. 20.21. (A) Contrast enhanced axial CT-scan in a 27-year-old woman shows a medium-sized pineoblastoma. (B) Postoperative CT-scan after total removal of the tumor.

More often, the callosal pathways are interrupted in the forceps major or in the paraventricular region (Damasio and Damasio, 1983). In either event, the patient is blind in the right half of each visual field by virtue of the left occipital lesion, and visual information reaches only the right occipital lobe; however, this information cannot be transferred, *via* the callosal pathways, to the cingular gyrus of the left (dominant) hemisphere.

A lesion deep in the white matter of the left occipital lobe at its junction with parietal lobe interrupts the projection from the intact visual cortex to the language areas but spares the geniculocalcarine pathway (Greenblatt, 1973).

This lesion, coupled with the one in the splenium, prevents all visual information from reaching the language areas, including the angular gyrus and Wernicke's area.

In yet other cases, the lesion is confined to the cingular gyrus, or the subjacent white matter. In such cases a right homonymous hemianopsia will also be absent but the alexia may be combined with agraphia, with anomic aphasia and other elements of the Gerstmann syndrome, i.e., right-left confusion, acalculia, and finger agnosia. The entire constellation of symptoms is referred to as the syndrome of the angular gyrus.

Alexia, with agraphia, is an acquired inability to read and write. The lesion is probably localised in the left angular gyrus of the parietal lobe (the left cerebral hemisphere is dominant for language in 95% of humans), corresponding to Brodmann's area 39. Such patients can comprehend spoken words. Alexia without agraphia is a rare and uncommon disorder, in which patients write fluently, but cannot read what they have written. They cannot read words or letters, but can read numbers. The injury usually involves the dominant medial occipital lobe. The intact right primary visual cortex has probably lost its connection with the intact dominant visual language area, particularly

1553

the angular gyrus. Patients see words, but cannot make the associations necessary for their identification. Some patients are able to learn to trace letters with their fingers or use ocular movements to identify these letters, and thus read, though slowly and inefficiently. Thus, the visual interhemispheric transfer is done especially through the splenium. A lesion of the splenium leads to alexia without agraphia (Geschwind, 1965).

After the posterior sectioning of the corpus callosum, although naming the stimuli in the left visual field is not possible, there are many high-degree informational transfers (Sidtis et al., 1981) as well as the possibility to integrate audio and visual information. Cerebral vascular strokes that produce partial callous lesions can lead to a tactile anomia and agraphia, which reveals the importance of fibres in the corpus callosum during language transfer between the two hemispheres (Baynes and Gazzaniga, 1997).

Pandya and Seltzer (1986) highlighted in monkeys a tract for interparietal fibres located just before the splenium (the isthmus of the corpus callosum), which, if sectioned, is enough to lead to disorders of a crisscross tactile localisation (Volpe et al., 1982). This area would also be critical for transferring audible information (Gazzaniga et al., 1975).

Complete callosotomy

When the corpus callosum is entirely sectioned at one sitting, the acute disconnection syndrome appears in about all respects as it is seen after a complete cerebral commissurotomy including the anterior commissure and massa intermedia (Bogen, 1987). This state after callosotomy includes transient mutism, hence, when this symptom follows a complete section it is not reasonably ascribed to the molestation of third ventricular structures.

Moreover, mutism does not necessarily follow a frontal commissurotomy that includes molestation of the third ventricular structures but spares the splenium. Thus, postcommissurotomy mutism requires an explanation on some other parts than third ventricle retraction. Staying out of the third ventricle does avoid same problems, including transient diabetes insipidus.

Experiments with monkeys have shown that if the anterior commissure is left intact it can compensate for the loss of the splenium with respect to interhemispheric transfer of certain kinds of visual information (Hamilton, 1982).

But the anterior commissure cannot compensate completely for splenial loss in humans because hemialexia usually is present after splenial section.

Indeed, most of the stabilized syndromes seen after a complete cerebral commissurotomy are also seen (i.e., have not been compensated) after a callosotomy sparing the anterior commissure (Gazzaniga and LeDoux, 1978; McKeever et al., 1981).

This is perhaps not surprising, because the anterior commissure is only 1/100 the size of the corpus callosum. On the other hand, we can appreciate how significant it might be when we consider the wealth of information that is conveyed over one optic nerve – the diameter of which is about the same as that of the anterior commissure.

This question is complicated by the fact that the size of the anterior commissure is quite variable; a diameter difference of 3 or 4 times has been reported (Yamamoto et al., 1981).

This discrepancy between monkeys (transfer of learning by the anterior commissure) and humans (inability of the anterior commissure to compensate for callosotomy) may reflect differences between recently acquired memories as opposed to long-standing ones. Current evidence suggests that memory deficits can be expected after a commissurotomy that includes the anterior commissure even when the splenium is spared (Zaidel and Sperry, 1974; Campbell et al., 1980; Milner, 1985).

The results originally suggested that a section of the corpus callosum prevented the spread of learning and memory from one hemisphere to the other. Each hemisphere existed independently and had a complete amnesia for the experience of the other (Sperry, 1962).

Extensions of these transfer studies in monkeys from visual to somesthetic and motor learning (Sperry, 1961, 1962; Gazzaniga, 1970) have indicated that the independence of the surgically separated hemispheres may be less clear cut than originally supposed.

Thus, both hemispheres may learn to discriminate simultaneously, one *via* a contralateral sensory system and the other by an ipsilateral sensory system (Gazzaniga, 1970).

Observations of the functional effects of surgical separation of the hemispheres in men (Gazzaniga et al., 1965; Gazzaniga and Sperry, 1967) by complete transection of the corpus callosum, anterior and hippocampal commissures, and of the thalamic adhesion (massa intermedia) have been reported.

These patients show a striking functional independence of the gnostic activities of the two hemispheres. Perceptual, cognitive, mnemonic, learned and volitional activities persist in each hemisphere, but each can proceed outside the realm of awareness of the other hemisphere.

Subjective experiences of each hemisphere are known to the other only indirectly through lower level and peripheral effects.

Disconnection of the hemispheres produces little disturbance of ordinary, daily behavior, temperament or intellect.

Functional deficits tend to be compensated for by the development of bilateral motor control from each hemisphere, as well as by the bilateralism of some sensory pathways.

Information perceived exclusively, or generated exclusively, in the minor (right) hemisphere could not be communicated in speech or in writing; it was expressed entirely by nonverbal responses.

There was no detectable impairment of speech or writing with reference to information processed in the major (left) hemisphere.

These authors found linguistic expression to be organized almost exclusively in the dominant hemisphere.

In contrast to the above, comprehension of language, both spoken and written, was found to be represented in both hemispheres, with the minor hemisphere a little less proficient.

In an analysis of the visual fields, with fixation assured, subjects verbally described only those small spots of light presented in the right half of the visual field (Gazzaniga, 1970). A similar light stimulus present in the left half of the visual field produced no verbal response.

With double field stimulation, only spots of light falling in the right visual field were reported. In these subjects, the visual fields stopped exactly in the midline and no macular sparing was evident.

Thus, it would appear that no visual information can be transferred from one hemisphere to the other after a section of the corpus callosum.

Certain lesions involving portions of the corpus callosum, or association areas of the cortex which give rise to commissural fibres, produce disturbances of higher brain functions collectively recognized as the disconnection syndrome (Geschwind, 1965, 1965a, 1970).

Word blindness without agraphia presumably results from lesions which interrupt fibres from the visual association area which cross in the splenium of the corpus callosum and project to the left angular gyrus.

Pure word deafness may result from subcortical lesions located in the left temporal lobe and which interrupt the left auditory radiation as well as callosal fibres from the contralateral auditory region. A similar syndrome manifested by various forms of agnosia or apraxia may result from lesions involving portions of the corpus callosum and the association fibre system (Carpenter, 1979).

Thus, after sectioning the corpus callosum, the two hemispheres are independent; each receives sensory input from all sensory systems, and each can control the muscles of the body, but the two hemispheres can no longer communicate with each other.

Because the functions in these separate cortices, or "split brain", are thus isolated, sensory information can be presented to one hemisphere and its function can be studied without the other hemisphere having access to the information.

So, information seen in a particular part of the visual world by both eyes is sent to only one hemisphere: input from the left side of the world (the left visual field) goes to the right hemisphere, whereas input from the right side of the world (the right visual field) goes to the left hemisphere. The two sides of the world are joined by a connection thorough the corpus callosum.

With the corpus callosum severed, the brain cannot relate the different views of the left and right hemispheres.

When the left hemisphere of a split-brain patient has access to information, it can initiate speech and hence communicate about the information. The right hemisphere apparently has reasonably good recognition abilities but is unable to initiate speech, because it lacks access to the speech mechanisms of the left hemisphere (Kolb and Whishaw, 2003).

The special capacities of the right hemisphere in facial recognition can also be demonstrated in split-brain patients.

Levy et al. (1972) devised the chimerical figures test, which consists of pictures of faces and other patterns that have been split down the centre and recombined in improbable ways. When the recombined faces were presented selectively to each hemisphere, the patients appear to be unaware of gross discordance between the two sides of the pictures. When asked to pick out the picture that they had seen, they chose the face seen in the left visual field (that is, by their right hemisphere), demonstrating that the right hemisphere has a special role in the recognition of face.

Thus, a surgical section of the corpus callosum cuts off direct interhemispheric communication (Bogen, 1985; Seymour et al., 1984; Baynes and Gazzaniga, 2000). When examined by special neuropsychological techniques (Zaidel et al., 1990), patients who have undergone a section of commissural fibres (commissurotomy) exhibit profound behavioral discontinuities between perception, comprehension, and response, which reflect significant functional differences between the hemispheres.

Probably because direct communication between two cortical points occurs less frequently than indirect communication relayed through lower brain centres, especially the thalamus and the basal ganglia, these patients generally manage to perform everyday activities quite well, including tasks involving interhemispheric information transfer (Myers and Sperry, 1985; Zaidel et al., 1990; Sergent, 1990, 1991) and emotional and conceptual information not dependent on language or complex visuospatial processes (Cronin-Golomb, 1986). In noting that alertness remains unaffected by commissurotomy and that emotional tone is consistent between the hemispheres, Sperry (1990) suggested that both phenomena rely on bilateral projections through the intact brain stem.

In sum, the results of careful studies of patients with commissurotomies provide clear evidence of the complementary specialization of the two cerebral hemispheres. It must be recognized, however, that, as interesting as these patients are, they represent only a very small population and their two hemispheres are by no means normal.

The right hand is superior in drawing fine, detailed featural information, and the left for the overall gestaltic interrelationships and general outline, in a manner analogous to the left - right dissociations noted in a constructional apraxia.

Similar hand differences appeared with respect to strategies adapted in tactually matching a viewed, unfolded, three-dimensional object: this led to the general conclusion that the right hemisphere has the synthetic ability to integrate unrelated parts into a meaningful whole, whereas the left hemisphere specializes in the analysis of component features.

Levy and Trevarthen (1976) concluded that each hemisphere has its own cognitive strategy, the right hemisphere synthesizing over space, the left hemisphere analyzing over time.

Callosal agenesis

Occasionally, individuals may be born with partial or complete absence of the corpus callosum. More and more instances of such "experiments of nature" are emerging with the development of new imaging techniques (Jeeves, 1990).

In large autopsy series their incidence is of 5.5% - 26 % (Jellinger et al., 1981). However, its clinics and pathogenicity remain partially obscure. Rohmer et al. (1960) claim that, although the agenesis of the corpus callosum had been described for the first time by Reil in 1812, its pathogenicity is little known.

Callosal deficits in such cases vary in degree, depending on the time after conception that the presumed causative insult occurred.

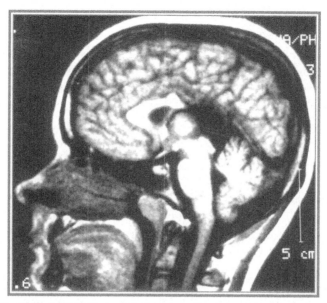

Fig. 20.22. Sagittal MRI, shows the posterior half agenesia of the corpus callosum.

Andermann et al. (1994) and Wisniewski and Jeret (1994) support the importance of the age-gestation factor, because the size of the malformation seems to be related to the moment in which the damaging factors enter in the course of foetal development. Thus, interrupting the development itself between the end of the first gestation month and the beginning of the forth month lead to a total absence of all neocortical commissures.

Interrupting the development during the fourth month leads to the agenesis of the corpus callosum with preservation of the anterior commissure. On the other hand, the development anomalies that appear after the forth month determine a partial agenesis, which especially affects the splenium (Fig. 20.22).

The splenium or rostrum are more likely to be absent, and the anterior commissure is usually still present, and is often hypertrophied due to the enclosure of heterotopic callosal fibres. The anterior commissure in fact is important in the extensive functional reorganization that seems to occur in such cases (Bradshaw and Mattingley, 1995). During the development, there can only occur an imperfect commissure and not a real agenesis, as the fibres of the corpus callosum are present, but instead of having a transversal projection they form the margins of the internal facets of the two hemispheres.

Therefore, from an anatomical point of view, the agenesis of the corpus callosum may be partial or total associated or not to craniofacial, either tumoural or constitutional (hydrocephalus, lack of septum pellucidum, microgyria etc.) (Lassonde, 1994).

Clinical manifestations. Ten percent of such cases are quite asymptomatic, coming to light by chance at necropsy, and other being recognized because of other neurological problems.

The symptoms in a callous agenesis may be discovered in a patient with normal intelligence or may be included in a major polimalformation syndrome. Because of this reason, different psychic disorders, mental debility, epilepsy etc. are related to the simultaneous presence of an extracallous pathology. Totally asymptomatic cases are discovered only in autopsy and are debatable.

However, many scientists tried to check for the presence of a disconnection syndrome, but the results were negative (Rohmer et al., 1960; Jeeves, 1979; Saul and Sperry, 1968; Sauerwein and Lassonde, 1983; Lassonde et al., 1981, 1984; Lassonde, 1994).

The absence of disconnection deficits led to more interpretation based on the use of some compensatory mechanisms (Jeeves, 1986, 1991, 1994) such as: (1) bilateralization of cerebral functions; (2) the use of subtle behavioral strategies (cross-cueing), that allow the non-stimulated hemisphere to use proprioceptive markers (a movement) derived from the answer provided by the other hemisphere. This ensures a bilateral distribution of information (Gazzaniga, 1970); (3) the overuse of ipsilateral sensitive and motor projection tracts, which allow each hemisphere to have a bimanual representation; (4) the maximum use of residual commissures (anterior and subcortical) in order to ensure an interhemispheric transfer.

The philogenetic, morphologic and functional characteristics of the anterior commissure show that it represents a single possible alternative for an interhemispheric transfer in case of a callous agenesis. In all situations in which this commissure is present it forms the main functional system capable of compensating the deficits induced by the absence of the corpus callosum (Guénot, 1998).

Moreover, there is a degree of anomalies in tests of interhemispheric transfer which correlates in case of a callous agenesis with the presence or absence of the anterior commissure which can sometimes be hypertrophic. Whichever the nature of the compensatory mechanisms used by subjects with an agenesis of the corpus callosum, they do not pass certain limits because the interhemispheric communication for these people has decreased (Lassonde et al., 1990, 1996).

According to Jeeves (1979), Sauerwein et al. (1994), Sylver and Jeeves (1994), and Lassonde et al. (1996), this decrease of interhemispheric commutation includes the following: slower motor tests, if bimanual coordination is needed; mostly severe difficulty of grabbing, well observed at the beginning of school age; slowness in performing certain visual tactile transfer tasks; difficulty in a crisscross localizing test for a tactile stimulus; difficulty of unimanual transfer (Geffen et al., 1994); deficit of median fusion observed at a discrimination test of two tactile stimulation points (Schiavetto et al., 1993); and deficit in the evaluation of distance between visual stimuli (Lassonde et al., 1981; Jeeves, 1991); and disorders of the ability to locate sound within the entire audio-field (Poirier et al., 1993).

Problems of phonologic analysis and video-constructive deficits have also been observed in children with normal intelligence (Temple and Ilsley, 1994). These deficits observed in persons with an agenesis of the corpus callosum are also seen in normal little children, because of the myelinization processes in the corpus callosum, which for them is not yet finished (Yakovlev and Lecours, 1967). As the growth process in the commissural system is ending, these aptitudes improve progressively (Lassonde et al., 1996).

Failure of the corpus callosum to develop (agenesis of the corpus callosum) may be accompanied by an absence of the anterior and hippocampal commissures.

Although some patients with this condition may experience focal seizures and have mental retardation, others live for many years with few or no obvious neurologic deficits.

These individuals frequently have developmental abnormalities in other parts of the nervous system.

Some persons with agenesis of the corpus callosum (a rare congenital condition in which the corpus callosum is insufficiently developed or absent altogether) are identified only when some other condition brings them to a neurologist's attention, as they normally display no neurological or neuropsychological defects (Harris, 1995; Zaidel et al., 2003) other than slowed motor performances, particularly of bimanual tasks (Lassonde et al., 1991).

Thus, persons who are born without a corpus callosum can perform interhemispheric comparisons of visual and tactile information. The interpretation of these results is that the patients have enhanced conduction in the remaining commissures (for example, for vision) and that they develop enhanced abilities to use their few uncrossed projections (for example, for tactile information) (Kolb and Whishaw, 2003)

There are a number of reports of poor transfer of information if stimuli are complex. Furthermore, nonspecific deficits in task performance have been reported in these patients.

Lassonde (1986) and Lassonde et al. (1991) presented pairs of stimuli to six patients with agenesis of the corpus callosum, asking them if the pairs were the same or different. Letters, numbers, colours or forms were used, either the pair was presented one on top of the other in one visual field (interahemispheric task) or one stimulus was presented in one visual field and the other stimulus in the other visual field (interhemispheric task).

The acallosal group was equally accurate in identifying same - different pairs under both conditions.

Their reactions, however, were very slow for both forms of presentation. Lassonde (1986) suggested that the callosum participates in hemispheric activation as well as in the transfer of information.

Thus, the acallosal group has alternative ways of obtaining the interhemispheric transfer of information but not of activation.

According to Jeeves (1986, 1990), one explanation of why language is lateralized to one hemisphere is that it gets a start there and then that hemisphere actively inhibits its development in the other hemisphere. In people with callosal agenesis, the opportunity for such an inhibitory process to work is much reduced. Yet the lateralization of language and other functions in most of these people is similar to that in the general population. Thus, the corpus callosum and other commissures are not necessary for the development of asymmetries.

They are clearly not indispensable, but may play the following roles (Jeeves, 1990):
1. Interhemispheric integration, updating, and information transfer;
2. Inhibition of ipsilateral pathways to avoid unnecessary competition;
3. Inhibition during development so as to facilitate hemispheric specialization.

4. Regulation and switching of attention and arousal levels;

5. Facilitation of information processing not only at an interhemispheric but even at an intrahemispheric level (Lassonde et al., 1996). Indeed, commissurotomy does not just stop seizure activity spreading to the other hemisphere, but also reduces it at the initial focus.

Stroke of the corpus callosum

A stroke involving the anterior cerebral artery may affect the anterior corpus callosum and result in apraxia (impairment of the capacity to execute various movements) of the left arm as a consequence of the isolation / disconnection of the language-dominant (left) hemisphere from the right motor cortex.

A stroke involving the posterior cerebral artery or a lesion involving the posterior corpus callosum on the left side, may result in alexia (the inability to recognize words or to read).

Visual input from the left visual field is relayed to the right, intact visual cortex, which is isolated / disconnected from the language dominant (left) hemisphere. If the basilar artery is affected, which gives rise to both the posterior cerebral arteries, the infarction of the visual cortex will be bilateral and will cause cortical blindness; however, the affected individual is unaware that he cannot see.

Tumors and degenerative diseases of corpus callosum

Open surgical approaches to lesions of the third and lateral ventricle are divided into 2 general categories: interhemispheric/transcallosal and transcortical. Each requires the violation of normal neural tissue *via* either a corticotomy or a callosotomy. Reported postoperative seizure rates after transcortical approaches, ranging from 26% to 70% (Fornari et al., 1981; Desai et al., 2002) have led some to advocate transcallosal over transcortical approaches when anatomic considerations would be conductive to either approach (Anderson et al., 2003). According to Milligan and Meyer (2010), although the 2 traditional approaches to the ventricular system had similar major complication rates, the transcallosal approach was associated with a significantly increased seizure risk.

The two main groups of tumors in the corpus callosum, lipomas and gliomas, represent between 1 and 5% of the intracranial neoplasias.

The lipomas of the corpus callosum are congenital tumors, which frequently appear in association to other callous malformations (hypoplasia or the agenesis of the corpus callosum) and other cerebral anomalies (cortical atrophy, microgyria etc.). They lead to few characteristic symptoms; therefore, the presence of these neoplastic processes is frequently discovered during autopsy. A patient with a corpus callosum lipoma and dysraphism was found to have trisomy 13 (Wainright et al., 1995).

The tendency for lipomas to occur in the midline and their frequent association with dysraphic anomalies have led some authors to believe that they are caused by an imperfection of neural tube closure, relating them to inclusion tumors (Gerber and

Plotkin, 1982; Hori, 1986). However, Zettner and Netsky (1960) believe that their pathogenesis lies in faulty differentiation of primitive meninx tissue in the intrahemispheric fissure, which may later interfere with the development of midline structures. More than 50% of patients with intracranial lipomas present with seizures. Almost 20% of patients have mentation defects (Clarici and Heppner, 1979). The symptoms are usually due to obstructive hydrocephalus.

The management of an intracranial lipoma should generally be conservative. Only in unusual cases does the tumor require debulking or removal. The tenacious attachments to surrounding structures may account for the poor results.

The gliomas of the corpus callosum (glioblastomas, oligodendrogliomas and astrocytomas) have a different symptomatology, which can be expressed even during the first days through headaches, epileptic seizures, neurologic disorders (lesions of cranial nerve, hemiparesis, walking disorders, and dysfunctions of the autonomous nervous system) and psychological changes (impulsivity, apathy, spatial or temporal disorientation, memory disorders etc.).

In this context, when the assembly in the callous territory and its neighbouring regions are invaded by the tumoural process, occurs a syndrome of callous disconnection. When there is a partial invasion of the corpus callosum, we find only some components of the disconnection syndrome (Fig. 20.23). Frontal lobe gliomas tend to invade the frontal lobe, crossing through the corpus callosum. Gliomas arising in the regions below the corpus callosum are largely confined and tend to invade the basal structures, such as the thalamus and peduncles along the corticospinal tracts.

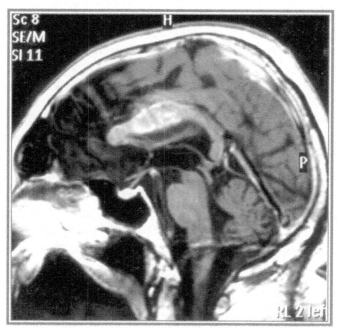

Fig. 20.23. Sagittal T1-weight gadolinium-enhanced magnetic resonance imaging scan from a patient with anaplastic astrocytoma of the corpus callosum.

T2-weight studies suggested that a larger proportion of tumors located close to the corpus callosum invade this white matter tract.

The spread of malignant gliomas through all the white matter tracts (i.e., corpus callosum, uncinate fasciculus, fasciculus longitudinalis and occipitofrontalis, auditive and visual bundle, and corona radiata) has been documented (Matsukado et al., 1961). The corpus callosum is the main white matter tract that leads to bilateral growth (Scherer, 1940; Salazar and Rubin, 1976). Grafted human glioma cells migrate along the glia limitans, the basement membrane-lined blood vessels and Virchow-Robin space, the subpial and subependymal space and the white matter fascicles of anatomic pathways, including the corpus callosum, internal capsule, optic tract, and other parallel and intersecting fibre tracts.

The intact vascular basement membrane is not penetrated by glioma cells (Bernstein and Woodard, 1995).

Marchiafava-Bignami disease

In 1903, Marchiafava and Bignami described a curious syndrome of selective demyelinisation of the corpus callosum in alcoholic Italians who indulged in large quantities of red wine.

The disease seems to affect severe and chronic alcoholics in their middle or late life, with a peak incidence between 40 and 60 years of age. A toxic cause, such as direct toxicity of ethanol or other constituents, seems equally plausible. Clinical observations of that three alcoholic patients were few and incomplete; in two of them, a chronic ill-defined psychosis had been present, and, in all three, seizures and coma had occurred terminally. In 1907, Bignami described a case in which the corpus callosum lesion was accompanied by a similar lesion in the central portion of the anterior commissure.

These early reports were followed by a spate of articles that confirmed and amplified the original clinical and pathological findings. About 40 cases of this disorder had been described in the Italian literature (Mingazzini, 1922). A clinical diagnosis is often difficult, because neurological presentation varies considerably. Many patients present in terminal coma, which often preludes a premortem diagnosis. Mental and motor slowing, other personality and behavior changes, incontinence, dysarthria, seizures, and hemiparesis occur to a varying extent. The most common picture on neurological evaluation is probably that of a frontal lobe or dementia syndrome.

Anterior corpus callosum vascular malformations

Anterior callosal arteriovenous malformations involve the corpus callosum, the cingulate gyrus and ventricular ependyma.

The blood supply comes from the pericallosal and callosal marginal arteries. Venous drainage occurs superiorly into the sagittal sinus and intraventricularly into the septal, thalamostriate, and eventually internal cerebral veins.

Larger lesions can involve the medial aspect of the striatum and anterior hypothalamus as well as the septal and preseptal regions. With lateral extension, the recurrent feeders of these malformations come from the recurrant artery of Heubner and

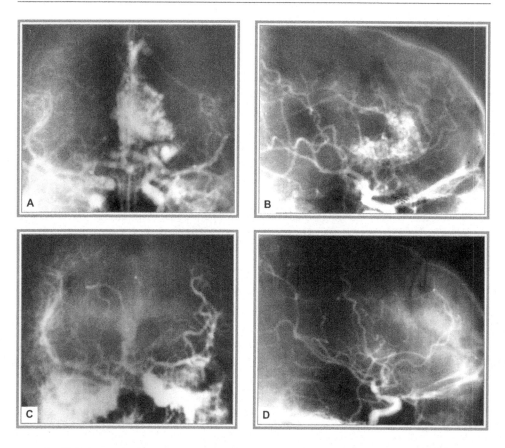

Fig. 20.24. Conventional anteroposterior and lateral angiographic view (A, B) show a large arteriovenous malformation that involve the anterior part of the corpus callosum, the cingulate girus and the right ventricular ependyma. Postoperative (C, D) carotid angiography demonstrates complete resection of that malformation with very good results.

from medial lenticulostriate arteries (Fig. 20.24). Blood supply also comes from perforators of the anterior cerebral arteries and anterior communicating artery (Dănăilă et al., 2010).

The approach uses a unilateral frontal craniotomy extending to the midline. The subfrontal approach allows identification and division of the feeding vessels from the anterior communicating complex and the anterior cerebral arteries. This can be followed by an anterior interhemispheric approach to follow A2 vessels distally.

Thus, these lesions can be resected by skeletonizing the pericallosal arteries as they pass through the lesion and taking only the side branches to the malformation. The dissection of the medial and intraventricular plane of the lesion is completed using an approach through the corpus callosum (Fig. 20.25).

Fig. 20.25. Preoperative (A, B, C) carotid angiography of a large interhemispheric arteriovenous malformation. This was approached through a large right frontoparietal craniotomy. Postoperative (D, E, F) carotid angiography demonstrates complete resection of that arteriovenous malformation. Postoperative evolution was excellent. ▶

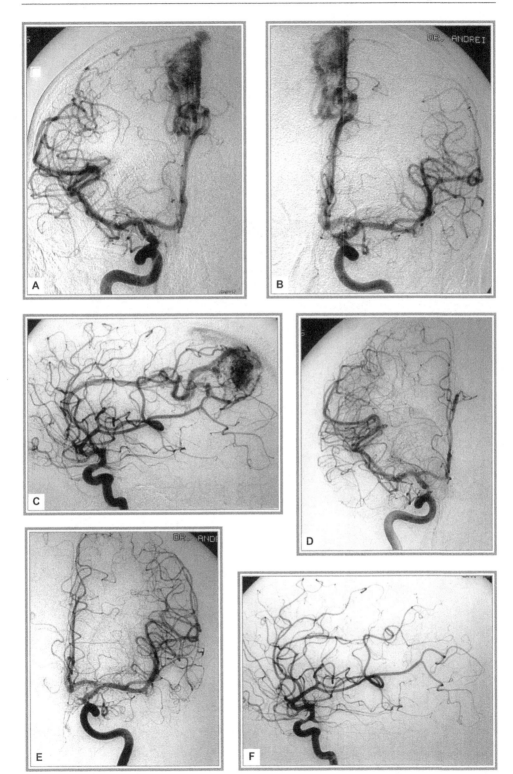

The AVMs of the splenium are supplied primarily by pericallosal branches of the posterior cerebral artery and distal pericallosal branches of the anterior cerebral artery as well as by medial and lateral choroid branches of the posterior cerebral artery. Drainage is usually into the internal cerebral vein and the vein of Galen (Fig. 20.26).

The surgical approach is parasagittal interhemispheric from the opposite side with division of the falx to have a more direct access to the lateral aspect of the lesion.

The lateral extent of the lesion is defined by splitting the splenium in the direction of the fibres.

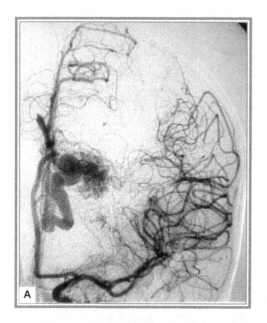
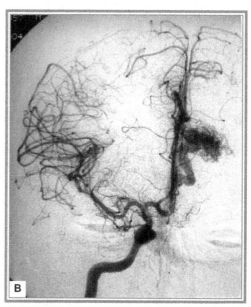
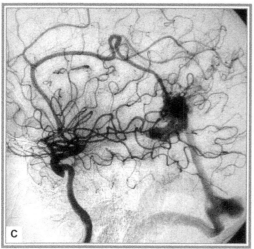
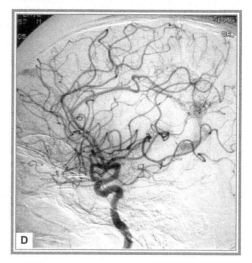

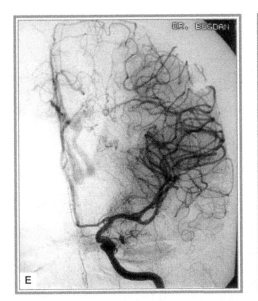
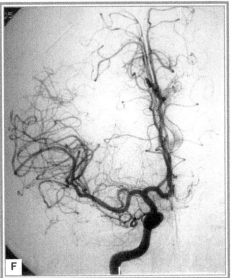

Fig. 20.26. Preoperative (A, B, C) carotid angiography of a splenial arteriovenous malformation. These AVMs of the splenium were supplied primarily by distal pericallosal branches of the anterior cerebral artery as well as by medial and lateral choroidal branches of the posterior cerebral artery. Drainage is into the internal cerebral vein and vein of Galen. The surgical approach was parasagittal interhemispheric from the right (opposite side with division of the falx to have more direct access to the left aspect of the lesion. Postoperative (D, E, F), carotid angiography demonstrates complete resection of the malformation. The evolution of the patient was excellent.

Summary

The loss of the ability to transfer information from the left hemisphere to the right hemisphere and vice-versa seems to have no impact on their overall psychological state.

However the question of the perceived unity of the world continues to interest scientists. The most spectacular finding in that respect has been the discovery that the corpus callosum can be cut in humans without changing the perceived unity of the world and of the self.

According to Baars (2007), the role of the two hemispheres in human cognition and mind-brain identity has been the subject of extensive studies, and we are still unfolding the subtle and not so subtle differences in the roles that the mirror-image hemispheres play in perception, language, thought, and consciousness.

For many years such callosotomies were performed to improve intractable epilepsy. This surgical procedure has proved to be effective in preventing seizures from being transferred from one cerebral hemisphere to the other (Fig. 20.27).

It was the introduction to lateralized procedures in early studies that led to that unique research opportunity presented by split-brain patients. Thus, more careful studies have provided evidence that a complete callosotomy does have subtle but long lasting effects. Because of this, a partial resection (callosectomy) is preferred.

There are some hemispheric differences that are fairly well understood, such as crossover wiring. Many aspects of sensory and motor processing entail the crossing over of input (sensory) or output (motor) information from the left side to the right, and vice-versa (Fig. 20.28).

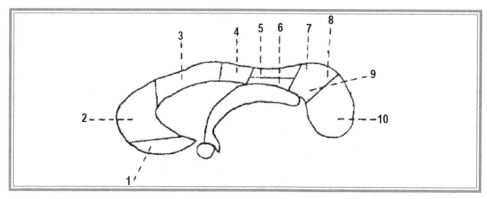

Fig. 20.27. The symptoms of callous disconnection and the location of the responsible lesions: 1. The fibres that pass through the rostrum and through the ventral area of the genu come from the ventral and medial region of the prefrontal cortex; 2. The arched fibres of the genu and the cingulate fibres that pass underneath the cortex of the cingulate gyrus are connected in the posterior area with the septal nucleus; 3. The fibres of the anterior half of the corpus callosum are destined to the fronto-frontal tracts; their lesion leads to the apraxia of the left hand without agraphia; 4. Fibres that connect the somato-sensorial cortex; their lesions lead to the left tactile anomia; 5. Fibres that connect the supramarginal gyrus; their lesions leads to the left ideomotor apraxia; 6. Fibres that connect the lateral temporal cortex; their lesions leads to a dichotic extinction in the left ear; 7. Fibres that connect the superior parietal lobe; their lesions leads to a diagnostic dyspraxia; 8. Fibres that connect the superior parietal lobe; their lesions leads to constructive disorders of the right hand and tactile anomia of the left hand; 9. Fibres that connect the angular gyrus; their lesions leads to agraphia of the left hand; 10. Fibres that connect the prestriate cortex; their lesions leads to left visual anomia and left hemialexia.

Only the olfactory nerve, which is a very ancient sensory system, stays on the same side of the brain on its way to the cortex.

The time lag between the two hemispheres working on the same task may be as short as 10 ms, or one-hundredth of a second (Handy et al., 2003).

Therefore, when the great information highway of the corpus callosum is intact, the differences between the hemispheres are not very obvious. But when it is cut, and the proper experimental controls are used to separate the input of the right and left half of each eye's visual field, suddenly major hemispheric differences become observable (Baars, 2007).

However, tactual testing of the right hand showed no significant impairment of the dominant but disconnected left hemisphere. Similar testing of the left hand indicated severe agnosia, anomia, and agraphia. Also, in tachistoscopic presentations, the results showed no abnormality in response to stimuli presented to the right visual field, but the patient was severely impaired with stimuli presented to the left visual field (Gazzaniga and Miller, 2009).

Severing the entire callosum blocks, the interhemispheric transfer of sensory, motor, perceptual, gnostic, and other forms of information in such a way that it allows us to study hemispheric differences and the unique ways in which the hemispheres interact with each other (Zaidel, 1990; Gazzaniga, 2000; 2005).

The most obvious hemispheric difference is the capacity to learn language. It had been known prior to split-brain research that the left hemisphere is dominant for language and, particularly, speech production (Broca, 1865; Wernicke, 1874).

Fig. 20.28. Liepmann's theory of apraxia resulting from lesions of the corpus callosum. (A) Normal response to a verbal command to move the left hand. The command is processed through the posterior speech zone (areas 22, 39, and 40) from the motor cortex of the left hemisphere through the corpus callosum to the motor cortex (area 4) of the right hemisphere to move the left hand. (B) Apraxic response. The jagged line through the callosal area indicates sectioning of the callosum. The verbal command has no way of informing the right-hemisphere motor cortex to move the left hand. Geschwind proposed that bilateral apraxia could result from a lesion disconnecting the posterior speech zone from the motor cortex of the left hemisphere because the verbal command cannot gain access to either the left or the right motor cortex. (after Kolb and Whishaw, 2003)

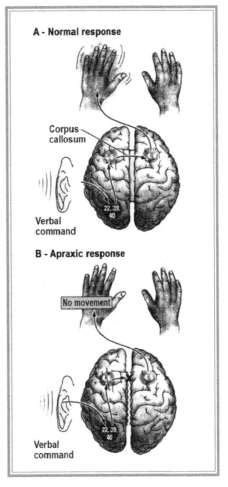

The left hemisphere is also specialized in written language. And, while the right hemisphere does have a limited capacity for reading and is able to read whole words (ideographic lexical / semantic access), it is unable to convert graphemes to phonemes as can the language-dominant left hemisphere (Zaidel and Peters, 1981; Zaidel et al., 1985).

Gazzaniga and Miller (2009) have a patient who generates spoken language exclusively from the left hemisphere, and the written language exclusively from the right hemisphere.

Previously, it had been assumed that spoken and written language shared the same neural mechanism but this patient demonstrates that the output of these two functions can be operated by independent modules (Baynes et al., 1998).

As much as cognitive styles and personal tastes and habits might seem to reflect the processing characteristics of one or the other hemisphere, these qualities appear to be integral to both hemispheres (Arndt and Berger, 1978; Sperry et al., 1979). "In the normal intact state, the conscious activity is typically a unified and coherent bilateral process that spans both hemispheres through the commissures" (Sperry, 1976).

However, very few tasks rely exclusively on one hemisphere. The interaction between hemispheres has important mutually enhancing effects. Complex mental tasks such as reading, arithmetic, and word and object learning are performing best when both hemispheres can be actively engaged (Rey, 1959; Moscovitch, 1979; Huettner et al., 1989; Gaillard, 1990; Belger and Banich, 1998; Weissman and Banich, 2000; Dănăilă and Golu, 2006).

Other mutually enhancing effects of bilateral processing show up in the superior memorizing and retrieval of both verbal and configurational material when simultaneously processed (encoded) by the verbal and configurational system (Milner, 1978; Moscovitch, 1979); in enhancing cognitive efficiency of normal subjects when hemispheric activation is bilateral rather than unilateral (Berger and Perret, 1986; Berger et al., 1987); and in better performances of visual tasks by commissurotomized patients when both hemispheres participate than when vision is restricted to either hemisphere (Zaidel, 1979; Sergent, 1991 a, b).

The cerebral processing of music illuminates the differences in how each hemisphere contributes, the complexities of hemispheric interactions, and how experience can alter hemispheric roles.

The left hemisphere tends to predominate in the processing of sequential and discrete tonal components of music (Gaede et al., 1978; Breitling et al., 1987; Botez and Botez, 1996).

The inability to use both hands to play a musical instrument (bimanual instrument apraxia) has been reported with left hemisphere lesions that spare motor functions (Benton, 1977).

The right hemisphere predominates in melody recognition and in melodic singing (Gordon and Bogen, 1974; Yamadori et al., 1977; Samson and Zatorre, 1988; Kumkova, 1990; Dănăilă and Golu, 2006). Its involvement with chord analysis is generally greatest in musically untrained persons (Gaede et al., 1978). Training can alter these hemispheric biases so that, for musicians, the left hemisphere predominates for melody recognition (Bever and Chiarello, 1974; Messerli et al., 1995), tone discrimination (Shanon, 1981; Mazziota et al., 1982), and musical judgments (Shanon, 1980, 1984).

Moreover, intact, untrained persons tend most to show lateralised effects for tone discrimination or musical judgments (Shanon, 1980, 1981, 1984). Taken altogether, these findings suggest that while cerebral processing of different components of music is lateralized with each hemisphere predominating in certain aspects, both hemispheres are needed for musical appreciation and performance (Bauer and McDonald, 2003).

The bilateral integration of cerebral function is most clearly exhibited by creative artists, who typically have intact brains. Excepting singing, harmonica playing, and the small repertoire of piano pieces written for one hand, making music is a two-handed activity.

Moreover, for instruments such as guitars and the entire violin family, the right hand performs those aspects of music that are mediated predominantly by the right hemisphere, such as expression and tonality, while the left hand interprets the linear sequence of notes best deciphered by the left hemisphere.

Thus, by its very nature, the artist's performance involves the smoothly integrated activity of both hemispheres (Lezak et al., 2004).

Although each hemisphere appears to have redundant knowledge structures that support basic functioning, the extent of the semantic systems in the right hemisphere is clearly impoverished compared to the left (Gazzaniga et al., 1984; Gazzaniga and Miller, 1989; Baynes et al., 1992; Reuter-Lorenz and Baynes, 1992), including a limited lexical organization in the right (Gazzaniga, 1983).

Kihlstrom and Klein (1997) have emphasized that the self is a knowledge structure, not some mystical entity. Severing the corpus callosum raises an interesting issue about whether a disconnected half brain will still have the same sense of self.

According to Turk et al. (2003), although it is very difficult to accurately assess the extent of the right hemisphere's knowledge (self and otherwise) given its limited language ability, there does appear to be hemispheric differences in the knowledge system that bias each hemisphere's responses.

Although the left hemisphere is clearly dominant for language, many problem-solving skills, and semantic knowledge (Gazzaniga, 2000), the right hemisphere does have some specialization as well. Studies with split-brain patients have revealed right hemisphere superiority for various tasks involving such components as part-whole relations (Nebes, 1972), spatial relationship (Nebes, 1973), apparent motion detection (Forster et al., 2000), mental rotation (Corballis and Sergent, 1988), spatial matching (Corballis et al., 1999) and mirror image discrimination (Funnell et al., 1999).

The right hemisphere also appears to be more veridical in its memory recollections (Phelps and Gazzaniga, 1992; Metcalfe et al., 1995) and to be better at illusory contour perception and amodal boundary completion (Corballis et al., 1999). One of the more compelling recent findings regarding the right hemisphere is its superiority in casual perception, although the left hemisphere was found to be superior at causal inference (Roser et al., 2005).

Understanding cause and effect is fundamental to making sense of the dynamic physical world, and the perception of spatial and temporal contiguity of the movements of colliding objects is a critical component of this basic understanding (Gazzaniga and Miller, 2009).

A well-known specialization of the right hemisphere is the detection of upright faces.

The term prosopagnosia was introduced by Bodamer (1947) for a type of visual defect in which the patient cannot identify a familiar face by looking at the person or a picture, even though he knows that a face is a face and can point out features. They may also be unable to interpret the meaning of facial expression or to judge the ages or distinguish the gender of faces. As a rule, other agnosias are present in such cases (colour agnosia, simultanagnosia), and there may be topographical disorientations, disturbances of body schema, and constructional or dressing apraxia. Visual field defects are nearly always present. The small number of cases that have been studied anatomically and by CT scanning and MRI indicate that prosopagnosia is associated with bilateral lesions of the ventromedian occipitotemporal regions (Damasio et al., 1982).

In their studies of split-brain patients Levy et al. (1972), Gazzaniga and Smylie (1983) and Miller et al. (2002), showed that the left hemisphere can perceive and recognize faces and it can perform just as well as the right with familiar faces, but the right hemisphere is superior in its ability to perceive and recognize unfamiliar faces.

However, while both hemispheres can generate spontaneous facial expression, only the dominant left hemisphere can generate voluntary facial expression (Gazzaniga and Smylie, 1990).

The expected right-hemispheric superiority in visuospatial functions has been demonstrated in callosotomy patients. The use of tactile information to built spatial representation of abstract shapes also appears to be better developed in the right hemisphere (Milner and Taylor, 1972).

Although the right hemisphere demonstrates superior levels of performance on a variety of perceptual and spatial tasks, the left hemisphere appears to have at least some competence in most areas and in some cases is essential for the solution of complex visual problems.

Verbal IQ appears to be stable following callosotomy, although performance IQ may decline (Zaidel, 1990).

However, the cognitive functioning of each hemisphere is quite redundant.

Both hemispheres are quite capable of encoding and retrieving of past events, despite a significant theory in the 1990s on the brain region underlying episodic memory function based on neuroimaging works. The theory, called HERA (hemispheric encoding / retrieval asymmetry), stipulated that episodic encoding was predominantly a left hemisphere process while episodic retrieval was predominantly a right hemisphere process (Tulving et al., 1994). The asymmetries observed in neuroimaging studies were based on the fact that most studies at the time used verbal material. Miller et al. (2002) found in split-brain patients that manipulating the encoding of words led to greater effects in the left hemisphere than the right, and that manipulating the encoding of faces led to greater effects in the right hemisphere than in the left.

Since that split-brain study, recent neuroimaging studies have confirmed that encoding and retrieval asymmetries are primarily due to the type of stimuli used and not the general hemispheric differences in processing (Wig et al., 2004).

Despite some unique specialization in the right hemisphere, breaking up the right hemisphere is not hard to do for the left hemisphere.

Although some effects due to the callosotomy surgery have been observed (e.g., Phelps et al., 1991, found impairments in free recall but not in recognition performance on some memory tasks that may be due to limitations in strategic and search processes imposed by the severing of the corpus callosum), most functions remain intact after the right hemisphere is disconnected from the left, including verbal IQ (Nass and Gazzaniga, 1987; Zaidel, 1990), and many problem-solving skills (LeDoux et al., 1977). However, in some cases, problems with higher order cognitive processes such as concept formation, reasoning, and problem solving with limited social insight have been observed (Brown and Paul, 2000).

The disconnection does not seem to affect another critical component of our conscious system, the "interpreter" (Gazzaniga and Miller, 2009).

Conclusions

Some authors consider the activity of the corpus callosum to have an inhibitory role (Eidelberg, 1969; Jeeves, 1986). It allows each hemisphere to apply an inhibiting action on its homologous, with the purpose of controlling a given function. This reciprocal inhibition avoids the duplication of functions (Dennenberg, 1981). The inhibiting model was suggested in order to explain the development of a domination of the contralateral tract over the ipsilateral fibres in motor and sensitive systems (Dennis, 1976).

However, the inhibiting role of the corpus callosum in the ontogenesis of hemispheric specialization has not yet been confirmed (Lassonde et al., 1990; Jeeves, 1994).

In the context of epilepsy pathogenesis, it was common to mention that the callous tract had a facilitating action (Bremer, 1966; Geoffroy et al., 1986). This affirmation supports the fact that a section of the corpus callosum determines not only the abolishment of bilateral propagation, but also a decrease or ceasing of epileptic discharge in the initial focal (Bogen and Vogel, 1962; Geoffroy et al., 1986; Lassonde et al., 1996). This is due to the fact that influxes from the intact hemisphere would moderate the activity of abnormal cells and the propagation of epileptic discharge to the healthy hemisphere through retroaction (Bremer, 1966, 1967; Lassonde, 1986).

On the other hand, clinical observations show that the corpus callosum is significantly involved in a functional reorganizing after a cerebral aggression. Thus, speech recovery, observed in patients with left hemispheric lesions is severely limited if produced at the same time as a lesion of the corpus callosum (Goldstein, 1948; Russel, 1963). As an assembly, these data suggest that the intact hemisphere could facilitate a better function of the damaged hemisphere through the effect of the corpus callosum (Lassonde et al., 1996).

In the case of patients with unilateral lesions and bilateral symptoms, the reciprocal transcallous facilitation may disrupt a well functioning intact hemisphere.

However, it is highly probable that the normal interhemispheric regulating process depends both on the inhibiting influences and on the stimulating ones (Lassonde et al., 1996). In this context, Berlucchi (1983) claims that the function of the corpus callosum is to equilibrate the activity of the two hemispheres and to allow an optimal integration of cortical activity.

The callous disconnection has an important role in the explanation of syndromes such as apraxia of limbs, pure alexia and unilateral agraphia.

The consequences of a callous lesion in adults are at the same time complex but relatively discrete. At first sight, they are not a major handicap and are compatible with a normal life and daily activity, if not associated with hemispheric lesions (Habib, 1996), ideomotor apraxia, left unilateral anomia and agraphia, right constructive apraxia, hemialexia and other manifestations given by a deficit of informational transfer between hemispheres that can pass unnoticed if not specifically searched for.

Consequently, even though after a callosotomy the behavior is almost unchanged, investigations revealed the capacity of each hemisphere and confirmed the hypothesis based on studies conducted on normal patients as well as those based on studies conducted on patients with focal lesions.

The most systematic investigations of hemispheric specialty and integration have been performed in patients with callosotomies (split-brain patients) in order to remove intractable epilepsy. Initial studies confirmed the affirmations of neurologists who claim that the left hemisphere is dominant for speech while the right hemisphere cannot name and "cannot describe objects presented visually or tactile", although it is capable of performing certain visual tasks. Experiments help with a better understanding of perceptual, cognitive, mnemonic and linguistic processes and with a better integration of these concepts in a coherent thinking and behavior.

The isolated right hemisphere cannot read, write or speak although it has an entire variety of conscious behaviours. A dissociation of the left hand by tactile anomia and agraphia indicates a minor linguistic capacity of the right hemisphere. The ability to understand visual and audio language can contribute to selecting aphasic and alexic patients.

Other observations show that the right hemisphere can participate in recovering aphasia in a long term, but the highest interest is represented by studying patients with callosotomies and investigating the basics of hemispheric cognition and integration of diverse perceptual sensorial and emotional information in a single behavioral plan. The independent function of hemispheres proved the important role played by the verbal left hemisphere in observing and interpreting of self action and recognizing emotional statuses.

It is worth noticing as far as the emotional functions, besides alexithymia, are concerned, that the callous lesion does not lead to obvious changes in affection and personality.

All in all, the callous syndrome remains a relatively homogenous entity, independent of the nature of the callous lesion.

REFERENCES

Aboitiz F, Scheibel AB, Fisher RS, Zaidel E, Fiber composition of the human corpus callosum. Brain Res 598; 143-153, 1992.

Adams RD, Victor M, Ropper AH, *Principles of Neurology*. Sixth Edition. McGraw-Hill, New York, St Louis, San Francisco etc.; 483, 1997.

Akelaitis AJ, Studies on the corpus callosum: Higher visual functions in each homonymous field following complete section of the corpus callosum. Arch Neurol Psychiatr 45; 788, 1941.

Akelaitis AJ, Studies on the corpus callosum. VII. Study of language function (tactile and visual lexia and graphia) unilaterally following section of the corpus callosum. Journal of Neuropathology and Experimental Neurology 2; 226-262, 1943.

Akelaitis AJ, A study of gnosis, praxis, and language following section of the corpus callosum and anterior commissure. J Neurosurg 7; 94-102, 1944.

Akelaitis AJ, Studies of the corpus callosum. IV. Diagnostic dyspraxia in epileptics following partial and complete section of the corpus callosum. Am J Psychiatr 101; 594-599, 1945.

Alexander MP, Warren RL, Localization of callosal auditory pathways: a CT case study. Neurology 38; 802-804, 1988.

Alpers BJ, Grant FC, The clinical syndromes of the corpus callosum. Arch Neurol Psychiatry 25; 67-86, 1931.

Andermann E, Andermann F, Nagy R, et al., Genetic studies of the Andermann syndrome. In: Lassonde, M, Jeeves MA (eds), *Callosal Agenesis – A Natural Split Brain? Advances in Behavioral Biology*. New York, London: Plenium Press; 31-38, 1994.

Anderson RC, Ghaton S, Feldstein NA, Surgical approaches to tumors of the lateral ventricle. Neurosurg. Clin N Am 14; 509-525, 2003.

Antunes JL, Louis, Ganti SR, Coloid cysts of the third ventricle. Neurosurgery 7; 450-455, 1980.

Apuzzo MLJ, Chikovani OK, Gott PS, et al., Transcallosal, interfornicial approaches for lesions affecting the third ventricle: Surgical considerations and consequences. Neurosurgery 10; 547-554 1982.

Arndt S, Berger DE, Cognitive mode and asymmetry in cerebral functioning. Cortex 14; 78-86, 1978.

Assal F, Schwartz S, Vuilleumier P, Moving with or without will: functional neural correlates of alien hand syndrome. Ann Neurol. 62; 301-307, 2007.

Augustine JR, *Human Neuroanatomy*. An introduction. Academic Press, Amsterdam, Boston, Heidelberg, etc., 2008.

Baars BJ, The brain. In: VJ Baars and NM Gage (eds). *Cognition, Brain, and Consciousness. Introduction to cognitive Neuroscience*. Academic Press. Elsevier. Amsterdam, Boston Heidelberg etc., 121-146, 2007.

Barbizet J, Duizabo P, Les syndromes de dysconexion interhemispheriques. Dans : *Abrégé de Neuropychologia*. 3ᵉ édition révisés. Paris: Masson: 115-126, 1985.

Bauer RM, McDonald, Auditory agnosia and amusia. In: TE Feinberg and MJ Farah (eds), *Behavioral neurology and neuropsychology*. New York: McGraw-Hill, 2003.

Baynes K, Gazzaniga MS, Callosal disconnection. In: TE Feinberg and MJ Farah (eds), *Behavioral Neurology and Neuropsychology* McGraw Hill. New York, St Louis, San Francisco, etc. 419-425, 1997.

Baynes K, Gazzaniga MS, Consciousness, introspection, and the split brain: the two minds / one body problem. In: MS Gazzaniga (ed.), *The new cognitive neurosciences (2nd ed)*, Cambridge; MA; MIT Press, 2000.

Baynes K, Tramo MJ, Gazzaniga MS, Reading with a limited lexicon in the right hemisphere of a callosotomy patient. Neuropsychologia 30; 187-200, 1992.

Baynes K, Funnell MG, Fowler CA, Hemispheric contributions to the integration of visual and auditory information in speech perception. Percept Psychophys 55; 633-641, 1994.

Baynes K, Wessinger CM, Fendrich R, Gazzaniga MS, The emergence of the capacity to name left visual field stimuli in a callosotomy patient implications for functional plasticity. Neuropsychologia 33; 1225-1242, 1995.

Baynes K, Eliassen JC, Lutsep H, Gazzaniga MS, Modular organization of cognitive systems masked by interhemispheric integration. Science 280; 902-905, 1998.

Belger A, Banich MT, Costs and benefits of integrating information between the cerebral hemispheres : A computational perspective. Neuropsychology 12; 380-398, 1998.

Benson DF, Alexia. In: Vinken PJ, Bruyn CW (eds). *Handbook of Clinical Neurology.* Amsterdam, Elsevier – Biomedical, 1985.

Bentin S, Sahar A, Moscovitch M, Intermanual information transfer in patients with lesions in the trunk of the corpus callosum. Neuropsychology 22; 601-611, 1984.

Benton AL, The amusias, In: M Critchley and RA Henson (eds), *Music and the brain.* London: William Heinemann, 1977.

Benton A, *Exploring the History of Neuropsychology.* Selected Papers. Oxford University Press, 2000.

Berger JM, Perret E, Interhemispheric integration in a surface estimation task. Neuropsychologia 24; 743-746, 1986.

Berger JM, Perret E, Zimmermann A, Interhemispheric integration of compound nouns: Effects of stimulus arrangement and mode of presentation. Perceptual and Motor Skills 65; 663-671, 1987.

Berlucchi G, Anatomical and physiological aspects of visual functions of the corpus callosum. Brain Res 37; 371-392, 1972.

Berlucchi G, Two hemispheres but one brain, Behav Brain Sci 6; 173-179, 1983.

Berlucchi G, Commissurotomy studies in animal. In: Boller F and Grafman J (eds), *Handbook of Neuropsychology.* Vol 4. Elsevier. Amsterdam; 9-49, 1990.

Berlucchi G, Filipo C, Di Stefano M, Tassinari G, Influence of spatial stimulus response compatibility on reaction time of ipsilateral and contralateral hand to lateralized light stimuli. Human perception and performance. J Exper Psychol 3; 505-517, 1977.

Bernstein JJ, Woodard CA, Glioblastoma cells do not introvasate into blood vessels. Neurosurgery 36; 124-132, 1995.

Bever TG, Chiarello RJ, Cerebral dominance in musicians and nonmusicians. Science 185; 537-539, 1974.

Bignami A, Sulle alteragione del corpo calloso e della commissura anteriore ritrovate in un alcoolista. Policlinico (sei part) 14; 460, 1907.

Biran I, Chatterjee A, Alien hand syndrome. Arch Neurol 61; 292-294, 2004.

Bodamer J, Die Prosopagnosie. Arch Psychiatr Nervenkr 179; 6, 1947.

Bogen J, Cerebral commissurotomy: a second case report. JAMA 194; 1328-1329, 1965.

Bogen JE, The other side of the brain: I. Dysgraphia and dyscopia following cerebral commissurotomy. Bull Los Angeles Neurp Soc 34; 73-105, 1969.

Bogen JE, Hemispherectomy and the placing reactions in cats. In: Kinsbourne M, Smith WL (eds); *Hemispheric Disconnection and Cerebral Function.* Springfield, IL, Charles C Thomas, 1974.

Bogen JE, Linguistic function in the short term following cerebral commissurotomy. In: Avakian -Whitaker H, Whitaker HA (eds), *Studies in Neurolinguistics*. Vol. 2. New York. Academic Press; 193-224, 1976.

Bogen JE, The callosal syndrome. In: Heilman KM, Valenstein E (eds), *Clinical Neuropsychology*. New York, Oxford University Press; 308-359, 1978.

Bogen JE, Split-brain syndrome. In: PJ Vinken, GW Bruyn, and HI Klawans (eds), *Handbook of clinical neurology*. New York : Elsevier, 1985 a.

Bogen JE, The stabilized syndrome of hemisphere disconnection. In: Benson DF, Zaidel E (eds); *The Dual Brain: Hemispheric Specialization in the Human*. New York. Guilford Press, 1985 b.

Bogen JE, Les callosal syndrome. In: KM Heilman, and E Valetein (eds), *Clinical Neuropsychology*. New York: University Press; 308-359, 1985.

Bogen JE, Psychological Consequences of complete or partial commissural section. In: Apuzzo LMI (ed.), *Surgery of the Third Ventricle*. Williams and Wilkins, Baltimore; 175-194, 1987.

Bogen JE, Vogel PJ, Cerebral commissurotomy in man. Bull Los Angeles Neurol Soc 27; 169-172, 1962.

Bogen JE, Gazzaniga MS, Cerebral commissurotomy in man: Minor hemisphere dominance for certain visuospatial functions. J Neurosurg 23; 394-399, 1965.

Bogen JF, Bogen GM, The other side of the brain: The corpus callosum and creativity. Bull Los Angeles Neurol Soc 34; 191-220, 1969.

Bogen JE, Campbell A, Thompson A, Long-term persistence of unilateral anomia following complete cerebral commissurotomy. Proc Soc Neurosci 7; 945, 1981.

Botez M, Bogen JE, The grasp reflex of the foot and related phenomena in the absence of other reflex abnormalities following cerebral commissurotomy. Acta Neurol Scand 54; 453-463, 1976.

Botez MI, Botez T, Les amusies. In : MI Botez (ed.), *Neuropsychologie clinique et neurologie du comportement* (2ᵉᵐᵉ ed). Montreal: Les Presses de l'Université du Montréal, 1996.

Bouchet A, Cuilleret J, Anatomice topographique descriptive et fonctionnelle. I. Le système nerveux controle la face, la tête et les organes de sens. Lyon, Villeurbaine, Paris: Simep 194-199, 1983.

Bradshaw JL, Nettleton NC, *Human Cerebral Asymmetry*. Englewood, Cliffs, NJ, Prentice-Hall, 1983.

Bradshaw JL, Mattingley JB, *Clinical Neuropsychology. Behavioral and Brain Science*. Academic Press. San Diego, Boston, New York etc. 187-205, 1995.

Breitling D, Guenther W, Rondot P, Auditory perception of music measured by brain electrical activity mapping. Neuropsychologia 25; 765-774, 1987.

Bremer F, Étude électrophysiologique d'un transfert interhémisphérique callosal. Arch Ital Biol 104; 1-29, 1966.

Bremer F, La physiologie du corps calleux à la lumière de travaux recents. Laval Medical 38; 835-843, 1967.

Brion S, Jedynak CP, Sémiologie calleuse dans les tumeurs et les malformations vasculaire. Dans: Michel F, Schott B (ed.), *Les syndromes de disconexion calleuse chez l'homme*. Lyon: Presses de l'imprimérie JP: 253-265, 1975.

Brion S, Jedynak CP, *Les troubles du transfer interhémisphérique*. Congrès de Psychiatrie et de Neurologie. Nîmes: Masson, Paris, 1975.

Broca P, Sur le siège de la faculté du language articulé. Bull Soc Anthrop (Paris) 6; 377-393, 1865.

Brodal A, *Neurological Anatomy* (3rd ed.) New York: Oxford University Press, 1981.

Brown WS, Paul LK, Cognitive and psychosocial deficits in agenesis of the corpus callosum with normal intelligence. Cognitive Neuropsychiatry 5; 135-137, 2000.

Cairns HR, Disturbances of consciousness with lesions of the brain stem and diencephalon. Brain 75; 109-146, 1952.

Campbell AL, Bogen JE, Smith A, Disorganization and reorganization of cognitive and sensorimotor functions in cerebral commissurotomy: Compensatory roles of the forebrain commissures. Brain 104; 493-511, 1980.

Carpenter MB, *Human Neuroanatomy.* Seventh Edition. The Williams and Wilkins Company. Baltimore, 1979.

Clarici C, Heppner F, The operative approach to lipoma of the corpus callosum. Neurochirurgia 22; 77-81, 1979.

Clark CR, Geffen GM, Corpus callosum surgery and recent memory. Brain 112; 165-175, 1989.

Clarke JM, McCann CM, Zaidel E, The corpus callosum and language. Anatomical - behavioral relationships. In: M Beeman and Chiarello (eds), *Right hemisphere language comprehension. Perspectives from cognitive neuroscience.* Mahwah, NJ: Erlbaum, 1998.

Colonier M, Notes on the early history of the corpus callosum with an introduction to the morphological papers published in this festschrift. In: F Lepore, M Ptito and H H Jasper (eds). *Two Hemispheres – One Brain.* New York : Liss, 1986.

Coltheart M, Deep Dyslexia: A right hemisphere hypothesis. In: Coltheart M, Patterson KF, Marshall JC (eds): *Deep Dyslexia.* London; Routledge, 1980.

Corballis MC, Sergent J, Imagery in a commissurotomized patient. Neuropsychologia 26; 13-26, 1988.

Corballis PM, Funnell MG, Gazzaniga MS, A dissociation between spatial and identity matching in callosotomy patients. Neuroreport 10; 2183-2187, 1999.

Corballis PM, Fendrich R, Shapley R, Gazzaniga MS, Illusory contours and amodal completion: Evidence for a functional dissociation in callosotomy patients. J Cogn Neurosci 11; 459-466, 1999.

Coslett HB, Saffran EM, Evidence for presumed reading in "pure alexia". Brain 112; 327-259, 1989.

Cronin-Golomb A, Subcortical transfer of cognitive information in subjects with complete forebrain commissurotomy. Cortex 22; 499-519, 1986.

Cusik CG, Kaas JH, Interhemispheric connections of cortical sensory and motor representations in primates. In: Lepore F, Ptito M, Jasper HH (eds), *Two hemispheres: One Brain: Functions of the corpus callosum.* Alen R Liss. New York; 83-102, 1986.

Damasio A, Pure alexia. Trends Neurosci 6; 93-96, 1983.

Damasio H, Damasio AR, Paradoxic ear extinction in dichotic listening: possible anatomic significance. Neurology 29; 644-653, 1979.

Damasio AR, Damasio H, The anatomic basis of pure alexia. Neurology 33; 1573-1583, 1983.

Damasio AR, Chui HC, Corbet J, Kassel N, Posterior callosal section in a nonepileptic patient. J Neurosurg Psychiatr 43; 351-356, 1980.

Damasio AR, Damasio H, van Goesen GW, Prosopagnosia: Anatomic basis and behavioral mechanisms. Neurology 32; 331, 1982.

Dănăilă L, Golu M, *Handbook of Neuropsychology,* Vol. II (Tratat de neuropsihologie) Editura Medicala, Bucharest, 2006.

Dănăilă L, Golu M, Tratat de neuropsihologie, Vol. 1, București, Editura Medicală, 2002.

Dănăilă L, Golu M, Role of the interaction of the two cerebral hemispheres in the integration of the language system. Rev Roum Sci Sociales - Série de Psychologie 31; 87-99 1987.

Dănăilă L, Petrescu AD, Rădoi MP, Tumors of the third ventricle. The 7th National Congress of Romanian Society of Neurosurgery. Cluj-Napoca, 28 Septembrie - 2 Octombrie Abstracts PC 13, 2010.

Degas JD, Gray F, Louarn T, et al., Posterior callosal infarction. Clinico-pathological correlation. Brain 110; 1155-1171, 1987.

Déjérine J, Contribution à l'étude anatomo-pathologique et clinique des différentes variétés de cécité verbale. Mémoires de la Société de Biologie 4, 61-90, 1892.

Déjérine J, Roussy G, Le syndrome thalamique. Rev Neurol 12; 521-532, 1906.

Dennenberg VH, Hemispheric laterality in animals and the effects early experience. Behav Brain Sci 4; 1-21, 1981.

Dennis M, Impaired sensory and motor differentiation with corpus callosum agenesis: a lack of callosal inhibition during ontogeny? Neuropsychologia 14; 455-469 1976.

Desai KI, Nadkarni TD, Muzumdar DP, Goel AH, Surgical management of colloid cyst of the third ventricle – a study of 105 cases. Surgical Neurology 57; 295-302, 2002.

Diamond SJ, Scammel RE, Brouwers EYM, Functions of the centre section (trunk) of corpus callosum in man. Brain 100; 543-562, 1977.

Di Stefano MR, Sauerwein HC, Lassonde M, Influence of anatomical factors and spatial compatibility on the stimulus response relationship in the absence of the corpus callosum. Neuropsychologia 302; 177-185, 1992.

Downer JL, Changes in visual gnostic functions and emotional behavior following unilateral temporal pole damage in the "split-brain" monkey. Nature 191; 50-51, 1961.

Duvernoy HM, *The human hippocampus*. Springer-Verlag, Berlin. Heidelberg, 1998.

Eidelberg E, Calosal and non-callosal connections between the sensory-motor cortices in cat and monkey. Electroenceph Clin Neurophysiol 26; 557-563, 1969.

Elberger AJ, The functional role of the corpus callosum in the developing visual system. A review. Prog Neurobiol 18; 15-79, 1982.

Efron R, Bogen JE, Yung EW, Perception of dichotic chords by normal and commissurotomized human subjects. Cortex 13; 137-149, 1977.

Ellenberg L, Sperry RW, Capacity for holding sustained attention following commissurotomy. Cortex 15; 421-438, 1979.

Erickson TC, "Spread of Epileptic Discharge", Archives of Neurology and Psychiatry 43; 429-452, 1940.

Eviator Z, Zaidel E, The effects of words length and emotionality on hemispheric contribution to lexical discution. Neuropsychologia 29; 415-428, 1991.

Fabri M, Polonara M, De Pesce A, et al., Posterior corpus callosum and interhemispheric transfer of somatosensory information: An fMRI and neuropsychological study of a partially callosotomized patient. Journal of Cognitive Neuroscience 13; 1071-1079, 2001.

Fantie B, Kolb B, Tasks traditionally used to assess callosal function reveal performance deficits associated with mild head injury. Neuroscience Abstracts 15; 132, 1989.

Ferguson SM, Some neuropsychiatric observations on behavioral consequences of corpus callosum section. In: Reeves A (ed): *Epilepsy and the corpus callosum.* New York Plenum, 1985.

Fergusson SM, Rayport M, Corrie WS, Neuropsychiatric observations on behavioral consequences of corpus callosum section for seizure control. In: Reeves AG (ed), *Epilepsy and the corpus callosum.* Plenum Press, New York; 501-514, 1985.

Forster BA, Corballis PM, Corballis MC, Effect of luminance on successiveness discrimination in the absence of the corpus callosum. Neuropsychologia 38; 441-450, 2000.

Fornari M, Savoiardo M, Morello G, et al., Meningiomas of the lateral ventricles. J Neurosurg 54; 64-74, 1981

Frith CD, Blakemore SJ, Wolpert DM, Abnormalities in the awareness and control of action. Philosophical Transactions of the Royal Society of London 355; 1771-1788, 2000.

Funnell MG, Corballis PM, Gazzaniga MS, A deficit in perceptual matching in the left hemisphere of a callosotomy patient. Neuropsychologia 38; 441-450, 1999.

Gaede SE, Parsons OA, Berters JH, Hemispheric differences in music perception: aptitude vs. experience. Neuropsychologia 16; 369-373, 1978.

Gaillard F, Synergie neuro-cognitive: Avantage dans les apprentissages en lecture et calcul. Approche Neuropsychologique des Apprentissages chez l'Enfant 2; 4-9, 1990.

Galin D, Diamond R, Herron J, Development of crossed and uncrossed tactile localization on the finger. Brain Lang 4; 588-590, 1977.

Galin D, Johnstone J, Nakell L, Herron J, Development of the capacity for tactile information transfer between hemispheres in normal children. Science 204; 1330-1332, 1979.

Gazzaniga MS, *The Bisected Brain.* Appleton Century Crafts. New York, 1970.

Gazzaniga MS, Right Hemisphere language following brain bisection: A 20 year perspective. Am Psychol 38; 525-537, 1983.

Gazzaniga MS, *Social Brain.* New York: Basic Books, 1985.

Gazzaniga MS, Cerebral Specialization and interhemispheric communication. Does the corpus callosum enable the human condition? Brain 123; 1293-1326, 2000.

Gazzaniga MS, Forty-five years of split-brain research and still going strong. Not Rev Neurosci 6; 653-659, 2005.

Gazzaniga MS, Sperry RW, Language after section of the cerebral commissure. Brain 90; 131-148, 1967.

Gazzaniga MS, LeDoux JE, *The Integrated Mind.* New York, Plenum, 1978.

Gazzaniga MS, Smylie CS, Facial recognition and brain asymmetries: Clues to underlying mechanisms. Ann Neurol 13; 536-540, 1983.

Gazzaniga MS, Miller GA, The recognition of antonymy by a language enriched right hemisphere. J Comp Neurosci 1; 187-193, 1989.

Gazzaniga MS, Smylie CS, Hemispheric mechanisms controlling voluntary and spontaneous facial expressions. J Cogn Neurosci 2; 239-245, 1990.

Gazzaniga MS, Miller MB, The left hemisphere does not miss the right hemisphere. In: Laureys S and Tononi G (eds), *The Neurology of Conciousness.* Academic Press. Elsevier Amsterdam, Boston, Heidelberg etc., 261-270, 2009.

Gazzaniga MS, Bogen JF, Sperry RW, Some functional effects on sectioning the cerebral commissures in man. Proc. Natl. Acad Sci USA 48; 1765-1769, 1962.

Gazzaniga MS, Bogen LE, Sperry RW, Observations on visual perception after disconnexion of the cerebral hemispheres in man. Brain 88; 221-236, 1965.

Gazzaniga MS, Bogen JE, Sperry RW, Dyspraxia following division of the cerebral commissures. Arch Neurol 16; 606-612, 1967.

Gazzaniga MS, Risse GL, Springer SP, et al., Psychologic and neurologic consequences of partial and complete cerebral commissurotomy. Neurology 25; 10-15, 1975.

Gazzaniga MS, Nass R, Reeves A, Roberts D, Neurologic perspectives on right hemisphere language following surgical section of the corpus callosum. Semin Neurol 4; 126-135, 1984.

Gazzaniga MS, Smylie CS, Baynes K, et al., Profiles of right hemisphere language and speech following brain bisection. Brain Lang 22; 206-220, 1984.

Gazzaniga MS, Kutas M, Van Patten C, Fendrich R, Human callosal function: MRI – verified neuropsychological functions. Neurology 39; 942-946, 1989.

Geffen G, Nilsson Quinn K, Teng EL, The effect of lesions of the corpus callosum on finger localization. Neuropsychologia 23; 497-514, 1985.

Geffen GM, Nilsson J, Simpson DA, Jeeves MA, The development of interhemispheric transfer of tactile information in cases of callosal agenesis. In: Lassonde M, Jeeves MA (eds), *Callosal Agenesis – A Natural Split Brain? Advances in Behavioral Biology*. New York, London: Plenium Press; 185-197, 1994.

Geoffroy G, Lassonde M, Jelisle F, Decarie M, Corpus callosotomy for control of intractable seizures in children. Neurology 33; 891-897, 1983.

Geoffroy G, Lassonde M, Saurwein H, Decarie M, Ellectivenes of corpus callosotomy for control of intractable epilepsy in children. In: Lepore F, Ptito M, Jasper HH (eds), *Two Hemispheres: One Brain*. New York: Alan Less; 361-368, 1986.

Gerber SS, Platkin B, Lipoma of the corpus callosum. J Neurosurg 57; 281-285, 1982.

Gersh F, Damasio AR, Praxis and writing of the left hand may be served by different callosal pathways. Arch Neurol 38; 634-636, 1981.

Geschwind N, Disconnection syndrome in animals and man. I. Brain 88; 237-294, 1965.

Geschwind N, Disconnection syndrome in animals and man. II. Brain 88; 585-644, 1965 a.

Geschwind N, The organization of language and the brain. Science 170; 940-944, 1970.

Geschwind N, Kaplan E, A human cerebral disconnection syndrome. Neurology 12; 675-685, 1962.

Geschwin N, Fusillo M, Color-naming defects in association with alexia. Arch Neurol 15; 137-146, 1966.

Giovannetti T, Buxbaum L J, Biran I, Chatterjee A, Reduced endogenous control in alien hand syndrome: Evidence from naturalistic action, Neuropsychologia 43; 75-88, 2005.

Goldberg G, Supplementary motor area structure and function. Review and hypotheses. Behav Brain Sci 8; 567-616, 1985.

Goldberg G, Goodwin ME, Alien hand syndrome. In: JS Kreutzer, J DeLuca, B Caplan (eds), *Encyclopedia of Clinical Neuropsychology*. Springer. New York, Dordrecht, Heidelberg, London, Vol. 1; 84-91, 2011.

Goldstein K, *Language and Language Disturbances*. New York: Grüne and Straton, 1948.

Gordon HW, Sperry RW, Lateralization of olfactory perception in the surgically separated hemispheres of man. Neuropsychologia 7; 111-120, 1968.

Gordon HW, Bogen JE, Sperry RW, Absence of disconnection syndrome in two patients with partial section of the neocommissures. Brain 94; 327-336, 1971.

Gordon HW, *Verbal and Nonverbal Cerebral Processing in Man for Audition*. Thesis. California Institute of Tehnology, 1973.

Gordon HW, Bogen JE, Hemispheric lateralization of singing after intracarotid sodium amylobarbitone. Journal of Neurology, Neurosurgery and Psychiatry 37; 727-738, 1974.

Greenblatt SH, Alexia without agraphia or hemianopsia. Brain 96; 307-316, 1973.

Greenblatt SH, Saunders RL, Culver CM, Bogdanowicz W, Normal interhemispheric transfer with incomplete section of the splenium. Arch Neurol 37; 567-571, 1980.

Guénot M, Transfer interhémisphérique et agénesie du corps calleux. Capacitées et limites de la commissure antérieure. Neurochirurgie 1 (suppl 44); 113-115, 1998.

Guillemot JP, Richer L, Prevost L, et al., Receptive field properties of somatosensory callosal fibers in the monkey. Brain Res 402; 293-302, 1987.

Guillemot JP, Lepore F, Prevost L, et al., Somatosensory receptive fields properties of fibres in the rostral corpus callosum of the cat. Brain Research 441; 221-232, 1988.

Haaland KY, Delaney HD, Motor deficit after left or right hemisphere damage due to stroke or tumor. Neuropsychologia 19; 17-27, 1981.

Habib M, Syndrome de déconexion calleuse et organisation fonctionnelle de corpus calleux chez l'adulte. Neurochirurgie 1 (suppl 44) 102-109, 1998.

Habib M, Pelletier J, Neuroanatomie functionnelle des relations interhémisphériques. Aspects théoriques et perspectives cliniques. I. organisation anatomo-fonctionnelle des connexions calleuses. Rev Neuropsychol 4; 69-112, 1994.

Habib M, Ceccaldi M, Poncet M, Syndrome de deconnexion calleuse par infarctus jonctionnel hémisphérique gauche. Revue Neurologique (Paris) 146; 19-24, 1990.

Hamilton CR, Mechanisms of interocular equivalence. In: Ingle D, Goodale M, Mansfield R (eds): *Advances in the Analysis of Visual Behavior*. Cambridge, MA, MIT Press; 693-717, 1982.

Hampson E, Kimura D, Hand movement asymmetries during verbal and nonverbal tasks. Can J Psychol 38; 102-125, 1984.

Handy TC, Gazzaniga MS, Ivry RB, Cortical and subcortical contribution to the representation of temporal information. Neuropsychologia 41; 1461-1473, 2003.

Hannequin D, Goulet P, Joanette Y, La contribution de l'hémisphère droit à la communication verbale. Raport de Neurologie, LXXXVᵉ Congrès de Psychiatrie et Neurologie de Langue Française. Masson, Paris, 1987.

Harris LJ, The corpus callosum and hemispheric communication. An historical survey of theory and research. In: FL Kitterle (ed.), *Hemispheric communication; Mechanisms and models*. Hillsdale, NJ, Erlboaum, 1995.

Hécaen H, Assal G, Revues Critiques: les relations interhémisphériques et le problème de la dominance cérébrale d'après les recherches sur les sections calleuses chez l'animal et chez l'homme. Année Psychol 73; 491-522, 1973.

Heilman KM, Apraxia. In: Heilman KM and Valenstein (eds), *Clinical Neuropsychology*. Oxford University Press. New York; 159-185, 1979.

Hommet CD, Billard C, Le syndrome calleux chez l'enfant. Neurochirurgie 1 (supl 44); 110-112, 1998.

Hoppe KD, Bogen JE, Alexinthymia in twelve commissurotomized patients. Psychotherapy and Psychosomatics 28, 148-155, 1977.

Hori A, Lipoma of the quadrigeminal plate region with evidence of congenital origin. Arch Pathol Lab Med 110; 851-951, 1986.

Huettner MIS, Rosenthal BL, Hynd GW, Regional cerebral blood flow (fCBF) in normal readers. Bilateral activation with narrative text. Archives of Clinical Neuropsychology 4; 71-78, 1989.

Imig TJ, Reale RA, Brugge JE, et al., Topography of cortico-cortical connections related to tonotopic and binaural maps of cat auditory cortex. In. Lepore F, Ptito M, Jasper HH (eds), *Two hemispheres: One Brain*. New York, Alen Liss; 75-81, 1986.

Innocenti GM, What is so special about callosal connections? In Lepore F, Ptito M, Jasper HH (eds) *Two hemispheres: One Brain*. New York, Alen Liss; 171-188, 1986.

Iwata M, Sugishita M, Toyokura Y, et al., Étude sur le syndrome de disconnexion visuo-linguale après la transection du splenium du corps calleux. J Neurol Sci 23; 421-432, 1974.

Jason GW, Hemispheric asymmetries in motor function: I. Left-hemisphere specialization for memory but not performance. Neuropsychologie 21; 35-45, 1983.

Jeeves MA, Some limits to interhemispheric integration in cases of callosal agenesis and partial commissurotomy. In: Russel IG, Von Hof MW, Berlucchi G (eds), *Structure and Functions of Cerebral Commissures*. Baltimore, University Park Press; 449-474, 1979.

Jeeves MA, Callosal agenesis: Neuronal and developmental adaptations. In: Lepore F, Ptito M, Jasper HH (eds), *Two hemispheres: One brain*. New York, Alen Liss, 403-422, 1986.

Jeeves MA, Agenesis of the corpus callosum. In: F Boller and J Grafman (eds), *Handbook of Clinical Neuropsychology*. Vol. 4, North Holland. Amsterdam: Elsevier; 9-47, 1990.

Jeeves MA, Stereoperception in callosal agenesis and partial callosotomy. Neuropsychologia 29; 19-34, 1991.

Jeeves MA, Callosal agenesis: A natural Split Brain? Overview. In: Lassonde M, Jeeves MA (eds), Advances in Behavioral Biology. New York, London: Plenum Press; 285-299, 1994.

Jellinger K, Gross H, Kaltenback E, Grisold W, Holoprosencephaly and agenesis of the corpus callosum frequency of associated malformations. Octa Neuropathol 55; 1-10, 1981.

Kazuis S, Sawanda T, Callosal apraxia without agraphia. Ann Neurol 33; 401-403, 1993.

Kihlstrom JF, Klein SB, Self-knowledge and self-awareness. In: Snodgrass JD and Thompson RL (eds). *The Self Across Psychology: Self Recognition, Self Awareness, and the Self Concept.* An NY Acad Sci 818, New York: New York Academy of science; 5-17, 1997.

Kimura D, Functional asymmetry of the brain in dichotic listening. Cortex 3; 163-178, 1967.

Kimura D, Archibold Y, Motor function of the left hemisphere. Brain 97; 337-350, 1974.

Kinsbourne M, The cerebral basis of lateral asymmetries in attention. Acta Psychol 33; 193-201, 1970.

Kinsbourne M, The control of attention by interaction between the hemispheres. In: S Konblum (ed), *Attention and Performance*. IV. Academic Press, London, 1973.

Klingler EL, *Atlas cerebri humani*. S. Karger (Suisse). New York, 1956.

Kolb B, Whishaw IQ, *Fundamentals of Human Neuropsychology*. Fifth Edition. Worth Publishers. United stated of America, 2003.

Kreuter S, Kinsbournt M, Trevarthen C, Are deconnected cerebral hemispheres independent channales? A preliminary study of the effect of unilateral loading on bilateral finger topping. Neuropsychologia 10; 453-461, 1972.

Kumkova E, Memory for birds' voices. Hemispheric specialization (abstract). Journal of Clinical and Experimental Neuropsychology 12; 42, 1990.

Kumar S, Short-term memory for a non-verbal tactual task after cerebral commissurotomy. Cortex 13; 55-61, 1977.

Lashley KS, In search of the enfram. Symposium of the Society of Experimental Biology. 4; 454-482, 1950.

Lassonde M, The facilitatory influence of the corpus callosum on intrahemispheric processing. In: F Lepore, M Ptito, HH Jasper (eds), *Two Hemispheres -- One Brain*. New York, Alen Liss, 1986.

Lassonde M, Disconnection syndrome in callosal agenesis. In: Lassonde M, Jeeves MA (eds), *Callosal agenesis. A natural Split Brain? Advances in Behavioral Biology*. New York, London, Plenum Press, 275-284, 1994.

Lassonde M, Lortie J, Ptito M, Geoffroy G, Hemispheric asymmetry in callosal agenesis as revealed by dichotic listening performance. Neuropsychologia 445-448, 1981.

Lassonde M, Ptito M, Laurencelle L, Étude tachistoscopique de la spécialization hémisphérique chez l'agenésie du corpus callosum. Rev Can Psychol 35; 527-536, 1984.

Lassonde M, Sauerwein H, Geoffroy G, Decarie M, Effects of early and late transection of the corpus callosum in children. Brain 109; 953-967, 1986.

Lassonde M, Ptito M, Lepore F, La plasticité du système calleux. Rev Can Psychol 44; 166-179, 1990.

Lassonde M, Sauerwein H, Chicoine AJ, Geoffroy G, Absence of disconnexion syndrome in callosal agenesis and early callosotomy: Brain reorganization of lack of structural specificity during antogeny? Neuropsychologia 29; 481-495, 1991.

Lassonde M, Lakmache Y, Ptito M, Lepore F, Funcţiile corpului calos. In: MI Botez (ed), *Neuropsihologie Clinică si Neurologia Comportamentului*. Ediţia a II-a. Editura Medicală Bucuresti, 253-272, 1996.

LeDoux JC, Gazzaniga MS, *The integral Mind*. New York: Plenum Press, 1978.

LeDoux JE, Risse GI, Springer SP, et al., Cognition and commissurotomy. Brain 100; 87-104, 1977.

Lepore F, Samson A, Molotchinikoff S, Effects of binocular activation of cells in visual cortex of the cat following transection of the optic tract. Expert Brain Res 50; 392, 1983.

Lepore F, Ptito M, Jasper H (eds), *Two hemispheres – One Brain*. New York: Alen Liss, 1986.

Lepore F, Ptito M, Guillemont JP, The role of the corpus callosum in midline fusion. In: Lepore F, Ptito M, Jasper HH (eds). *Two hemispheres: One brain*. New York, Alan Liss, 211-230, 1986.

Lepore F, Lassonde M, Poirier P, et al., Midline sensory integration in callosal agenesis. In: Lassonde M, Jeeves A (eds), *Callosal agenesis: A Natural Split Brain*. New York, Plenum Press; 155-169, 1994.

Levy J, Cerebral asymmetries as manifested in split-brain man. In: Kinsbourne M, Smith WL (eds.), *Hemispheric Disconnection and Cerebral Function*. Springfield. IL. Thomas, 1974.

Levy J, Trevarthen C, Metacontrol of hemispheric function in human split-brain patients. Journal of Experimental Psychology: Human Perception and Performance 2; 299-312, 1976.

Levy J, Nebes RB, Sperry RW, Expressive language in the surgically separated minor hemisphere. Cortex 7; 49-58, 1971.

Levy J, Trevarthen C, Sperry RW, Perception of bilateral chimeric figures following hemispheric deconection. Brain 95; 61-78, 1972.

Lezak MD, Howieson DB, Loring DW, *Neuropsychological Assessment*. Oxford University Press; 39-85, 2004.

Liepmann H, Das Krankheitsbild der Apraxie (motorishen Asymbolie). Monatsschr Psychiatr Neurol 8; 15-44, 102-132, 182-197, 1900.

Liepmann H, Kleine Hilfsmittel bei der Unterschung von Gehirnkrankheiten. Itsch. Med. Wachenschr 38; 1, 1905.

Liepmann H, Maas O, Fall von linkseitiger Agraphie und Apraxia bei rechtseitiger Lahmung. J Psychol Neurol 10; 214-227, 1907.

Long DM, Leibrock L, The transcallosal approach to the anterior ventricular system and its application in the therapy of cranopharyngioma. Clin Neurosurg 27; 160-168, 1980.

Luessenhop AJ, Interhemispheric commissurotomy: (The split brain operation) as an alternate to hemispherectomy for control of intractable seizures. Am Surg 36; 265-268, 1970.

Lutsep HL, Wessinger CM, Gazzaniga MS, Cerebral and callosal orgànization in a right hemisphere dominant "split-brain" subject. J Neurol Neurosurg Psychiatry 59; 50-54, 1995.

Manzoni T, Barharesi P, Bellardinelli E, Cominitti R, Callosal projections from the two body midlines. Exp Brain Res 39; 1-9, 1980.

Marchiafava E, Bignami A, Sopra un alterazione del corpo calloso osservata in soggeti alcoolisti. Rev Patol Nerv. 8; 544, 1903.

Maspes PE, Le syndrome expérimental chez l'homme de la section du splénium du corps calleux: Aléxie visuelle pure hémianopsique. Rev Neurol 80; 100-113, 1948.

Matsukado Y, MacCarty CS, Kernahan JW, The growth of glioblastoma multiforme (astrocytomas, grade 2 and 4) in neurosurgical practice. J Neurosurg 18; 636-644, 1961.

Mayer E, Koenig O, Ponshaud A, Tactual extinction without anomia: evidence of attentional factors in a patient with a partial callosal disconnection. Neuropsychologia 26; 851-868, 1988.

Mazziota JC, Phelp ME, Carson RE, Kuhl DE, Tomographic mapping of human cerebral metabolism : Auditory stimulation. Neurology 32; 921-937, 1982.

McKeever WF, Sullivan KF, Ferguson SM, Rayport M, Typical cerebral hemisphere disconnection deficits following corpus callosum section despite sparing of the anterior commissure. Neuropsychologia 19; 745-755, 1981.

McKeever WF, Sullivan KF, Ferguson SM, Rayport M, Right hemisphere speech development in the anterior commissure-spared commissurotomy patient: A second case: Clin Neuropsychol 4; 17-22, 1982.

McKenna TM, Whitsel BL, Dreyer DA, Metz CB, Organization of cat anterior parietal cortex. Relation among cytoarchitecture single neuron functional properties and interhemispheric connectivity. J Neurophysiol 45; 667-697, 1981.

Mendoza JE, Split-brain. In: JS Kreutzer, J De Luca, B Caplan (eds), *Encyclopedia of Clinical Neuropsychology*. Springer. New York. Vol. 4; 2359-2360, 2011.

Messerli P, Pegma A, Sorder N, Hemispheric dominance for melody recognition in musicians and non-musicians. Neuropsychologia 33; 395-405, 1995.

Mesulam MM, Large-scale neurocognitive network and distributed processing for attention language, and memory. Ann Neurol 28; 597-613, 1990.

Metcalfe J, Funnell M, Gazzaniga MS, Right-hemisphere memory superiority: Studies of a split-brain patient. Psychol Sci 6; 157-164, 1995.

Meyers RE, Function of corpus callosum in interocular transfer. Brain 79; 358-363, 1956.

Michel F, Peronnet F, Extinction gauche au test dichotique: Lésion hémisphérique ou lésion commissurale? In : Michel F, Schott B (eds). *Les Syndromes de Disconnexion Calleuse chez l'Homme*. Lyon, Hopital Neurologique, 1975.

Michel F, Henaff MA, Intriligator J, Two different readers in the same brain after a posterior callosal lesion. Neuroreport 7; 786-788, 1996.

Milligan BD, Meyer FD, Morbidity of transcallosal and transcortical approaches to lesions in and around the lateral and third ventricles: a single-institution experience. Neurosurgery 67; 1483-1496, 2010.

Milner B, Clues to the cerebral organization of memory. In: PA Buser and A Rougeul-Ouser (eds), *Cerebral Correlates of conscious Experience*. INSERM Symposium 6. Amsterdam. Elsevier/North-Holland, 1978.

Milner B, Analysis of memory disorder after cerebral commissurotomy. In: Trevarthen C (ed), *Essays in Honour of RW Sperry*. Cambridge, Cambridge University Press, 1985.

Milner B, Taylor L, Right hemispheric superiority in tactile pattern recognition after cerebral commissurotomy. Evidence for non-verbal memory. Neuropsychologia 10; 1-15, 1972.

Milner AD, Lines CK, Interhemispheric pathways in simple reaction time to lateralized light flash. Neuropsychologia 20; 171-179, 1982.

Milner B, Taylor L, Sperry RW, Lateralized suppression of dichotically presented digits after commissural section in man. Science 161; 184-186, 1968.

Miller MB, Kingstone A, Gazzaniga MS, Hemispheric encoding asymmetries are more apparent than real. J Cogn Neurosci 14; 702-708, 2002.

Mingazzini G, *Der Balken*. Berlin, Springer Verlag, 1922.

Mishkin M, Analogous neural models for tactile and visual learning. Neuropsychologia 17; 139-152, 1979.

Mitchel GF, Self-generated experience and the development of lateralized neurobehavioral organization in infants. Advances in the Study of Behavior 17; 61-83, 1987.

Moscovitch M, Information processing and the cerebral hemisphere. In: MS Gazzaniga (ed), *Handbook of behavioral neurobiology*, II. Neuropsychology. New York: Plenum Press, 1979.

Musier FE, Reeves AG, Effects of partial and complete corpus callosotomy an central auditory function. In: Lepore F, Ptito M, Jasper HH (eds), *Two hemispheres: One Brain*. New York. Alen Liss, 1986.

Mountcastle VB (ed) *Interhemispheric Relations and Cerebral Dominance*. Johns Hopkins Press, Baltimore, 294, 1962.

Myers RE, Functions of the corpus callosum in interocular transfer. Brain 57; 358-363, 1956.

Myers JJ, Sperry RW, Interhemispheric communication after section of the forebrain commissures. Cortex 21; 249-260, 1985.

Nakamura KK, Mishkin M, Blindness in monkeys following non-visual cortical lesions. Brain Research. 188; 572-577, 1980.

Nass RD, and Gazzaniga MS, Cerebral lateralization and specialization of human central nervous system. In: Mountcastle VB, Plum F and Geiger SR (eds), *Handbook of Physiology*, Vol. 5, Bethesda (MD): American Physiological Society. Sect 1, PT. 2; 701-761, 1987.

Nebes R, Superiority of the minor hemisphere in commissurotomized man on a test of figural unification. Brain 95; 633-638, 1972.

Nebes R, Perception of spatial relationship by the right, and left hemispheres of a commissurotomized man. Neuropsychologia; 733-349, 1973.

Nebes RD, Hemispheric specialization in commissurotomized man. Psychol Bull 81; 1-14, 1974.

Nieuwenhuys R, Meek J, The telencephalon of actinopterygion fishes. In: EG Jones and A Peters (eds). *Comparative structure and evolution of cerebral cortex*. Part I, Plenum Press. New York; 31-73, 1990.

Njiokiktjien C, Driessen M, Habraken L, Development of supination - pronation movements in children. Human Neurobiol 5; 199-203, 1986.

Ozgur MH, Johnson T, Smith A, Bogen JE, Transcallosal approach to third ventricle tumor. Case report. Bull Los Angeles Neurol Soc 42; 57-62, 1977.

Pack BC, Stewart KJ, Diamond PT, Gale SD. Posterior-variant alien hand syndrome: clinical features and response to rehabilitation. Disabil Rehabil 24; 817-818, 2002.

Pandya DN, Seltzer B, The topography of commissural fibres. In: F Lepore, M Ptito, and HH Jasper (eds.), *Two Hemispheres – One Brain*. New York: Alen Liss, 1986.

Patestas MA, Gartner LP, *A Textbook of Neuroanatomy*. New Age International Publishers. Blackwell Publishing. Main Street, Malden, USA, 2008.

Phelps EA, Gazzaniga MS, Hemispheric differences in mnemonic processing: The effects of left hemisphere interpretation. Neuropsychologia 30; 293-297, 1992.

Phelps EA, Hirst W, Gazzaniga MS, Deficits in recall following partial and complete commissurotomy. Cereb Cortex 1; 492-498, 1991.

Poirier P, Lassonde M, Lepore F, Sound localization in a callosal human listeners. Brain 116; 53-69, 1993.

Poncet M, Les séparations des hémisphères cérebraux, Neurologie 33; 539-544, 1983.

Poncet M, Habib M, Robillard A, Deep left parietal lobe syndrome: conduction aphasia and other neurobehavioral disorders due to a small subcortical lesion. J Neurosurg Psychiatr. 50; 709-713, 1987.

Powell TPS, Certain aspects of the intrinsic organization of the cerebral cortex. In: O. Pompeiano and CA Marson (eds). *Brain mechanism of perceptual awareness and purposeful behavior.* Raven Press, New York; 1-19, 1981.

Preilowski BFB, Possible contribution of the anterior forebrain commissures to bilateral motor coordination. Neuropsychologie 10; 267-277, 1972.

Preilowski B, Bilateral Motor interactions: Perceptual motor performance of partial and complete „split-brain" patients. In: KJ Zulch, O Creutzfeldt, and GC Galbraith (eds), *Cerebral localization.* Berlin and New York: Springer, 1975

Preilowski B, Intermanual transfer. Interhemispheric interaction and handedness in man and monkey. In: Trevarthen CB (eds), *Brain Circuits and Functions of the Mind.* University Press. Cambridge; 168-180, 1990.

Ptito M, Lepore F, Interocular transfer in cats with early callosal transection. Nature 301; 513-515, 1983.

Purves SJ, Woadhurst WB et al., Result of anterior corpus callosum section in 24 patients with medically intractable seizures. Neurology 38; 1194-1201, 1988.

Quin K, Geffen G, The development of tactile transfer of information. Neuropsychologia 24; 793-804, 1986.

Ramackers G, Nijokiktjien C, Pediatric Behavioral. Neurology. Vol. 3: *The child corpus callosum.* Amsterdam, Duyi Publication, 1991

Rayport M, Ferguson SM, Corrie WS, Outcomes and indications of corpus callosum section for intractable seizure control. Appl Neurophysiol 46; 47-51, 1983.

Rayport M, Carrie WS, Ferguson SM, Results of two-stage corpus callosum section for seizure control in clinically and electroencephalographically defined cases. In: Reeves A (ed); *Epilepsy and the Corpus Callosum.* New York. Plenum, 1985.

Reeves A (ed), *Epilepsy and the corpus callosum.* New York, Plenum, 1985.

Reeves AG, Behavioral changes following corpus callosotomy. In Smith D, Treiman D, Trimble M (eds). *Advances in Neurology*, Vol. 55, Raven Press, New York, 1991.

Reil JC, Mangel des Mittleren, Freyen. Theils des Balkens in Menschengehirn. Arch Physiol 11; 314-344, 1812.

Reuter-Lorenz PA, Baynes K, Modes of lexical access in the callosotomized brain. J Cogn Neurososci 4; 155-164, 1992.

Rey A, Sollicitation de la mémoire de fixation par des mots et des objects presentés simultanément. Archives de Psychologie 37; 126-139, 1959.

Risse GL, LeDoux JC, Springer SP, et al., The anterior commissure in man: Functional variation in a multisensory system. Neuropsychologia 16; 23-31, 1978.

Risse GL, Gates J, Lund G, et al., Interhemispheric transfer in patients with incomplete section of the corpus callosum: Anatomic verification with magnetic resonance imaging. Arch Neurol 46; 437-443, 1989.

Rivest J, Mitchell T, Intriligator J, Perceptual learning in the visual and auditory systems with and without attention. The Association for Research in Vision and Ophthalmology, 37, 180, 1996.

Rohmer F, Wackenheim A, Vrousos G, Les agénésies du corps calleux. In: Cossa P (ed), Comptes rendus du Congrès de Psychiatrie et de Neurologie de langue française. LVII session. Tours: Masson, 1960.

Roser ME, Fugelsang JA, Dunbar KN, et al., Dissociating causal perception and causal inference in the brain. Neuropsychology 19; 591-602, 2005.

Ross ED, Stewart RM, Akinetic mutism from hypothalamic damage: Successful treatment with dopamine agonists. Neurology (NY) 31; 1436-1439, 1981.

Ross MK, Reeves AG, Roberts DW, Postcommissurotomy mutism. Ann Neurol 16; 114, 1984.

Rudy JW, Stadler-Morris S, Development of interocular equivalence in rats trained on a distal-cue navigation task. Behavioral Neuroscience 101; 141-143, 1987.

Rugg MD, Lines CA, Milner AD, Visual evoked potentials to lateralized visual stimuli and the measurement of interhemispheric transmission time. Neuropsychologia 22; 215-225, 1984.

Russel WR, Some anatomical aspects of aphasia. Lancet 1; 1173-1177, 1963.

Salazar OM, Rubin P, The spread of glioblastoma multiforme as a determining factor in the radiation volume. Int J Radiol Oncol Biol Phys 1; 627-637, 1976.

Samson S, Zatorre RJ, Melodic and harmonic discrimination following unilateral cerebral excision. Brain and Cognition 7; 348-360, 1988.

Saul RE, Sperry RW, Absence of commissurotomy symptoms with agenesis of the corpus callosum. Neurology 18; 307, 1968.

Sauerwein H, Lassonde M, Intro- and interhemispheric processing of visual information in callosal agenesis. Neuropsychologia 21, 167-171, 1983.

Sauerwein H, Nolin P, Lassonde M, Cognitive functioning in callosal agenesis. In: Lassonde M and Jeeves MA (eds), *Callosal agenesis – A natural split brain? Advances in Behavioral Biology.* New York. London; Plenum Press, 221-233, 1994.

Scepkowski LA, Cronin-Golomb A, The alien hand: cases, categorizations, and anatomical correlates. Behav Cogn Neurosci Rev. 2; 261-277, 2003.

Schiavetto A, Lepore F, Lassonde M, Somesthetic discrimination there should be in the absence of corpus callosum. Neuropsychologia 31; 695-707, 1993.

Scherer HJ, The forms of growth in gliomas and their practical significance. Brain 63; 1-34, 1940.

Schmidt J, De oblivione lectionis ex. apoplexia salva scriptione. Miscellanea curiosa medicophysica. Academiae naturae curiosorum; 4; 195-197, 1676.

Schrift MS, Bandla H, Shah Pond, Taylor MA, Interhemispheric transfer in major psychoses. Journal of Nervous and Mental Disease 174; 203-207, 1986.

Sergent J, A new look at the human split brain. Brain 110; 1375-1392, 1987.

Sergent J, Furtive incursion into bicameral minds. Integrative and coordinating role of subcortical structures. Brain 113; 537-568, 1990.

Sergent J, Judgment of release position and distance on representations of spatial relations. Journal of Experimental Psychology: Human Perception and Performance 91; 762-780, 1991 a.

Sergent J, Processing of spatial relations within and between the disconnected cerebral hemispheres. Brain 114; 1025-1043, 1991 b.

Sergent J, Myers JJ, Manual blowing, and verbal reactions to lateralized flashes in commissurotomized patients. Perception Psychophys 37; 571-578, 1985.

Seymour SE, Reuter-Lorenz PA, Gazzaniga MS, The disconnection syndrome. Basic findings reaffirmed. Brain 117; 105-115, 1994.

Shanon B, Lateralization effects in musical decision tasks. Neuropsychologia 18; 21-31, 1980.

Shanon B, Classification of musical information presented in the right and left ear. Cortex 17; 583-596, 1981.

Shanon B, Asymmetries in musical aesthetic judgments. Cortex 20; 567-573, 1984.

Shucart WA, Stein BM, Transcallosal approach to the anterior ventricular system. Neurosurgery 3; 339-343, 1978.

Sidtis JJ, Volpe BT, Wilson DH, et al., Variability in right hemisphere language function after callosal section: Evidence for a continuum of generative capacity. J Neurosci 1; 323-331, 1981.

Sidtis JJ, Volpe BT, Hotzman JD, et al., Cognitive interaction after staged callosal section: Evidence for transfer of semantic activation. Science 212; 344-346, 1981.

Sparks R, Geschwind N, Dichotic listening in man after section of neocortical commissures. Cortex 4; 3-16, 1968.

Sparks R, Goodglass H, Niskel B, Ipsilateral versus contralateral extinction in dichotic listening from hemispheric lesions. Cortex 6; 249-260, 1970.

Spencer SS, Spencer DD, Williamson PD, et al., Corpus callosum for epilepsy. II. Neuro-psychologicial outcome. Neurology 38; 24-28, 1988.

Sperry RW, Neural basis of the spontaneous optokinetic response produced by visual inversion; I. Camp Physiol Psychol 43; 482-489, 1950.

Sperry RW, Cerebral organization and behavior. Science 1933; 1949 -1757, 1961.

Sperry RW, Some general aspects of interhemispheric integration. In: VB Mountcastle (ed.). *Interhemispheric Relations and Cerebral Dominance*. John Hopkins Press. Baltimore. Ch 3, 43-49, 1962.

Sperry RW, Lateral specialization in the surgically separated hemispheres. In: FO Schmitt and FG Worden (eds), *Neurosciences: Third Study Program*. Cambridge, MA: MIT Press, 1974.

Sperry RW, Changing concepts of consciousness and free will. Perspectives in Biology and Medicine 20; 9-12, 1976.

Sperry RW, Consciousness, personal identity, and the divided brain. In: F Lepore, M Ptito, HH Jasper (eds) *Two hemispheres: One brain*. New York, Alen Liss; 3-20, 1986.

Sperry RW, Forebrain commissurotomy and conscious awareness. In: CB Trevarthen and RW Sperry (eds), *Brain circuits and functions of the mind*. Cambridge : Cambridge University Press, 1990.

Sperry RW, Gazzaniga MS, Bogen JE, Interhemispheric relationship: The neocortical commissure: syndrome of hemisphere disconnection. In: Vinken PJ, Bruyn GW (eds), *Handbook of Clinical Neurology*. Vol. 4. Amsterdam. Elsevier; 273-290, 1969.

Sperry RW, Zaidel E, Zaidel D, Self – recognition and social awareness in the deconnected minor hemisphere. Neuropsychologia 17; 153-166, 1979.

Springer S, Gazzaniga MS, Dichotic testing of partial and complete commissurotomized patients. Neuropsychologia 13, 341-346, 1975.

Sugishita M, Toyokura Y, Yoshioka M, Unilateral agraphia after section of the posterior half of the truncus of the corpus callosum. Brain Lang 9; 215-225, 1980.

Sugishita M, Shinohara A, Shimoji T, Does a posterior lesion of the corpus callosum cause hemialexia? In: Reeves A (ed.), *Epilepsy and the Corpus Callosum*. New York, Plenum Press, 1985.

Sumner P, Husain M, At the edge of consciousness: automatic motor activation and voluntary control. The Neuroscientist 14, 474-486, 2008.

Sylver PH, Jeeves MA, Motor coordination in callosal agenesis. In: Lassonde M, Jeeves MA (eds). *Callosal agenesis – A natural split-brain? Advances in Behavioral Biology*. New York. London: Plenum Press, 207-219, 1994.

Tanaka Y, Yoshida A, Kawahata N, Hashimoto R, Obayashi T, Diagnostic dyspraxia. Clinical characteristics, responsible lesion and possible underlying mechanism. Brain 119; 859-873, 1996.

Temple CM, Ilsley J, Sounds and shapes: Language and spatial cognition in callosal agenesis. In: Lassonde M, Jeeves MA (eds). *Callosal agenesis – A natural split-brain? Advances in Behavioral Biology*. New York. London: Plenum Press; 261-273, 1994.

Teng EL, Dichotic ear difference is a poor index for the functional asymmetry between the cerebral hemispheres. Neuropsychologia 19; 235-240, 1981.

Ten Houten W, Hoppe K, Bogen J, Walter D, Alexinthymia: an experimental study of cerebral commissurotomy patients and normal control subjects. Am J Psychiatry, 143, 312-316, 1986.

Trescher JR, Ford FR, Colloid cyst of the third ventricle. Report of a case, operative removal with section of posterior half of corpus callosum. Arch Neurol Psychiat 37; 959-973, 1937.

Trevarthen C, Hemispheric specialization. In: *Handbook of Physiology – The Nervous System III*. Washington DC, American Society of Physiology; 1129-1190, 1984.

Tulving E, Kapur S, Craik EM, et al., Hemispheric encoding / retrieval asymmetry in episodic memory: Positron emission tomography findings. Proc Natl Acad Sci USA 91; 2016-2020, 1994.

Turk DJ, Heatherton TF, Macrae CN, et al., Out of contact, out of mind: The distributed nature of self. Ann NY Acad Sci 1001; 65-78, 2003.

Van Gijn J, *Plantar Reflex*. Rotterdam Krips Repro-Meppel, 1977.

Van Wagenen WP, Herren RY, Surgical division of commissural pathways in the corpus callosum. Relation to spread of an epileptic seizure. Arch Neuro Psychiatr 44; 470-759, 1940.

Velut S, Destrieux C, Kakou M, Anatomie morphologique du corps calleux. Neurochirurgie 1 (suppl 44); 17-30, 1998.

Versalius A, De humani corporis fabrica librarum epitome. Baselieae: Joannis Opporini, 1543.

Volpe BT, Sidtis JJ, Hotzman JB, et al, Cortical mechanisms involved in praxis. Observations following partial and complete section of the corpus callosum in man. Neurology 32; 645-650, 1982.

Wainright H, Bowen R, Radcliffe M, Lipoma of corpus callosum associated with dysraphic lesions and trisomy 13. Am J Med Genet 57; 10-13, 1995.

Watson RT, Heilman KM, Callosal apraxia. Brain 106; 391-403, 1983.

Wechsler AF, Transient left hemialexia. Neurology (NY) 22; 628-633, 1972.

Weissman DH, Banich MT, The cerebral hemispheres cooperate to perform complex but not simple tasks. Neuropsychology 14; 41-59, 2000.

Wernicke C, *Der Aphasische Symptomencomplex*. Breslau: Cohn und Weigert, 1874.

Wig G, Miller MB, Kingstone A, Kelley W, Separable routes to human memory formation: Dissociating task and material contributions in prefrontal cortex. J Cogn Neurosci 16; 139-148, 2004.

Wilson DW, Culver C, Waddington M, Gazzaniga M, Disconnection of the cerebral hemisphere: an alternative to hemispherectomy for the control of intractable seizures. Neurology 25; 1149-1153, 1975.

Wilson DH, Reeves A, Gazzaniga M, Culver C, Cerebral commissurotomy for control of intractable seizures. Neurology (NY) 27; 708-715, 1977.

Winkler PA, Weis S, Buttner A, et al., The transcallosal interforniceal approach to the third ventricle: Anatomic and microsurgical aspects. Neurosurgery 40; 973-982, 1997.

Winston KR, Cavazzuti A, Arkins T, Absence of neurological and behavioral abnormalities after anterior transcallosal operation for third ventricular lesions. Neurosurgery 4; 386-393, 1979.

Wisniewski KE, Jeret JS, Callosal agenesis: A review of the clinical, pathological and cytogenetic features. In: M Lassonde and MA Jeeves (Eds.), *Callosal agenesis: A natural split brain?* (1-6). New York: Plenum Press, 1994.

Witelson SF, Wire of the mind: Anatomical variation in the corpus callosum in relation to hemispheric specialization and integration. In: F Lepore, M Ptito, and HH Jasper (eds). *Two Hemispheres – One Brain*. New York: Alen Liss, 1986.

Witelson SF, Hand and sex differences in the isthmus and genu of human corpus callosum: A postmortem morphological study. Brain 112; 799-835, 1989.

Witelson SF, Neuroanatomical bases of hemispheric functional specialization in the human brain: Possible developmental factors. In: FL Kitterle (ed), *Hemispheric communication: Mechanisms and models*. Hillsdale NJ: Erlbaum, 1995.

Yakovlev PI, Lecours AR, The myelogenetic cycles of regional maturation of the brain. In: A Minkowski (ed.), *Regional Development of the Brain in Early Life*. London: Blackwell 3-65, 1967.

Yamamoto J, Rhoton AL, Peace DA, Microsurgery of the third ventricle: Part I. Neurosurgery 8; 334-356, 1981.

Yamadori A, Osumi Y, Masuhara S, Okubo M, Preservation of singing in Broca's aphasia. Journal of Neurology, Neurosurgery and Psychiatry 40; 221-224, 1977.

Young PA, Young PH, *Basic Clinical Neuroanatomy*. Williams and Wilkins, Baltimore: Lippincott, 1997.

Zaidel E, Lexical organization in the right hemisphere. In: Buser, Rougeul – Buser A (eds), Cerebral Correlates of Conscious Experience. Amsterdam. Elsevier, 1978.

Zaidel E, Performance on the ITPA following cerebral commissurotomy and hemispherectomy. Neuropsychologia 17; 259-280, 1979.

Zaidel E, Disconnection syndrome as a model for laterality effects in the normal brain. In: Hellinge J (ed), *Cerebral Hemisphere Asymmetry Methods. Theory and Application*. New York: Praeger, 1983.

Zaidel E, Language functions in the two hemispheres following complete commissurotomy and hemispherectomy. In: Boller F, Grafman G (eds.); *Handbook of Neuropsychology*. New York: Elsevier. Vol. 4; 115-150, 1990.

Zaidel D, Sperry RW, Memory impairment after commissurotomy in man. Brain 97; 263-276, 1974.

Zaidel D, Sperry RW, Some long-term motor effects of cerebral commissurotomy in man. Neuropsychologia 15; 193-204, 1977.

Zaidel E, Peters AM, Phonological encoding and ideographic reading by the disconnected right hemisphere. Two cases studies. Brain Lang 14; 205-234, 1981.

Zaidel E, Benson DF, Zaidel E. *The Dual Brain,* 205-231. New York Guilford, 1985.

Zaidel E, Zaidel DW, Bogen JE, Testing the commissurotomy patient. Neuromethods 17; 147-201, 1990.

Zaidel E, Clarke J, Suyenobu B, Hemispheric independence: a paradigm case for cognitive neuroscience. In: AB Scheibel and AF Wechsler (eds), *Neurobiology of higher cognitive function*. New York: Guilford; 297-352, 1990.

Zaidel E, Iacoboni M, Zaidel DW, Bogen JE, The callosal syndromes. In: Heilman and E Valenstein (eds) *Clinical neuropsychology* (4th ed), New York Oxford University Press, 2003.

Zettner A, Netsky MC, Lipoma of the corpus callosum. J Neuropathol Exp Neurol 19; 305-319, 1960.

Chapter 21

CEREBRAL CORTEX

Introduction

Anatomists use the term cortex (from the Latin for "bark", as in a tree's bark) to refer to any outer layer of cells. In neuroscience, the terms cortex and neocortex (new cortex) are often used interchangeably to refer to the outer part of the forebrain, and so by convention "cortex" refers to "neocortex" unless otherwise indicated. So, most of the cortex that covers the cerebral hemispheres is neocortex, defined as the cortex that has six cellular layers, or laminae. Each layer comprises more or less distinctive populations of cells based on their different densities, sizes, shapes, inputs, and outputs. Despite an overall uniformity, regional differences based on these laminar features have long been apparent, allowing investigators to identify numerous subdivisions of the cerebral cortex. The cortex is the part of the brain that has expanded the most in the course of evolution; it comprises 80% by volume of the human brain (Kolb and Whishaw, 2003).

The human neocortex has an area as large as 2 500 cm² but a thickness of only 1,5 to 3,0 mm. It consists of four to six layers of cells (gray matter) and is heavily wrinkled. This wrinkling is nature's solution to the problem of confining the huge neocortical surface within a skull that is still small enough to pass through the birth canal. Just as crumpling a sheet of paper enables it to fit into a smaller box than it could when flat, the folding of the neocortex permits the human brain to fit comfortably within the relatively fixed volume of the skull (Kolb and Whishaw, 2003).

According to Baars (2007), we usually see the brain from the outside, so that the cortex is the most visible structure. But the brain grew and evolved from the inside out, very much like a tree, beginning from a single seed, then turning into a thin shoot, and then mushrooming in three directions: upward, forward and outward from the axis of growth. That point applies both to phylogenesis – how species evolved – and ontogenesis – how the human brain grows from the foetus onward.

The mature brain reveals that pattern of growth and evolution. It means, for example, that lower regions like the brain stem are generally more ancient than higher regions, such as the frontal cortex. Basic survival functions like breathing are controlled by neural centres in the lower brain stem, while the large prefrontal cortex in humans is a late addition to the basic mammalian brain plan. It is located the farthest upward and forward in the neural axis. Thus, local damage to the prefrontal cortex has little impact on basic survival functions, but it can impair sophisticated abilities like decision-making, self-control and even personality (Baars, 2007).

The cerebral cortex of the cerebral hemispheres, the convoluted outer layer of gray matter composed of tens of billions of neurons and their synaptic connections, (Fig. 21.1) is the most highly organized correlation centre of the brain, but the specificity of cortical structures in mediating behavior is neither clear-cut nor circumscribed (Collins, 1990; Franckowiak et al., 1997). The bulk of the cerebral cortex is comprised of the neocortex. The phylogenetically older parts of the cortex include the paleocortex (olfactory cortex, entorhinal and periamygdaloid areas) and the archicortex (the hippocampal formation). The tens of billions of neurons send, in all directions, a large number of axons, covered by supportive myelin. These form the white matter of the cortex that fills the large subcortical space.

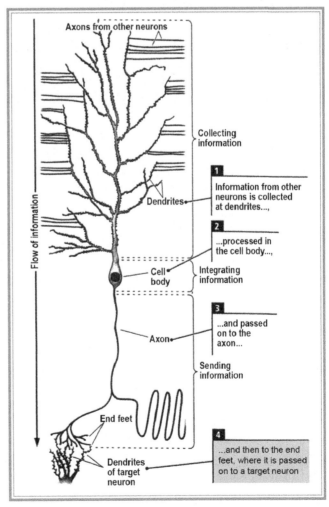

Fig. 21.1. A schematic representation of information flow in neuron (after Kolb and Whishaw, 2003).

Because the brain involves hundreds of millions of years of evolutionary layering on top of older layers, the more recent levels hide the older ones.

That is particularly true for the fast-ballooning neocortex in primates and humans, called the "new cortex" because it is more recent, and has six layers rather than the four or five layers of the reptilian and early mammallian brain (Baars, 2007).

Other large mammals have bigger muscles and greater speed, but humans have an exceptionally big and flexible brain, specialized for excellent vision and hearing, language and social relationships, and for manual control and flexible executive control. The human brain makes culture and technology possible (Baars, 2007).

The cerebral cortex receives sensory information from the internal and external environments of the organism, processes this information and then decides on and carries out a response to them. To receive information regarding the external and internal milieu and to generate commands to control the muscles and organs, the cerebral cortex has both direct and indirect connections with all other regions of the brain and spinal cord.

Multiple cortical and subcortical areas are involved to some degree in the mediation of complex behavior (Fuster, 1995; Mesulam, 2000), and specific regions are typically multifunctional (Lloyd, 2000).

The boundaries of functionally definable cortical areas, or zones, are vague. Cells subserving a specific function are highly concentrated in the primary area of a zone, thin out, and overlap with other zones as the perimeter of the zone is approached (Polyakov, 1966; Goldberg, 1989, 1995).

While the cortex is vital for cognitive functions, it interacts constantly with major satellite organs, notably the thalamus, basal ganglia, hypothalamus, cerebellum, brain stem and limbic regions, among others.

Different regions of the cerebral cortex have modular specific functions (somatic sensory and motor, visceral sensory and motor, integrative cognitive functions, speech functions etc.) responsible for the high-order cognitive processing of the conscious mind. These correspond to the Brodmann areas, as well as to each of the four cerebral lobes (frontal, parietal, temporal and occipital).

Modules are dynamic structures which, in neural terms, roughly coincide with neuronal assemblies and the connections between the neurons. Modular view of functional neocortical organization is in favour of the distributed-emergent principle of functional cortical organization.

The nature of cortical modules is distributed as well as localized. Modules can be considered unitary in the sense that they are in charge of action, both external and internal, and work to integrate such factors as time, novelty, complexity, and possibly ambiguity. So, the term modular or functional localization is used to indicate that certain functions can be localized in a particular area of the cerebral cortex. The mapping of cortical functions began with the inference made from the deficits produced by cortical lesions in humans.

Cognitive functions are represented by information exchange within and between modules.

Partial or total lesions of same Brodmann specialized areas or one of the lobes leads to a modular loss of consciousness. When all the cerebral cortex is destroyed as well as the white matter, the patient becomes unconsciousness.

The majority of the human cerebral cortex is devoted to tasks that transcend encoding primary sensations or commanding motor actions.

Collectively, the association cortices mediate these cognitive functions of the brain, broadly defined as the ability to attend to, identify, and act meaningfully in response to complex external or internal stimuli.

Descriptions of patients with cortical lesions, functional brain imaging of normal subjects, and behavioral and electrophysiological studies of non-human primates have established the general purpose of the major association areas.

Subsequently, techniques such as single-cell recording and electrical stimulation of cells in the cerebral cortex have been used in animals, non-human primates, as well as humans undergoing surgery for diseases such as epilepsy and Parkinson's disease to map out functional areas of the brain (Jones, 2000).

Functional neuroimaging techniques such as positron emission tomography (PET), functional magnetic resonance imaging (fMRI), and magnetoencephalography (MEG) have been used to confirm previous knowledge about the localization of functions within the cerebral cortex as well as to conduct studies in healthy human subjects that were previously not possible.

Even those functions that are subserved by cells located within relatively well-defined cortical areas have a significant number of components distributed outside the local cortical centre (Brodal, 1981; Paulescu et al., 1997).

In this way, effortful tasks show a wider spread of brain activity, even beyond the executive regions of the frontal cortex. For example, in a classic study, Smith and Jonides (1998) found dramatically expanded cortical activity as a function of memory load. The difficulty level rises very quickly with the number of items to be kept in mind.

What we cannot see yet, even with advanced brain recording methods, is the strength of connections between brain cells. Mental effort changes connection strengths, the neural signalling density between cortical localizations. Cognitive efforts is one of the biggest factors in brain functioning.

The neural firing or brain metabolism is not a direct measure of the complexity of some mental processes. It seems to indicate the recruitment of neuronal resources that are needed to work together to perform a task that is new or unpredictable. Once even very complex processes are learned, they seem to require less cortical activity. Automaticity also involves a loss of conscious access and voluntary control as assessed by behavioral measures (Schneider, 1995; Baars, 2002).

Cortical involvement appears to be a prerequisite for awareness of experience (Fuster, 1995; Kohler and Moscovitch, 1997; Roth, 2000).

Patterns of functional localization in the cerebral cortex are broadly organized along two spatial planes. The lateral plane cuts through homologous areas of the right and left hemispheres. The longitudinal plane runs from the front to the back of the cortex, with a relatively sharp demarcation between functions that are primarily localized in the forward portion of the cortex and those whose primary localization is behind the central sulcus or fissure of Rolando (Lezak et al., 2004).

In the newborn, the two cerebral hemispheres weigh approximately 402 g in the male and 380 g in the female. By the end of the first year, the weight of the brain has doubled, and by the end of the sixth year, it has tripled to at least 90% of its adult weigh at that time. This increase in weight is due mainly to an increase in the number of blood vessels, myelin layers, and supporting or glial elements (Schmitt et al., 1981; Roland and Zilles, 1996; Steinmetz, 1996; Zilles, 2004).

The role of glia, in among other examples, synapse formation, synapse maturation and plasticity, and rapid conduction of action potentials, as well as their immunological functions in the nervous system, have by now been unequivocally established (Stern, 2010). The molecular mechanisms underlying astrocyte specifications and growth and the interaction with other cell types to assemble the nervous system are still not completely understood. Another type of glial cell, oligodendrocytes, is central to the brain's myelination, which ensures the efficiency and speed of action potentials (Emery, 2010). Microglia are another fascinating subpopulation of glial cells. They sense pathological tissue alternation and they can develop into brain macrophages and perform immunological functions (Graeber, 2010).

Lee at al. (2010) report that tonic inhibition in the cerebellum is due to GABA being released from glial cells by permeation through the Bestrophin 1 anion channel. Ginhoux et al. (2010) investigate the developmental origin of microglia and show that adult microglia derive from primitive myeloid progenitor cells that arise before embryonic day 8.

In a perspective, Fields (2010) presents his hypothesis that white matter, which consists mostly of myelinated axons, may play a role in brain plasticity and learning.

In adults, the cerebral hemispheres weight about 1 450 g in males with a normal range of 1 200 to 1 600 g. In females, the cerebral hemispheres weight about 1 350 g, with a normal range between 1 100 and 1 500 g. The brain of an elephant weighs about 5 000 g and that of the blue whale weighs about 6 800 g.

The surface of the brain is folded such that two-thirds of its surface area lies buried and out of view in the depths of the cerebral fissures or sulci.

When one considers the surface area of the brain per lobe, about 41% of the human brain consists of the frontal lobe, 17% consists of the occipital lobe, 21% consists of the temporal lobe, and the parietal and insular lobes make up about 21% of the surface area of the brain (Roland and Ziels, 1996; Steinmetz, 1996; Augustine, 2008).

The surface gray matter of the cerebral hemispheres, or cerebral cortex, average about 2.5 mm in thickness, with variations from one brain region to another. The primary visual cortex (area 17 of Brodmann) is about 1.5 mm in depth whereas the primary motor cortex (area 4 of Brodmann) is about 4.5 mm. There is a variation in the thickness of the cerebral cortex, with it being thinner in the depths of the fissures than at the upper margins of the fissures. Some 10^{12} neurons may be present in both cerebral hemispheres ($10^{12} = $ = 1 trillion or 1 million × 1 million) (Augustine, 2008).

The total area of the cerebral cortex is about 2 500 cm^2.

Fissures, sulci, and gyri

The wrinkled surface of a neocortex consists of clefts and ridges. A cleft is called a fissure if it extends deeply enough into the brain to indent the ventricles, whereas it is a sulcus (plural: sulci) if it is shallower.

A ridge is called a gyrus (plural: gyri).

There is some variation in the location of these features on the two sides of a single individual's brain, and substantial variation in the location, size, and shape of the gyri and sulci in the brains of different individuals.

Adjacent gyri differ in the way that cells are organized within them; the shift from one kind of arrangement to another is usually at the sulcus. There is some evidence that gyri can be associated with specific functions.

There are four major gyri in the frontal lobe: the superior frontal, middle frontal, inferior frontal and precentral (which lie in front of the central sulcus).

Lateral organization

The two mirror-image halves of the cortex have puzzled people for centuries. Why are there two hemispheres? If we have but one mind, why do we have two hemispheres?

The two cerebral hemispheres are nearly symmetrical. The primary sensory and motor centres are homologously pozitioned within the cerebral cortex of each hemisphere in a mirror-image relationship. With certain exceptions, such as the visual and auditory systems, the centres in each cerebral hemisphere predominate in mediating the activities of the contralateral (other side) half of the body.

Thus, an injury to the primary somesthetic or somatosensory area of the right hemisphere results in decreased or absent sensations in the corresponding left-sided body part; an injury affecting the left motor cortex results in a right-sided weakness or paralysis (Lezak et al., 2004).

The hemispheres are completely separate, divided by the longitudinal fissure that runs between the two hemispheres from the anterior to the posterior part of the brain.

But, how do the two hemispheres "talk" to each other? The answer lies in the fibre tract (corpus callosum), a large arch of white matter that runs from the front to the back of the brain, linking the two hemispheres.

Although the two hemispheres are similar in appearance and structure, they are not biologically identical and they have different information processing abilities and propensities.

The corpus callosum, with at least 200 million nerve fibres, is the largest tract that connects the two cerebral hemispheres. Although there are no cortical landmarks that divide the corpus callosum, it is generally the cause that different regions of the corpus callosum contain fibres originating in different cortical areas. That is, the anterior portion of the corpus callosum contains primarily fibres that originate in promotor and frontal regions of the cortex, middle portion contain fibres that originate in motor and somatosensory regions and so forth. In addition, many callosal fibres are homotopic; that is they connect homologous areas of the two hemispheres. The corpus callosum also contains fibres that originate in a specific region of one hemisphere and terminate in a completely different region of the opposite hemisphere.

Comparisons of split-brain patients with intact individuals provide a clear indication that the corpus callosum is critical to normal interhemispheric interactions, especially interactions that require the transfer of information about the identity or name of a stimulus.

The corpus callosum has been hypothesized to play two important but very different roles: transferring information between the hemispheres and creating a kind of inhibitory barrier that minimized maladaptive cross talk between the complementary processes for which each hemisphere is dominant. Anyhow, same types of information can be transferred subcortically, and subcortical structures can also play a role in producing unified behavioral responses. Studies of perceptual processing in normal individuals provide important insights about the factors that determine when it is more efficient for the two hemispheres to operate collaboratively than to operate independently (Ivry and Roberts, 1998).

A major difference in the sources of innervation of the association cortices is the enrichment in direct projections from other cortical areas called corticocortical connections. These connections form the majority of the input to the association cortices. Ipsilateral corticocortical connections arise from primary and secondary sensory and motor cortices, and from other association cortices within the same hemisphere. Corticocortical connections also arise from both corresponding and noncorresponding cortical regions in the opposite hemisphere *via* the corpus callosum and anterior and posterior commissure, which together are referred to as interhemispheric connections.

In the association cortices of humans and other primates, corticocortical connections often form segregates bands or columns in which interhemispheric projection bands are interdigitated with bands of ipsilateral corticocortical projections (De Felipe and Jones, 1988; Garey, 1994; Posner and Raiche, 1994; Purves et al., 2004).

One general conclusion suggested by this research is that distributing information across both hemispheres becomes more beneficial as the task becomes more demanding of attentional resources. That is, when the processing demands are minimal, there is often a within-hemisphere advantage. However, when the processing demands are increased (as much as indicating whether two letters of different cases have the same name or whether both are vowels), there is typically an across-hemisphere advantage (Gazzaniga, 2000).

Interhemispheric collaborations can have emergent properties that are impossible to deduce from the sum of the parts provided by the two individual hemispheres.

Longitudinal organization

Although no two human brains are exactly alike in their structure, all normally developed brains share the same major distinguishing features. The external surface of each half of the cerebral cortex is wrinkled into a complex of ridges or convolutions called gyri (sing.: gyrus), which are separated by two deep fissures and many shallow clefts, the sulci (sing.: sulcus).

The two prominent fissures and certain of the major sulci divide each hemisphere into four lobes, the occipital, parietal, temporal and frontal lobes (Brodal, 1981; Mesulam, 2000; Dănăilă and Golu, 2006).

Point-to-point representation on the cortex

A consistent theme in neuroanatomy throughout the past century is that cortical regions can be categorized as primary sensory cortex, primary motor cortex, and association cortex. The last of these categories, the association cortex, is usually also categorized as secondary cortex, which elaborates information coming from primary areas, and as higher-order areas, which may combine information from more than one system. This idea can be traced to Flechsig (1920) and his studies of the development of myelin in the cortex.

Flechsig (1920) divided cortical regions into: 1) an early-myelinating primordial zone including the motor cortex and a region of visual, auditory, and somatosensory cortex; 2) a field bordering the primordial zone that myelinates next; and 3) a late-myelinating zone, which he called the "association zone".

Flechsig hypothesized psychological functions for his hierarchy, with the general idea being that the primary zones perform simple sensorimotor functions, whereas the association areas conduct the highest mental analyses. Flechsig's ideas greatly influenced neurological thinking throughout the twentieth century.

According to Lezak et al. (2004), the organization of both the primary sensory and primary motor areas of the cortex provides for a point-to-point representation of the body. The amount of cortex identified with each body portion or organ is proportional to the number of sensory or nerve endings in that part of the body rather than to its size. For example, the areas connected with sensation and movement of the tongue or fingers are much more extensive than the areas representing the elbow or back.

The visual system is also organized on a contralateral plan, but it is one-half of each visual field that is projected onto the contralateral visual cortex. The precise point-to-point arrangement of projection fibres from the retina to the visual cortex permits an especially accurate localization of lesions within the primary visual system (Sterling, 1998). Visual recognition is mediated by (at least) two different systems: one system processes visuospatial analysis, and one is dedicated to pattern analysis and object recognition. Movement perception may involve a third system (Zihl et al., 1983; Iwata, 1989).

An adult-onset lesion limited to the primary visual cortex produces loss of visual awareness (cortical blindness, blind sight) while reasoning ability, emotional control, and even the ability for visual conceptualization may remain intact (Farah and Weiskrantz, 1986; Guzeldere et al., 2000; Farah, 2003).

A majority of nerve fibres transmitting auditory stimulation from each ear are projected to the primary auditory centres in the opposite hemisphere; the remaining fibres go to the ipsilateral auditory cortex. Thus, the contralateral pattern is preserved to a large degree in the auditory system, too. So, destruction of one of the primary auditory centres does not result in loss of hearing in the contralateral ear. A point-to-point relationship between sensory receptors and cortical cells is also laid out on the primary auditory cortex, with a cortical representation arranged according to pitch, from high tones to low ones. So, these areas that receive projections from structures outside the neocortex or send projections to it are called primary projection areas. Nevertheless, the primary projection areas of the neocortex are small relative to the total size of the cortex.

Destruction of a primary cortical sensory or motor area results in specific sensory or motor deficits but generally has little effect on the higher cortical functions. Some mild decrements in movement speed and strength of the hand on the same side as the lesions in the motor cortex have been reported (Smutok et al., 1989; Cramer et al., 1999).

Association areas of the cortex

When Penfield and Boldrey (1958) stimulated the motor and somatosensory strips of their patients, they identified two regions of the parietal cortex that appeared to represent localised body parts such as the leg, hand, and face. These regions called homunculi were seen as the areas of the cortex responsible for basic tactile sensations such as touch, pressure, and temperature.

Subsequent investigations of nonhuman subjects led to the identification of analogous maps of the visual and auditory worlds as well.

Thus, the human cortex was generally believed to be occupied by complex mental analyses that we might loosely call cognition.

Doubt about this simple view of cortical organisation arose in the late 1970s and the 1980s, however, as more refined physiological and anatomical research techniques began to reveal literally dozens of maps in each sensory modality, rather than just one or two. For example, between 25 and 32 regions in the monkey cortex have roles in visual functioning, depending on the definition used (Kolb and Whishaw, 2003).

Although the somatosensory and auditory maps are less numerous, from about 10 to 15 cortical maps in each of these modalities, do not duplicate the original maps but rather process different aspects of sensory experience. For example, visual areas are specialised for analysing basic features such as form, colour, and movement. Furthermore, many psychological processes, such as visual object memory and visually guided movements, require visual information (Kolb and Whishaw, 2003).

Cortical representation of sensory or motor nerve ending in the body takes place on a direct point-to-point basis, but stimulation of the primary cortical area gives rise only to meaningless sensations or nonfunctional movements (Luria, 1966; Brodal, 1981). Modified and complex functions involve the cortex adjacent to the primary sensory and motor centres (Goldberg, 1990; Passingham, 1997; Paulescu et al., 1997).

According to Purves et al. (2004), the connectivity of the association cortices is appreciably different from that of the primary and secondary sensory and motor cortices, particularly with respect to inputs and outputs. For instance, two thalamic nuclei that are not involved in relaying primary motor or sensory information provide much of the subcortical input to the association cortices: the pulvinar projects to the parietal association cortex, while the medial dorsal nuclei project to the frontal association cortex. Several other thalamic nuclei, including the anterior and ventral anterior nuclei, innervate the association cortices as well.

So, signals coming into the association cortices *via* the thalamus reflect sensory and motor information that has already been processed in the primary sensory and motor areas of the cerebral cortex.

Unlike the thalamic nuclei that receive peripheral sensory information and project to primary sensory cortices, the input to these association cortex-projecting nuclei comes from other regions of the cortex. The primary sensory cortices receive thalamic information that is more directly related to peripheral sense organs and to the basal ganglia and cerebellum.

In any case, the primary sensory areas send projections into the areas adjacent to them, and the motor areas receive fibres from areas adjacent to them. These adjacent areas, less connected with the sensory receptors and motor neurons, are referred to as secondary areas. The secondary areas are thought to be more engaged in interpreting perceptions or organising movements than are the primary areas.

Neurons in these secondary cortical areas integrate and refine raw percepts or simple motor responses.

Tertiary association or overlap zones are areas peripheral to the functional centres where the neuronal components of two or more different functions or modalities are interspersed. The posterior association cortex, in which the supramodal integration of perceptual functions takes place, has also been called the multimodal (Pandya and Yeterian, 1990) or heteromodal (Strub and Black, 1988; Mesulam, 2000) cortex.

So, the areas that lie between the various secondary areas are referred to as tertiary areas. Often referred to as association areas, tertiary areas serve to connect and coordinate the functions of the secondary areas. Tertiary areas mediate complex activities such as language, planning, memory, and attention. These processing areas are connected in a "stepwise" manner so that information-bearing stimuli reach the cortex first in the primary sensory centres. They then pass through the cortical association areas in order of increasing complexity, interconnecting with other cortical subcortical structures along the way to the frontal and limbic system association areas and finally comes the expression through action, thought, and feelings (Pandya and Yeterian, 1998; Mesulam, 2000; Arciniegas and Beresford, 2001).

Another important source of innervation to the association areas is subcortical, arising from the dopaminergic nuclei in the midbrain, the noradrenergic and serotonergic nuclei in the brain stem reticular formation, and cholinergic nuclei in the brain stem and basal forebrain.

This diffuse input projects to different cortical layers and, among other functions, determines the mental state along a continuum that ranges from deep sleep to high alert (Mc Cormick, 1992; Mc Carley, 1995; Provencio et al., 2000; Willie et al., 2003).

Generally, each association cortex is defined by a distinct subset of thalamic, cortico-cortical, and subcortical connections. As a result, inferences about the function of human association areas continue to depend critically on the observation of patients with cortical lesions. Damage to the association cortices in the parietal, temporal, and frontal lobes, respectively, results in specific cognitive deficits; this indicates much about the operations and purposes of each of these regions (Purves et al., 2004).

These projection systems have both forward and reciprocal connections at each step in the progression to the frontal lobes; and each sensory association area makes specific frontal lobe connections which, too, send their reciprocal connections back to the association areas of the posterior cortex (Rolls, 1998).

Generally, there are identified areas that function in more than one modality (for example, vision and touch). These areas, known as the multimodal or polymodal cortex, presumably function to combine characteristics of stimuli across different modalities. For example, we can visually identify objects that we have only touched, which implies some common perceptual system linking the visual and somatic system (Kolb and Whishaw, 2003). Insight into the function of these cortical regions has come primarily from the observations of human patients with damage to one or another of these areas. Noninvasive brain imaging of normal subjects, functional mapping during neurosurgery, and electrophysiological analysis of comparable brain regions in non-human primates have generally confirmed the clinical deduction. There are four distinct regions of multimodal cortex, one in each of the occipital, parietal, temporal and frontal lobes. These areas imply that more than one process requires polymodal information.

Different regions could take part in different memory processes, object perception, emotion, movement control, and so on.

Anyhow, it is now clear that virtually the entire cortex behind the central fissure has some kind of sensory function.

The multimodal cortex appears to be of two general types, one type related to the recognition and related processing of information and the other type controlling movement related to the information in some manner (Kolb and Whishaw, 2003). This concept suggests that we have parallel cortical systems: one system functions to understand the world, whereas the other system functions to move us around in the world and allows us to manipulate our world. According to Kolb and Whishaw (2003), the cortex is fundamentally an organ of sensory perception and related motor processes. Jerison (1991) suggested that our knowledge of reality is related directly to the structure and number of our cortical maps. As the number of maps possessed by an animal brain increases, more of the external world is known to the animal and more behavioral options are available to it. For instance, animals such as rats and dogs, whose brain does not have a cortical region analysing colour, perceive the world in black and white. This lack must limit their behavioral options, at least with respect to colour.

Jerison (1991) suggested that cortical maps determine reality for a given species. Furthermore, he noted that, the more maps a species has, the more complex the internal representation of the external world must be.

Thus, if humans have more maps than dogs, then our representation of reality must be more complex than that of a dog. Similarly, if dogs have more maps than mice then a dog's understanding of the world is more complex than that of a mouse. This viewpoint suggests that the relative intelligence of different mammallian species may be related to the number of maps that the cortex uses to represent the world.

Dogs would have more olfactory maps than people and would thus be more intelligent about smells, but the total number of maps in all sensory regions taken together is far greater in humans than in dogs.

This referred to the cognition, which is the process by which we came to know the world.

More specifically, cognition refers to the ability to attend to external stimuli or internal motivation: to identify the significance of such stimuli and to make meaningful responses. So, the association cortices receive and integrate information from a variety of sources, and they influence a broad range of cortical and subcortical targets.

Unlike damage to primary cortical areas, a lesion involving association areas and overlap zones typically does not results in specific sensory or motor defects; rather, the behavioral effects of such damage will more likely appear as a pattern of deficits running through related functions or as impairment of a general capacity (Goldberg et al., 1989; Goldberg, 1995).

Thus, certain lesions that are implicated in drawing distortions also tend to affect the ability to do computations on paper; lesions of the auditory association cortex do not interfere with hearing acuity per se but with the appreciation of patterned sounds.

In sum, the association cortex includes most of the cerebral surface of the human brain and is largely responsible for the complex processing that goes on between the arrival of input in the primary sensory cortices and the generation of behavior.

The diverse functions of the association cortices are loosely referred to as cognition, the process by which we came to know the world (Mountcastle et al., 1975; Platt and Glimcher, 1999).

Inputs to the association cortices include projections from the primary and secondary sensory and motor cortices, the thalamus, and the brain stem. Outputs from the association cortices reach the hippocampus, the basal ganglia and cerebellum, the thalamus, and other association cortices.

So, different regions of the neocortex have different functions. Some regions receive information from sensory systems, other regions command movements, and yet other regions are the sites of connections between the sensory and the motor areas, enabling them to work in concert (Penfield and Boldrey, 1958; Truex and Cerpenter, 1969; Elliott, 1969).

Overall, the neocortex can be conceptualized as consisting of a number of fields: visual, auditory, body senses, and motor. Because vision, audition and body senses are functions of the posterior cortex, this region of the brain (parietal, temporal, and occipital lobes) is considered to be largely sensory; and because the motor cortex is located in the frontal neocortex, that lobe is considered to be largely motor.

Finally, because each lobe contains one of the primary projection areas, it can roughly be associated with a function (Kolb and Whishaw, 2003).

Frontal lobes: motor

Parietal lobes: body senses

Temporal lobes: auditory function

Occipital lobes: visual functions

On the other hand, all studies indicate that, among other functions, the frontal association cortex is especially important for the planning of appropriate behavioral responses, the parietal association cortex is especially important for attending to stimuli in the external and internal environment, and the temporal association cortex is especially important for identifying the nature of such stimuli.

Anyhow, these parts of the brain are responsible for encoding sensory information (primary sensory cortices), and commanding movements (primary motor cortex). But these regions account for only a fraction (perhaps a fifth) of the cerebral cortex. Much of the remaining cortex is concerned with attending to complex stimuli, identifying the relevant features of such stimuli, recognizing related objects, and planning appropriate responses as well as storing aspects of this information. Collectively, these integrative abilities are referred to as cognition, and it is evidently the association cortices in the frontal, parietal and temporal lobes that make cognition possible.

The extrastriate cortex of the occipital lobe is equally important in cognition; its functions, however, are largely concerned with vision. These other areas of the cerebral cortex are referred to collectively as the association cortices (Tanji and Shima, 1994; Garey, 1994; Glimcher, 2003).

Connections between cortical areas and binding problems

According to Kolb and Whishaw (2003), the various regions of the neocortex are interconnected by three types of axon projections: (1) relatively short connections between one part of a lobe and another, (2) longer connections between one lobe and another, and (3) interhemispheric connections or commissures, between one hemisphere and another.

Most of the interhemispheric connections link homotopic points in the two hemispheres – that is, contralateral points that correspond to one another in the brain's mirror-image structure. Thus, the commissures act as a zipper to link the two sides of the neocortical representation of the world and of the body together.

The two main interhemispheric commissures are the corpus callosum and the anterior commissure.

The cortex also makes other types of connections with itself. Cells in any area may send axons to cells in a subcortical area such as the thalamus, and the cells there may then send their axons to some other cortical area. These types of relations are more difficult to establish anatomically than are those based on direct connections (Curtis, 1972; Passingham, 1979).

The various connections between regions of the cortex are of considerable functional interest, because damage to a pathway can have consequences as severe as damage to the functional areas connected by the pathway.

As we saw, the cortex has multiple anatomically segregated and functionally specialised areas. But, according to Kolb and Whishaw (2003), how does brain organization translate into our perception of the world as a gestalt – a unified and coherent whole?

When you look at the face of a person, why do shape, colour, and size combine into a coherent, unchanging image? This question identifies the binding problem, which asks how sensations in specific channels (touch, vision, hearing, and so forth) combine into perceptions that translate as a unified experience that we call reality (Kolb and Whishaw, 2003).

Various researchers (Pandya and Yeterian, 1985, Fellemen and van Essen, 1991; Zeki, 1993) have tried to determine the rules of connectivity, but they did not succeed.

In reality, only about 40% of the possible intercortical connections within a sensory modality are actually found, which leads us to the flowing solution: intracortical networks of connections among subsets of cortical regions. This idea has considerable appeal.

First, all cortical areas have internal connections among units with similar properties. These connections link neurons that are neighbours and synchronise their activity.

Second, through a mechanism called re-entry, any cortical area can influence the area from which it receives input. This remarkable, interactive aspect of cortical connectivity means that, when area A sends information to area B, area B reciprocates and sends a return message to area A (Kolb and Whishaw, 2003). Zeki suggested that an area could actually modify its inputs from another area before it even receives them. An important point is that the connections from area A and B do not originate from the same layers, suggesting they play different roles in influencing each other's activity. Computer modelling suggests that the primary function of neural connections is to coordinate activity within and between areas in order to produce a globally coherent pattern, known as integration, over all areas of the perceptual system (Kolb and Whishaw, 2003). This concept of cortical organisation is likely to be foreign to many readers.

Jerison (1991) related the binding problem to his analogy of multiple cortical maps. The evolutionary expansion of the cortex in area has implications for the brain with multiple neurosensory channels that are trying to integrate information into a single reality. Because so many different kinds of sensory information reach the cortex, it is necessary somehow discriminate equivalent features in the external world.

Suppose that the brain creates labels to designate objects and a coordinate system to locate objects in the external world – that is, in space and time. Suppose also that sensory information must be tagged to persist through time and must be categorized to be retrieved (remembered) when needed.

Labels, coordinates, and categories are products of cognition (knowledge and thought). Viewed in this way, jerison's analogy of multiple cortical maps provides a basis for thinking about how the information that is arriving to the cortex is integrated into perception and organized as knowledge and thought.

It should not be a surprise that injuries to discrete cortical areas alter the way people perceive the self and the environment and the way they think about them.

One form of sensory deficit is agnosia. It renders a partial or complete inability to recognize sensory stimuli.

Histology of the cerebral cortex

The gray matter of the cerebral cortex is composed of neuron cell bodies of variable sizes and shapes, intermixed with myelinated and unmyelinated fibres. These cell bodies may be visualized with stains that bind to the rough endoplasmic reticulum (Nissl substance). Such stains leave the axons and dendrites almost invisible.

Yet another way of looking at cortical cells is to immerse small blocks of tissue in dilute silver salts, which precipitate on the membranes of the entire neuron. This reaction causes the cell body, its dendrites, and portions of the axon to become visible; this technique is called the Golgi method (Lunch, 2006).

The pattern of distribution of neuron cell bodies, is, generally, called cyto-architecture.

There are five neuronal types in the human cerebral cortex. These include the characteristic neuron of the cerebral cortex, the **pyramidal neuron** which measures some 10 to 70 μm in diameter. The majority of neurons in the human cerebral cortex are pyramidal neurons. These excitatory neurons project to other pyramidal neurons forming networks among themselves. A single pyramidal cell may have up to 200 synapses from other neurons on its cell body but upwards of 40,000 synapses on its axon and dendrites.

Pyramidal cells are found in all layers of the cortex with the exception of molecular layer I, and they are the predominant cell type in layers II, III and V.

Pyramidal cells are characterized by a roughly triangular cell body, a single large apical dendrite that arises from the apex of the cell body and usually extends towards the molecular layers, giving off branches along the way, an array of basal dendrites that run in a predominantly horizontal direction, and an axon that originates from the base of the soma leaves the cortex, and passes through the white matter.

The largest pyramidal neurons, called the giant pyramidal cell of Betz, are found almost exclusively in the primary motor cortex, which is located in the precentral and anterior paracentral gyri. Betz cells are most common in the region of the motor cortex that projects to the anterior horn of the lumbar spinal cord and hence are concerned with the control of leg movement.

Apical and basal dendrites of pyramidal cells are characterized by membrane specialization called dendritic spines that give the impression of thorns on a rose bush. Pyramidal neurons represent virtually the only output pathway for the cerebral cortex. Axons of pyramidal cells may terminate in another region of the cortex in the same hemisphere (**association fibres**), decussate in the corpus callosum to terminate in the cerebral cortex of the opposite hemispheres (**callosal fibres**), or course through the white matter to any of the numerous subcortical targets in the forebrain, brain stem, or spinal cord (**projection fibres**) (Lynch, 2006).

Pyramidal cells display a laminar organization, with the cell bodies in a given layer projecting to specific neural targets (Fig 21.2). Generally, pyramidal neurons in layers II and III give rise to association and callosal fibres. Pyramidal cell in layers V project to many subcortical structures, including the spinal cord, as projection fibres. The neurons in layer VI send their axons to a variety of locations, including the thalamic nuclei and other regions of the cortex. Within the cortex, the axons of pyramidal cells send off an extensive and relatively dense array of axon collaterals. These collaterals terminate in all cortical layers and extend through a horizontal area covering several millimetres around the cell body (Fig. 21.3). Pyramidal cells use an excitatory aminoacid, either glutamate or aspartate, as their neurotransmitter.

The **stellate** or **granule neuron** is another neuronal type found in the cerebral cortex. These cells are small, polygonal or triangular in shape and have dark-staining nuclei and scanty cytoplasm. These neurons, ranging from 4 to 8 μm, have a number of dendrites passing in all directions and a short axon which ramifies close to the cell body (Golgi type II).

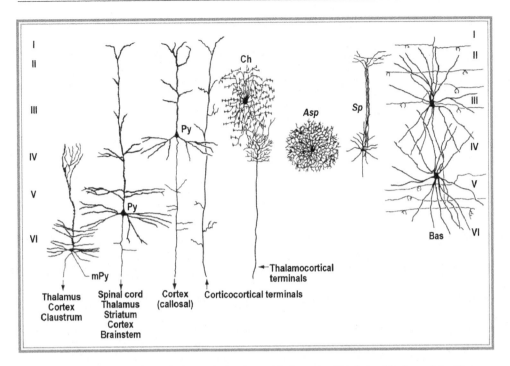

Fig. 21.2. Representative cell types in the cerebral cortex and the layers in which their cell bodies and dendrites are found. Dendrites of pyramidal cells (Py) of layers II, III, and V extended into layer I, whereas those of modified pyramidal cells (mPy) in layer VI extend only to about layer IV. Chandelier cells (Ch) are restricted almost entirely to layer III. The somata of aspiny and spiny stellate neurons (Asp, Sp) are in layer IV, although their processes extend into other layers. Basket cells (Bas) have processes that collectively extend into all cortical layers from cell bodies located mainly in layers III and V. (Adapted from Hendry SHC, Jones EG: Size and distributions of intrinsic neurons incorporating tritiated GABA in monkey sensory motor cortex. J. Neurosci. 1; 390-408, 1981, and from Jones EG: Laminar distribution of cortical efferent cells. In: Cerebral Cortex, vol. 1, New York, Plenum Press, 1984, pp. 521-553.

Other larger stellate cells have longer axons which may enter the medullary substance. Some resemble the pyramidal cells in that they have an apical dendrite which extends to the surface. These cells are known as stellate or star pyramidal cells (Lorente de Nó, 1949). Stellate cells are found throughout all layers of the cortex but are especially numerous in layer IV.

This neuronal type has a wide distribution and is probably correlative in function, interrelating different cortical layers.

Spiny stellate cells are the second most numerous cell type in the neocortex. Several primary dendrites, profusely covered in spines, radiate for a variable distance from the cell body. Their axons ramify within the grey matter predominantly in the vertical plane. Spiny stellate cells probably use glutamate as their neurotransmitter.

The smallest group comprises the heterogeneous non-spiny or sparsely spinous stellate cells. All are interneurones and their axons are confined to the grey matter. However, there is not a single class of cells, but a multitude of different forms, including basket, chandelier, double bouquet, neurogliaform, bipolar / fusiform and horizontal cells.

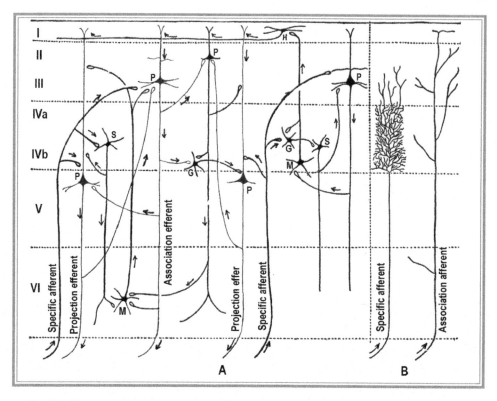

Fig. 21.3. Diagram showing some of the intracortical circuits. Sinaptic junction are indicated by loops; Afferent thalamocortical fibres; efferent cortical neurons, intracortical neurons; G, granule cell; H, horizontal cell; M, Martinotti cell; P, pyramidal cell; S, stellate cell; B, mode of termination of afferent cortical fibres.
(Based on data by Lorente de Nó, 1949).

These types may have horizontally, vertically or radially ramifying axons. The principal recognisable neuronal type is the neurogliaform or spiderweb cell. These small spherical cells, 10 to 12 μm in diameter, are found mainly in laminae II to IV, depending on cortical area. Seven to ten dendrites typically radiate out from the cell soma, some branching once or twice to form a spherical dendritic field of approximately 100 to 150 μm in diameter. The slender axon arises from the cell body or a proximal dendrite. It branches profusely within the vicinity of the dendritic field to give a spherical axonal arbour up to 350 μm in diameter (Crossman, 2008).

The **horizontal cells of Cajal** are located in the superficial cortical layers. These small neurons correlate adjoining areas with each cerebral hemisphere and have axons and dendrites that run parallel to the cortical surface.

The **cells of Martinotti**, present in practically all cortical layers, are small triangular cells whose axons are directed towards the surface. Some fibres arborize in the same layer; others send collaterals to a number of layers.

The **fifth cortical neuronal type** is the polymorph, multiform, or pleomorphic neuron. These essentially modified pyramidal neurons are associative in function and occur in the innermost cortical layers (Augustine, 2008).

The majority of non-spiny or sparsely spinous non-pyramidal cells probably use GABA as their principal neurotransmitter. This is almost certain in case of basket, chandelier, double bouquet, neurogliaform and bipolar cells. Some are characterised by the coexistence of one or more neuropeptides, including neuropeptide Y, vasoactive intestinal polypeptide, cholecystokinin, somatostatin and substance P.

Acetylcholine is present in a subpopulation of bipolar cells, which may additionally be GABAergic and contain vasoactive intestinal polypeptide (Toga et al., 2006; Crossman, 2008).

Inhibitory interneurons in the neocortex

The neocortex contains two major classes of neurons: glutamatergic excitatory neurons and gamma-aminobutyric acid – (GABA)-ergic – inhibitory interneurons. Proper functioning of the neocortex critically depends on the production of a correct number of excitatory and inhibitory neurons, which largely occurs during the embryonic stages (Brown et al., 2011).

Clones of neocortical excitatory neurons originating from the same progenitor cell provided a comprehensive view of excitatory neuron neurogenesis in the developing of the neocortex. These cells are spatially organized and contribute to the formation of functional microcircuits.

In contrast, little is known about the production and organization of neocortical interneurons (Brown et al., 2011) especially inhibitory interneurons (Brown et al., 2011). Most, if not all, neocortical interneurons are generated in the developing ventral (i.e., subcortical) telencephalon, including the ganglionic eminence (GEs) and the preoptic area (PoA), and migrate tangentially over long distances to reach their destination in the neocortex (Wonders and Anderson, 2006; Batista-Brito and Fishell, 2009; Gelman and Marin, 2010).

Different regions of the GEs generate distinct interneuron subgroups that differ in morphology, expression of neurochemical markers, biophysical properties and synaptic connectivity (Butt et al., 2005; Flames et al., 2007; Fogarty et al., 2007; Wonders et al., 2008; Miyoshi et al., 2010; Xu et al., 2010).

Distinct temporal origin of physiologically defined interneuron subgroups have also been reported (Butt et al., 2005; Miyoshi et al., 2007).

However, little is known about the cellular processes that produce neocortical interneurons.

The neocortex is thought to be functionally organized into columns consisting of excitatory neurons and inhibitory interneurons (Mountcastle, 1997). Clonal analysis of neocortical excitatory neuron production and migration has revealed that individual radial glial progenitor cells in the ventricular zone of the dorsal telencephalon undergo consecutive rounds of asymmetric cell division, producing a number of lineage-related sister excitatory neurons (Noctor et al., 2001). Despite some lateral dispersion during migration (Walsh and Cepko, 1993; Reid et al., 1995; O'Rourke et al., 1995), clonal related sister excitatory neurons are often spatially organized into vertical clusters and, to a lesser extent, horizontal arrays in the mature neocortex (Rakic, 1988; Price and Thurlow, 1988; Kornack and Rakic, 1995; Yu et al., 2009). Moreover, specific chemical synapses preferentially form between vertically aligned sister excitatory neurons, suggesting that spatially organized ontogenetic clones of excitatory neurons contribute to the formation of functional columnar microcircuits in the neocortex (Yu et al., 2009).

Whether inhibitory interneurons are spatially organized with respect to the formation of repetitive functional columns in the neocortex remains an outstanding question (Brown et al., 2011).

However, neocortical interneurons are remarkably diverse and often classified by distinctive morphologies, expression of neurochemical markers, firing pattern, and synaptic connectivity (Markram et al., 2004; Huang et al., 2007; Ascoli et al., 2008). Proper production of a correct number of each of these different subgroups of neocortical interneurons is essential for constructing a functional neocortex.

Brown et al. (2011) found that neocortical inhibitory interneurons were produced as spatially organized clonal units in the developing ventral telencephalon.

Furthermore, clonally related interneurons did not randomly disperse but formed spatially isolated clusters in the neocortex. Individual clonal clusters consisting of interneurons expressing the same or distinct neurochemical markers exhibited clear vertical or horizontal organization.

These results suggest that the lineage relationship plays a pivotal role in the organization of inhibitory interneurons in the neocortex (Brown et al., 2011).

Proper production of each of these different subgroups of neocortical interneurons is essential for constructing a functional neocortex. Radial migration of daughter cells along the mother radial glial cell has been extensively characterized in the dorsal telencephalon during excitatory neuron neurogenesis and migration. Brown et al. (2011) showed that before tangential migration differentiating daughter cells in the medial GE (MGE) and the PoA, which include neocortical interneurons, migrate radially along the mother radial glial progenitor cell. The physiological importance of this initial radial migration is unclear (Brown et al., 2011). It may allow proper neuronal differentiation of the daughter cells before they begin migrating tangentially to reach the neocortex (Brown et al., 2011).

It has been suggested that direct contact with the radial glia promotes GABAergic interneuron differentiation (Li et al., 2008). Consistent with this, Brown et al. (2011) found that cells within individual clones with the most pronounced neuronal characteristics are located furthest away from the ventricular zone. They possess the typical bipolar morphology of a tangentially migrating interneuron, indicating that they are poised for tangential migration. Cells with less pronounced neuronal characteristics are located close to the ventricular zone (Brown et al., 2011).

Neocortical interneurons generated in the MGE and PoA undertake complex migration routes to reach their final destination in the neocortex (Corbin et al., 2001; Mariss and Rubenstein, 2003).

They migrate tangentially over long distances to enter the neocortex through the marginal zone or the intermediate and subventricular zones before turning radially to reach their ultimate location in the neocortex. Similar to excitatory neurons, inhibitory interneurons generated in the MGE and PoA display a birth date-dependent laminar distribution in the neocortex (Ang et al., 2003; Batista-Brito and Fishell, 2009; Miyoshi and Fishell, 2011), thereby arguing for a regulated process of interneuron migration. However, the long-distance tangential migration of interneurons has been considered to be mostly random (Ang et al., 2003; Tanaka et al., 2009).

Brown et al. (2011) found that clonally related interneurons do not randomly disperse but form spatially organized vertical and horizontal clusters in the neocortex.

Nearly all neocortical neuronal circuits are composed of excitatory neurons and inhibitory interneurons.

Similar to excitatory neurons, inhibitory interneurons in the neocortex develop highly specific synaptic connections for the assembly of functional circuits (Gupta et al., 2000; Yoshimura and Callaway, 2005; Thomson and Lamy, 2007; Fino and Yuste, 2011).

The synaptic connections from local inhibitory interneurons to excitatory neurons exhibit a stereotypic spatial pattern (Kätzel et al., 2011), suggesting a high degree of spatial and functional organization of neocortical interneurons (Brown et al., 2011).

Cortical layers

Although the cerebral cortex contains an enormous number of cells, the number of cell types is small (Colonnier, 1967).

Based on cell size and packing density (cytoarchitectonics) each cortical region is divisible into six cellular layers, with three of these layers being subdivided based on their architectural features.

This six-layered cellular arrangement is characteristic of the entire neopallial cortex, which is referred to as **neocortex**, **isocortex** (Vogt and Vogt, 1919) or homogenetic cortex (Brodmann, 1909).

Two regions of the cerebral cortex have fewer than six layers. The first contains only three layers, is classified as **archicortex**, and includes the hippocampal formation. The second contains from three to five layers, is classified as **paleocortex**, and includes the olfactory sensory area and the nearby entorhinal and periamygdaloid cortices.

On the other hand, those cortical areas with six definite layers are termed **homotypic areas.**

Homotypical variants, in which all six laminae are found, are called frontal, parietal and polar.

Those cortical areas in which six layers are obscure, such as in the primary motor cortex (where there appears to be only five layers) or where seven layers are identifiable, such as in the primary visual cortex, are termed **heterotypic areas.**

The two types of cortex, granular and agranular, are regarded as virtually lacking certain laminae, and are referred to as heterotypical.

The agranular type is considered to have diminished, or absent, granular laminae (II and IV), but always contains scattered stellate somata. Large pyramidal neurones are found in the greatest densities in the agranular cortex, which is typified by the numerous efferent projections of pyramidal cell axons. Agranular cortex occurs in areas 4, 6, 8, and 44 and parts of the limbic system.

In the granular type of cortex the granular layers are maximally developed, and it contains densely packed stellate cells, among which small pyramidal neurons are dispersed.

Layers III and IV are poorly developed or unidentifiable. This type of cortex is particularly associated with afferent projections.

However, it does receive efferent fibres, derived from the scattered pyramidal cells, although they are less numerous than elsewhere.

Granular cortex occurs in the postcentral gyrus (somatosensory area), striate area (visual area) and superior temporal gyrus (acoustic area), and in small areas of the parahippocampal gyrus. Despite its very high density of stellate cells, it is almost the thinnest of the five main types.

The other three types of cortex are intermediate forms. **In the frontal type**, large numbers of small- and medium-sized pyramidal neurons appear in laminae III and V, and granular layers (II and IV) are less prominent.

The parietal type of cortex contains pyramidal cells, which are mostly smaller in size than those found in the frontal type.

In marked contrast, the granular laminae are wider and contain more stellate cells: this kind of cortex occupies large areas in the parietal and temporal lobes.

The polar type is classically identified with small areas near the frontal and occipital poles and is the thinnest form of cortex. All six layers are represented, but the pyramidal layers (III) are reduced in thickness and not as extensively invaded by stellate cells as is the granular type of cortex. The multiform layers (VI) are more highly organised than other types.

However, these six cortical layers include the: (I) molecular layer, (II) external granular layer, (III) external pyramidal layer, (IV) internal granular layer, (V) internal pyramidal layer, and (VI) multiform layer.

Layer (I) – the molecular layer contains very few neuron cell bodies and consists primarily of axons running parallel (horizontal) to the surface of the cortex. Within it are found the terminal dendritic ramifications of the pyramidal and fusiform cells from the deeper layers, and the axonal endings of the Martinotti cells.

Layer (II) – the external granular layers are composed of a mixture of small neurons called granule cells and slightly larger neurons, which are called pyramidal cells based on the shape of their cell body.

The apical dendrites of these pyramidal cells extend into layer I and their axons descend into, and through the deeper cortical layers. This layer is poor in myelinated fibres. Myelin fibre stains show mainly vertically arranged processes traversing the layer.

Layer (III) – the external pyramidal layers are composed mainly of well formed pyramidal neurons. The size of the pyramidal cells is smallest in the most superficial part of the layer and greatest in the deepest part. Two sublayers are recognized: a superficial layer of medium-sized pyramidal cells, along with some neurons of other types, and a deeper layer of larger ones. Their apical dendrites go to the first layer, while most of their axons enter the white matter, chiefly as association or commissural fibres. Intermingled with the pyramidal neurons are granules and Martinotti cells. In the most superficial part of the layer, a number of horizontal myelinated fibres constitute the band of Kaes-Becherew.

Layer (IV) – the internal granular layer is usually the narrowest of the cellular laminae and is composed almost exclusively of smooth (aspiny) stellate neurons and spiny stellate neurons many of which have short axons ramifying within the layer. By the 1950s it had become customary to refer to virtually all intrinsic cortical neurons as stellate cells, even though many were not actually star shaped.

Now, a number of distinct morphologic types are recognized. Some of the more important are the spiny and aspiny stellate cells, basket cells, and chandelier cells.

Three types of intrinsic neurons receive thalamocortical axon terminals in layer IV: the small spiny cells, the aspiny stellate cells, and dendrites of the large basket cells. Of these, the spiny cells are believed to be excitatory, whereas basket cells and aspiny stellate cells use the neurotransmitter GABA and are thus considered to be inhibitory interneurons. Most other intrinsic neurons are presumed to be inhibitory (Lynch and Tian, 2005).

This layer is free of pyramidal-shaped cells. It can be divided into an outer (IV a) and inner (IV b) portion in many neocortical areas and into three portions (IV a, IV b, IV c) in the primary visual cortex.

Layer IV is the primary target for ascending sensory information from the thalamus (Lynch, 2006).

Layer (V) – the internal pyramidal (ganglionic) layer, consists of medium-sized and large pyramidal neurons intermingled with granule and Martinotti cells. The apical dendrites of the larger pyramids ascend to the molecular layer; dendrites of the smaller pyramids ascend only to layer IV.

The large pyramidal cells of this layer are a major source of cortical efferent fibres including axons to the basal nuclei, brain stem, and spinal cord. Some corticocortical axons also originate in layer V. These are probably collateral branches of axons that are projecting to some subcortical targets. A considerable number of callosal fibres is furnished by the smaller pyramidal cells. The horizontal fibre plexus in the deeper portion of this layer constitutes the internal band of Baillarger.

Layer VI – the multiform (or fusiform / pleomorphic) layer, contains an assortment of neuron types including some with pyramidal, ovoid and fusiform cell bodies. These spindle-shaped cells have their axes perpendicular to the cortical surface. Like the pyramidal neurons of layer V, the spindle cells vary in size; the longer ones send a dendrite into the molecular layer, while the dendrites of the smaller ones ascend to layer IV, or arborize within the fusiform layer. Thus, the dendrites of many pyramidal and spindle cells from layers V and VI come into direct relation with the endings of sensory thalamocortical fibres, which ramify chiefly in the internal granular layer (Mountcastle, 1997).

The axons of the cells of this layer project to subcortical targets, such as the thalamus, and to other cortical regions as corticocortical connections.

Many of the short arcuate association fibres connecting adjacent convolutions are furnished by the deep stellate cells of layer VI (Lorente de Nó, 1949).

Cortical connectivity

Different cortical areas have widely different afferent and efferent connections.

Afferent connections

The widely separated but functionally interconnected areas of cortex share common patterns of connections with subcortical nuclei and within the neocortex. Thus, contiguous zones of the striatum, thalamus, claustrum, cholinergic basal forebrain, superior colliculus and pontine nuclei connect with anatomically wide areas of the prefrontal and parietal cortex, which are themselves interconnected.

In contrast, other functionally distinct regions, e.g., areas in the temporal and parietal cortex, do not share such contiguity in their subcortical connections.

All the various nonpyramidal neurons of the cerebral cortex function as cortical interneurons, because their axons do not leave the immediate region of the cell body (Jones 1975; Lynch and Tian 2005).

With the help of the Golgi technique, the distribution of dendritic and axonal terminals has been worked out by a number of investigators, notably Cajal (1909-1911).

Lorente de Nó (1949) has given a detailed account for the elementary pattern of cortical organization that is applicable to the parietal, temporal and occipital isocortex. According to this investigator, the arrangement of the axonal and dendritic branchings forms the most constant feature of cortical structure.

The afferent fibres to the cortex include projection fibres from the thalamus, association fibres from other cortical areas of the same side and commissural fibres from the opposite side.

The thalamocortical fibres, especially the specific afferent ones from the ventral tier thalamic nuclei and the geniculate bodies, pass unbranched to layer IV. Here, the axons form a dense terminal plexus (Colonnier, 1967); some of these fibres extend to layer III where they arborize. Specific afferent fibres in layer IV establish both axodendritic and axosomatic synapses upon stellate neurons which are fantastically profuse on some cells (Colonnier, 1968).

Fibres of the so-called nonspecific thalamocortical system, related to the intralaminar thalamic nuclei and indirectly to the ascending reticular activating system, also reach the cerebral cortex. Histological data concerning the origin, course and termination of these afferent fibres, have been meagre (Hanberry and Jasper, 1953; Nauta and Whitlock, 1954; Bowsher, 1966).

Jones and Leavit (1974) and Jones (1984) have been shown that the intralaminar thalamic nuclei, which project mainly to the striatum, project collateral fibres diffusely to broad regions of the cerebral cortex.

Thus, the cerebral cortex receives inputs, called diffuse inputs, and it consists of fibres that branch extensively and end diffusely over a wide area of cortex without respect for the cytoarchitectural boundaries. These inputs arise from the nonspecific nuclei of the thalamus (for example, the ventral anterior, central lateral, and midline nuclei), the locus ceruleus, and the basal nucleus (of Meynert). These structures are generally concerned with regulating overall levels of cortical excitability and the associated phenomena of arousal, sleep, and wakefulness (Lynch, 2006).

According to Jasper (1960), the synaptic termination of fibres of this nonspecific system in the cortex is chiefly axodendritic and widely distributed in all layers, but the principal physiological effects appear to be within the superficial layers.

The association of callosal fibres give off some collaterals to layer V and VI and ramify mainly in layer II and III, and to a lesser extent in layer IV (Carpenter, 1979). Thus, thalamocortical axons terminate primarily in layer IV and to a lesser extent in layers III and VI. In layer IV, they terminate on excitatory and inhibitory interneurons as well as on dendrites from neurons in other layers. The axons of interneurons, in turn, may end on dendrites of pyramidal cells or of other interneurons.

Generally, the details of intrinsic circuitry of the cerebral cortex are very complex. A single neuron may also receive synaptic contacts from thousands of other neurons. The basic framework of cortical circuitry consists of afferent fibres, local circuits for the processing of this afferent information, and efferent fibres that convey the processed information to another site.

The local processing of information culminates in connections to pyramidal cells, which carry the information to other cortical and subcortical regions. A copy of the information also goes to neurons in the immediate vicinity *via* axon collaterals. Generally, the termination of corticocortical axons is quite different from that of thalamocortical axons. Corticocortical axons branch repeatedly and make synaptic contacts on neurons in all layers of the cortex (Lynch, 2006).

Thalamocortical relationship

According to Lynch (2006) the cortex of the frontal lobe encompasses Brodmann's areas 4, 6, 8 to 12, 32 and 44 to 47. The primary somatomotor cortex (area 4) and the premotor and supplementary motor cortices (area 6) receive input mainly from the ventral lateral nucleus of the thalamus and subserve important motor functions.

The lateral, medial, and orbital aspects of the frontal lobe receive thalamocortical fibres mainly from the dorsomedial and anterior nuclei of the thalamus.

These latter cortical areas relate primarily to functions of the limbic system through a variety of direct and indirect connections. Of particular note are the pars orbitalis and pars triangularis of the inferior frontal gyrus, damage to which results in Broca aphasia.

Areas 3, 1, 2, 5, 7, 39, 40 and 43 are located in the parietal lobe. The primary somatosensory cortex (areas 3, 1 and 2) receives inputs from the ventral posterolateral and ventral posteromedial nuclei.

These thalamic nuclei receive a full range of somatosensory inputs through synaptic relays in the spinal cord and brain stem and transmit this information to the cerebral cortex. The inferior parietal lobule comprises, in general, areas 39 and 40. Along with area 22, these areas are the cortical regions associated with Wernicke aphasia.

The occipital and temporal lobe encompass areas 17 to 22, 36 to 38, and 41 and 42. These areas of the cortex, plus portions of the parietal lobe, have extensive connections with the pulvinar nucleus of the thalamus and are involved in the processing of visual and auditory information at several different functional levels. In this area are the primary sensory cortices for vision and hearing. Area 17, on the bank of the calcarine sulcus, is the primary visual cortex; areas 41 and 42, in the depth of the lateral fissure in the transverse temporal gyri, constitute the primary auditory cortex.

These cortical areas receive inputs from the lateral and medial geniculate nuclei of the thalamus, respectively.

The limbic lobe, which forms the most medial edge of the hemisphere, contains areas 23 to 31 and 33 to 35. The cingulate cortex receives fibres primarily from the anterior nucleus of the thalamus but also from the lateral dorsal nucleus.

Other regions of the limbic lobe have some connections with the dorsomedial nucleus. However, many of the subcortical targets of the parahippocampal and uncal cortices are structures such as the hippocampal formation. These are, in turn, projects to a variety of thalamic and basal forebrain targets (Lynch, 2006).

Major afferents to the cortical area tend to terminate in layers I, IV and VI. Quantitatively lesser projections end either in the intervening laminae II / III and V, or sparsely throughout the depth of the cortex. Numerically, the largest input to a cortical area tends to terminate mainly in layer IV. This pattern of termination is seen in the major thalamic inputs to visual and somatic sensory cortex.

Generally, non-thalamic subcortical afferents to the neocortex, which are shared by wide spread areas, tend to terminate throughout all cortical layers, but the laminar pattern of their endings still varies considerably from area to area (Crossman, 2008).

Generally, all cortical areas receive topographically organized cholinergic projections from the basal forebrain, noradrenergic fibres from the locus ceruleus, serotoninergic fibres from the midbrain raphe nuclei, dopaminergic fibres from the ventral midbrain, and histaminergic fibres from the posterior hypothalamus.

Efferent connections

All neocortical areas have axonal connections with other cortical areas on the same side (**association fibres**), the opposite side (**commissural fibres**), and with subcortical structures (**projection fibres**). The pyramidal cells are the efferent neurons of the cerebral cortex.

Thus, all neocortical areas are connected with subcortical regions although their density varies between areas. First among these are connections with the thalamus. All areas of the neocortex receive afferents from more than one thalamic nucleus, and all such connections are reciprocal.

The vast majority, if not all, of the cortical areas project to the striatum, tectum, pons and brain stem reticular formation. Additionally, all cortical areas are reciprocally connected with the claustrum; the frontal cortex connects with the anterior part and the occipital lobe with the posterior part (Crossman, 2008).

The primary somatosensory, visual and auditory cortices give rise to ipsilateral corticocortical connections to the association areas of the parietal, occipital and temporal lobes, respectively, which then progressively project towards the medial temporal limbic areas, notably the parahippocampal gyrus, entorhinal cortex and hippocampus.

Thus, the first (primary) somatosensory area (SI) projects to the superior parietal cortex (Brodmann's area 5), which in turn projects to the inferior parietal cortex (area 7). From here, connections pass to the cortex in the walls of the superior temporal sulcus, and so on to the posterior parahippocampal gyrus, and into the limbic cortex.

Similarly, for the visual system, the primary visual cortex (area 17) projects to the parastriate cortex (area 18), which in turn projects to the peristriate region (area 19). Information then flows to the inferotemporal cortex (area 20), to the cortex in the walls of the superior temporal sulcus, then to the medial temporal cortex in the posterior parahippocampal gyrus, and so to limbic areas. The auditory system shows a similar progression from the primary auditory cortex to the temporal association cortex and so to the medial temporal lobe (Crossman, 2008).

The primary somatosensory cortex (SI) in the postcentral gyrus is reciprocally connected with the primary motor cortex (area 4) in the precentral gyrus.

The superior parietal lobule (area 5) is interconnected with the premotor cortex (area 6), that in turn is connected with area 7 in the inferior parietal lobule. This has reciprocal connections with the prefrontal association cortex on the lateral surface of the hemisphere (areas 9 and 46), and the temporal association areas, which connect with more anterior prefrontal association areas, and, ultimately in the sequence, with the orbitofrontal cortex. Similar stepwise links exist between areas on the visual and auditory association pathways in the occipitotemporal lobe and areas of the frontal association cortex.

The connections between sensory and association areas are reciprocal (Crossman, 2008). Generally, short corticocortical fibres arise more superficially, and long corticocortical (both association and commissural) axons come from cells in the deeper parts of the layer III.

The internal pyramidal lamina, layer V, gives rise to cortical projection fibres, most notably corticostriate, corticopontine, corticobulbar, and corticospinal axons. In addition, a significant proportion of feedback corticocortical axons arise from cells in this layer, as do some corticothalamic fibres. Layer VI, the multiform lamina, is the major source of corticothalamic fibres.

Supragranular pyramidal cells, predominantly from layer III, but also lamina II, give rise primarily to both association and commissural corticocortical pathways.

Myeloarchitectonics

Based on the types of fibres present (radial, oblique, and horizontal fibres), their distribution, layering, and amount of myelin, collectively termed **myeloarchitectonics**, six major cortical fibre layers are identifiable in the human cerebral cortex.

Related to layer II is the **stria of the external granular layer**. This layer of fibres is associative in function with many association and commissural fibres. The stria of **the**

internal granular layer in layer IV, receives inputs from various specific thalamic nuclei.

Finally, the **stria of the internal pyramidal layer** is located in the deep part of layer V (Fig. 21.4).

The infragranular cortical layers have their output through the stria in layer V (Jones, 1984; Braitenburg and Schüz, 1998; Zielles and Palomero-Gallagher, 2001; Augustine, 2008).

Thus, two features of the myelinated fibres in the neocortex are noteworthy. First, there are prominent plexuses of horizontally running myelinated fibres in layers IV and V. These are called the **outer** and **inner bands of Baillarger**, respectively. In the primary visual cortex, bordering on the calcarine sulcus the outer band of Baillarger is greatly expanded. This band can be seen with the naked eye in fresh and stained sections and is called the **stria (line) of Gennari**.

Second, in most regions of the neocortex, there are many radially oriented bundles of axons passing between the subcortical white matter and various parts of the cortex or between the inner and outer cortical layers (Fig. 21.5).

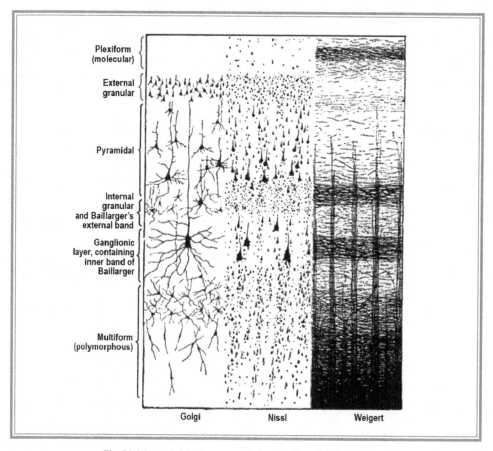

Fig. 21.4. Layers of the human cerebral cortex (from Standring, 2005).

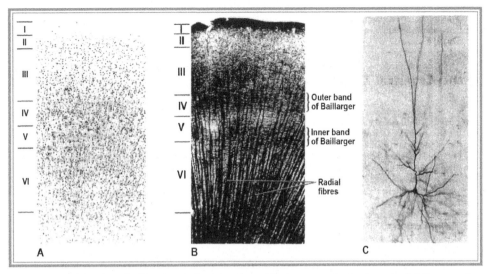

Fig. 21.5. Nissl (A) and myelin (B) stains of adjacent sections of the human cerebral cortex and a Golgi impregnation (C) of a pyramidal neuron in the primate neocortex. (A and B by courtesy of Drs. Grazyna Rajkowska and Patricia Goldman-Rakic, University of Mississippi Medical Center and Yale University; C by courtesy of Dr. José Rafols, Wayne State University).

Cortical columns spots and stripes (microarchitecture)

Although the most striking feature of Nissl-stained sections of the cerebral cortex is its horizontal lamination, physiological studies of the somatosensory and visual cortex indicate that a vertical column of cells, extending across all cellular layers, constitutes the elementary functional cortical units (Mountcastle, 1957; Powell and Mountcastel, 1957, 1959 a; Hubel and Wiesel, 1962, 1963).

This conclusion is supported by the following evidence: (1) neurons of a particular vertical column are all related to the same, or nearly the same, peripheral receptive field, (2) neurons of the same vertical column are activated by the same peripheral stimulus, and (3) all cells of a vertical column discharge at more or less the same latency following a brief peripheral stimulus.

Thus, the cell size and packing density of the cerebral cortex (cytoarchitectonics), permits the identification of cortical layers and cortical parcellation into regions and areas. In addition, there is also a columnar cortical organisation (microarchitecture).

The term "**column**" refers to the observation that all cells encountered by a microelectrode penetrating and passing perpendicularly through the cortex respond to a single peripheral stimulus, a phenomenon first identified in the somatosensory cortex.

The columns display variations in size and cross-sectional area, and the receptive field axis of orientation varies in a continuous manner as the surface of the cortex is traversed. Anatomically, an elementary functional unit of the cortex, represented by a column of cells, must contain the afferent, efferent and internuncial fibre system necessary for the formation of a complete cortical circuit. In the basic columnar unit, the internal circuitry must vary with differences in cytoarchitecture.

The convergence of specific afferents upon specific cells in the columnar units appears to imprint a specific modality which is relayed by intracortical connections to other cells in the column. The complex axonal branching suggests that intracortical circuits involve cells in all parts of the column. These vertical circuits are interconnected by short neuronal links represented primarily by the short axons of granule cells whose processes arborize within a single layer.

Through these short links, cortical excitation may spread horizontally and involve a progressively larger number of vertical units.

Thus, in one cortical region, all neurons might have receptive fields for a finger, whereas, in a nearby region, the neurons might have receptive fields for the wrist. Within a cortical region in which all neurons had about the same receptive field, the neurons responded to different sensory submodalities. Some neurons are activated by light touch on the skin, others by joint rotation, and still others by strong pressure on deep tissue (Lynch, 2006).

So, neurons in the somatosensory cortex are located in vertical columns at right angles to the surface and extend through all cortical layers; they often share similar receptive fields and have specific functions. The width of these cortical columns has an upper limit in primates of about 5 mm. Columns in SI are functionally interrelated by intrinsic corticocortical connections and by direct horizontal connections between columns. These intrinsic connections serve to connect parts of the cerebral cortex having different response properties, yet lying in regions of similar regional representation (Augustine, 2008). Thus, a specific afferent fibre may not only fire vertical columns of cells in its immediate vicinity, but may reach other units through Golgi type II cell relays (Lorente de Nó, 1949).

According to Cajal (1909, 1911) the unique morphological feature of the human cortex is the enormous number of Golgi type II cells considered to interrelate vertical cell columns.

The topographical pattern present on the cortical surface extends throughout its depth. Studies of the visual (striate) cortex demonstrate similar discrete functional columns extending from the pial surface to the white matter that are responsive to a specific kind of retinal stimulation in the form of long narrow rectangles of light ("slits"), dark bars against a light background, or straight-line borders, all of which must have a particular axis of orientation (Hubel and Wiesel, 1962, 1963).

Thus, in the visual cortex, narrow (50 µm) vertical strips of neurons respond to a bar stimulus of the same orientation (orientation columns) and wider strips (500 µm) respond preferentially to stimuli detected by one eye (ocular dominance columns). Adjacent orientation columns aggregate within an ocular dominance column to form a hypercolumn, responding to all orientations of a stimulus for both eyes for one point in the visual field (Lynch, 1980; Peters and Jones, 1999; Casanova Manuel, 2005; Crossman, 2008).

Thus, in the visual cortex, at least three types of regularly repeating features are superimposed on the laminar patterns of neurons: the stimulus orientation columns, the ocular dominance columns, and the cytochrome oxidaze-rich blobs.

The ocular dominance columns in the visual cortex provide a clear example of the role of thalamic inputs in columnar organization.

Neurons in the layers of the lateral geniculate nucleus that receive inputs from the right eye send their axons to layer IV of the right eye-dominant columns. Here, the axons terminate predominantly on spiny and aspiny stellate cells, which, in turn, project to pyramidal cells. Collaterals of pyramidal cell axons provide one pathway by which neural signals can spread from one column to influence activity in adjacent columns.

This influence may be either excitatory *via* direct connections, or inhibitory *via* interneurons.

The right eye has a direct and strong influence on neurons in right-eye-dominant columns and an indirect and weaker influence on neurons in the adjacent left-eye-dominant columns (Lynch, 2006).

When a microelectrode was inserted at right angles to the surface of the cortex, all of the neurons encountered were activated by only one of these submodalities (Fig 21.6, B).

In contrast, when a microelectrode was moved parallel or obliquely relative to the surface of the cortex, it encountered neurons of different submodalities as it moved from one functionally related group of neurons to another (Fig. 21.6, A) (Lynch, 2006).

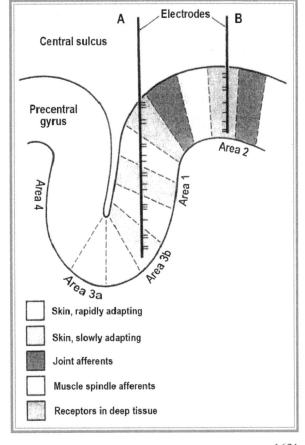

Fig. 21.6. Diagramatic section through the precentral and postcentral gyri showing the organization of columns in the somatosensory cortex. The columns are shown as compartments oriented, generally, perpendicular to the surface of the cortex. An electrode (at A) passing parallel to the surface of the cortex will pass through several columns with resultant recordings of the several modalities represented by the types of afferent information arriving at each column. An electrode passing through one column (at B) passing perpendicular to the surface of the cortex penetrates only a single column. Therefore, it records activity related to the single submodality received by that column (after Lynch, 2006).

If all of the cells in one column respond to maintained pressure on the skin, the cells in an adjacent column respond to joint position.

Similar columnar organization has been described in widespread areas of the neocortex, including the motor cortex and association areas.

According to Kolb and Whishaw (2003), most interactions between the layers of the cortex take place within the cells directly above or below the adjacent layers.

There have been many terms for the vertical organization of the cortex, two of the most common being column and module. Although these terms are not always interchangeable, the underlying idea is that groups of 150 to 300 neurons form little circuits ranging from about 0.5 to 2.0 mm wide, depending on the cortical region. Evidence for some kind of modular unit comes from two principal sources: staining and probing (Purves et al., 1992).

If a radioactive aminoacid is injected into one eye of a monkey, the radioactivity is transported across synapses to the primary visual cortex. The radioactivity is not evenly distributed across the cortex, however, in that it travels only to places that connect with the affected eye. Thus, the pattern of radioactivity seen in the primary visual cortex (area 17) is a series of stripes, much like those on a zebra (Purves et al., 1992).

A different pattern is seen in the same visual cortex when a different technique is used. If the cortex is stained with cytochrome oxidaze, which shows areas of high metabolic activity by staining mitochondria, the visual cortex appears spotted. These spots, known as "blobs", have a role in colour perception (Fig. 21.7, A and B) (Purves et al., 1992).

Curiously, if the same stain is applied to area 18, which is an adjacent visual region, the staining pattern looks more like stripes (Fig. 21.7, C) than like spots (Purves et al., 1992).

Finally, if the primary somatosensory cortex of a rat is stained with succinic dehydro-genaze, the cortex shows a pattern of spots that are known as "barrels" (Fig. 21.7, D). Each barrel corresponds to one of the vibrissae on the face of the rat (Purves et al., 1992).

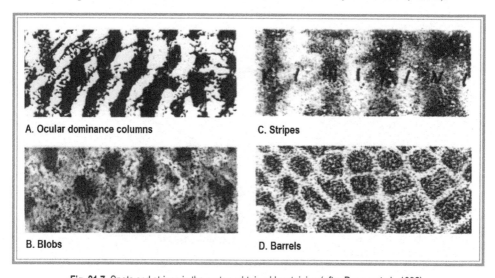

A. Ocular dominance columns

C. Stripes

B. Blobs

D. Barrels

Fig. 21.7. Spots and stripes in the cortex, obtained by staining (after Purves et al., 1992).

As these examples illustrate, there appear to be many types of modules, and even the same stain shows a different modular organization in different regions.

A second way to demonstrate modular organization is shown physiologically in the sensory cortex. According to Kolb and Whishaw (2003), if a microelectrode is moved vertically through the sensory cortex from layer I to layer VI, all the neurons encountered appear to be functionally similar. The functional similarity of cells across all six layers at any point in the cortex suggests that the simplest functional unit of the cortex is a vertically orientated column of cells that composes a minicircuit. Groups of these columns may be organized in somewhat larger units as well. If an electrode samples the cells of area 17 (visual cortex), all the cells in a column will respond to a line of a given orientation (for example, 45°). If the electrode is moved laterally across the cortex, adjacent columns will respond to successively different orientations (for example, 60°, 90°, and so on) until all orientations over 360° are sampled. Thus, in the visual cortex, columns are arranged in larger modules (Fig. 21.8).

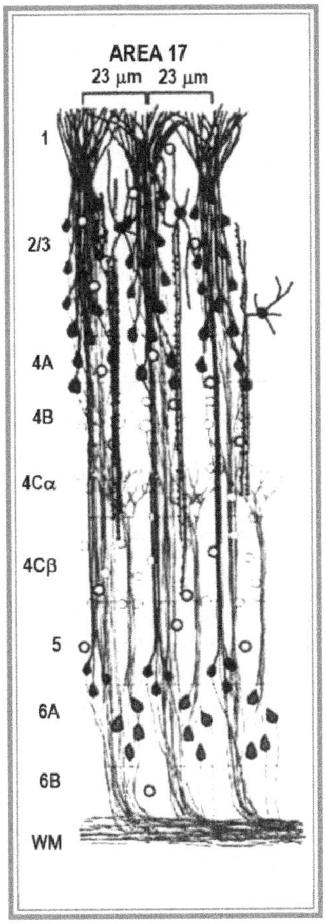

One problem is that, although modules are apparent in primary sensory regions, they are less apparent in the association or motor areas of the cortex. The stripes and spots are also a problem because they differ greatly in size. Furthermore, closely related species often have very different patterns of spots and stripes, which seem strange if they are fundamental units of cortical functions.

Zeki (1993) suggested that the search for the basic module of cortical organization is akin to the physicist's search for the basic unit of all matter.

Fig. 21.8. The six major layers of cortex in cross section. The figure shows three columns in Area 17, also called V1, the first visual projection area to the cortex (source Squire et al., 2003).

The underlying assumption is that the cortical module might be performing the same basic functions throughout the cortex. In this view, the evolutionary expansion of the cortex corresponds to an increase in the number of basic units, much as one would add chips to a computer to expand its memory or processing speed.

Anyhow, we are left wandering what the basic function and operation of the cortical module might be.

Purves and his colleagues (1992) have offered a provocative answer. They noted that the spots and stripes on the cortex resemble the markings on the fur of many animals. They suggested that, even though these patterns may provide camouflage or broadcast sexual signals, these functions are secondary to fur's fundamental purpose of maintaining body temperature. Pursuing this analogy, the researcher proposed that same modular patterns in the cortex may well correspond to secondary functions of cortical organization. One suggested that the cortex forms its intrinsic connections to process information; one efficient pattern of connectivity is the vertical module.

The module certainly conforms to an important aspect of cortical connectivity, but it does not cause cortical connectivity. There must be an alternative way (or ways) of organizing complex neural activity that does not require a constant module. Although a cortical organization with columns is a useful arrangement, it is not the only way to organize a brain (Kolb and Whishaw, 2003).

The organization of the cells of the cortex

Nerve cells can be easily distinguished in the cortex as spiny neurons or aspiny neurons by the presence or absence, respectively, of dendritic spines.

Dendritic spines serve as functional compartments for chemicals as well as a location for synaptic connections with other cells (Kolb and Whishaw, 2003).

About 95% of all excitatory synapses on spiny neurons occur on the spines (Peters and Jones, 1984, 1999).

Spiny neurons include pyramidal cells, which have pyramid-shaped cell bodies and generally send information from one region of the cortex to some other brain area, and spiny stellate cells, which are smaller, star-shaped interneurons whose processes remain within the region of the brain in which the cell body is located. Spiny neurons are excitatory and are likely to use glutamate or aspartate as transmitters. The pyramidal cells, which constitute the largest population of cortical neurons (70%-85%), are the efferent projection neurons of the cortex (Peters and Jones, 1984, 1999).

They are found in layers II, III, V, and VI. Generally, the largest cells send their axons the furthest.

The pyramidal cells of layer V are the largest, projecting to the brain stem and spinal cord. Those in layer II and III are smaller and project to other cortical regions.

The neurons of the neocortex are arranged in about six layers. The six horizontal layers of cortex are organized in cortical columns, vertical barrel-shaped slices. These often contain closely related neurons, such as visual cells that respond to different orientations of a single light edge in just one part of the visual field.

Columns may be clustered into hypercolumns, which may be part of an even larger cluster. Thus, the cortex has both a horizontal organization into six layers, and a vertical one, into columns, hypercolumns, and eventually entire specialized regions. These six layers can be separated into three groups of functions (Everett, 1965; Elliot, 1969; Passingham, 1979).

1. The output cell layers, layers V and VI, send axons to other areas. Both of these layers and the cells of which they are composed are particularly large and distinctive in the motor cortex, which sends projections to the spinal cord. Large size is typical for cells that send information to long distances.

2. The input cell layer, layer IV, receives axons from the sensory system and other cortical areas. This layer features large numbers of small, densely packed cells in the primary areas of vision, somatosensation, audition, and taste-olfaction, which receive large projections from their receptive sensory organs.

3. The association cell layers, layers I, II, and III, receive input mainly from layer IV and are quite well developed in the secondary and tertiary areas of the cortex.

In short, sensory areas have many layer IV cells, motor areas have many layer V and VI cells, and association areas have many layer I, II and III cells.

Some cortical neurons send their axons to the thalamus, while others receive input from thalamic neurons. Millions of cortical nerve cells go to the opposite hemisphere, while many others project their axons to the same hemisphere. However, the densest connections are to neighbouring neurons. Cortical layer I consists largely of dendrites (input fibres) that are so densely packed and interconnected that this layer is sometimes called a "feltwork", a woven sheet of dendrites. These connection patterns in the cortex undergo major changes in human development and throughout the lifespan.

Aspiny neurons are interneurons with short axons and no dendritic spines. They are diverse in appearance, with different types named largely on the basis of the configurations of their axons and dendrites. One type of aspiny stellate cell is called a basket cell because its axon projects horizontally, forming synapses that envelop the postsynaptic cell like a basket.

Another, the double-bouquet type, has a proliferation of dendrites on either side of the cell body, much as if bouquets of flowers were aligned stem to stem. Despite differences in shape, all aspiny neurons are inhibitory and are likely to use GABA as a transmitter.

Aspiny neurons also use many other transmitters; virtually every classical transmitter and neuropeptide has been colocalized with GABA in aspiny cells. Thus, not only are aspiny cells morphologically diverse, but they also show a remarkable chemical diversity (Kolb and Whishaw, 2003).

Cortical layers, afferents and efferents

According to Kolb and Whishaw (2003), each of the four to six layers of the cortex has different functions, different afferents (inputs), and different efferents (outputs). The cells from the middle layers of the cortex (especially in and around layer IV) constitute a zone of sensory analysis in that they receive projections from other areas of the cortex and other areas of the brain. The cells from layers V and VI constitute a zone of output in that they send axons to other cortical areas or other brain areas (Fig. 21.9).

Therefore it is hardly surprising that the somatosensory cortex has a relatively large layer IV and a small layer V, whereas the motor cortex has a relatively large layer V and a small layer IV.

Anyhow, different cortical layers can be distinguished by the neuronal elements they each contain, and by the thickness of the layers, which also corresponds to their function.

Afferents to the cortex are, specific and nonspecific:

1) Specific afferents bring information (sensory information, for example) to an area of the cortex and terminate in relatively discrete cortical regions, usually in only one or

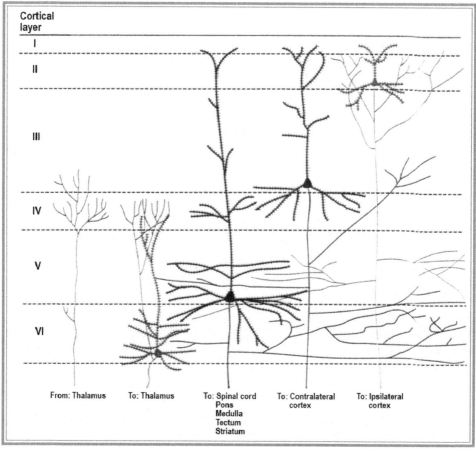

Fig. 21.9. A schematic drawing of the six layers of cortex, the gray matter. Note that some cortical neurons send axons to the thalamus, while other receive input from thalamic neurons. Ipsilateral = same side of the cortex; Contralateral = opposite side.

two layers. Specific afferents include projections from the thalamus as well as from the amygdala. Most of these projections terminate in layer IV, although projections from the amygdala and certain thalamic nuclei may terminate in more superficial layers.

2) Nonspecific afferents presumably serve general functions, such as maintaining a level of tone or arousal, so that the cortex can process information. They terminate diffusely over large regions of the cortex – in some cases, over all of it. Nonspecific afferents even release their transmitter substances into the extracellular space. The norepinephrinergic projections from the brain stem, the cholinergic projections from the basal forebrain, and the projections from certain thalamic nuclei are examples of nonspecific afferents (Kolb and Whishaw, 2003).

Despite significant variations among different cytoarchitectonic areas, the circuitry of all cortical regions has some common features. First, each cortical layer has a primary source of inputs and a primary output target. Second, each area has connections in the vertical axis (called columnar or radial connections) and connections in the horizontal axis (called lateral or horizontal connections). Third, cells with similar functions tend to be arrayed in radially aligned groups that span all of the cortical layers and receive inputs that are often segregated into radial or columnar bands. Finally, interneurons within specific cortical layers give rise to extensive local axons that extend horizontally in the cortex, often linking functionally similar groups of cells. The particular circuitry of any cortical region is a variation on this canonical pattern of inputs, outputs and vertical and horizontal patterns of connectivity (Purves et al., 2004).

Mapping the human cortex

The cortex can be divided by topographic maps, which are based on various cytoarchitectonic areas. These cytoarchitectonic areas are histologically defined subdivisions, which a zealous band of neuroanatomists has painstakingly mapped over the years in humans and in some of the more widely used laboratory animals. Early in the twentieth century, cytoarchitectonically distinct regions were identified with little or no knowledge of their functional significance. However, studies of patients in whom one or more of these cortical areas had been damaged, supplemented by electrophysiological mapping in both laboratory animals and neurosurgical patients, supplied this information. This work showed that many of the regions neuroanatomists had distinguished on histological grounds are also functionally distinct. Thus, cytoarchitectonic areas can sometimes be identified by the physiological response properties of their constituent cells, and often by their patterns of local and long-distance connections (Milner, 1963; Lezak, 1995). The first complete cortical map of the human brain was published in 1905 by Campbell, and it was based on both cell structure and myelin distribution.

Soon after, several alternative versions emerged, the most notable belonging to Brodmann.

In 1909, Korbinian Brodmann published a treatise "Localisation in the Cerebral Cortex" on histological localization in the cerebral cortex. He described his work in the introduction: "Localisation which uses exclusively anatomical features as the basis for investigation, in contrast to physiological or clinical aspects" (Garey, 1994). The lasting result of this work was a scheme for the parcellation of the cerebral cortex into 52 distinct areas based on common anatomical features (Fig. 21.10).

About 100 Brodmann's areas are now recognized, and it is therefore convenient to take this as a rough estimate of the number of specialized regions of the cortex. The Brodmann areas correspond well to different specialized functions of the cortex such as the visual and auditory areas, motor cortex, and areas involved in language and cognition.

Brodmann's map represents differences in the density of different kind of neocortical neurons. In Brodmann's map, the different areas are numbered, but the numbers themselves have no special meaning. To do his analysis, Brodmann divided the brain at the central sulcus and then examined the front and back halves of the brain separately, numbering new conformations of cells as he found them but without following a methodical path over the surface or through the layers. Thus, he found areas 1 and 2 in the posterior section, then switched to the anterior section and found area 3 and 4, and then switched back again, and then looked somewhere else.

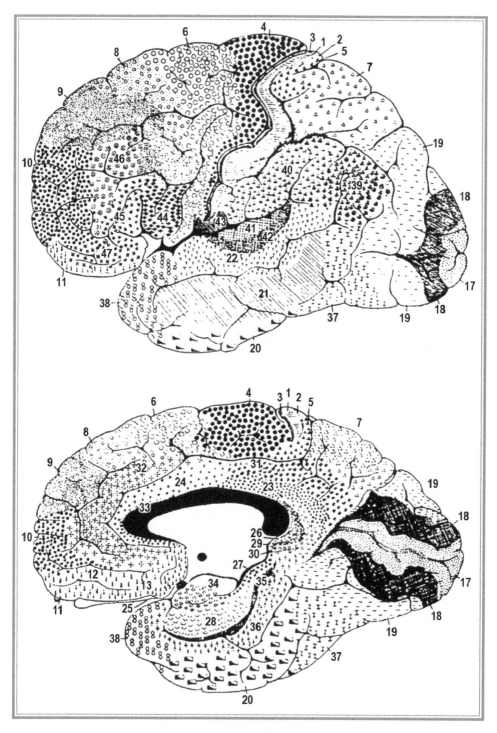

Fig. 21.10. Cerebral hemispheres of the human with Brodmann's areas applied. From Vergleichende Lokalisationsliehre der Grosshirnrinde in ihren Prinzipien dargestellt auf Grund der Zellenbaues.

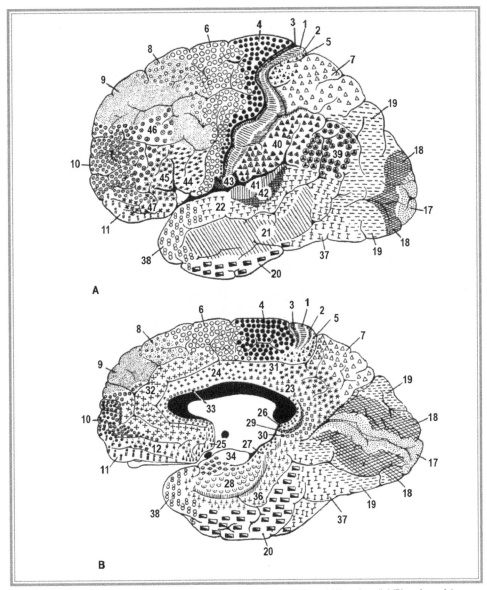

Fig. 21.11. Cytoarchitectural map showing Brodmann areas on the lateral (A) and medial (B) surface of the hemisphere. (Modified after Brodmann K from Carpenter MB, Sutin J: Human Neuroanatomy. Baltimore, Williams and Wilkins, 1983.)

Brodmann's map is very useful because the regions depicted in it correspond quite closely with regions discovered with the use of noncytoarchitectonic techniques. Figure 21.11 summarises some of the relations between areas on Brodmann's map and areas that have been mapped according to their known functions (Brodmann, 1909; Everett 1965; Elliot, 1969). For example, area 17 corresponds to the primary visual projection area, whereas areas 18 and 19 correspond to the secondary visual projection areas. Area

1629

4 is the primary motor cortex. Broca's area related to the articulation of words is area 44, areas 6 and 8 (eye movement) correspond to secondary areas. The motor territory corresponds to areas 9, 10, 11, 45, 46 and 47.

Areas 1, 2 and 3 correspond to the primary body senses projection areas, areas 5 and 7 correspond to the secondary body senses projection areas, and areas 7, 22, 37, 39, and 40 correspond to the territory sensory projection areas.

One of the problems with Brodmann's map is that new, more powerful analytical techniques have shown that many Brodmann's areas actually consist of two or more architectonically distinct areas. For this reason, the map is continually being updated and now consists of an unwieldy mixture of numbers, letters, and names (Kolb and Whishaw, 2003).

Anyhow, Brodmann's areas (BA) are distinct areas of the cerebral cortex based on the organization of cells or the cytoarchitecture of the human brain. A functional distinction of brain regions correlates remarkably well with this neuroanatomic differentiation.

Some of these are so important that we will call them modules (high functional areas). These modules are widely used today when discussing the results of neuroimaging studies.

At a microscopic level of description, we have the Brodmann areas.

When the surface layers of the cortex are carefully studied under a microscope, small regional differences can be seen in the appearance of cells in the layers and their connections (Baars, 2007).

However, about 70% of the human cerebral cortex is buried in sulci which complicate our ability to visualize its extent from a surface view or topographic map. A surface view of the brain thus hides the source of the majority of activation in imaging studies. This problem is solved by the flat map, which allows images to visualize the entire surface area of a hemisphere in a single view.

Van Essen and Drury (1997) used the MRI analysis of the Visible Man, a digital atlas of the human body, to generate flat maps of the human cortex. Figure 21.12, A shows a surface view of the Visible Man's two hemispheres with the lobes, identified by different shadings. Flat maps display the sulci and gyri in an alternative format (Fig. 21.12, B), in which buried cortex (not visible from the exterior of the hemisphere) is shown in darker shades.

The location of brain areas in a whole brain can be calculated by using a three-dimensional atlas. Sections are taken at regular intervals (typically 4 mm in the human brain). So, van Essen and Drury were able to identify the coordinates for the regions in their flat map. Their coordinate system makes it possible to identify the location of activations in imaging studies with respect to cortical surface.

Neurotransmitters of the cerebral cortex

According to Lynch (2006), there are a variety of neuroactive substances associated with neurons of the cerebral cortex.

Principal among these are glutamate, aspartate, and **gamma-aminobutyric acid** (GABA). Pyramidal cells are the efferent neurons of the cerebral cortex. They are predominantly **glutaminergic** and excitatory to their targets.

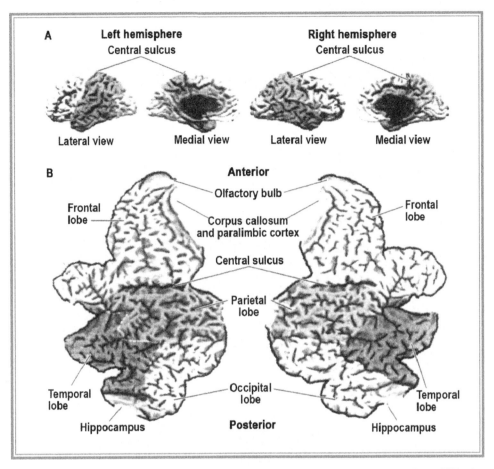

Fig. 21.12. Cortical maps. (A) A digital surface map. (B) The cortex has been "flattened" so that all tissues hidden in sulci are visible. Flat maps provide a perspective on the relative size of various cortical regions and on the amount of tissue dedicated to different functions, as detailed in the table (after van Essen and Drury, 1997).

The pyramidal cells of the cortex, and therefore the output of the cortex, are modulated by a variety of cortical afferents. The influence of these afferent fibres is to act on pyramidal cells either directly or *via* interneurons. Most interneurons within the cortex are GABAergic and inhibitory.

A variety of **neuropeptides** (monoamines) are also found in the cerebral cortex; they influence not only populations of neurons but also local metabolic activity and vascular smooth muscle. The most important monoamines in the cortex are (1) norepinephrine, which originates from the locus ceruleus of the pons and distributes sparsely to all cortical layers, (2) dopamine, which arises from the substantia nigra – pars compacta and the adjacent ventral tegmental area and is found in moderate amounts in layers I and VI and sparsely in II-V, and (3) serotonin, which arises from the raphe nuclei and distributes heavily to all cortical layers (Vogt et al., 1997; Mesulam, 2004; Lynch, 2006).

Cortical areas

The cerebral cortex does not have a uniform structure. It has been mapped and divided into a number of distinctive areas that differ from each other in total thickness, in the thickness and density of individual layers and in the arrangement and number of cells and fibres.

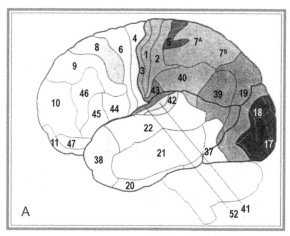

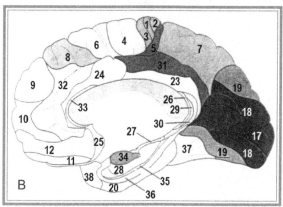

Fig. 21.13. A) The Brodmann classification of the regions in the left hemisphere, shown a lateral view. B) The Brodmann classification of the regions in the right hemisphere, shown a medial view.

In 1905, Campbell defined some 20 cortical fields in the human cerebral cortex.

In 1909, Brodmann published a monograph that continues to guide the study of neuroscience even today. The cerebral cortex was originally classified by Brodmann into 52 different cytoachitectural areas (Fig. 21.13), but he did not assign a function to each area at that time. He numbered them 1 to 52, which reflects the order in which he examined and mapped them. Additional studies have provided information correlating a function to many of these areas.

The anatomical / functional correlation, however, is not as accurate as was thought in the past.

Some of these areas are commonly referred to by both name and number, and should be known by the student. These are: the primary somatosensory cortex (Brodmann's areas 3, 1, and 2), motor cortex (Brodmann's areas 4, 6, and 8), secondary sensory cortex

(Brodmann's areas 5 and 7), visual cortex (Brodmann's areas 17, 18 and 19), and auditory cortex (Brodmann's area 41 and 42). The functional areas of the cerebral cortex are shown in figures 21.14 and 21.15.

Vogt and Vogt (1919) parcelled the human cerebral cortex into more than 200 areas based on cellular patterns. The Vogts were leaders in this field, defining some 229 cortical areas. Von Economo (1929) divided it into 109. Thus, according to von Economo (1929), all cortical structure is reducible to five fundamental types (Fig. 21.16), based primarily on the relative development of granule and pyramidal cells. Types 2, 3 and 4, known respectively as the frontal, parietal, and polar types, are homotypical and constitute by far the largest part of the cortex.

Type 1 (agranular) and 5 (granular) are heterotypical and limited to smaller specialized regions (Fig. 21.17).

Even the last numbers are apparently insufficient, since other investigators have found a number of distinctive cytoarchitectural fields in regions previously considered homogeneous (Beck, 1929; Rose, 1935).

The brain map of Bailey and von Bonin (1951) utilizes various colours to distinguish distinctive cytoarchitectural features. These authors felt that the concept of absolutely sharp areal boundaries has been carried to absurd lengths and that most brain maps failed to properly represent transitional areas.

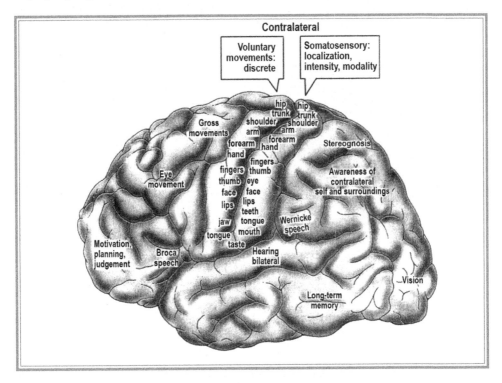

Fig. 21.14. Lateral view of the cerebral hemisphere showing the functional areas of the cerebral cortex. (Modified from Young PA, Young PH (1997), Basic Clinical Neuroanatomy. Williams and Wilkins, Baltimore.)

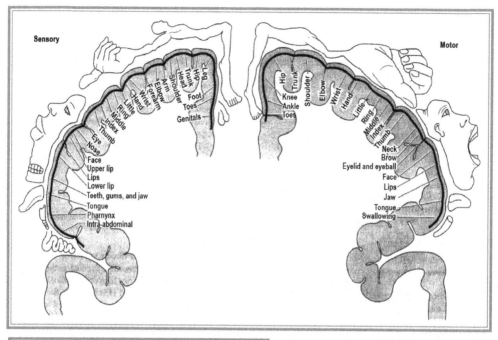

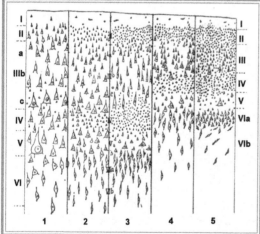

Fig. 21.15. Coronal section through the cerebral hemisphere showing homunculi of the primary somatosensory cortex (left) and the primary motor cortex (right) (after Patestas and Gartner, 2008).▲

Fig. 21.16. The five fundamental types of cortical structure. 1, agranular; 2, frontal; 3, parietal; 4, polar; 5, granulous (koniocortex) (von Economo, 1929). ◄

However, such cortical fields or areas are a morphological expression of functional differences between the various regions of the cerebral hemispheres. Cotemporary methods of cortical parcellation have used a combination of anatomy, neurochemistry, and function (Schüz and Miller, 2002).

Functional aspects of the cerebral cortex

Flechsig (1920) was the first to suggest that anatomical criteria could be used to delineate a hierarchy of cortical areas, but Luria (1973) fully developed the idea in the 1960s. Luria divided the cortex into two functional units.

Fig. 21.17. Distribution of the five fundamental types of cortex over the convex (A) and the medial (B) surface of the hemisphere. 1, agranular; 2, frontal; 3, parietal; 4, polar; 5, granulous (koniocortex) (von Economo, 1929).

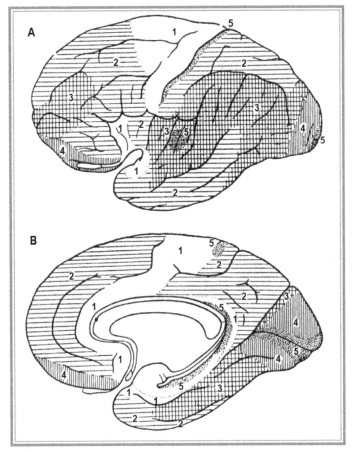

The posterior part of the cortex is the sensory unit. It receives sensations, processes them, and stores them as information.

The anterior cortex (the frontal lobe) is the motor unit. It formulates intentions, organizes them into programs of action, and executes the programs. Both cortical units have a hierarchical structure with three cortical zones arranged functionally one above the other. The first zone corresponds to Flechsig's primary cortex; the second corresponds to the slower-developing cortex bordering the primary cortex, which Luria labelled secondary cortex; and the third, the slowest-developing cortex, which Luria labelled tertiary cortex.

Luria conceives of the cortical units as working in concert along zonal pathways.

Sensory input enters the primary sensory zones, is elaborated in the secondary zones, and is integrated in the tertiary zones of the posterior unit. To execute an action, activation is sent from the posterior tertiary sensory zones to the tertiary motor zone for formulation, to the secondary motor zone for elaboration, and then to the primary frontal zone for execution.

Information in the tertiary sensory zone activates the paralimbic cortex for memory processing and the amygdala for emotional assessment. A lesion in the primary visual zone would produce a blind spot in some part of the visual field. A lesion in the secondary visual zone might produce a perceptual deficit, making the person unable to recognize the activity. A lesion in the tertiary sensory zone might make it impossible to recognize the significance of the activity in its abstract form (somebody lost his money).

Damage to the paralimbic cortex would leave no memory of the event, and damage to the amygdala would render the person unresponsive to the event's emotional significance. A lesion in the tertiary motor area might prevent the formation of the intention. A lesion in the secondary motor zone might make it difficult to execute the sequences of movements required in an activity. A lesion in the primary zone might make it difficult to execute a discrete movement required in an action.

Luria (1973) based his theory on three assumptions:

1) The brain processes information is serially – that is, one step at a time. Thus, information from sensory receptors goes to the thalamus, then to the primary cortex, then to the secondary cortex, and finally to the tertiary sensory cortex. Similarly, the output goes from tertiary sensory to tertiary motor, then to secondary motor, and finally to primary motor.

2) Serial processing is hierarchical; that is, each level of processing adds complexity that is qualitatively different from the processing in the preceding levels. The tertiary cortex could be considered a "terminal station" in so far as it receives input from the sensorimotor and perceptual areas and performs higher cognitive processes on that input.

3) Our perceptions of the world are unified and coherent entities. So, the same active process creates each percept, and naturally the simplest way to do so is to form it in the tertiary cortex.

According to Kolb and Whishaw (2003), a strictly hierarchical processing model requires that all cortical areas be linked serially, but this serial linkage is not the case. All critical areas have reciprocal (reentrant) connections with the regions to which they connect, which means that there is no simple "feed forward" system. Only about 40% of the possible connections among different areas in a sensory modality are actually found.

Then, Zeki (1993) made the interesting point that, because a zone of cortex has connections with many cortical areas, it follows that each cortical zone is probably undertaking more than one operation, which is subsequently relayed to different cortical areas. In addition, the results of the same operation are likely to be of interest to more than one cortical area, which would account for multiple connections.

These principles can be seen in the primary visual cortex, which appear to make calculations related to colour, motion, and form. These calculations are relayed to specific cortical regions for these processes. And the same calculation may be sent to cortical as well as to subcortical regions. This implies that cortical processing can bypass Luria's motor hierarchy and go directly to subcortical motor structures.

So, an area such as the primary visual cortex, which is processing colour, form, and movement, might be considered more complex than an area that processes only colour (Kolb and Whishaw, 2003).

Finally, Luria assumed that his introspection about perception being a unitary phenomenon was correct.

There are two logical possibilities to put this knowledge together in a meaningful way to see organization in the cortex. According to Kolb and Whishaw (2003), one possibility is that there is no hierarchical organization but rather some sort of nonordered neural network. As individual organisms gain experiences, this network becomes ordered in some way and so produces perceptions, cognitions, and memories. The results of a wealth of perceptual research suggest that the brain filters and orders sensory information in a species-typical fashion.

Felleman and van Essen (1991) suggested that cortical areas are hierarchically organized in some well-defined sense, with each area occupying a specific position relative to other areas, but with more than one area being allowed to occupy a given hierarchical level. Felleman and van Essen (1991) proposed that the pattern of forward and backward connections could be used to determine hierarchical position.

Thus, ascending (or forward) connections terminate in layer IV whereas descending (or feedback) connections do not enter layer IV, usually terminating in the superficial and deep layers (Fig. 21.18).

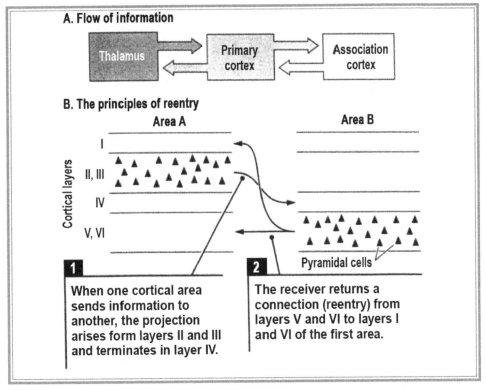

Fig. 21.18. Inter- and intraareal connections. (A) The flow of information to and from the cortex. Information from the thalamus goes to the primary cortex, which then projects to the association cortex. Note the reciprocal connections at each level, representing feedback loops. (B) The principle of the reentry. When one cortical area sends information to another, the projection arises from layers II and III and terminates in layer IV. The receiver returns a connection (reentry) from layers V and VI to layers I and VI of the first area. In this way, a receiving cortical area can modify the inputs that it is getting. This reentry principle holds for all levels of cortical connectivity (after Kolb and Whishaw, 2003).

They also recognize a third type of connection, which is columnar in its distribution and terminating in all layers. This type of connection is uncommon but provides a basis for placing areas in the same location in the hierarchy.

By analysing the patterns of connectivity among the visual, auditory, and somatosensory areas, Felleman and van Essen (1991) found evidence of what they call a distributed hierarchical system.

The cerebral cortex is the organ of thought. More than any other part of the nervous system, the cerebral cortex is the site of the intellectual functions that make us human and that make each of us a unique individual. These intellectual functions include the ability to use language and logic, and to exercise imagination and judgment (Lynch, 2006). Although other brain structures, including the thalamus, corpus striatum, claustrum, and cerebellum contribute to these functions, the multimodal association cortex is closely linked to the most complex intellectual functions, such as logical analysis, judgment, language and imagination.

Neurons in the cortex receive input from many subcortical structures by way of the thalamus and also from other regions of the cortex *via* association fibres.

Cortical neurons, in turn, project to a wide range of neural structures, including other areas of the cerebral cortex, the thalamus, the basal nuclei, the cerebellum *via* the pontine nuclei, many of the brain stem nuclei, and the spinal cord.

The cerebral cortex is divided into distinct functional areas, some of which are devoted to the processing of incoming sensory information, others to the organization of motor activity, and still others primarily to what are considered "higher intellectual functions".

These functions include memory, judgment, the planning of complex activities, processing of language, mathematical calculations, and the construction of an internal image of an individual's surroundings. Thus, in discussing functions of the cortical areas in humans, it is essential to understand that we are not dealing with properties inherent in the cerebral cortex itself, but we are dealing with complete neuronal arcs or chains of neurons that project their impulses from specific areas of the nervous system to their terminations.

The functional features of any cortical area are dependent on the connections to and from that area and the interrelations that exist between the various primary and secondary sensory receptive areas, the motor projection areas and the primary, secondary, and tertiary association areas (Augustine, 2008).

Cerebral dominance refers to the observation that one cerebral hemisphere of the brain is more involved in certain functions such as language, handedness, musical talents, visual-spatial abilities, attention, and emotion. (Amunts et al., 1996; Braitenburg and Schuz, 1998; Augustine, 2008).

In some cases, there is a functional lateralization and, in other cases, there is an accompanying structural asymmetry in the brain. The early studies of Broca and Wernicke demonstrated the lateralization of language function to the left hemisphere.

Subsequent studies demonstrated a structural asymmetry in the temporal language region termed the planum temporale which corresponds to the posterior superior surface of the superior temporal gyrus.

This asymmetry in a region corresponding to the core of Wernicke's region, an auditory association area, was greater in right-handers than in left-handers.

Both macroscopic and microscopic structural asymmetry exists in the primary motor area in humans with regard to handedness (Amunts et al., 1996).

In right-handers, MR morphometry reveals a deeper central sulcus on the left than on the right and vice versa in left-handers (Moore et al., 2000; Schüz and Miller, 2002). Correspondingly, at the microscopic level the neuropil volume is Brodmann's area 4 is larger on the left than on the right.

These anatomical asymmetries may reflect increased connectivity in area 4 along with an increase in the intrasulcal length of the posterior bank of the precentral gyrus in the left hemisphere of right-handers (Amunts et al., 1996; Geyer et al., 1996).

The functional areas of the cerebral cortex

There are different types of functional areas of the cerebral cortex including **receptive areas** and **projection areas.** According to this view, the cerebral cortex can be divided into four general functional categories: sensory, motor, unimodal association cortex, and multimodal association cortex.

The receptive areas relate to specific sensory modalities and include the primary somatosensory, primary visual, primary gustatory, primary olfactory, primary vestibular, and primary auditory areas of cerebral cortex. The primary sensory areas, except that for olfaction, receive thalamocortical fibres from diencephalic relay nuclei that are functionally related to each modality.

In addition to primary and some well-defined secondary sensory receptive or motor projection areas, there are also **cortical association areas** related to correlating, interrelating, and interpreting information that reaches the cerebral cortex.

The association areas receive impulses from various cortical regions. In the association areas are the ultimate functional capacities of the human brain. An association area may be under the influence of only one type of impulse from a single neighbouring projection (a primary association area) or receptive area, or it may correlate two different types of sensory information (a secondary association area).

The remaining portion of the cerebral cortex that is classified as a tertiary or multimodal association area in the human brain forms regions of integration, association, and correlation. These areas receive information from several different sensory modalities and create for us a complete experience of our surroundings.

Multimodal association areas are critical to our ability to communicate using language, to use reason, to extrapolate future events on the basis of present experience, to make complex and long-range plans, and to imagine and create things that have never existed.

Indeed, in terms of the associations that underlie the most complex of human capabilities there may well be heteromodal and supramodal association areas that provide the anatomical basis for our ability to read, write, speak, learn, think, reason, remember, and ultimately create new concepts and ideas.

Summary

Knowledge of the world is constructed by the brain. To Jerison, this knowledge is mind. The levels of function in the brain are hierarchically organized and then focused on the structure and functional organization of the cortex.

The cortex comprises spiny and aspiny neurons organized into about six layers (sensory, motor and associational). The vertical organization of the cortex is referred to as columns or modules. There are many cortical maps. As cortical maps develop, the brain must also develop the mind to organize the maps in such a way as to produce knowledge of the external world. The next step in mental development is language. After all, language is the way of representing knowledge. Multiple representations of sensory and motor functions exist in the cortex. One evolutionary change in mammals has been an increase in the number of representations. The cortex processes information about the world, in multiple representations, and these representations are not formally connected; yet we perceive the world as a unified whole.

This conundrum is the "binding problem" (Kolb and Whishaw, 2003).

The connections among cortical areas in a sensory system constitute only a part of all cortical connections. The four other principal connections in the cortical hierarchy are with the frontal lobe, paralimbic cortex, (phylogenetically the older cortex), multimodal cortex, and subcortical connections and loops.

Sensory regions do not connect directly with the motor cortex but may project to either the premotor or prefrontal cortex. Connections to the premotor cortex participate in ordering movements in time and controlling hand, limb, or eye movements with respect to specific sensory stimuli. Projections to the prefrontal cortex take part in the control of movements in time and short-term memories of sensory information.

The paralimbic cortex is adjacent and directly connected to the limbic structures and it comprises roughly three layers. It can be seen in two places: 1) on the medial surface of the temporal lobe, where it is known as the piriform cortex, entorhinal cortex, and para-hippocampal cortex; and 2) just above the corpus callosum, were it is referred to as the cingulate cortex. The paralimbic cortex plays a role in the formation of long-term memories.

Sensory inputs from subcortical structures are received by the cortex, from the thalamus or indirectly through midbrain structures, such as the subcortical loops.

Each level interacts and is integrated with higher and lower levels by ascending and descending connections. Subcortical loops connect the cortex, thalamus, amygdala, and hippocampus; an indirect loop with the striatum connects with the thalamus (Kolb and Whishaw, 2003).

Subcortical loops are presumed to play some role in amplifying or modulating cortical activity. The amygdala adds affective tone to visual input. In absence of the amygdala, laboratory animals display absolutely no fear of threatening objects.

Cortical areas controlling motor activity

Corticofugal fibres arise from all regions of the cerebral cortex. These projections convey impulses concerned with motor functions, modifications of muscle tone and reflex activity, modulation of sensory input and alterations of awareness and of the state of consciousness (Carpenter, 1979).

Corticofugal fibres originating largely from the deeper layers of the cerebral cortex, are projected to parts of the corpus striatum, the brain stem nuclei at all levels, and the spinal cord.

Cortical efferent fibres projecting to other cortical areas of the same hemisphere are designated as associational, while those projecting to cortical areas of the opposite hemisphere are commissural. The frontal lobe is the rostral region of the hemisphere, anterior to the central sulcus and above the lateral fissure. The precentral gyrus runs parallel to the central sulcus on the superolateral surface, extends into the medial surface, and is limited anteriorly by the precentral sulcus.

The motor activity of the entire opposite side of the body is controlled by the motor areas of the cerebral cortex (area 4) that are located anterior to the central sulcus. Fibres arise from the primary motor cortex (MI), the secondary motor cortex (MII), and the primary somatosensory (somesthetic) cortex (SI) of the frontal and parietal lobes to terminate in the motor nuclei of the brain stem and spinal cord. Cytoarchitecturally area 4 represents a modification of the typical six-layered isocortex in which the pyramidal cells in layers III and V are increased in number and the internal granular layer is obscured. For this reason this cortex is called agranular.

THE PRIMARY MOTOR AREA

The primary motor area is located superior to the lateral sulcus and in front of the central sulcus in the frontal lobe. In this region are many significant functional areas. This includes the primary motor cortex corresponding to Brodmann's area 4, which occupies the precentral gyrus on the lateral surface of the hemisphere.

It is broad at the superior border of the hemisphere, where it spreads over a considerable part of the precentral gyrus, then it narrows inferiorly and, at the level of the inferior frontal gyrus, it is practically limited to the anterior wall of the central sulcus.

On the medial surface of the hemisphere it comprises the anterior portion of the paracentral lobule.

The unusually thick cortex of the motor area (3.5 to 4.5 mm) is agranular in structure, and its ganglionic layer contains the giant pyramidal cells of Betz, whose cell bodies may reach a height of 60 to 120 μm. These cells are the largest in the paracentral lobule and the smallest in the inferior opercular region. The density of Betz cells also varies in different parts of area 4 (Lassek, 1940). Approximate percentages of Betz cells in different topographical subdivisions of area 4 are: 75% in the leg area, 18% in the arm area, and 7% in the face area. According to Lassek (1940, 1947), 34,000 giant pyramidal cells with cross-sectional areas between 900 and 4100 μm^2 have been counted in area 4 of the human brain. Neurons in area 4 are responsive to peripheral stimulation, and have receptive fields similar to those in the primary sensory cortex. Cells located posteriorly in the motor cortex have cutaneous receptive fields, whereas more anteriorly situated neurons respond to stimulation of deep tissues (Crossman, 2008).

Thus, nerve cells in the primary motor cortex are organized into groups, each group sending its axons to the cranial nerve motor nuclei, or the reticular formation, or the gray matter of the spinal cord, where they control the motor activity of a single muscle.

The rostral border of area 4 has been distinguished physiologically as a distinct subdivision, referred to as area 4S (Hines, 1936, 1937). Ablation of this narrow strip of cortex along the rostral border of area 4 in monkeys was said to produce a transient spastic paralysis, and stimulation of this area was reported to inhibit extensor muscle tone. Subsequent studies indicated that area 4S was one of a number of cortical areas from which suppressor effects could be obtained in response to stimulation (Dusser de Barenne and Mc Culloch, 1939).

Thus, on the lateral surface of the brain, the precentral sulcus bounds the precentral gyrus anteriorly and the central sulcus bounds it posteriorly. However, on the medial surface of the brain there is no reliable anatomical landmark for the anterior border of area 4.

The primary motor cortex (Brodmann's area 4) plays an important role in the execution of distinct, well defined, voluntary movements. The precentral gyrus of the right cerebral hemisphere controls movement of the left side of the head and body, whereas that of the left cerebral hemisphere controls the right side of the head and body (Passingham, 1993).

Studies in primates have demonstrated two spatially separate motor representations of the arm and hand in area 4 (Amunts et al., 1996; Augustine, 2008). The long axes of these representations are oriented approximately parallel to the central sulcus. Stimulation in both areas causes the same movements and activates the same muscles at similar strengths. This phenomenon is termed the **double representation hypothesis.** These two different areas or subareas of area 4 differ with regard to their somatosensory input. The caudal area relates to movements that use tactile feedback for their execution whereas the rostral area relates to movements that use proprioceptive feedback for their execution.

These findings along with cytoarchitectural observations and quantitative distributions of transmitter-binding sites have led to the suggestion that area 4 in humans includes **area 4 anterior (4a)** and **area 4 posterior (4p)** (Augustine, 2008).

In addition to the motor representation across area 4, tactile and proprioceptive maps occur in 4a and 4p as well. Thus, the primary motor area in humans can be subdivided based on anatomy, neurochemistry, and function.

The thumb, index, and middle fingers have a representation in both 4a and 4p (Augustine, 2008).

The primary motor cortex (MI) corresponds to the precentral gyrus (area 4), and is the area of cortex with the lowest threshold for eliciting contralateral muscle contraction by electrical stimulation.

It contains a detailed topographically organized map (**motor homunculus**) of the opposite body half, with the head represented most laterally, and the leg and foot represented on the medial surface of the hemisphere in the paracentral lobule (Fig. 21.19) (Penfield and Rasmussen, 1950).

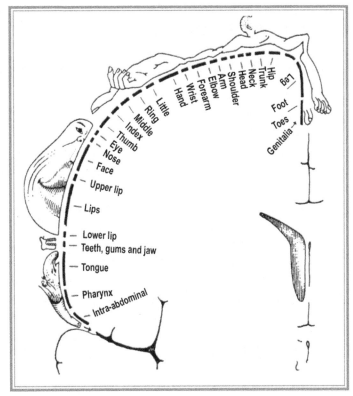

Fig. 21.19. The motor homunculus across the precentral gyrus and paracentral lobule (after Penfield and Rasmussen, 1950).

Electrical stimulation of the motor area evokes discrete isolated movements on the opposite side of the body. Usually, the contraction involves the functional muscle groups concerned with a specific movement, but individual muscles, even a single interosseous, may be contracted separately.

Flexion or extension at a single finger joint, twitchings at the corners of the mouth, elevation of the palate, protrusion of the tongue and even vocalization, expressed in involuntary cries or exclamation, all may be evoked by careful stimulation of the proper areas. Charts of motor representation, which are in substantial agreement, have been furnished by a number of investigators (Foerster 1936 a, 1936 b; Penfield and Boldrey, 1937; Scarff, 1940; Penfield and Rasmussen, 1950; Penfield and Jasper, 1954).

The location of centre specific movements may vary from individual to individual, but the sequence of motor representation appears constant. Ipsilateral movements have not been observed in men, but bilateral responses occur in muscles of the eyes, face, tongue, jaw, larynx and pharynx. According to Penfield and Boldrey (1937), the centre for the pharynx (swallowing) lies in the most inferior opercular portion of the precentral gyrus; it is followed, from below upward, by centres for the tongue, jaw, lips, larynx, eyelid and brow, in the order named. Next come the extensive areas for finger movements, the thumb being lowest and the little finger highest; these are followed by areas for the hand, wrist, elbow and shoulder. Finally, in the most superior part, are the centres for the hip, knee, ankle and toes. The last named are situated at the medial border of the hemisphere and extend into the paracentral lobule, which also contains the centres for the anal and vesicle sphincters.

There has been considerable controversy regarding the location of representation of the lower extremity, due mainly to difficulties in stimulating the medial surface. According to Foerster (1936 a), the paracentral lobule contains foci related to the foot, the toes, the bladder and the rectum. Penfield and Boldrey (1937) reported leg movements in 23 cases produced by the stimulation of superior portions of the precentral gyrus, but Scarff (1940) was unable to elicit any leg movements by stimulating the lateral surface of the hemisphere. According to Scarff (1940), the leg, as a rule, is represented only on the medial surface of the hemisphere (i.e., in the paracentral lobule). The threshold in different topographical parts of area 4 varies. The region of the thumb appears to have the lowest threshold, while the face area has the highest threshold.

Motor cortical neurons are active in relation to the force of contraction of agonist muscles; their relation to amplitude of movement is less clear. Their activity precedes the onset of electromyographic activity by 50 to 100 milliseconds, suggesting a role for cortical activation in generating rather than monitoring movement (Passingham, 1993).

A striking feature is the disproportionate representation of body parts in relation to their physical size: large areas represent the muscle of the face and hand, which are capable of finely controlled or fractionated movements. The hand area is on the middle third of the human precentral gyrus. The size of its representation reflects its extraordinary capabilities to sense temperatures, to participate in the active sense of touch in exploring the world around us, as well as carry out complex fine skilled movements including communicating with our hands. **In sum**, the representation of the knee, leg, ankle, foot and bladder begin on the edge of each cerebral hemisphere and pass over onto the anterior paracentral lobule.

The bladder region is just anterior to the region representing the ankle and the toes.

The part of the precentral gyrus controlling movement of the toes is located near its superior aspect, whereas the part of the precentral gyrus controlling movement of the tongue, mouth, and larynx is located near its inferior aspect (bordering the lateral fissure). Half of it is associated with motor activity of the hands, tongue, lips, and larynx – reflecting the manual dexterity and ability for speech that humans possess.

Prior to the onset of movement, the primary motor cortex receives instructions and information about the pattern of the intended movement from the other motor areas of the cortex.

The ipsilateral somatosensory cortex (SI) projects in a topographically organized way to area 4, and the connection is reciprocal. The projection to the motor cortex arises in areas 1 and 2, with little or no contribution from area 3b. SI fibres terminate in layers II and III of area 4, where they contact mainly pyramidal neurons. Evidence suggests that neurons activated, monosynaptically, fibres from SI, as well as those activated polysynaptically, make contact with layer V pyramidal cells, including Betz cells, which give rise to corticospinal fibres (Passingham, 1993; Bodegard et al., 2000; Geyer et al., 2000; Kaas, 2004). Movement-related neurons in the motor cortex which can be activated from SI tend to have a late onset activity, mainly during the execution of movement. It has been suggested that this pathway plays a role primarily in making motor adjustments during a movement. Additional ipsilateral corticocortical fibres to area 4 from behind the central sulcus come from the second somatic sensory area (S II) (Burton et al., 1995; Amunts et al., 1996; Geyer et al., 1999; Disbrow et al., 2000; Bodegord et al., 2000; Parsons et al., 2005).

The motor cortex receives major frontal lobe association fibres form the premotor cortex and the supplementary motor area and also fibres from the insula (Augustine, 1985; 1996; Geyer et al., 1996; Kaas, 2004).

It is probable that these pathways modulate motor cortical activity in relation to the preparation, guidance and temporal organization of movements. Area 4 sends fibres to, and receives fibres from its contralateral counterpart, and also projects to the contralateral supplementary motor cortex (Crossman, 2008).

Apart from its contribution to the corticospinal tract, the motor cortex has diverse subcortical projections. The connections with the thalamus, striatum, pontine nuclei and the subthalamic nucleus are strong.

Thus, the major thalamic connections of area 4 are with the ventral posterolateral nucleus (VPL), which in turn receives afferents from the deep cerebellar nuclei. The VPL nucleus also contains a topographic representation of the contralateral body, which is preserved in its point-to-point projection to area 4, where it terminates largely in lamina IV.

Other thalamic connections of area 4 are with the centromedian and parafascicular nuclei. These appear to provide the only route through which output from the basal ganglia, routed *via* the thalamus, reaches the primary motor cortex, since the projection of the internal segment of the globus pallidus to the ventrolateral nucleus of the thalamus is confined to the anterior division, and there is no overlap with cerebellothalamic territory.

The anterior part of the ventrolateral nucleus projects to the premotor and supplementary motor areas of the cortex with no projection to area 4 (Crossman, 2008).

Corticospinal tract. The corticospinal tract, which is considered to transmit direct impulses for highly skilled volitional movements to lower motor neurons, arises mainly from area 4. The larger corticospinal fibres are probably the axons of giant pyramidal cells, for these cells undergo chromatolysis following a section of the pyramid (Holmes and May, 1909; Levin and Bradford, 1938).

Since the number of fibres in the human corticospinal tract at the level of the pyramid is approximately 1,000,000, axons of the giant cells of Betz could account for only a little over 3% of these fibres, assuming that each cell gives rise to a single corticospinal fibre (Lassek, 1940). Studies of the fibre spectrum of the human corticospinal tract, indicating about 30,000 fibres with diameters between 9 and 22 μm (Lassek and Rasmussen, 1939, 1940; Lassek, 1954), strongly support the view that these fibres are the parent axons of the giant pyramidal cells.

Approximately 90% of the fibres of the corticospinal tract range from 1 to 4 μm in diameter. Of the total number of fibres in the tract, about 40% are poorly myelinated.

The more numerous small fibres of the corticospinal tract are considered to arise from smaller cells in this and other cortical regions.

Interruption of the corticospinal tract also gives rise to chromatolytic cell changes in small pyramidal cells in layers III and V, not only in area 4, but also in areas 3, 1, 2 and 5 (Levin and Bradford, 1938). Ablations of area 4 in monkeys cause degeneration of 27 to 40% of the corticospinal tract, including virtually all of the large myelinated fibres (Lassek, 1942, 1954). Other authors have reported smaller percentages of degenerated fibres after similar ablations (Häggqvist, 1937), but more reported complete degeneration of the corticospinal tract (Mettler 1944 a; Welch and Kennard, 1944).

Ablations of the parietal cortex (areas 3, 1, 2, 5 and 7) also produce degeneration of myelinated fibres in the corticospinal tract (Minkowski, 1923-1924; Peele, 1942).

Combined ablations of the precentral and postcentral gyri cause degeneration of 50 to 60% of the fibres in the corticospinal tract (Lassek, 1942, 1942 a; Russell and De Myer, 1961).

A quantitative study of the origin of corticospinal fibres in monkeys based on silver staining methods (Russell and De Myer, 1961) indicates that virtually all fibres of the corticospinal tract arise from area 4, area 6 and parts of the parietal lobe.

Approximate percentages of corticospinal fibres arising from these areas are as follows: (1) area 4, 31%; (2) area 6, 29%; and (3) parietal lobe, 40%. Complete decortication, or hemispherectomy, causes all fibres of the corticospinal tract to degenerate in men (Lassek and Evans, 1945) and in monkeys (Mattler, 1944 a; Russel and De Myer, 1961).

Thus, the corticospinal fibres arise from the pyramidal cells in layer V and give rise to the largest corticospinal axons in diameter. There is also a widespread origin from other parts of the frontal lobe, including the premotor cortex and the supplementary motor area. Many axons from the frontal cortex, notably the motor cortex, terminate in the ventral horn of the spinal cord. In cord segments mediating dexterous hand and finger movements they terminate in the lateral part of the ventral horn, in close relationship to the motor neuronal group. A small percentage establishes direct monosynaptic connections with alpha motor neurons.

Between 40 and 60% of pyramidal tract axons arise from parietal areas, including area 3a, area 5 of the superior parietal lobe, and S II in the parietal operculum. The majority of parietal fibres to the spinal cord terminate in the deeper layers of the dorsal horn.

The motor cortex also projects to the subthalamic nucleus. The motor cortex sends projections to all nuclei in the brain stem, which are themselves the origin of descending pathways to the spinal cord, namely the reticular formation, the red nucleus, the superior colliculus, the vestibular nuclei and the inferior olivary nucleus.

Ablation of the motor cortex in mammals produces increasingly greater neurological deficits at progressively higher levels of the phylogenetic scale (Walker and Fulton, 1938).

In cats, the removal of the motor cortex, or even hemidecortication, do not impair the animal's ability to walk upon recovery from anesthesia.

Ablations of area 4 in monkeys produce a contralateral flaccid paralysis, marked hypotonia and areflexia. Within a relatively short time myotatic reflexes reappear, along with withdrawal responses to nociceptive stimuli (Fulton and Keller, 1932). Recovery of movement begins in the proximal musculature and progresses distally, but the digits tend to remain permanently paralysed. Studies by Travis (1955) in monkeys confirm these things, except that recovery of motor function in the distal parts of the extremity was as rapid as that in proximal parts.

However, skilled movements were performed slowly and with some deliberation. The atrophy present in the paretic limbs during the period of greatest disuse disappeared after maximal functional recovery. No significant spasticity developed in these animals. Other results (Denny-Brown and Botterell, 1948; Denny-Brown, 1960) differ from the above in that some degree of spasticity accompanying by the paretic manifestations after all lesions of the precentral gyrus in monkeys. Relatively mild spasticity developed first in proximal muscle groups and was described as most enduring following total ablation (Carpenter, 1979).

Because the precentral gyrus gives rise to a large number of nonpyramidal fibres, and is the source of only a part of the corticospinal tract, it is instructive to compare the motor deficits described above with those which follow a surgical section of the pyramids.

Selective pyramidotomy in monkeys and chimpanzees, accomplished by an anterior approach, produces a contralateral paresis which is somewhat more severe in chimpanzees than in monkeys (Tower, 1940, 1949). The usage which survives is stripped of all the finer qualities which contribute to the skill, precision and versatility of motor performance.

A pyramidotomy is associated with hypotonia and loss of superficial abdominal and cremasteric reflexes.

The myotatic reflexes are increased in threshold and somewhat pendular. Tonic neck reflexes are absent, and clonus does not occur. A forced grasp reflex is prominent and may be so severe as to interfere with climbing.

Observation of monkeys with bilateral pyramidal lesions by Lawrence and Kuypers (1968) also indicate that considerable recovery of independent limb movements occurs, but recovery of individual finger movements never returns. All movements are slower and the muscles fatigue more rapidly than in normal animals. These findings indicate that the corticospinal pathway conducts impulses concerned with speed and agility of movement, and fractionation of movements, as exemplified by individual finger movements. Motor function remaining after bilateral pyramidotomy must be mediated by brain stem pathway projections to spinal levels.

Lesions of the motor cortex in men produce neurological deficits similar to those described in primates (Foerster, 1936 a; Bucy, 1949, 1959; Penfield and Rasmussen, 1950). Ablation limited to the "arm" or "leg" area of the precentral gyrus results in a paralysis of a single limb. The ultimate loss of movement is always greatest in the distal muscle groups, but motor recovery in the affected limb usually is more complete than that associated with nearly total lesions of the motor area (Bucy, 1949).

According to Bucy (1949), the spasticity is not severe and is less intense than that commonly associated with hemiplegias resulting from large capsular lesions.

Although there is considerable restitution of function in proximal muscle groups, relatively little recovery of skilled motor function occurs in the smaller distal muscles of the extremities.

However, immediately after complete or partial lesions of the precentral gyrus, there is a flaccid paralysis of the contralateral limbs or limb, marked hypotonia and loss of superficial and myotatic reflexes. Within a relatively short time, the Babinski sign can be elicited. The myotatic reflexes generally return early in an exaggerated form.

The total cortical area that mediates motor activity of a particular body region is proportional to the complexity of the movements produced in that region.

Secondary motor cortex

The secondary motor cortex consists of four regions: the premotor cortex, supplementary motor cortex, the frontal eye field, and the posterior parietal motor area (Fig. 21.20).

The first three of these motor cortical areas reside in the frontal lobe (rostral to the central sulcus); the posterior parietal motor area is located in the parietal lobe.

The principal function of the secondary motor cortex is the programming of complex motor activity, which is then relayed to the primary motor cortex where the execution of motor activity is initiated.

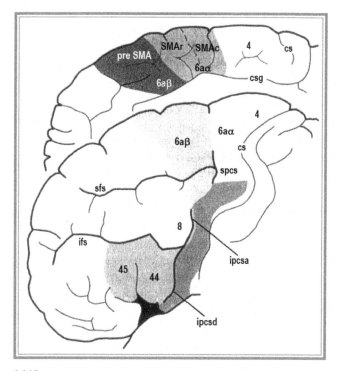

Fig. 21.20. Several Brodmann's areas in the frontal lobe of the human brain: primary motor area 4, premotor area 6, Broca's motor speech region (areas 44 and 45) (from Paxinos and Mai, 2004).

The primary motor cortex then translates this information into execution of movement, and relays it mainly to the brain stem or spinal cord. Most of the nerve signals that arise in the secondary motor cortex mediate complex movements produced by groups of muscles performing a particular task, unlike the discrete muscle contractions elicited by the stimulation of the primary motor cortex (Patestas and Gartner, 2008).

PREMOTOR CORTEX

Immediately in front of the primary motor cortex lies Brodmann's area 6. It extends onto the medial surface, where it becomes contiguous with area 24 in the cingulate gyrus, anterior and inferior to the paracentral lobule. Near the superior border it is quite broad and includes the caudal portion of the superior frontal gyrus. The rostral border of area 6 on both medial and lateral surfaces of the human brain is unclear. On the medial surface of the brain, area 6 extends inferiorly to the cingulate sulcus where its caudal border is Brodmann's area 24, part of the anterior cingulate cortex.

Inferiorly the premotor area narrows, and near the operculum, it is limited to the precentral gyrus. Its histological structure resembles that of the motor area; it is composed principally of large well formed pyramidal cells, but there are no giant cells of Betz. The presence of pyramidal cells in layers III and V and the narrowness of layer V make it difficult to distinguish an internal granular layer (Campbell, 1905).

For this reason, area 6, like area 4, is referred to as the agranular frontal cortex.

Area 6 has been subdivided into various portions (Fig. 21.21) (Foerster, 1936 b). According to this parcellation, area 6aα lies immediately rostral to area 4 along the convexity of the hemisphere, while area 6aβ occupies the region of the superior frontal gyrus on both the lateral and medial surfaces of the hemisphere. A small area called 6b lies in front of the face area.

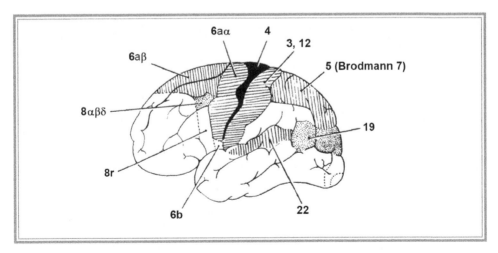

Fig. 21.21. The areas of electrically excitable cortex on the lateral surface of the human brain. The motor area is shown in black, and the so-called "extrapyramidal areas" are hatched except for the eye fields, which are stippled (after Foerster, 1936 b).

Electrical stimulation of area 6aα in men produces responses similar to those obtained from area 4, although stronger stimuli are required (Foerster, 1931, 1936 a). It is probably area 6aα that discharges *via* the corticospinal tract.

Stimulation of area 6aβ elicits more general movement patterns characterized by rotation of the head, eyes and trunk to the opposite side, and synergic patterns of flexion or extension in the contralateral extremities.

These general movements appear independent of area 4, since they can be obtained after its removal.

Portions of area 6aβ on the medial aspect of the hemisphere are considered to constitute part of the supplementary motor area. Stimulation of area 6b is reported to produce rhythmic coordinated movements of a complex type involving facial, masticatory, laryngeal and pharyngeal musculature (Foerster, 1931, 1936 a).

Unilateral ablations of area 6, including portions on the medial aspect of the hemisphere, produce transient grasp reflexes in monkeys (Richter and Hines, 1932).

Bilateral removals of area 6 produce more enduring grasp reflexes (Kennard and Fulton, 1933; Welch and Kennard, 1944).

The unilateral destruction of area 6aβ in men produces little or no motor deficits (Foerster, 1936 a). Only lesions involving the supplementary motor areas produce grasping phenomena (Erickson and Woolsey, 1951; Travis, 1955 a).

Combined ablations of areas 4 and 6 produce a contralateral spastic paralysis (Kennard and Fulton, 1933; Fulton and Kennard, 1934; Kennard, 1949). Similar findings were reported in men following ablations of area 6, which undoubtedly included parts of area 4, as well as the so-called area 4 S (Kennard et al., 1934).

Ablations of the posterior part of area 4 result in a contralateral flaccid paresis. Subsequent investigations (Travis, 1955 a) explain the spasticity resulting from combined lesions of areas 4 and 6 on the basis of simultaneous destruction of precentral and supplementary motor areas, which are known to produce a contralateral spastic paralysis. According to Crossman (2008) the premotor cortex is divided into a dorsal and ventral area on functional ground, and on the basis of ipsilateral corticortical association connections.

The premotor cortex receives axon terminals from the cerebellum *via* a relay in the ventral lateral (VLp) nucleus of the thalamus, and fibres from the cortical association areas. Input from the cerebellum assists the premotor cortex in its role in movement.

The major thalamic connections of the premotor cortex are with the anterior division of the ventrolateral nucleus and with the centromedian, parafascicular and contralateral components of the intralaminar nuclei. (Passingham, 1993; Toga et al., 2006; Crossman, 2008).

Subcortical projections to the striatum and pontine nuclei are prominent, and this area also projects to the superior colliculus and the reticular formation.

Area 6 contributes to the corticospinal tract. Commissural connections are with the contralateral premotor, motor and superior parietal (area 5) cortex.

Ipsilateral corticocortical connections with area 5 in the superior parietal cortex, and inferior parietal area 7b are common to both dorsal and ventral subdivisions of the premotor cortex, and both send a major projection to the primary motor cortex.

The dorsal premotor area also receives fibres from the posterior temporal cortex and projects to the supplementary motor cortex.

The frontal eye field (area 8) projects to the dorsal subdivision. Perhaps the greatest functionally significant difference in connectivity between the two premotor area subdivisions is that the dorsal premotor area receives fibres from the dorsolateral prefrontal cortex, whereas the ventral subdivision receives fibres from the ventrolateral cortex. All of these association connections are likely to be or are known to be, reciprocal (Crossman, 2008).

The main function of this area is the motor control of axial and proximal limb musculature. It also plays a role in orienting the body and upper limbs in the direction of a target. Once a motor task has been initiated, activity in the premotor cortex diminishes, reflecting its key function in the planning phase of motor activity.

A motor pattern exists across the premotor cortex with responses that are contralateral, but not as discrete as the responses that follow stimulation of the primary motor cortex.

Neuronal activity in the premotor cortex in relation to both preparation for movement and movement itself has been extensively studied experimentally. Thus, according to Crossman (2008) direction selectivity for movements is a common feature of many premotor neurons. In behavioral tasks, neurons in the dorsal premotor cortex show anticipatory activity and task-related discharge as well as direction selectivity, but little or no stimulus-related changes.

The dorsal premotor cortex is probably important in establishing a motor set or intention, contributing to motor preparation in relation to internally guided movements. In contrast, the ventral premotor cortex is more related to the execution of externally (especially visually) guided movements in relation to a specific external stimulus (Crossman, 2008).

According to Roland and Zilles (1996), Zilles (2004), and Augustine (2008), the premotor cortex is an extrapyramidal motor area in that it supplements the activity of the primary motor cortex. The premotor cortex is also termed the frontal aversive field in that stimulation of this area causes rotation of the head, eyes, and trunk to the opposite side with complex synergistic movements of flexion and extension of the contralateral arm and leg. In addition to the motor representation across area 6, a tactile map occurs across this area as well.

Injury to the premotor cortex produces a **motor apraxia.** This purely cortical concept refers to the inability to carry out a sequence of motor activities in the presence of intact motor and sensory paths. Motor apraxia is evident through clumsiness in writing or drawing (Augustine, 2008).

A grasp reflex is likely to appear as well. Following damage to the primary motor cortex, the premotor cortex is able to substitute to some degree.

This region also participates in cortical automatic associated movements that accompany fine skilled voluntary movements. The grasp reflex (grasping of the examiner's hand) is elicited by firmly stroking the palm fingers of the patient's hand in an outward direction. The grasp tends to persist, and the more force exerted, the greater the intensity of the grasp. Unlike a normal grasp, the thumb usually remains extended.

A grasp reflex appearing in newborns and disappearing at two to four months is likely to be marked by suspending a child by his grasp. In older individuals, the primary motor cortex inhibits this reflex.

Supplementary motor area (SMA)

Observations by early investigators indicated that responses in different parts of the body could be elicited by electrical stimulation of the medial surface of the frontal lobe rostral to the primary motor area (Carpenter, 1979). This motor area, identified in the human brain, has been designed as the supplementary motor area (Penfield and Rasmussen, 1950).

The supplementary motor area lies medially to area 6, and extends from the most superolateral part of the medial surface of the hemisphere. Area 24 in the cingulate gyrus adjacent to area 6 contains several motor areas, which are termed cingulate motor areas. An additional functional subdivision, the pre-SMA, lies anteriorly to the supplementary motor area on the medial surface of the cortex. These additional medial motor areas are included in the supplementary motor cortex (Crossman, 2008).

SMA is divisible into a rostral, **pre-SMA** and a caudal region **(the SMA proper)** (Augustine, 2008).

Detailed descriptions of somatotopic representations within the supplementary motor area of the monkey have been provided by Woolsey et al. (1951).

The threshold for stimulation of the supplementary motor area in men and monkeys is slightly higher than for the precentral region, but the motor effects are not due to the spreading of excitation across the cortex.

SMA receives axon terminals from the basal ganglia (the globus pallidus and the pars reticulate of the substantia nigra) *via* a relay in the ventral lateral (VLa) nucleus of the thalamus.

Subcortical connections, other than with the thalamus, pass to the striatum, subthalamic nucleus and pontine nuclei, the brain stem reticular formation and the inferior olivary nucleus. Additional thalamic afferents are form the ventral anterior nucleus, the intralaminar nuclei, notably the centrolateral and centromedial nuclei, and also from the mediodorsal nucleus. The connections with the thalamus are reciprocal. The supplementary motor cortex receives connections from widespread regions of the ipsilateral frontal lobe, including from the primary motor cortex, the dorsal premotor area, the dorsolateral and ventrolateral prefrontal, medial prefrontal and orbitofrontal cortex and the frontal eye field. These connections are reciprocal, but the major ipsilateral efferent pathway is to the motor cortex (Crossman, 2008).

Parietal lobe connections of the SMA are with the superior parietal area 5 and possibly inferior parietal area 7b. Contralateral connections are with the SMA, and motor and premotor cortices of the contralateral hemisphere (Crossman, 2008).

The SMA makes a substantial contribution to the corticospinal tract, contributing as much as 40% of the figures from the frontal lobe (Passingham, 1993; Toga et al., 2006; Crossman, 2008).

The SMA contains a representation of the body in which the leg is posterior and the face anterior, with the upper limb between them. According to Augustine (2008), SMA is somatotopically organized in humans with index finger responses anterior and dorsal to shoulder responses.

Unilateral ablations of the SMA in men produce no permanent deficit in the maintenance of posture or the capacity of movement (Penfield and Rasmussen, 1950; Penfield and Welch, 1951).

According to Travis (1955), unilateral ablations of the supplementary motor area in monkeys produce weak transient grasp reflexes in the contralateral limbs, and moderate bilateral hypertonia of the shoulder muscles, but no paresis.

Bilateral simultaneous ablations of this area result in disturbances of posture and tonus, but produce no paresis. Gradually increasing hypertonia, resulting in muscle contracture, develops in a period of 2 to 4 weeks.

The hypertonia is mainly in flexor muscles. Myotatic reflexes are hyperactive, and clonus can be demonstrated. Ablations of the SMA and the precentral motor area on the same side result in an immediate contralateral hypotonic paresis with impaired myotatic reflexes. Within a period of 2 weeks, the hypotonus changes to hypertonus and the myotatic reflexes become exaggerated.

All evidence indicates that the SMA is a bilaterally functioning entity concerned primarily with mechanisms of posture and movement. Following bilateral simultaneous ablations of the SMA in monkeys indicate that such lesions produce a milder increase in muscle tone, inconsistent reflex changes and no evidence of joint contracture (Coxe and Landau, 1965).

According to Bertrand (1956), ablations of the SMA do not produce degeneration passing to the spinal cord, but electrical stimulation of the SMA in monkeys evokes potentials bilaterally in the region of the corticospinal tracts at spinal cord levels. The bilateral features of this system are striking and appear to explain why unilateral lesions of the SMA cause only minor deficits.

Penfield and Jasper (1954) report that motor responses from the SMA can be elicited after the removal of the precentral gyrus. Stimulation of this motor area in men, following hemispherectomy, induces ipsilateral movements similar to those which can be produced voluntarily (Bates, 1953).

According to Augustine (2008), complex motor tasks activate the rostral SMA whereas simple motor tasks activate the caudal SMA proper. Pre-SMA is involved in the acquisition of new motor sequences whereas SMA proper participates in the acquisition of motor sequences that are essentially automatic.

Activation of SMA occurs during imagined movements whereas regional cerebral blood flow increases in this area during complex sequential movements (Gelnar, 1998; Bodegård et al., 2000; Fuster, 2001; Kaas, 2004).

According to Crossman (2008), the role of the SMA in the control of movement is primarily in complex tasks which require temporal organization of sequential movements and in the retrieval of motor memory. Input from the basal ganglia assists the SMA in its role in the programming phase of the patterns and sequences of complex movements, and the coordination of bilateral movements. The SMA mediates muscle contractions of the axial (trunk) and proximal limb (girdle) musculature (i.e., the muscle controlling movements of the arm and thigh). Stimulation of the supplementary motor area in conscious patients has been reported to elicit the sensation of an urge to move, or of anticipation that a movement is about to occur. A region anterior to the SMA for face representation (area 44, 45) is important in vocalization and speech production.

In sum, the traditionally defined supplementary motor area includes two separate regions: a caudal region (SMA proper) that has reciprocal connections with the primary motor area and project to the spinal cord, and a rostral region (presupplementary motor area) that receives projections from the prefrontal and cingulate cortices. Basal ganglia input reaches the caudal region, whereas cerebellar input reaches the rostral region. Neuronal responses to visual stimuli prevail in the rostral region, whereas somatosensory responses prevail in the caudal region. The urge to initiate movement in humans is elicited only from the rostral region (Wise, 1985; Tanji and Kurata, 1989; Tanji, 1994; Gallese et al., 1996).

Posterior parietal motor area

The posterior parietal motor area corresponds to Brodmann's areas 5 and 7. Area 5 is involved in tactile discrimination (the ability to perceive a subtle distinction by the sense of touch) and stereognosis (the recognition of the three-dimensional shape of an object by the sense of touch), as well as statognosis in relation to reaching and guiding movements.

Area 7 is involved with movements that require visual guidance. Thus, when one reaches for a glass of cold water, visual guidance (turning the body and aiming the upper limb in the direction of the glass) and tactile sensation (which in this case helps to realize that the glass is slippery and must be grasped firmly), both play a role in accomplishing a desired motor task (Patestas and Gartner, 2008).

Extrapyramidal cortical areas in the parietal and occipital lobes influence ocular movements, particularly following of automatic movements of the eyes.

Frontal eye field

Because the direction of gaze often indicates the visual stimuli to which a subject attends, the study of eye movement control is also producing important insights into the mechanisms of visual attention and other higher-order cognitive processes (Corbetta et al., 1998). Much of what is known about eye movement control has been learned from combined eye movement and single-cell electrophysiological recordings from awake, behaving monkeys.

Two types of eye movements are studied most often in human and nonhuman primates: saccades and smooth pursuit. Saccades are shifts of gaze that serve to maintain an image on the fovea, the area of the retina with the highest visual acuity. Saccades can be reflexive, or voluntary.

Smooth pursuit allows for continuous, undistorted vision of objects moving across the visual field by matching the velocity of eye movements with the velocity of a target. Smooth pursuit likely requires a more complicated neural network, and more processing in cortical, basal ganglia, brain stem, and cerebellar regions for proper functioning (Krauzlis, 2004).

Because the generation of saccades can be largely automatic and independent of cortical structures, study of "top-down" control of saccades can be used to model cognitive aspects of motor control (Stuphorn and Schall, 2002).

Multiple regions within the frontal cortex and subcortical nuclei are involved in the generation of eye movements. For saccades, it is believed that the frontal lobe oculomotor regions are most important for voluntary saccades, whereas accurate reflexive saccades can be generated with little input from the frontal lobes (Pierrot-Deseilligny et al., 2004).

Data from both monkeys and humans support the roles for the frontal lobes in both movement perception and representation (Rizzolati and Luppino, 2001) as well as planning and execution of movements.

The first intraoperative stimulation studies in humans resulted in a broad region for the frontal eye fields because eye movements were elicited from various areas encompassing Brodmann's areas 6, 8, 9 and 46 (Foerster, 1936; Penfield and Boldrey, 1937; Smith, 1944). The latest studies, in which smaller current intensities have been used, restricted the frontal eye fields to the anterior portion of the motor strip, in the upper portion of the facial area (Woolsey et al., 1979; Lüders et al., 1988; Godoy et al., 1990). However, the sulcal cortex could not be investigated with large subdural electrodes, and the mediolateral position of frontal eye fields remains imprecise. Positron emission tomography studies also have been utilised to improve our knowledge of the localization and function of the frontal eye fields (Fox et al., 1985; Anderson et al., 1994; O'Sullivan et al., 1995; Petit et al., 1996; Sweeney et al., 1996).

The results of these studies have indicated that human frontal eye fields are located more posteriorly in the frontal lobe than expected by a comparison with monkey frontal eye fields.

In humans, fMRI imaging, with its increased spatial resolution, has provided new insights into the functional anatomy of frontal eye fields (Darby et al., 1996; Petit et al., 1997; Luna et al., 1998; Corbetta et al., 1998).

Contrary to studies performed using subdural electrodes, intracerebral electrical stimulation enables localized stimulation of almost any part of the cortex, including the sulcal cortex (Munari et al., 1993, 1994).

Lobel et al. (2001) used intracerebral electrical stimulation in 38 patients with epilepsy prior to surgery, and frontal regions where stimulation induced versive eye movement were identified. These studies showed that two distinct oculomotor areas could be individualized in the region classically corresponding to the frontal eye fields. One oculomotor area was consistently at the intersection of the superior frontal sulcus with the fundus of the superior portion of the precentral sulcus. The second oculomotor area was located more laterally and close to the surface of the precentral gyrus. Lobel et al.

(2001) compared results obtained from fMRI imaging with those obtained using intracerebral electrical stimulation.

These two areas are anatomically distinct (mean distance from each other is 19 mm).

The deep oculomotor areas are the regions of the human frontal lobe where eye movements can be most easily elicited by electrical stimulation. It is located more posteriorly in the frontal lobe, apparently within Brodmann's area 6. The most remarkable feature is the specific anatomical link between the deep oculomotor areas and the intersection of the superior frontal sulcus.

Anatomy. The frontal eye field in men occupies principally the caudal part of the middle frontal gyrus (corresponding to parts of area 8) and extends into contiguous portions of the inferior frontal gyrus (Carpenter, 1979).

According to Boxer (2007), in the frontal lobes, three regions are most involved in eye movement control: the **frontal eye field,** the **supplementary eye fields,** and the **dorsolateral prefrontal cortex** (Fig. 21.22). These frontal eye movement control regions are strongly connected to regions in the dorsal parietal lobe involved in eye movement control, particularly in the vicinity of the lateral intraparietal sulcus, the basal ganglia, and brain stem structures.

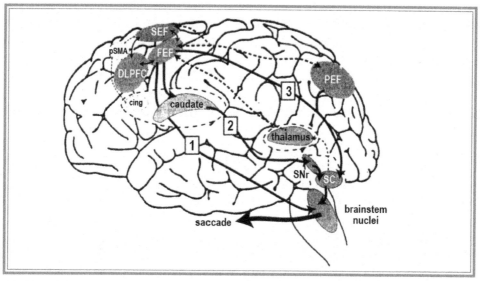

Fig. 21.22. Brain regions involved in saccade control. In the frontal lobes, frontal eye field (FEF) is a critical node for initiation of voluntary saccades. It receives input from the parietal eye fields (PEFs) and thalamus, which provide visual information. The supplementary eye field (SEF) monitors and supervises FEF activity, and the dorsolateral prefrontal cortex (DLPFC) likely exerts a direct modulatory influence on the FEF, as well as on downstream structures in the brain stem. Other regions in the medial frontal lobes, including the pre-supplementary motor area (pSMA) and anterior cingulate (cing), may also exert modulatory influences on the FEF *via* the SEF and DLPFC. There are three main pathways from the FEF to the primary and secondary motor neurons in the brain stem nuclei that generate saccades: (1) a direct connection between the FEF and the brain stem oculomotor nuclei; (2) a pathway through the caudate eye field and substantia nigra pars reticulata (SNr), which helps to suppress saccades; and (3) a direct connection between the FEF and superior colliculus (SC), which is finely tuned for saccade programming and can generate reflexive saccades independently of the FEF (after Boxer, 2007).

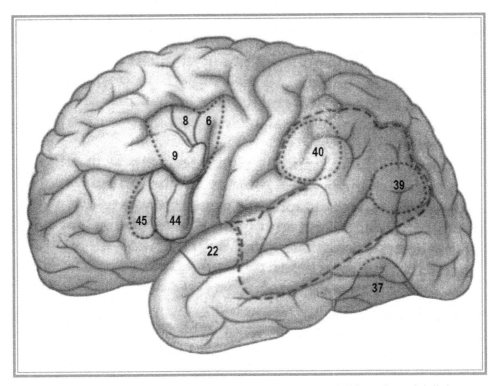

Fig. 21.23. Lateral surface of the left cerebral hemisphere showing the frontal eye field (parts of areas 6, 8, 9), the motor speech (Broca's) area (areas 44, 45) and Wernicke's area. The perimeter of these areas is delineated by an interrupted line to indicate uncertainly as to their precise extent. Wernicke's area is variously depicted by different authorities as encompassing a large parietotemporal area which includes areas 39 and 40. Areas 22 and 37 are considered by some to be respectively auditory and visuo-auditory areas associated with speech and language (after Crossman, 2008).

According to Augustine (2008) and Crossman (2008), there are **primary** and **secondary eye fields** that occupy parts of Brodmann's areas 6, 8 and 9 (Fig. 21.23). The primary frontal eye field is in the posterior part of the middle frontal gyrus. The secondary frontal eye field is in the dorsal part of the inferior frontal gyrus. Cytoarchitecturally, area 8 is a typical six layered isocortex of the frontal type in which the granular layers are distinct.

Processes of neurons in the eye fields project their fibres through the corticobulbar path to nuclei of the ocular muscle. The primary eye fields project fibres to agonist muscles, whereas neurons in the secondary eye fields project fibres to antagonist muscles. Voluntary ocular movements obviously involve the cooperative action of eye field in both cerebral hemispheres (Paus, 1996; Lebel et al., 2001).

Frontal eye field. The frontal eye field is located in the rostral bank of the arcuate sulcus in macaque monkeys (Stuphorn and Schall, 2002). In humans, high-resolution fMRI studies have localized the frontal eye field to the anterior wall of the precentral sulcus, near the caudal end of the superior frontal sulcus, a region homologous to the location of the frontal eye field in monkeys (Rosano et al., 2002).

The frontal eye field can be further subdivided into two regions, one involved in the generation of saccades, which is located in the upper portion of the anterior wall of the precentral sulcus, and a smooth pursuit-related area, which is found deeper along the anterior wall, extending in some subjects to the fundus or deep posterior wall. Using histopathological markers from postmortem specimens, these regions have been demonstrated to be structurally similar to other regions of the motor cortex (Rosano et al., 2003).

Electrical stimulation of the frontal eye field in men causes conjugate deviation of the eyes, usually to the opposite side (Foerster, 1931; Penfield and Rasmussen, 1950). Stimulation here causes occasionally upward movements, convergence, divergence of the eyes and pupillary changes. Movements of the head and pupillary changes usually accompany movements of the eyes.

Unilateral stimulation of the frontal eye fields in humans usually produces bilateral opening or closing of the lids (Paus, 1996; Lobel et al., 2001; Milea et al., 2002).

Based on electrical stimulation studies of human subjects prior to brain surgery, the saccade-generating portion of the frontal eye field is found 1-2 cm anterior to the primary motor cortical regions involved in finger and hand movements, a region in close agreement to that identified in fMRI studies (Yamamoto et al., 2004).

Similarly, cortical stimulation experiments in humans confirm that the smooth pursuit region is located more posteriorly than the saccade region (Blanke and Seeck, 2003).

The frontal eye field receives connections that convey both visuosensory information and motor information to its neurons. Importantly, regions within the frontal eye field receive information from both the ventral visual stream (the "what" pathway) and the dorsal visual stream (the "where" pathway; Schall et al., 1995). The neurons of the frontal eye field that receive connections from the ventral stream generate shorter saccades than those innervated by dorsal stream neurons. This is consistent with the expected size of saccades necessary to explore visually a small object of the face (in detail) versus those necessary to characterize distant aspects of a subject's spatial environment.

The frontal eye field also receives information from the supplementary eye fields, the dorsolateral prefrontal cortex, the thalamus, and the substantia nigra pars reticulata. According to Crossman (2008), the frontal eye field receives its major thalamic projection from the parvocellular mediodorsal nucleus, with additional afferents from the medial pulvinar, the ventral anterior nucleus and the suprageniculate-limitans complex, and connects with the paracentral nucleus of the intralaminar group.

The thalamocortical pathways to the frontal eye field form part of a pathway from the superior colliculus, the substantia nigra and the dentate nucleus of the cerebellum.

Neurons in the cerebellum are critical for maintaining smooth pursuit eye movements and may help to refine certain types of saccades.

The frontal eye field has extensive ipsilateral corticocortical connections, receiving fibres from several visual areas in the occipital, parietal and temporal lobes, including the medial temporal area (V5) and area 7a.

There are also projections from the superior temporal gyrus, which is auditory rather than visual in function. From within the frontal lobe, the frontal eye field receives fibres from the ventrolateral and dorsolateral prefrontal cortices.

These inputs can positively and negatively modulate the activity of neurons within the frontal eye field.

From the frontal eye fields fibres descend in the corticobulbar path, enter the genu of the internal capsule, the cerebral crus at the base of the midbrain, and descend into the brain stem. Along the way, a few fibres turn off oculomotor nuclear levels to supply the oculomotor nucleus as the remaining fibres descend and end in the abducens nucleus.

This area contains cell bodies whose axons join the corticonuclear tract and descend to terminate in the eye movement control centres located in the midbrain reticular formation and the paramedian pontine formation. In turn, they transmit information to the motor nuclei of cranial nerves III, IV, and VI, which control voluntary eye movements.

The frontal eye field projects to the dorsal and ventral premotor cortices and to the medial motor area, probably, to the supplementary eye field adjacent to the supplementary motor area proper. It projects prominently to the deeper layer of the superior colliculus *via* a transtegmental projection (Kuypers and Lawrence, 1967). However, the most substantial and highly organized projections to the superior colliculus arise from the visual cortex (Garey et al., 1968). These fibres mainly enter the stratum opticum *via* the brachium of the superior colliculus. In the brain stem, the superior colliculus plays a dominant role in organizing many aspects of eye movement control through its connections with other nuclei in the dorsal midbrain (for vertical eye movements) and the pons (for horizontal eye movements). Although the superior colliculus does not project direct fibres to the nuclei of the extraocular muscles, it has projections to both the reticular formation and the accessory oculomotor nuclei (Carpenter, 1971).

Thus, the frontal eye field projects to the pontine gaze centre within the pontine reticular formation, and to other oculomotor related nuclei in the brain stem.

Studies in nonhuman primates suggest that in normal subjects most of the control of saccades by the frontal eye movement regions is mediated by the superior colliculus (Sparks, 2002).

Under conditions of superior colliculus damage, other cortical and brain stem regions can partially compensate for the lost superior colliculus functions; however, saccades are much less accurate in time and space.

Neurons that have saccade-related activity in the intermediate and deep layers of the superior colliculus are arranged topographically and fire bursts of activity before an eye movement, be it a saccade or smooth pursuit (Krauzlis and Dill, 2002).

Thus, the activation of rostral cells generates small-amplitude eye movements, and the activation of caudal cells generates larger-amplitude saccades. Electrical stimulation of the rostral pole of the superior colliculus inhibits saccades, consistent with an important role for maintaining fixation on a target.

These neurons have monosynaptic excitatory inputs neurons in the brain stem that inhibit eye movements (Leigh and Kennard, 2004). Upward saccades are represented medially, and downward saccades, laterally, within the superior colliculus (Sparks, 2002).

Neurons that are located downstream of these signals in midbrain and pontine oculomotor nuclei, have firing rates that directly correlate with the speed and amplitude of saccades. *Via* a basal ganglia circuit, which includes the oculomotor portions of the caudate nucleus, with projections to the substantia nigra pars reticulata, the superior colliculus integrates information regarding the reward value of saccades to specific locations (Hikosaka et al., 2000).

Impairments in memory-guided and predictive saccades in neurodegenerative disease with basal ganglia damage may in part arise from damage to this circuit (Leigh and Kennard, 2004).

Nicotinic cholinergic inputs from the pedunculopontine nucleus to the superior colliculus may also have important effects on attention and motivation for saccades through a stimulatory effect on the superior colliculus (Kobayashi et al., 2001). Decreased attention and visual search efficiency (Doffner et al., 1992; Mosimann et al., 2004) and difficulties with saccade programming (Shafiq-Antonacci et al., 2003) in Alzheimer's disease may be in part explained by damage to this cholinergic circuit.

In addition to, and as part of, their roles in generating saccades, the neurons of the frontal eye field represent the behavioral relevance of objects within the visual field; thus, the activity over portions of the frontal eye field can be said to represent a visual saliency map (Thompson and Bichot, 2005).

After the presentation of a visual stimulus, over time, activity within the frontal eye field evolves to represent the behavioral significance of the stimulus. This behavioral significance can be read out as a saccade to the novel stimulus, but it may be represented as a covert shift of attention without an actual eye movement (Boxer, 2007).

However, this cortical field is believed to be a centre for voluntary eye movements not dependent upon visual stimuli. The conjugate eye movements commonly are called "movements of command", since they can be elicited by instructing the patient to look to the right or left (Cogan, 1956).

Some studies in men and primates suggest a double representation of specific eye movements in each frontal eye field (Crosby, 1953; Lemmen et al., 1959; Crosby et al., 1962).

Unlike the frontal eye field, the occipital eye centre is not localized to a small area. Eye responses can be obtained from a wide region of the occipital lobe in monkeys, but the lowest threshold is found in area 17 (Walker and Weaver, 1940). The occipital eye centres are presumed to subserve movements of eyes induced by visual stimuli, such as following moving objects. These pursuit movements of the eyes are largely involuntary, although they are not present in young infants.

Electrophysiological recordings in monkeys and lesion studies in humans have shown that brain stem structures, the basal ganglia, thalamus, cerebellum, and within the cortex, the parietal eye fields, supplementary eye field, and frontal eye fields are involved in the execution and control of saccades (Leigh and Zee, 1991; Pierot-Deseiligny et al., 1995).

However, two regions of the cerebral cortex in humans influence ocular movements. At the posterior end of the middle frontal gyrus and corresponding to Brodmann's areas 8 and 9 is a region responsible for voluntary eye deviation called the **primary eye field.**

There is also a **secondary motor eye field** at the posterior end of the inferior frontal gyrus on its dorsal part.

Stimulation of the human primary eye fields yields deviations of the eyes, including divergence, horizontal conjugate deviation to the contralateral side, and deviation up and to the contralateral side.

The pattern on the secondary eye field is a mirror image of that on the primary eye field. The secondary eye fields permit relaxation of the antagonistic muscles during voluntary eye deviations.

Thus, the frontal eye field plays a role in the coordination of eye movements, particularly those mediating voluntary visual tracking of a moving object *via* conjugate deviation of the eyes.

Supplementary eye fields. According to Boxer (2007), the supplementary eye field is located on the medial surface of the superior frontal gyrus, in the dorsal aspect of the paracentral sulcus. An oculomotor area in the frontal cortex, separated from the frontal eye field, was defined by Schlag and Schlag-Rey in 1987. It is located rostrally to the supplementary motor area (M II) on the medial surface of the hemisphere. The supplementary eye fields receive connections form the frontal eye field, the dorsolateral prefrontal cortex, the anterior cingulate cortex and the posterior part of the cerebral hemisphere. The supplementary eye field projects to the frontal eye field and to the subcortical nuclei involved in eye movements (superior colliculus and reticular formation).

The supplementary eye field is involved in programming sequences of saccades or combined saccade-body movements and likely has important preparatory roles in more complex eye movements (spatiotopic saccades), (Isoda and Tanji, 2003).

Functional imaging studies in humans suggest that the supplementary eye field is activated prior to both simple and more complex saccade tasks (Gagnon et al., 2002), suggesting that it may have a supervisory role over neurons in the frontal eye field (Schall et al., 2002).

Dorsolateral prefrontal cortex. The dorsolateral prefrontal cortex is involved in multiple aspects of saccade programming, including making decisions to initiate voluntary saccades and maintaining spatial working memory for target locations (Funahashi et al., 1993; Pierrot-Deseilligny et al., 2002, 2003; Cisek and Kalaska, 2004). The regions of the dorsolateral prefrontal cortex that are most important for the control of eye movements are located in the middle frontal gyrus in Brodmann's areas 46 and 9.

The suppression of unwanted reflexive saccades likely involves a direct inhibitory projection from dorsolateral prefrontal cortex neurons to the brain stem saccade-generating circuitry, including the superior colliculus (Condy et al., 2004).

Experiments with monkeys suggest that there are neurons in the vicinity of the dorsolateral prefrontal cortex whose activity signals the suppression of a reflexive saccade or the command "Don't look" (Hasegawa et al., 2004). Activity from these neurons may be crucial for the ability of the dorsolateral prefrontal cortex ability to help select one behaviorally relevant saccade over a range of other visually salient targets.

Nyffeler et al. (2002) confirmed the roles of the dorsolateral prefrontal cortex in spatial memory, first identified in nonhuman primates by Constantinidis et al. (2001).

Thus, studies of the voluntary control of eye movements, particularly saccades, are revealing important principles about the mechanisms of motor control by the frontal lobes.

Thus, three cortical areas not involved directly in triggering of saccades play important roles in planning, integration, and chronologic ordering of saccades.

The prefrontal cortex (Brodmann's area 46) plays a role in planning saccades to remembered target locations. The inferior parietal lobe is involved in visuospatial integration. Bilateral lesions in this area result in Balint's syndrome (optic ataxia, ocular apraxia, psychic paralysis of the visual fixation).

The hippocampus appears to control the temporal working memory required for chronologic order of saccade sequences (Afifi and Bergman, 2005).

Smooth-pursuit movements are slow eye movements initiated by a moving object. Unlike saccades, smooth-pursuit movements cannot occur in darkness.

Cortical areas involved in smooth pursuit include the temporooccipital region and the frontal eye field. Each of these areas has direct projections to brain stem neurons that drive pursuit. The temporooccipital region is driven by input from the primary visual cortex. The posterior parietal and the superior temporal cortices may also contribute to smooth pursuit indirectly through visual attention.

Lesions in the temporooccipital cortex in humans associated with smooth-pursuit deficits correspond to Brodmann's areas 19, 37, and 39. Lesions in the frontal eye field also have been associated with deficits in smooth pursuit.

A corticofugal pathway for smooth-pursuit courses from the temporooccipital cortex through the posterior limb of the internal capsule to the dorsolateral pontine nucleus in the mid-pons. The second courses from the frontal eye field to the dorsolateral pontine nucleus and the nucleus reticularis tegmenti pontis (Afifi and Bergman 2005).

Cortical areas for smooth pursuit also project to the flocculus of the cerebellum after relaying in the dorsolateral pontine nucleus. The flocculus, in turn, projects on the vestibular nuclei, which project to the cranial nerve nuclei of extraocular movement (CN III, IV, IV) (Leichnetz et al., 1981; Morrow and Sharpe, 1990; Tijsen et al., 1991; Gaymard et al., 1993; Sharp et al., 1995; Lekwuuwa and Barnes, 1996; Deseilligny et al., 1996; Morecraft and Yeterian, 2000; Pierrot-Deseilligny et al., 1995; Pryse-Phillip, 2003; Afifi and Bergman, 2005). Cerebral hemisphere lesions impair ocular pursuit ipsilaterally, or laterally whereas posterior fossa lesions impair ocular pursuit either contralaterally or ipsilaterally.

The antisaccade task. According to Boxer (2007), the antisaccade task has two components: suppression of a reflexive saccade towards a target, and programming of a new saccade in the opposite direction. Due to its ease of performance, this task has been used extensively to investigate aspects of voluntary motor control. The ability to perform antisaccades accurately develops in late childhood (Klein, 2001) and decline in normal elderly subjects in parallel to other cognitive measures of frontal lobe function (Klein et al., 2000).

Early studies in patients with **frontal lobe lesions** showed that the antisaccade task is exquisitely sensitive to frontal lobe damage (Guitton et al., 1985).

The anatomy of antisaccade dysfunction has been elicited in subjects with focal brain lesions and shown to involve a dorsolateral prefrontal cortex internal capsule – the superior colliculus brain stem circuit – in which damage to any component of the circuit results in a difficulty of reflexive saccade suppression (Pierrot-Deseilligny et al., 2003; Condy et al., 2004).

The antisaccade function is abnormal in attention-deficit / hyperactivity disorder in both children (Mostofsky et al., 2001) and adults (Feifel et al., 2004). In contrast, subjects with Tourette's syndrome have enhanced ability to perform this task, possibly consistent with the subjects' necessity to suppress unwanted movements (Munoz et al., 2002).

A large number of studies have described the prominent antisaccade abnormalities associated with schizophrenia (Huton and Kennard, 1998). The antisaccade task is exquisitely sensitive to first-episode schizophrenia and correlates with disease severity and working memory impairments (Nieman et al., 2000). Antisaccade impairments may serve as a marker of an endophenotype or genetic risk factor for schizophrenia (Thaker et al., 2000). More recently, antisaccade performance has been used as an outcome measure in trials of therapeutic agents for this disease (Ettinger et al., 2003; Wonodi et al., 2004).

Impairment on the antisaccade task is a sensitive marker of human immuno-deficiency virus (HIV) dementia (Johnston et al1996), and is present in subjects with Alzheimer's disease (Abel et al., 2002; Shafiq-Antonacci et al., 2003).

Antisaccade impairment is also associated with the presence of dementia in subjects with Parkinson's disease but not in cognitively normal patients with Parkinson's disease (Mosimann et al., 2005).

Injuries to the frontal eye fields in humans are either **irritative** or **destructive**. Irritative injuries result in deviations of the eyes to the contralateral side, whereas destructive injuries result in deviation of the eyes to the same side. Ablation of the frontal eye field will result in deviation of the eyes to the side of ablation as a result of the unopposed action of the intact frontal eye field. Such a condition is encountered in patients with occlusion of the middle cerebral artery, which supplies the bulk of the lateral surface of the hemisphere, including the frontal eye field. Such patients manifest paralysis of the face and limbs (upper limbs more than lower) contralateral to the side of the arterial occlusion and conjugate the deviation of the eyes towards the cortical lesion.

In humans, conjugate eye deviation occurs more frequently after lesions in the right hemisphere than after lesions in the left hemisphere because it is related to the neglect syndrome associated more frequently with right hemisphere lesions. Conjugate deviation of the eyes with pupillary dilation of the abducting eye may appear with the onset of seizures. Such cases localize the epileptogenic focus to the contralateral frontal lobe (Augustine, 2008). Conjugate eye deviations have been observed with lesions that spare the frontal eye field but that interrupt the connections between the posterior parietal and frontal eye fields or their subcortical projections.

Subjects with brain lesions involving the dorsolateral prefrontal cortex have difficulty in suppressing unwanted reflexive saccades and in generating predictive saccades to targets presented in a predictable sequence in time and space (Pierrot-Deseilligny et al., 2003).

There is evidence from studies in nonhuman primates and humans performing a simple voluntary saccade paradigm, such as countermanding and antisaccade tasks, that the same brain region and patterns of activity are involved in deciding to initiate or cancel an eye movement (Boxer, 2007). Data from human subjects with local brain lesions or neurodegenerative syndromes suggest that the integrity of these circuits is necessary for accurate voluntary saccade initiation (Boxer, 2007).

Motor speech region

The posterior parts of the frontal lobe have been more directly implicated in language processing per se. In fact, the left posterior inferior frontal lobe (often referred to as "Broca's area") likely has a role in all aspects of language – in comprehension and production of both spoken and written language.

Broca's region for motor speech occupies the triangular and opercular parts of the posterior end of the inferior frontal gyrus of the left cerebral hemisphere in 95% of humans. There exists a wealth of evidence about a great deal of individual variability in the cytoarchitectural fields, as well as the shape and size of sulci and gyri, of the human brain. Much of the evidence for this individual variability has in fact come from studies of Broca's area, which often (but not always) has been assumed to encompass Brodmann's areas 44 and 45 (pars opercularis and pars triangularis). Area 44 or the pars opercularis (which is a dysgranular cortex) is separated from area 45 or pars triangularis (which is a granular cortex) by the ascending or vertical ramus of the lateral sulcus whereas the anterior ramus of the lateral sulcus divides the pars triangularis from pars orbitalis (area 47).

This region, corresponding to Brodmann's areas 44 and 45, has connections with the primary motor cortex, especially with those parts of area 4 that supply muscles concerned with speech (Grodzinsky and Amunts, 2006)

The left posterior inferior frontal cortex has diverse roles in both production and comprehension of language. This area appears to be critical for phonological discrimination and segmentation, processing of morphosyntactic structure, and / or working memory functions needed for syntax processing, retrieval of modality-specific lexical forms (especially in particular grammatical categories – such as verbs or particular morphological forms – for spoken and written output), motor programming of speech articulation, and selecting letter-specific motor programs for writing (Hillis, 2007).

Nearby regions are also engaged in various aspects of semantic tasks, including controlled retrieval from semantic memory and response selection, although they are not critical for decoding the meanings of individual words (Hillis, 2007).

In general, Broca's area is involved in the planning of motor activity that is necessary in order for words to be produced. Broca's area projects this information to the premotor cortex where activity is planned and relayed to the primary motor cortex, which initiates the movements necessary to produce speech. A lesion in Broca's area will disrupt Broca's area input to the premotor cortex.

Injury to the motor speech area causes an expressive or motor aphasia also described as Broca's aphasia or Broca's loss of "articulated speech". While there is no paralysis of the muscles related to speech, there is a loss of coordination of those muscles leading to a difficulty in expressing oneself.

Broca's aphasia, also termed expressive aphasia or nonfluent aphasia, consists of a loss of the ability to speak fluently.

Patients with the most severe form of Broca's aphasia are unable to speak (mutism), although they are able to swallow and breathe normally and make guttural sounds. Here is a difficulty in turning a concept or thought into a sequence of meaningful sounds. In less severe cases, or in patients during the recovery process, limited speech is possible.

In Broca's aphasia, there is a low fluency associated with relatively well-preserved comprehension.

The patient is likely to be unable to speak or continually repeats the last word said before the injury occurred. There may be difficulty with certain sounds or letters. However, speech is slow and laboured, enunciation is poor, and nonessential words are commonly omitted (telegraphic speech).

Broca's area is involved in the planning of motor activity that is necessary for words to be produced. Broca's aphasia also impairs an individual's ability to express a thought or concept by writing it down. So, affected persons typically have as much difficulty with writing (agraphia) as with speaking. Although the patient is able to understand spoken or written language and can communicate verbally to some degree, the extremely laborious nature of the process of communication causes considerable frustration. Under particular emotional stress, patients may use inappropriate or vulgar words or phrases to express their distress.

Mild aphasia without other deficits indicates that the damage affects only cortical areas. However, full-blown Broca's aphasia indicates that the damage extends beyond the Broca area of the cortex to include insular cortex and subjacent white matter.

Patients typically have contralateral motor signs and symptoms, such as weakness (paresis of the lower part of the face, lateral deviation of the tongue when protruded, and weakness of the arm (Lynch, 2006).

The resulting deficit depends on the size, depth, severity, timing, and whether the cerebral hemisphere is dominant for language (the left cerebral hemisphere in approximately 95% of humans).

Most patients with Broca's aphasia are able to sing, although they do not speak well. It is likely that the right cerebral hemisphere is dominant over the left for singing capacity.

If injury leading to aphasia takes place at an early age, it is possible to build up speech patterns in the other cerebral hemisphere. This is an example of the plasticity of the nervous system and its ability to compensate when injured (Grodzinsky and Amunts, 2006).

The most common causes of Broca's aphasia are tumors and occlusions of frontal M4 branches of the middle cerebral artery.

Aphasia plus motor problems suggest an occlusion of branches from the proximal parts of the middle cerebral artery (M1), including the lenticulostriate arteries, which serve the internal capsule.

The mirror system: ventral premotor and parietal cortex

One of the most interesting findings in recent years related to the human cerebral cortex is that some cortical motor areas that are active during the planning and execution of movements are also active when viewing the motor actions of others. This phenomenon is termed "mirror representation" of the actions of others.

Thus, a special class of neurons was discovered in the inferior frontal cortex of the macaque brain. These neurons were found in area F5, the rostral sector of the ventral premotor cortex (Matelli et al., 1985).

Area F5 is connected with the rostral part of the inferior parietal lobule (area PF). Mirror neurons have also been observed in area PF (Fogassi et al., 2005; Shmuelof and Zohary, 2006).

Thus, the mirror neurons system in macaques is composed of two major centres – one in the posterior inferior frontal cortex and the other in the rostral inferior parietal cortex, that are strongly interconnected. The anterior part of the human intraparietal sulcus is involved in visually guided grasping as well as during the observation of other actions. There is a complex network of cortical regions in the frontal, parietal and temporal lobes forming this mirror system in the human brain.

The premotor neurons fire not only when the monkey performs goal-directed actions, such as grasping objects, but also when holding, tearing, manipulating, and so forth.

These neurons also fire when the monkey is simply watching somebody else performing goal-directed actions (di Pellegrino et al., 1992; Gallese et al., 1996).

Because of these properties, these neurons were dubbed "mirror" neurons (Gallese et al., 1996). There is generally a good congruence between the action coded motorically and the action coded visually by mirror neurons; that is, if a mirror neuron fires during a monkey's execution of a precision grip, it will likely fire when the monkey sees a precision grip rather than a whole-hand prehension.

Mirror neurons fire even when the sight of the hand grasping the object is occluded, as long as the monkey can see the initial movement of the hand towards the object (Umilta et al., 2001). Moreover, they also fire when the monkey – in complete darkness – hears the sound associated with an action, for instance, breaking a peanut (Kohler et al., 2002).

Mirror neurons also code for mouth actions, some of which are communicative actions for monkeys, such as lip smacking (Ferrari et al., 2003).

Several brain-imaging techniques have addressed the properties of the human homologue of the macaque mirror neuron system. In good accordance with the monkey data, areas with mirror properties have been described in the posterior inferior frontal and rostral inferior parietal cortex in humans (Iacoboni et al., 1999, 2005; Buccino et al., 2004).

These findings suggest that mirror neurons may implement very abstract representations of actions, now that they can map actions of others into actions of the self, a fundamental functional step for understanding other people (Geschwind and Iacoboni, 2007).

In terms of their laterality, the single-unit data do not offer striking asymmetries. However, with regard to the laterality of the human mirror neuron system, robust lateralized responses have been observed in some cases.

In one of the original reports (Gallese et al., 1996), some interesting laterality patterns were observed. About 40% of the mirror neurons tested demonstrated a discharge influenced by the laterality of the observed hand.

The majority of these neurons responded more strongly when the observed hand was ipsilateral to the recorded hemisphere (i.e., a left-hand action triggered stronger discharge in mirror neurons in the left ventral premotor cortex, compared to a right-hand action).

Another finding was related to the direction of the observed reach-and-grasp action. About two-thirds of the mirror neurons tested demonstrated directional preference. More than 80% of these neurons preferred the direction towards the recorded side, that is, from right to left for mirror neurons in the left hemisphere (Gallese et al., 1996).

Iacoboni et al. (1996) described that the human left inferior frontal area responded to action observation, action execution, and even more during action imitation. In light of the evolutionary hypothesis of a link between mirror neurons and language (Rizzolatti and Arbib, 1998), the left lateralization report in this study has been often taken as suggesting that the whole mirror neuron system in humans is left-lateralized (Corballis, 2003).

In that study, right-hand actions imitated left-hand observed actions. Even the monkey data would have predicted a left-lateralized pattern in this case (Iacoboni et al., 1999).

In fact, a reanalysis of seven fMRI studies of imitation adapting various forms of hand imitation has shown a fairly bilateral activation pattern in the posterior inferior frontal cortex (Molnar-Szakacs et al., 2005).

A highly reproducible effect that is likely due to the mirror neuron system is the increase in the excitability of the motor corticospinal system during action observation. When a transcranial magnetic stimulation (TMS) pulse is applied over the primary motor hand area, a motor response is evoked in the contralateral hand. If subjects are also watching somebody else's actions, this motor evoked response is much stronger when compared to watching some visual control stimuli (Fadiga et al., 1995; Aziz-Zadeh et al., 2002; Fadiga et al., 2005).

This effect is likely due to the activation of mirror neurons in the premotor cortex that feed directly onto primary motor regions (Cerri et al., 2003; Shimazu et al., 2004).

When subjects are listening to action sounds, their corticospinal excitability is facilitated (Aziz-Zadeh et al., 2004).

This effect, likely mediated by mirror neurons that respond to the sound of an action (Kohler et al., 2002), is completely lateralized to the left hemisphere in humans (Aziz-Zadeh et al., 2004).

This strong left-hemisphere lateralization suggests that a fundamental step in the hypothesized evolutionary progression from action recognition to language may be the multimodal representation of action that only the left hemisphere appears to have in humans (Geschwind and Iacoboni, 2007).

Right-hemisphere lateralization was observed during imitation and observation of facial emotional expression (Carr et al., 2003).

A strongly lateralized response in a mirror neuron area was observed in an action observation task in which the context of the actions provided the observers information to predict the intention of the actor, in other words, to predict the following (unseen) action (Iacoboni et al., 2005). This suggests a link between the right hemisphere and the capacity to "read the mind" of other people (Winner et al., 1998; Happe et al., 1999).

Thus, the laterality findings in the human mirror neuron system suggest that this system is not lateralized to the left or right hemisphere, but that asymmetries may emerge in the system on the basis of the function tapped by specific tasks (Geschwind and Iacoboni, 2007).

PREFRONTAL CORTEX

The prefrontal cortex makes up about a third of the human neocortex and corresponds to three major regions on the various surfaces of the frontal lobe. Collectively these three regions forming the prefrontal cortex constitute a complex association area that provides the structural basis for the most complex intellectual and moral functions of which humans are capable (Markowitsch et al., 1979; Morecraft and Yeterian, 2000)

The lateral prefrontal cortex

The prefrontal cortex on the lateral surface of the hemisphere (**the lateral prefrontal cortex**) which involves the superior, middle, and inferior frontal gyri anterior to the premotor cortex, comprises Brodmann's areas 8, 9, 10, 11, 45, 46, and 47 (Fuster, 2001). Areas 44 and 45 are particularly notable in men since, in the dominant hemisphere, they constitute the motor speech area (Broca's area).

In nonhuman primates, two subdivisions of the lateral prefrontal cortex are recognized, a dorsal area equivalent to area 9, and perhaps including the superior part of area 46, and a ventral area, consisting of the inferior part of area 46 and area 45.

According to Crossman (2008), both the dorsolateral and ventrolateral prefrontal areas receive their major thalamic afferents from the mediodorsal nucleus, and there are additional contributions from the medial pulvinar nucleus, the ventral anterior nucleus, and from the paracentral nucleus of the anterior intralaminar group.

The dorsolateral area receives long association fibres from the posterior and middle superior temporal gyrus (including auditory association areas), from parietal area 7a, and from much of the middle temporal cortex. From within the frontal lobe it also receives projections from the frontal pole (area 10), the medial prefrontal cortex (area 32) and the medial surface of the hemisphere. It projects to the supplementary motor area, the dorsal premotor cortex and the frontal eye field. All these thalamic and corticocortical connections are reciprocal. Commissural connections are with the homologous area, and with the contralateral inferior parietal cortex (Crossman, 2008).

The ventrolateral prefrontal area receives long association fibres from both area 7a and area 7b of the parietal lobe, from auditory association areas of the temporal operculum, from the insula and from the anterior part of the lower bank of the superior temporal sulcus. From within the frontal lobe it receives fibres from the anterior orbitofrontal cortex and projects to the frontal eye field and the ventral premotor cortex.

It connects with the contralateral homologous area *via* the corpus callosum. These connections are probably all reciprocal (Crossman, 2008).

The cortex of the frontal pole (area 10) receives thalamic inputs from the mediodorsal nucleus, the medial pulvinar nucleus and the paracentral nucleus. It is reciprocally connected with the cortex of the temporal pole, the anterior orbitofrontal cortex, and the dorsolateral prefrontal cortex.

The inferior or orbital prefrontal cortex

The inferior or orbital prefrontal cortex of the frontal lobe includes Brodmann's areas 10, 11, 13, and 47 (Fig. 21.24).

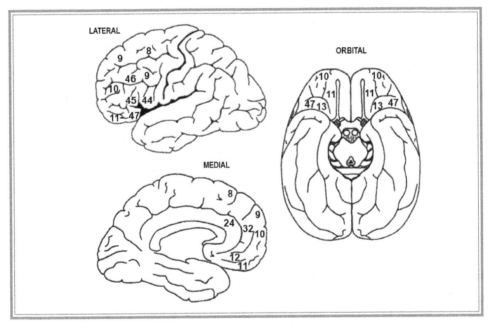

Fig. 21.24. Human prefrontal areas numbered according to Brodmann (from Fuster, 2001).

The orbitofrontal cortex connects with the mediodorsal, anteromedial, ventral anterior, medial pulvinar, paracentral and midline nuclei of the thalamus.

Cortical association pathways come from the inferotemporal cortex, the anterior superior temporal gyrus and the temporal pole. Within the frontal lobe it has connections with the medial prefrontal cortex, the ventrolateral prefrontal cortex and medial motor areas. Commissural and other connections follow the general pattern for all neocortical areas.

The medial prefrontal cortex

The medial surface of the frontal lobe involves in part the anterior cingulate gyrus and includes Brodmann's areas 8, 9, 10, 11, 12, 24 and 32 (Fuster, 2001).

The medial prefrontal cortex is connected with the mediodorsal, ventral anterior medial pulvinar, paracentral, midline and suprageniculate-limitans nuclei of the thalamus.

It receives fibres from the anterior cortex of the superior temporal gyrus. Within the frontal lobe, it has connections with the orbitofrontal cortex, and the medial motor areas of the dorsolateral prefrontal cortex (Crossman, 2008).

SENSORY AREAS OF THE CEREBRAL CORTEX

Primary sensory areas

The primary sensory areas are involved in distinguishing and integrating sensory input relayed there primarily by the thalamic nuclei. Although certain aspects of sensation probably enter consciousness at thalamic levels, the primary sensory areas are concerned especially with the integration of sensory experience and with the discriminative qualities of sensation. The organization of the thalamus is such that all of the specific sensory relay nuclei are located caudally in the ventral tier. The cortical projections of the specific sensory relay nuclei are localized in areas of the parietal, occipital and temporal lobes (Carpenter, 1979).

Established primary sensory areas in the cerebral cortex are: (1) the somesthetic area, consisting of the postcentral gyrus and its medial extension in the paracentral lobule (areas 3, 1 and 2); (2) the visual or striate area, located along the lips of the calcarine sulcus (area 17); and (3) the auditory area, located on the two transverse gyri (Heschl; areas 41 and 42). The gustatory area appears to be localized to the most ventral part (opercular) of the postcentral gyrus (area 43). The primary olfactory area consists of the allocortex of the prepyriform and periamygdaloid regions and has not assigned numbers under Brodmann's parcellation. A vestibular projection to the human cerebral cortex has not been established (Carpenter, 1979).

Primary somatosensory (somesthetic) cortex (S I)

A significant area in the parietal lobe is the primary somatosensory cortex, or S I, that corresponds to Brodmann's areas 3, 1 and 2 on the postcentral gyrus (Fig 21.25). The primary somatosensory cortex also comprises the posterior part of the paracentral lobule, which resides and is visible only on the medial surface of the cerebral hemisphere.

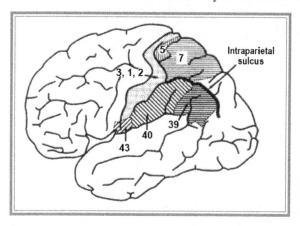

Fig. 21.25. Brodmann's areas in the human parietal lobe (from Paxinos and Mai, 2004).

Area 1 is on the crown of the postcentral gyrus, area 2 intrasulcal in position forming the anterior wall of the postcentral sulcus, area 3 is divisible into areas 3a and 3b in nonhuman primates and humans, with area 3b being intrasulcal but forming the posterior wall of the central sulcus. Area 3a, also intrasulcal, forms the floor of the central sulcus, is a transition region between primary motor area 4 along the precentral gyrus and area 3b on the posterior bank of the central sulcus. Thus, there are four strep-like somatosensory areas in the human primary somatosensory area of the postcentral gyrus of the parietal lobe (Geyer et al., 1999, 2000; Augustine, 2008).

The primary somatosensory cortex contains within it a topographical map of the contralateral half of the body. The face, tongue and lips are represented inferiorly, the trunk and upper limb are represented on the superolateral aspect, and the lower limb on the medial aspect of the hemisphere, giving rise to the familiar "homunculus" map (Fig. 21.26). Thus, the body is represented on the somatosensory cortex by an upside-down homunculus. The foot is represented on the superior medial surface of the hemisphere, the leg, thigh, trunk, shoulder, arm, and forearm on the superior surface of the postcentral gyrus, whereas the hand, head, teeth, tongue, larynx, and pharynx are on the lateral surface of the postcentral gyrus. The total cortical area representing a body part is proportional to the discriminative capability of the body part.

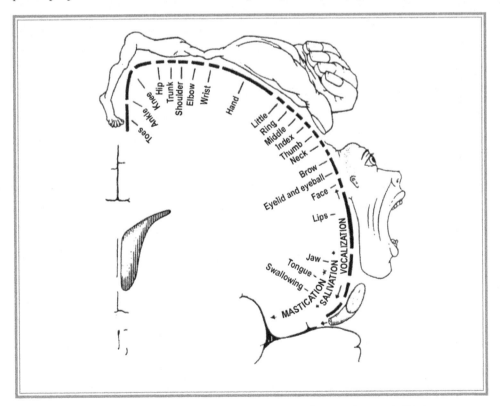

Fig. 21.26. The sensory homunculus across the postcentral gyrus and paracentral lobule (after Penfield and Rasmussen, 1950).

Cutaneous areas of the greatest sensitivity have corresponding larger cortical representation. Hence, the size of the parts of the homunculus is a reflection of the cortical area devoted to individual parts of the body. The sensory homunculus has the same order as the motor homunculus in the frontal lobe.

Certain aspects of the human sensory homunculus are of special interest. The toes, foot, ankle and leg have their representation in the posterior part of the paracentral lobule on the medial surface of the brain.

The representation of the thigh or hip occurs at the medial to superolateral surface junction followed in order by the trunk, neck, shoulder, arm, forearm, and hand across the superolateral surface of the brain (Sutherling et al., 2002).

The genitalia and perineum likely have their representation on the medial surface of the human brain just ventral to the representation of the toes.

Recent recording of cerebrocortical potentials evoked by stimulation of the dorsal nerve of the penis in humans suggest a representation of the penis with the hip and upper leg near the junction of the medial to superolateral surface (Bradley et al., 1998). The anal and genital regions are represented in the most ventral portion of the medial surface just above the cingulate gyrus. All five fingers have a separate medial to lateral representation along the wall of the central sulcus not on the lateral surface (Gelnar et al., 1998; Overduin and Servos, 2004). The anterior surfaces of the body face the central sulcus.

Experimental studies of the face area of S I in nonhuman primates demonstrate that oral soft tissues (gingiva, inner aspect of the lips) have their representation near the surface of the postcentral gyrus with the dental pulp along the floor of the central sulcus, coinciding with area 3a (Urasaki et al., 1994).

Stimulation of dental pulp in humans causes painful sensations that are accurately localized suggesting involvement of the primary somatosensory cortex for localization of painful sensations (Geyer et al., 1996; Gelnar et al., 1998; Bodegård et al., 2000; Disbrow et al., 2000; Overduin and Servos, 2004).

The face area, occupying most of the lower half of the postcentral gyrus, receives trigeminal impulses including those from the face and mouth.

The back of the head has its representation caudal in the postcentral gyrus; the face faces the central sulcus.

The primary sensory cortex also includes Brodmann's area 3a, which is buried in the central sulcus. This area receives sensory input from muscle receptors. Some of the cells residing in the primary somatosensory cortex give rise to fibres that descend to terminate in the brain stem and spinal cord gray matter. There they influence motor activity, not by synapsing with motoneurons, but instead by modulating the transmission of sensory inputs from peripheral structures into the brain stem and spinal cord.

In addition to the four cytoarchitectonic subdivisions of S I, there is also a columnar cortical organization (microarchitecture) in the postcentral gyrus.

Neurons in S I are organized in vertical columns at right angles to the surface and extend through all cortical layers; they often share similar receptive fields and have specific functions. Columns in S I are functionally interrelated by intrinsic corticocortical connections and by direct horizontal connections between columns. These intrinsic connections serve to connect parts of the cerebral cortex having different response properties yet lying in regions of similar regional representation. (Gelnar et al., 1998; Geyer et al., 1999; Bodegård et al., 2000; Disbrow et al., 2000; Overduin and Servos, 2004; Augustine, 2008).

However, the somatosensory properties of S I depend on its thalamic input from the ventral posterior nucleus of the thalamus, which in turn receives the medial lemniscal, spinothalamic and trigeminothalamic pathways. Within, the ventral posterior nucleus, neurons in the central core respond to cutaneous stimuli and those in the most dorsal anterior and posterior parts, which arch as a "shell" over this central core, respond to deep stimuli (Jones, 2007).

This is reflected in the differential projections to S I: the cutaneous central core projects to 3b, the deep tissue-responsive neurons send fibres to areas 3a and 2, and an intervening zone projects to area 1. Thus, ventral posterior nucleus is the principal thalamic relay for the somatosensory pathways. It consist of two major divisions, the ventral posterolateral and ventral posteromedial nuclei. The ventral posterolateral nucleus receives the medial lemniscal and spinothalamic pathways (information from the trunk and limb) and the ventral posteromedial nucleus receives the trigeminothalamic pathway in which the head is represented. These fibres convey general sensory (touch, pain, and temperature) as well as proprioceptive sensory modalities (position, vibration, and two-point discrimination).

The laminar termination of thalamocortical axons from the ventral posterior nucleus is different in the separate cytoarchitectonic subdivisions of S I in 3a and 3b; these axons terminate mainly in layer IV and the adjacent deep part of layer III, whereas in area 1 and 2 they end in the deeper half of layer III avoiding lamina IV. Additional thalamocortical fibres to S I arise from the intralaminar system, notably the centrolateral nucleus (Jones, 2007; Crossman, 2008).

Corticospinal pyramidal cells are found in layer V of S I. The topographical representation in the cortex is preserved in terms of the spinal segments to which different parts of the postcentral gyrus project. Thus, the arm representation projects to the cervical enlargement, the leg representation to the lumbosacral enlargement, and so on. Within the grey matter of the spinal cord, fibres from S I terminate in the dorsal horn, in Rexed's laminae 3 to 5: fibres from 3b and 1 end more dorsally, and those from area 2 more ventrally (Jones, 2007; Crossman, 2008).

S I has ipsilateral corticocortical association connections with a second somatosensory area S II; area 5, in the superior parietal lobe; area 4, in the motor cortex, in the precentral gyrus; and the supplementary motor cortex in the medial part of area 6 of the frontal lobe.

So, although the primary somesthetic area is concerned basically with sensory modalities, it is possible to elicit motor responses following its stimulation.

In addition to thalamic afferents, the primary somesthetic cortex receives commissural fibres through the corpus callosum from the contralateral primary somesthetic cortex and short association fibres from the adjacent primary motor cortex. Callosal fibres in S I arise mainly from the deep part of layer III and terminate in layer I to IV.

Thus, efferents from the primary somesthetic cortex project to the motor cortex, the opposite primary somesthetic cortex, and the association somatosensory cortex (area 5 and 7) in the posterior parietal cortex (Fig. 21.27).

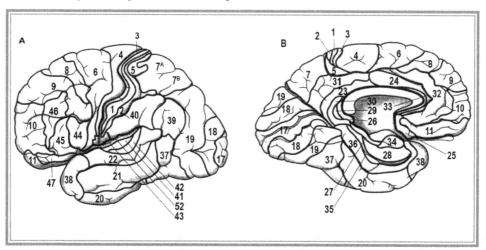

Fig. 21.27. The lateral (A) and medial (B) surfaces of the left cerebral hemisphere depicting Brodmann's areas (after Crossman, 2008).

The primary and secondary areas are reciprocally interconnected. In addition, projection fibres descend within the internal capsule to the ventral posterior nuclei of the thalamus, posterior column nuclei of the medulla oblongata, and dorsal horn of the spinal cord. Thus, S I had reciprocal subcortical connections with the thalamus and claustrum, and receives afferents from the basal nucleus of Meynert, the locus ceruleus and the midbrain raphe. Corticostriatal fibres, arising in layer V, pass mainly to the putamen on the same side. Corticopontine and corticotectal fibres from S I arise in layer V. S I projects to the main pontine nuclei, and to the pontine tegmental reticular nucleus. In addition, axons arising in S I pass to the dorsal column nuclei and the spinal cord (Ramansky et al., 1979; Brodal, 1978; Brouwer and Ashby, 1991; Iwatsubo et al., 1990; Jones, 2007; Crossman, 2008).

The ability to recognize, localize and assess pain and thermal sensation require cortical participation. Although sensations of thermal extremes and superficial pain enter consciousness at a thalamic level in humans, the primary somatosensory cortex is capable of discriminating and comparing qualities of pain and slight variations in temperature, accurately localizing these tactile and proprioceptive sensations (Augustine, 2008).

Although impulses for visceral pain likely reach consciousness at a thalamic level, areas of the cerebral cortex are also involved in visceral sensation. The intralaminar nuclei, part of the "diffuse thalamocortical projection system", relay visceral impulses to the cerebral cortex. Their diffuseness presumably accounts for the poor localization of visceral pain. Electrical stimulation reveals that visceral sensory areas in the cerebral cortex in humans include the lower end of the primary somatosensory cortex and part of the insular lobe (Augustine, 2008).

In a study of the speed of moving stimuli across the skin of the hand, there was primarily activation in area 1 and secondary in area 3b of the somatosensory cortex. In another study, the discrimination of caricatures or objects rich in curvatures led to an increase in regional cerebral blood flow outside of area 1 but perhaps in area 2 on the posterior bank of the postcentral sulcus.

Positron emission tomography, cytoarchitectonic mapping, and a combination of sensory stimuli (passive or active touch, brush velocity, edge length, curvature, and roughness) reveal the probable hierarchical processing of tactile shape in sensory areas of the human brain. This involves areas 3b and 1 as the first steps in the process, area 2 being the next step, and the anterior part of the cortex lining the intraparietal sulcus and the adjacent part of the supramarginal gyrus being the final step. The anterior part of the human intraparietal sulcus is involved in visually guided grasping (Augustine, 2008). Lastly, in a fourth study, a pleasant and soft touch to the hand elicited by using velvet in comparison to a neutral stimulus produces activation in the orbitofrontal cortex. This suggest that the pleasant or rewarding aspects of touch ("that feels good") as well as the pleasant rewarding aspect of taste ("that tastes good") or smell ("that smells good") all of which are represented in different parts of the orbitofrontal cortex, collectively contribute to our state of emotion (Badegård et al., 2000 a, b, 2001; Augustine, 2008).

Functional imaging studies of the human S I show that multiple digit representations occur in the four subdivisions (3a, 3b, 1 and 2) resembling a multiple representation hypothesis that is present in nonhuman primates (Kaas et al., 1999, 2004).

Neurophysiologic studies of the somesthetic cortex have revealed the following information: (1) the functional cortical unit appears to be associated with a vertical column of cells that is modality specific. Neurons within a cortical unit are activated by the same peripheral stimulus and are related to the same peripheral receptive field. (2) Area 3b is activated by cutaneous stimuli and areas 2 and 3a by proprioceptive impulses, whereas area 1 is activated by either cutaneous or proprioceptive impulses. Area 2 appears to represent predominantly deep receptors, including those signalling the position of joints and other deep body sensations, whereas area 3a represents sensory input from muscles (Burton et al., 1995).

(3) Somatosensory neurons responding to joint movement show a marked degree of specificity in that they respond to displacement in one direction. (4) Fast- and slow-adapting neuronal pools have been identified in response to hair displacement or cutaneous deformation. (5) Fibres mediating cutaneous sensations terminate rostrally, whereas those mediating proprioceptive sensations terminate more caudally in the somesthetic area (Afifi and Bergman, 2005).

The cortical representation along the postcentral gyrus reflects a composite of somatotopically organized areas instead of a continuous homunculus.

Stimulation of the primary somesthetic cortex in conscious patients elicits sensations of numbness and tingling, a feeling of electricity, and a feeling of movement without actual movement. These sensations are referred to the contralateral half of the body, except when the face area is stimulated. The face and tongue are represented bilaterally (Penfield and Boldrey, 1937; Penfield and Rasmussen, 1950; Urasaki et al., 1994).

Ablation of the postcentral gyrus will result, in the immediate postoperative period, in loss of all modalities of sensation (touch, pressure, pain, and temperature). Soon, however, pain and temperature sensation will return. It is believed that pain and temperature sensation are determined at the thalamic level, whereas the source, severity, and quality of such sensations are perceived in the postcentral gyrus.

Thus, the effects of postcentral gyrus lesions would be (1) complete loss of discriminative touch and proprioception; and (2) crude awareness of pain, temperature, and light touch (Penfield and Rasmussen, 1950; Afifi and Bergman, 2005).

Thermal and painful auras. Loss of discriminative pain or thermal sensation may result from cortical injury. Thermal and painful sensations foreshadow the onset of an epileptic seizure, a phenomenon known as an aura.

Sensory Jacksonian seizures. An analysis of seizure patterns involving subjective sensory experiences without objective signs has shown that such episodes, or sensory Jacksonian seizures, involve abnormal, localizable, cutaneous sensations without apparent prior stimulation. Seizures arise from discharges in the cerebral cortex. The behavioral manifestations of a seizure are determined by the normal functions of the region of cortex in which neurons fire abnormally. A diversity of potential mechanisms exist by which a small region or focus of cortex could become hyperexcitable after injury, and it seems likely that different mechanisms may operate in different patients or even at different stages of the disease in the same patient.

The sensation spreads or progresses to adjacent cutaneous areas, in the body or along a limb, reflecting propagation of an epileptic discharge – an abnormal firing of neurons in the postcentral gyrus. Thus, sensory disorder is usually described as numbness, tingling, or a "pins-and-needles" feeling and occasionally as a sensation of crawling (fornication), electricity, or movement of the part. Pain and thermal sensation may occur but are infrequent. In the majority of cases, the onset of the sensory seizure is in the lips, fingers, or toes, and the spread to adjacent parts of the body follows a pattern determined by sensory arrangements in the postcentral (post-rolandic) convolution of the parietal lobe. If the sensory symptoms are localized to the head, the focus is in, or adjacent to the lowest part of the convolution, near the sylvian fissure. If the symptoms are in the leg or foot, the upper part of the convolution, near the superior sagittal sinus or on the medial surface of the hemisphere, is involved.

Secondary somatosensory cortex (S II)

Near each primary receptive area there are cortical zones which may receive sensory inputs directly, or indirectly, from the thalamus. These cortical zones, adjacent to primary sensory areas, but outside of the principal projection area, of the specific sensory relay nuclei of the thalamus, are referred to as the secondary sensory areas (Carpenter, 1979). These areas have been defined and mapped in experimental animals by recording evoked potentials in response to peripheral stimulation (Adrian, 1940, 1941; Woolsey and Walzl, 1942; Woolsey and Fairman, 1946; Thompson et al., 1950). Studies of these secondary sensory areas indicate that sequential representation of parts of the body, or of the tonotopic pattern in the case of the auditory areas, is not the same as in the primary areas (Woolsey, 1958; Rose and Woolsey, 1958).

Adjoining the primary somatosensory cortex or S I is a smaller region, the secondary somatosensory cortex or S II, on the superior bank of the lateral sulcus, continuing onto the parietal operculum of the human brain and corresponding to Brodmann's area 43. (Eickhoff et al., 2006 a, b). S II contains a somatotopic representation of the body, with the head and face most anteriorly, adjacent to S I, and the sacral regions most posteriorly. Thus, body representation in this area is bilateral, with contralateral predominance, and is reverse of that in the primary area so that the two face areas are adjacent to each other. The secondary somatosensory area in animals appears to coincide with the so-called secondary motor area (Welker et al., 1957; Disbrow et al., 2000).

The secondary sensory area contains neurons with receptive fields that are large, poorly demarcated, overlap extensively, and often have bilateral representation.

Representation of the body form in the secondary somatosensory area (II) is nearly as detailed as that in the postcentral gyrus (Woolsey, 1958), and single unit analysis (Carreras and Levitt, 1959) has revealed many cells in this area to both mode and place specific. Although a detailed somatotopic organization exists in S II, with the exception of parts of the digit representation, neighbouring neurons in S II do not form a precise body map comparable to that in S II of nonhuman primates.

In S II, there is a split in the representation for the face, thumb, and foot causing a dual presentation of the same body part in the composite map of S II (Krubitzer et al., 1995; Kaas, 2004).

Within the cortex, S II is reciprocally connected with S I in a topographically organized manner, and projects to the primary motor cortex. S II also projects in a topographically organized way to the lateral part of area 7 (area 7b) in the superior parietal lobe, and makes connections with the posterior cingulate gyrus. Both right and left S II areas are interconnected across the corpus callosum, although distal limb representations are probably excluded. There are projections to S II and area 7b (Crossman, 2008).

The secondary somesthetic area contains no cells sensitive to join movement or join position.

The S II is reciprocally connected with the ventral posterior nucleus of the thalamus in a topographically organized fashion. Some thalamic neurons probably project to both S I and S II *via* collaterals. Other thalamic connections of the S II are with posterior groups of nuclei and with the intralaminar central lateral nucleus. S II also projects to laminae IV to VII of the dorsal horn of the cervical and thoracic spinal cord, the dorsal column nuclei, the principal trigeminal nucleus, and the periaqueductal grey matter of the midbrain.

S II in nonhuman primates receives fibres from the ventral posterior medial nucleus and the caudal part of the ventral posterior lateral nucleus. Reciprocal corticothalamic fibres occur from S II in nonhuman primates to the ventral posterior nucleus. Output from S II is to S I, to the primary motor cortex (Brodmann's area 4), and the premotor cortex (Brodmann's area 6).

Lesions interrupting connections between the secondary somesthetic area, posterior parietal cortex, and ventral posteromedial and centrolateral thalamic nuclei have been associated with pseudothalamic pain syndrome. The pain is spontaneous and characterized as burning or icelike and is associated with impairment of pain, and temperature appreciation (Déjérine 1900; Schmahmann and Leifer, 1992).

The unilateral or bilateral removal of area S II in monkeys causes a profound defect of tasks requiring tactile learning and retention. Even in the face of injury to the primary association cortex in the parietal lobe, patients are still able to recognize two points as two points and to identify the position of the parts of their body.

However, the patient will be unable to name an object placed in the affected hand, based on somatosensory information. There are disturbances mainly of the discriminative sensory function of the opposite leg, arm, and side of face without impairment of the primary modalities of sensation. The lack of recognition of shape and form is frequently a manifestation of cortical disease. Thus, astereognosis, connotes an inability to identify an object by palpation, even though the primary sense data (touch, pain, temperature, and vibration) are intact. Astereognosis is either right-, or left-sided, and is the product of a lesion in the opposite hemisphere, involving the sensory cortex, particularly S II, or thalamoparietal projections. With this deficit, (cortical astereognosis) patients lose the ability to use the somatosensory information.

Part of the parietal lobe including the primary (area 3, 1, and 2) and secondary somatosensory cortex (area 43) is often termed the anterior parietal cortex. The entire parietal cortex behind S I and S II is often termed the posterior parietal cortex. Posterior parietal cortex, in turn, is divisible in the superior parietal lobule and the inferior parietal lobule.

The superior parietal lobule lies superior to the intraparietal sulcus and includes Brodmann's areas 5 and 7a and 7b, whereas the inferior parietal lobule lies inferior to the intraparietal sulcus and includes Brodmann's areas 39 and 40.

Based on the serial processing of sensory information from secondary sensory areas, the superior parietal lobule is likely to be a **tertiary somatosensory association area in terms of its higher order processing.**

Area 5 receives a dense feedforward projection from all cytoarchitectonic areas of S I in a topographically organized manner. The thalamic afferents to this area come from the lateral posterior nucleus and from the central lateral nucleus of the intralaminar group. Ipsilateral corticocortical fibres from area 5 go to area 7, the premotor and supplementary motor cortices, the posterior cingulate gyrus, and the insular granular cortex.

Commissural connections between both sides of area 5 tend to avoid the areas of representation of the distal limb. The response properties of cells in area 5 are more complex than in S I, with larger receptive fields and evidence of submodality convergence. Area 5 contributes to the corticospinal tract (Crossman, 2008).

Areas 5 and 7 receive their inputs mainly from the primary somatosensory areas but also have reciprocal connections with the pulvinar and lateral posterior nucleus of the thalamus. Such connections permit the reinforcement, correlation, and integration of sensory information. The superior parietal lobule is involved in spatial orientation.

In monkeys area 7a is not related to the cortical pathway for somatosensory processing but instead forms part of a dorsal cortical pathway for spatial vision. The major ipsilateral corticocortical connections to area 7a are derived from visual areas in the occipital and temporal lobes. In the ipsilateral hemisphere, area 7a has connections with the posterior cingulate cortex (area 24) and with area 8 and 46 of the frontal lobe. Commissural connections are with its contralateral homologue. Area 7a is connected with the medial pulvinar and intralaminar paracentral nuclei of the thalamus.

In experimental studies, neurons within area 7a are visually responsive: they relate largely to the peripheral vision, respond to stimulus movement, and are modulated by eye movement (Crossman, 2008).

In monkeys, area 7b receives somatosensory inputs from area 5 and S II. Connections pass to the posterior cingulate gyrus (area 23), insula and temporal cortex. Area 7b is reciprocally connected with area 46 in the prefrontal cortex and the lateral part of the premotor cortex. Commissural connections of area 7b are with the contralateral homologous area, and with area S II, the insular granular cortex and area 5. Thalamic connections are with the medial pulvinar nucleus and the intralaminar paracentral nucleus (Crossman, 2008).

Neuronal responses in the tertiary somatosensory association areas involve the integration of a number of cortical and thalamic inputs. The processing of multisensory somatosensory inputs in these areas allows for the perception of shape, size and texture, and the identification of objects by contact (stereognosis).

The tertiary somatosensory association areas project to multimodal nonprimary association areas (areas 39 and 40) in the inferior parietal lobule that receive inputs from more than one sensory modality and serve intermodal integration and multisensory perception.

Single-cell recording in area 5 in monkeys suggests that this area is essential for the proper use of somatosensory information, for goal-directed voluntary movements, and for the manipulation of objects (Lüders et al., 1985).

Single-cell recording in area 7 indicates that this area plays an important role in the integration of visual and somatosensory stimuli, which is essential for the coordination of the eyes and hands in visually guided movements (Godoy et al., 1990; Pierrot-Deseilligny and Gaymard, 1990; Pierrot-Deseilligny et al., 1995).

Injuries to the parietal tertiary somatosensory association areas often lead to rare visual illusions that are modifications of the normal position of objects. The world appears upside down and the chair, table or other objects also appear upside down.

Such phenomena do not have any emotional component to them, as do such illusions that occur after injury to the temporal lobe.

Loss of the body schema often results because such patients do not recognize a body part as belonging to themselves. This agnosia can occur for a digit, hand, or half of the face. This condition, most frequently results from an extensive lesion in the superior aspect of the nondominant parietal lobe (areas 5, 7, 40, and 39). The individual does not recognize certain parts of the body as being his and show unilateral unawareness of denial defects on one side of the body (anosognosia).

In milder cases, patients may show an inappropriate **lack of concern for their deficits** (anosodiaphoria). Tests such as line bisection, drawing, copying, and visual search tasks may provide useful clinical screening procedures (Robertson and Marshall, 1993).

Apraxia is a deficit in the voluntary use of the limbs to carry out a series of movements in which each step depends on the preceding movement. Injuries to the dominant parietal lobe often result in the phenomena of ideational apraxia. Ideational apraxia is impairment of familiar and well-practiced movements (pick up a cup, pour water in it, drink the water etc.).

Sensory extinction is a subtle symptom of parietal lobe injury due to perceptual rivalry so that the injured area loses out, and the sensation coming from that side of the body is extinguished.

The inferior parietal lobule includes the supramarginal gyrus and the angular gyrus corresponding to Brodmann's areas 40 and 39. The intraparietal sulcus forms the dorsal border of the inferior parietal lobule. The supramarginal gyrus caps the posterior tip of the lateral sulcus (Fig. 21.28), whereas the angular gyrus caps the posterior tip of the superior temporal sulcus. The angular gyrus, corresponding to Brodmann's area 39, is functionally involved in language.

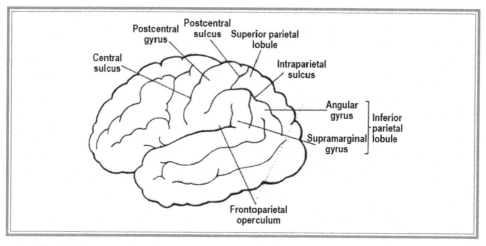

Fig. 21.28. Superolateral surface of the left cerebral hemisphere including the boundaries, major sulci, and gyri of the parietal lobe (after Augustine, 2008).

A unilateral lesion involving Brodmann's areas 39, 40, 22 and 37, results in Wernicke's (receptive) aphasia. Because this area plays a role in the comprehension and formulation of language, an individual with a severe form of this condition has difficulty in comprehending the spoken words. These patients cannot name an object they are able to see, although they know how to use it, and have a condition termed alexia without agraphia or the inability to read, although the ability to write remains.

Sentence comprehension impairments are usually observed in the context of tasks requiring a precise understanding of the grammatical relationships among words in a sentence. In 1906, Pierre Marie first noted that this type of test was very sensitive to mild degrees of language deficit.

Injury to the supramarginal gyrus, particularly in the left hemisphere corresponding to Brodmann's area 40, causes the loss of the ability to express oneself in language, a condition called conduction apraxia. Speech is broken but comprehension is good. In classic conduction aphasia, phonemic errors are more common in repetition tasks than in spontaneous speech. In transcortical motor aphasia, repetition may be spared, but spontaneous speech is contaminated by phonemic errors.

The major association cortex is connected with all the sensory cortical areas and, thus, functions in higher-order and complex multisensory perception. The major association cortex refers to supramarginal and angular gyri in the inferior parietal lobule which corresponds to areas 39 and 40 of Brodmann. Its relation to the speech areas in the temporal and frontal lobes gives it an important role in communication skills. Patients with lesions in the major association cortex of the dominant hemisphere present a conglomerate of manifestations that include receptive and expressive aphasia, inability to write (agraphia), inability to synthesize, correlate, and recognize multisensory perceptions (agnosia), left - right confusion, difficulty in recognizing different fingers (finger agnosia), and the inability to calculate (acalculia). These symptoms and signs are grouped together under the term Gerstmann's syndrome (Afifi and Bergman, 2005).

Involvement of the major association cortex in the nondominant hemisphere is usually manifested by disturbances in drawing (constructional apraxia) and in the awareness of body image. Such patients have difficulty in drawing a square or circle or copying a complex figure. They often are unaware of a body part and thus neglect to shave half of face or dress half the body (Afifi and Bergman, 2005).

Primary vestibular cortex

According to Brandt and Dieterich (1999) and Augustine (2008), the primary vestibular cortex, along the upper lip of the intraparietal sulcus (Fig 21.29), has the cytoarchitectural appearance of area 2 (Guldin and Grüsser, 1998). The cognitive perception of motion and spatial orientation arise through the convergence of information from the vestibular, visual, and somatosensory systems at the thalamocortical level. Neurons in the superior, lateral, and inferior vestibular nuclei project bilaterally to two thalamic areas. The first is located in the ventral posterolateral (VPL) nucleus and includes adjacent cells in the ventral posteroinferior (VPI) nucleus. The second is the posterior nuclear group, located near the medial geniculate body (Baloh and Honrubia, 1990; Goldberg, 1991; Highstein et al., 1996; Yates and Miller, 1996; Dickman et al., 2000; Dickman, 2006).

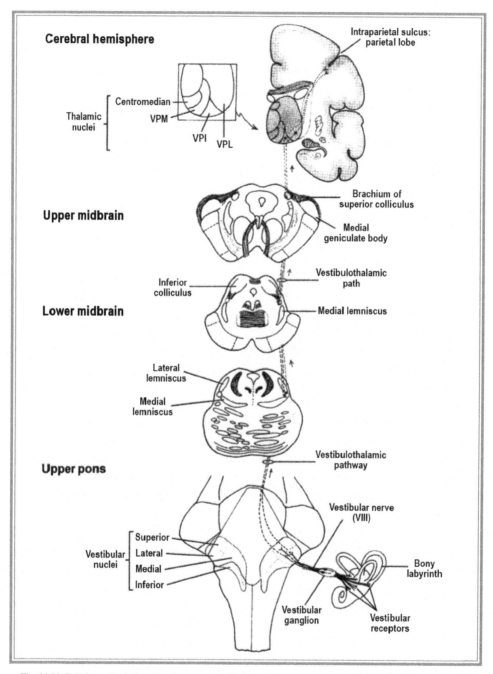

Fig. 21.29. Path for vestibular impulses from receptors in the peripheral vestibular apparatus to the primary vestibular cortex of the parietal lobe. This path is presumably bilateral in that there is never any direction of movement of the head that does not stimulate both sets of vestibular receptors. The thalamic termination of this path includes the oral part of the ventral posterior lateral nucleus (VPLo), caudal part of the ventral lateral nucleus (vLc) and dorsal part of the ventral posterior inferior nucleus (VPId). Some authors include VPI in the borders of the ventral posterior lateral nucleus (VPL) of the dorsal thalamus. The few primary fibres that reach the cerebellum are not shown (after Augustine, 2008).

Thalamic VPL and posterior nucleus neurons constitute separate, parallel pathways transmitting vestibular information from the brain stem to the cortex, because their connections with cortical areas are distinct. In addition, vestibular signals indirectly project to the anterior thalamic nuclei, where cells respond only when facing a preferred heading direction. These neurons are thought to be involved in spatial navigation and lose their directional selectivity through vestibular ablation (Baloh, 1990; Yates and Miller, 1996; Guldin and Grusser, 1998).

According to Dickman (2006), two cortical areas respond to vestibular stimulation (Fig. 21.30). One region, **area 2v,** lies at the base of the intraparietal sulcus just posterior to the hand and mouth representation in the postcentral gyrus. This region functions in vestibular consciousness – the awareness of position or movement of our body caused by the effects of gravity and acceleration and deceleration. Other than vertigo (the abnormal sensation of self-motion or of the motion of external objects often described as "dizziness"), there is no easily definable, discrete vestibular sensation. Cells in area 2v receive visual and proprioceptive inputs. Thus, area 2v is probably involved with motion perception and spatial orientation, because it has reciprocal connections with other parietal regions involved in similar functions (e.g.: area 5 and 7) (Kahane et al., 2003; Dickman, 2006).

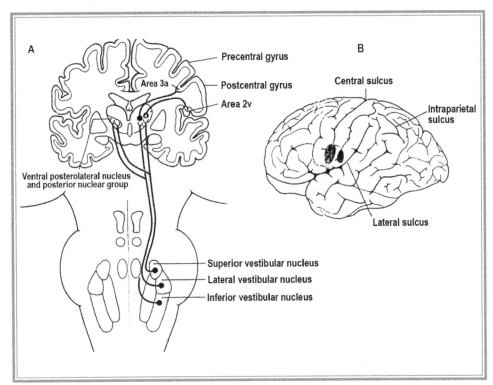

Fig. 21.30. The vestibulo-thalamo-cortical pathway. Vestibular input arises from the vestibular nuclei as vestibulothalamic fibres and is relayed to the cortex as thalamocortical fibres. (A) Areas 3a and 2v (B) are the main cortical regions that receive this input (after Dickman, 2006).

It appears that vestibular stimuli integrate with visual and somatosensory modalities. In the process of this integration, vestibular stimuli seem to lose their original, pure character. This overlap of vestibular and visual with other somatosensory modalities often allows each to compensate for a deficiency in the other (Leigh, 1994; Brand and Dieterich, 1999; Augustine, 2008).

Electrical stimulation of area 2v in humans produces sensations of moving, spinning, or dizziness. Area 2v neurons respond to head movements and receive projections from the posterior thalamic nucleus.

Lesions of parietal cortical areas result in confusion in spatial awareness. Injuries along the intraparietal sulcus lead to dizziness and a subjective feeling that the world is whirling about the patient. There is the illusion of rotation or of flouting.

The second cortical area responding to vestibular stimulation, **area 3a**, lies at the base of the central sulcus, adjacent to the motor cortex, and receives input from the VPL or VPI thalamic nuclear neurons. In addition, area 3a cell receives inputs from the somatosensory system. Because these cells project to areas of the motor cortex, it is believed that one of their function is to integrate motor control of the head and body. (Leigh, 1994; Kahane et al., 2003).

Visual disorientation and the disorder of spatial (topographic) localization is another syndrome. Spatial orientation depends upon visual, tactile, and kinesthetic perceptions. There are instances where the deficit in visual perception predominates. Patients with this disorder, in distinction to those with environmental agnosia, are unable to orient themselves in an abstract spatial setting (topographagnosia). Such patients cannot draw the floor plan of their house or a map of their town, and cannot describe a familiar route, from their home to their place of work, or find their way in familiar surroundings. In brief, they have lost topographic memory. This disorder is almost invariably caused by lesions in the dorsal convexity of the right parietal lobe, which is of interest, since it suggests that there are two separate processes for spatial orientation – one for the actual space (environmental) and one for the abstract topography of space.

Awareness of voluntary action and the parietal cortex

Voluntary action implies a subjective experience of the decision and the intention to act, as well as neural control of motor execution. For willed action to be a functional behavior, the brain must have a mechanism for matching the consequences of the motor act against the prior intention (Sirigu et al., 2004).

It is widely thought that the brain uses internal anticipatory models for this purpose (Wolpert et al., 1995; Kawato, 1999).

Estimating the time of a conscious intention presumably requires access to an internal representation of the desired movement. Internal motor representation, or internal models predict the future outcome of a given action (Wolpert and Ghahramani, 2000).

Several studies suggest that the parietal cortex is important in activating and maintaining such internal models (Sirigu et al., 1996; Desmurget and Grafton, 2000).

For instance, when the parietal cortex is damaged, patients lose the ability to predict through mental simulation the time necessary to perform various hand movements (Sirigu et al., 1996, 2004), indicating that this region is involved in generating conscious motor images. According to some reports (Wolpert et al., 1995; Kawato, 1999; Blakemore et al., 2001), another brain region, the cerebellum, is also involved in predicting the future state of a motor act.

For example, when lifting an object, subjects anticipate the increase in load force and accordingly adapt their grip force to hold the object (Flanagan and Wing, 1997). However, these processes may not be available to conscious awareness. Sirigu et al. (2004) found that cerebellar patients, similar to normal control subjects, were able to report when they first intended to move, whereas patients with parietal damage could not. These results suggest that the parietal cortex is involved in monitoring awareness of one's movements.

Sirigu et al. (2004) show that patients with parietal lesions could report when they started moving, but not when they first became aware of their intention to move. This stands in contrast with the performance of cerebellar patients who behaved as normal subjects. Thus, Sirigu et al. (2004) propose that when a movement is planned, activity in the parietal cortex, as part of a corticocortical sensorymotor processing loop, generates a predictive internal model of the upcoming movement. This model might form the neural correlate of motor awareness.

Sirigu et al. (2004) suggest that the brain may contain several internal models used for predictive control of voluntary action. An implicit module in the cerebellum would provide fast processing for execution of action and predicting their sensory consequences (Blakemore et al., 2001; Wolpert et al., 2001). A second system, in the parietal cortex, would monitor intentions and motor plans at a higher level, detecting when actions match their desired goals. These processes typically involve conscious experience (Sirigu et al., 2004).

Primary visual cortex (V1)

The occipital lobe comprises almost entirely Brodmann's areas 17, 18 and 19. Area 17, the striate cortex, is the primary visual cortex (V1). A host of other distinct visual areas resides in the occipital and temporal cortex. The functional subdivisions V2, V3 (dorsal and ventral) and V3A lie within Brodmann's area 18. Other functional areas at the junctions of the occipital cortex with the parietal or temporal lobes lie wholly or partly in area 19.

The primary visual cortex is located mainly in the medial surface of the occipital lobes on the banks of the **calcarine fissure**, although it extends into their posterolateral surface.

The primary visual cortex is the thinnest cortex of the entire brain. Layer IV of this cortex is prominent due to a thick layer of myelinated fibres, the **external band of Baillarger.** This band is characteristically so thick in this cortex that it gives the primary visual cortex a grossly visible striped appearance, and is referred to as the **stripe of Gennari.** In sections of fresh cortex, area 17 of Brodmann is characterized by the appearance of a prominent band of white matter that can be identified by the naked eye and is named the band of Gennari, after the Italian medical student who described it in

1782. This band of Gennari represents a thickened external band of Baillarger in layer IV of the cortex.

In myelin preparations, the band of Gennari appears as a prominent dark band in the visual cortex, also known as the striate cortex. The term striate refers to the presence in unstained preparations of the thick white band of Gennari.

It occupies the upper and lower lips and depths of the posterior part of the calcarine sulcus and extends into the cuneus and lingual gyrus.

The primary visual cortex receives **afferent** fibres from the lateral geniculate nucleus *via* the optic radiation. The latter curves posteriorly and spreads through the white matter of the occipital lobe. Its fibres terminate in strict point-to-point fashion in the striate area.

The superior lip of the calcarine sulcus receives fibres projecting from the superior retinal quadrants whereas the inferior lip of the calcarine sulcus receives projections from the inferior retinal quadrants.

Thus, the lateral geniculate nucleus projects visual information to the primary visual cortex (V1) (Brodmann's area 17). This cortical area receives input arising from the contralateral visual field: the temporal half of the ipsilateral retina and the nasal half of the contralateral retina. The cortex of each hemisphere receives impulses from two hemiretinas, which represent the contralateral half of the binocular visual field.

The superior and inferior retinal quadrants are connected with corresponding areas of the striate cortex. Thus, the superior retinal quadrants (representing the inferior half of the visual field) are connected with the visual cortex above the calcarine sulcus, and the inferior retinal quadrants (representing the upper half of the visual field) are connected with the visual cortex below the calcarine sulcus. Thus, fibres originating from the superior half of the retina terminate in the superior part of the visual cortex; those from the inferior half of the retina terminate in the inferior part. The peripheral parts of the retina activate most anterior parts of the visual cortex.

Geniculocalcarine fibres pass in the external sagittal stratum which is separated from the wall of the inferior and posterior horns of the lateral ventricle by the internal sagittal stratum and by fibres of the corpus callosum designed as the tapetum. Fibres of the internal sagittal stratum are corticofugal fibres passing from the occipital lobe to the superior colliculus and the lateral geniculate body (Altman, 1962; Garey et al., 1968).

The macular fibres project most posteriorly along the calcarine sulcus around the occipital pole, followed by fibres from the paramacular areas. The macular representation in the primary visual cortex is much larger than that of other areas of the retina, reflecting the high visual acuity of the macula.

Unilateral injury to the calcarine sulcus will lead to a contralateral homonymous hemianopsia in which there is blindness in the ipsilateral nasal field and the contralateral temporal field.

Lesions involving portions of the visual cortex, such as the inferior calcarine cortex, produce a homonymous quadrantanopsia, in which blindness results in the superior half of the visual field contralaterally. Similarly, lesions limited to the upper calcarine cortex produce a lower contralateral quadrantanopsia in which blindness is limited to the contralateral lower quadrant of the visual field (Fig. 21.31).

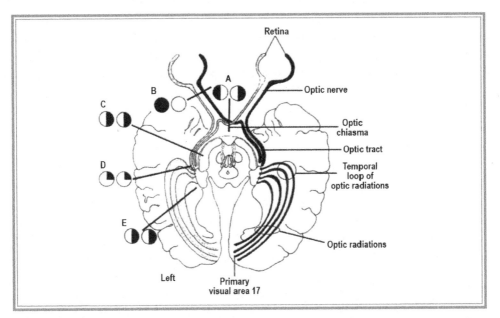

Fig. 21.31. Visual field deficits caused by interruption or transection of fibres at certain points along the visual path. A. Section of the optic chiasma with a resulting bitemporal hemianopia (loss of vision in the temporal parts of both right and left visual fields). B. Section of the left optic nerve with blindness in the left visual field and a normal right visual field. C. Section of the optic tract causing a contralateral homonymous hemianopia. D. Section of the optic radiations in the temporal lobe with an incongruous visual field defect. The temporal part of the right visual field is affected, as is the superior nasal quadrant of the left visual field – a superior quadrantanopia. E. Section of the optic radiations in the parietal lobe with a resulting contralateral homonymous hemianopia (modified from Harrington, 1981).

A bilateral destruction of the striate areas causes total blindness in men, but other mammals, such as dogs and monkeys, retain the ability to distinguish light intensities after ablations of the visual cortex (Klüver, 1942; Glees, 1961; Snyder et al., 1966). If the destructive lesion is of vascular origin as occurs in occlusions of the posterior cerebral artery, central (macular) vision in the affected visual field is spared. This phenomenon is known clinically as macular sparing and is attributed to the contralateral arterial supply of the posterior visual cortex (macular area) from the patent middle cerebral artery.

The striate cortex is granular. Layer IV, bearing the stria of Gennari, is commonly divided into three sublayers. Passing from superficial to deep, these are IV A, IV B (which contains the stria) and IV C. The densely cellular IV C is further subdivided into a superficial IV Cα and a deep IV Cβ. Layer IV B contains only sparse mainly non-pyramidal neurons.

Thus, the primary visual cortex occupies about 21 cm² in each cerebral hemisphere. Area 17 in young adults has about 35,000 neurons per mm³.

The primary visual cortex (Area 17 / V1) is thin, averages 1,8 mm in thickness, and sums up to about 3% (range 2-4%) of the entire cerebral cortex. Although it resembles other cortical areas, being arranged in six layers (I to VI), extensive quantitative analyses and correlation studies in humans have identified at least ten layers in the primary visual cortex: layer I, II, III, IVa, IVb, IVc, Va, Vb, VIa and VIb. Layer IVc, in turn, is divisible into IVc-α and IVc-β. Neurons in each layer have a distinctive size, shape, density, and response to visual stimuli (Zilles et al., 1986; Glickstein, 1988; Zeki et al., 1991; Zilles, 1995, 2004). The input to area 17 from the lateral geniculate nucleus terminates predominantly in IV A and IV C (Paxinos, 1990; Lee et al., 2000).

Other thalamic afferents from the inferior pulvinar nucleus and the intralaminar group pass to layers I and IV. Geniculocortical fibres terminate in alternating bands. Axons from the geniculate lamina which receives information from the ipsilateral eye (laminae 2, 3 and 5) are segregated from those of laminae which receive input from the contralateral eye (laminae 1, 4 and 6).

Neurons within layer IV C are monocular, i.e., they respond to stimulation of either the ipsilateral or contralateral eye, but not both.

This horizontal segregation forms the anatomical basis of the ocular dominance column in that neurons encountered in a vertical strip from below the pia to the white matter, although binocular outside layer IV, exhibit a preference for stimulation of one or the other eye (Lee et al., 2000; Crossman, 2008).

Thus, the primary visual cortex is arranged into columns oriented perpendicularly to the cortical surface, extending from the cortical surface (under the pia mater) to the subcortical white matter. Nerve cells, in a particular cortical column, are functionally similar. Columns in the primary visual cortex include the **ocular dominance columns,** the site where fibres relaying information from the ipsilateral or the contralateral eye terminate, and the **orientation columns**, where nerve cells are responsive to visual stimuli that have a comparable spatial orientation.

Layers II and III of the primary visual cortex also contain vertically oriented aggregates of nerve cells that are responsive to colour.

The striate cortex, anatomically far more complex than the retina or lateral geniculate body, does not have cells with concentric receptive fields. Cells of the striate cortex show marked specificity in their response to restricted retinal stimulation (Hubel and Wiesel, 1959, 1963). A given cell responds vigorously when an appropriate stimulus is shone on its receptive field, or moves across it, provided the stimulus is presented in a specific orientation.

Thus, all cells within each column have the same receptive field axis of orientation. The receptive field axis of orientation differs from one cell column to the next, and may be vertical, horizontal or oblique. Thus for each stimulated area of the retina, each line and each orientation of the stimulus, there is a particular set of "**simple**" striate cortical cells that respond.

Changing any of the stimulus arrangements will cause an entirely new and different population of "simple" striate cells to respond (Hubel and Wiesel, 1962).

"**Complex**" type cells, like "simple" cells, respond best to "slits", "bars", or "edges", provided the orientation is suitable. Unlike "simple" cells, these cells respond with sustained firing as the slits of light are moved across the retina, preserving the same receptive field axis of orientation (Hubel and Wiesel, 1962). There is a relationship between the complexity of response and the position of cells in relation to the cortical laminae. Simple cells are mainly in layer IV and complex and hypercomplex cells predominate in either layers II and III or layers V and VI.

Since columns of cells constitute the fundamental functional units of the cortex, each small region of the visual field must be represented in the striate cortex many times, in column after column of cells with different receptive field orientation.

The receptive fields of all binocularly influenced cortical cells occupy corresponding sites in the two retinas. About 80% of the cells in the striate cortex are influenced independently by the two eyes (Hubel and Wiesel, 1962).

Considerable evidence indicates that early visual experience can change the distribution of the selective orientation of striate cortical units (Hirsch and Spinelli, 1970; Blakemore and Cooper, 1970).

Cells of the striate cortex in kittens with controlled visual deprivation appear to adapt functionally to the restricted visual orientations to which they have exposed during the early critical period (Pettigrew et al., 1973).

Studies of controlled, visually deprived kittens, that permitted normal binocular viewing after the critical period, show a dramatic increase in the number of striate cells which are binocularly activated (Spinelli et al., 1972).

The other major functional basis for visual cortical columnar organization is the orientation column. Thus, an electrode passing through the depth of the cortex at right angles to the plane from below the pia to the white matter, encounters neurons that respond preferentially to either a stationary or a moving straight line of a given orientation within the visual field. Cells with simple, complex and hypercomplex receptive fields occur in area 17. **Simple cells** respond optimally to lines in a narrowly defined position. **Complex cells** respond to lines anywhere within a receptive field, but with a specific orientation. **Hypercomplex cells** are similar to complex cells except that the length of the line or bar stimulus is also critical for an optimal response. Thus, the visual cortex units are of two varieties: simple and complex. Simple units respond only to stimuli in corresponding fixed retinal receptive fields. Complex and hypercomplex units are connected to several simple cortical units. It is presumed that the complex units represent an advanced stage in cortical integration.

Thus, the visual cortex is organized into units, and, for each unit, a particular orientation of the stimulus is most effective. Some units respond only to vertically oriented stripes, while others respond only to horizontally oriented stripes. Some units respond at onset of illumination, while others respond at cessation of illumination.

Units that respond to the same stimulus and orientation are grouped together in repeating units referred to as columns. Two general varieties of functional columns have been described: ocular dominance and orientation columns. Thus, the striate cortex is organized into vertical and horizontal columns. The vertical columnar system is concerned with retinal position, line orientation, and ocular dominance. The horizontal system segregates cells of different orders of complexity. Simple cells located in layer IV are driven monocularly, while complex and hypercomplex cells, located in other layers, are driven by impulses from both eyes (Afifi and Bergman, 2005).

Ocular dominance columns are parallel columns arranged perpendicularly to the cortical surface and reflect eye preference (right versus left) of cortical neurons. Alternating ocular dominance columns are dominated by inputs from the left and right eye. Orientation columns comprise a sequence of cells that have the same receptive field axis orientation (Hubel and Wiesel, 1962; Hirsch and Spinelli, 1970; Pettigrew et al., 1973; Spinelli et al., 1972; Afifi and Bergman, 2005). Visual units respond optionally to moving stimuli. Most cortical units receive fibres from corresponding receptive fields in both retinas, thus allowing for single-image vision of corresponding points in the two retinas. Thus, units in the primary visual secondary areas are of the complex and hypercomplex types.

The output from the primary visual cortex. Ipsilateral corticocortical fibres pass from area 17 to a variety of functional areas in areas 18 and 19 and in the parietal and temporal cortices. Fibres from area 17 pass to area 18 (which contains visual areas V2, V3 and V3a), area 19 (which contains V4), the posterior intraparietal and the parieto-occipito areas, and to parts of the posterior temporal lobe, the middle temporal area and the medial superior temporal area (Livingstone and Huber, 1984; Crossman, 2008).

The main output from the primary visual cortex follows two pathways or streams: a **dorsal stream** to the occipitoparietal cortex (the "where" pathway) and a **ventral stream** to the occipitotemporal cortex (the "what" pathway). Bilateral lesions in the "where" pathway, result in the inability to direct the eyes to a certain point in the visual field despite intact eye movements (Balint syndrome).

Balint's syndrome consists of (1) an inability to look voluntarily into and to scan the peripheral field, despite the fact that the eye movements are complete (psychic paralysis of fixation or gaze); (2) a failure to precisely grasp or touch an object under visual guidance, as though hand and eye were not coordinated (inappropriately called optic ataxia); and (3) visual inattention (disorientation) affecting mainly the periphery of the visual field, attention to other sensory stimuli being intact.

Bilateral lesions in the "what" pathway result in the inability of patients, with normal visual perception, to comprehend the meaning of nonverbal visual stimuli (**visual agnosia**).

Subcortical efferents of the striate cortex pass to the superior colliculus, pretectum and parts of the brain stem reticular formation.

Projections to the striatum (notably, the tail of the caudate nucleus), and to the pontine nuclei, are sparse.

Geniculo- and claustrocortical projections are reciprocated by prominent descending projections, which arise in layer IV (Crossman, 2008).

Secondary visual cortex (V2)

Adjoining the primary visual cortex is an extrastriate cortex which consists of the secondary and tertiary visual cortical areas. They include areas 18 and 19 of Brodmann on the lateral and medial aspects of the hemisphere. Areas 20, 21, and 37 in the inferior temporal cortex are also dedicated to visual information processing. Area 18 corresponds to the second (V2) and area 19 to the third (V3) visual areas. V4, in humans, is probably located in the inferior occipitotemporal area, in the region of the lingual or fusiform gyrus. V5 in humans is probably located in area 19 of Brodmann. V2 like V1 is retinotopically organized. V3 is associated with form, V4 with color, and V5 with motion.

Area 18, also termed the parastriate area, has connections with the primary visual cortex and with area 19 in the occipital lobe through short association fibres. Area 18 has connections with areas 18 and 19 in the contralateral cerebral hemisphere by way of commissural fibres. Long association fibres connect area 18 with the frontal lobe permitting this region to receive sensory, motor, and auditory impulses as well as those from the insular and temporal lobes (Augustine, 2008). The importance of the existence of long association fibres, that interrelate the frontal lobe with the occipital lobe, is evident in a patient who has an injury in the middle frontal gyrus and saw stars and flashes of light. This suggests that the occipital lobe was being stimulated when in fact the lesion irritated fibres in the frontal lobe that interrelate the frontal and the occipital lobes (Augustine, 2008).

Thus, the primary visual cortex projects to the visual association area where information is processed and subsequently relayed to the tertiary visual areas (areas V3, V4, and the middle temporal area) of the cortex. So, the major ipsilateral corticocortical feedforward projection to V2 comes from V1. Areas 18 and 19 do not have a visible stripe of fibres in layer IV. Area 18, the secondary visual cortex or area V2, surrounds V1, connects with it, and lacks a specialized layer IV. More than 30 extrastriate association areas are identifiable in the temporal, parietal and occipital lobes of primates (Huck et al., 2002; Zilles, 2004).

Feedforward projections from V2 pass to several other visual areas (and are reciprocated by feedback connections) including the third visual area (V3) and its various subdivisions (V3 / V3 d; VP / V3v; V3a), the fourth visual area (V4), areas in the temporal and parietal association cortices, and the frontal eye field (Crossman, 2008).

Thus, primary visual area 17 sends many fibres to the extrastriate visual area 18 and area 19 that have an especially well-differentiated system of intracortical and myelinated fibres. Area 18, in turn, has reciprocal connections with other extrastriate areas.

Thalamic afferents to V2 come from the lateral geniculate nucleus, the inferior and lateral pulvinar nuclei and parts of the intralaminar group of nuclei. Subcortical efferents arise predominantly in layers V and VI. They pass to the thalamus, claustrum, superior colliculus, pretectum, brain stem reticular formation, striatum and pons.

As for area 17, the callosal connections of V2 are restricted predominantly to the cortex, which contains the representation of the vertical meridian (Crossman, 2008).

Area 18 interprets, associates, and facilitates the understanding of impulses that reach area 17. Information from area 18 in the dominant cerebral hemisphere correlates with that from area 18 in the nondominant cerebral hemisphere. Area 18 participates in colour vision in humans (Hurlbert, 2003). Area 18 and 19 in the parietal lobe are involved with following of automatic eye movements. Stimulation of area 18 in humans yields unformed images, wheels, flashing lights, streaks, flickering light, and coloured spots (Fox et al., 1987; Zeki et al., 1991; Huck et al., 2002; Goodale and Westwood, 2004).

Injury to area 18 will result in the loss of following eye movements towards the contralateral side. Although the patient is still able to see because the primary visual cortex is intact, they often present with a visual agnosia – the loss of power to recognize the import of visual stimuli in the absence of visual defects.

Connections of the secondary visual cortex to the angular gyrus (area 39) play a role in recognition of visual stimuli. Lesions interrupting this connection result in visual agnosia (De Renzi, 2000).

The third visual area (V3)

It is a narrow strip adjoining the anterior margin of V2, probably still within area 18 of Brodmann. V3 has been subdivided into dorsal (V3 / V3d) and ventral (VP / V3v) regions on the basis of its afferents from area V1, myeloarchitecture, callosal and association connections, and receptive field properties (Zilles, 2004).

The dorsal subdivision receives afferent from V1, whereas the ventral does not (Burkhalter and Bernardo, 1989).

Functionally, the dorsal part shows less wavelength selectivity, greater direction selectivity and smaller receptive fields than does the ventral subdivision.

Both areas receive a feedforward projections from V2 and are interconnected by association fibres.

A further visual area, area V3a, lies anterior to the dorsal subdivision of V3. It receives afferent association connections from V1, V2, V3 / V3d and VP / V3v and has a complex and irregular topographic organization.

All subdivisions project to diverse visual areas in the parietal and temporal cortices, including V4, and to the frontal eye fields (Zilles, 2004; Crossman, 2008).

Thus, extrastriate area 19 is the most rostral part of the visual cortex in the occipital lobe. This latter area is not homogenous but is divisible into a number of visual areas. It is likely a tertiary visual area.

Current concepts of visual processing in inferior temporal and temporoparietal cortices suggest that two parallel pathways (dorsal and ventral) emanate from occipital lobe. The dorsal pathway, concerned primarily with visuospatial discrimination, project from V1 and V2 to the superior temporal and surrounding parietotemporal areas and ultimately to area 7a of the parietal cortex.

The fourth visual area (V4)

This visual area lies within area 19 anterior to the V3 complex. Visual area V4 is in the collateral sulcus or lingual gyrus of the occipital lobe. It receives input from the parvicellular layers of the lateral geniculate in nonhuman primates, and a major ipsilateral feedforward projection from V2. In humans, this extrastriate visual area is specialized for different aspects of object recognition including colour and shape. Colour selectivity as well as orientation selectivity may be transmitted to V4 and bilateral damage causes achromatopsia (Hurlbert, 2003; Goodale and Westwood, 2004; Zilles, 2004).

V4 is more complex than a simple colour discrimination area because it is also involved in the discrimination of orientation, form and movement (Goodale and Milner, 1992; Goodale and Westwood, 2004; Crossman, 2008).

It sends a feedforward projection to the inferior temporal cortex and receives a feedback projection.

It also connects with other visual areas that lie more dorsally in the temporal lobe, and the parietal lobe. Thalamocortical connections are with the lateral and inferior pulvinar and the intralaminar nuclei.

Other subcortical connections conform to the general pattern for all cortical areas.

Callosal connections are with the contralateral V4 and other occipital visual areas (Glickstein and Whitteridge, 1987; Fox et al., 1987; De Yoe et al., 1994; Zilles, 2004; Crossman, 2008).

Thus, **afferents** to areas 18 and 19 are mainly from the primary visual area (area 17) but include some direct thalamic projections from the lateral geniculate nucleus and pulvinar nucleus. The primary visual area projects bilaterally and reciprocally to areas 18 and 19. The projections from the pulvinar nucleus constitute important extrageniculate links to the visual cortex (Burkhalter and Bernardo, 1989).

Outputs from areas 18 and 19 project to the posterior parietal cortex (area 7) and to the inferotemporal cortex (areas 20 and 21) (Livingstone and Hubel, 1984; Ishai et al., 2000; Hurlbert, 2003; Lennie, 2003; Zilles, 2004).

The projection to area 7 is concerned with stereopsis (depth perception and movement (Goodale and Milner, 1992; Goodale and Westwood, 2004). The inferotemporal projection is concerned with the analysis of form and colours (Hurlbert, 2003).

The fourth visual area, V4, is a key relay station for the ventral pathway, which is related to perception and object recognition. Its connections pass sequentially along the inferior temporal gyrus in a feedforward manner, from V4 to the posterior, intermediate, and then anterior, inferior temporal cortices. Ultimately they feed into the temporal polar and medial temporal areas and so interface with the limbic system (Burkhalter and Bernardo, 1989; De Yoe et al., 1994; Goodale and Westwood, 2004; Zilles, 2004; Crossman, 2008).

Thus, information travels first to the primary visual cortex and then relays in serial fashion through a series of increasingly complex visual association areas (the extrastriate visual area).

This "what" and "where" model of vision in nonhuman primates includes a ventral stream ("what" path), the occipito-temporo-prefrontal path for perception, identification, and recognition of visually presented objects (object vision, faces, and words) based on features like colour, texture and contours. The occipitotemporal cortex includes Brodmann's areas 19 and 37. Area 37, behind area 21, at the occipitotemporal junction contains modules devoted to recognition of faces.

Colour vision is localized inferiorly in the inferior occipitotemporal cortex (V4). No colour representation is found in the superior association visual cortex. Thus, in unilateral inferior association visual cortex lesions, the patient loses colour vision in the contralateral half of field **(central hemiachromatopsia)**.

Cerebral achromatopsia results from bilateral damage to the V4/V4 α region of the colour centre. If patients experience complete ablation of V4, they lose colour vision in the entire visual field. Thus, cerebral achromatopsia arises following brain damage to V4/V4 α located in the ventral medial region of the occipital lobe, typically caused by a tumor, haemorrhage, or some sort of brain trauma. Because V4 is located in the vicinity of the fusiform gyrus and the lingual gyrus, known to process faces, the comorbidity between **achromatopsia** and **prosopagnosia** is extremely high (Kanwisher et al., 1997; Bouvier and Engel, 2006).

In less extreme cases, known as **dyschromatopsia**, patients lose the ability to perceive selective colour and / or colour constancy (Glickstein and Whitteridge, 1987; Goodale and Milner, 1992; Bartels and Zeki, 2000; Bouvier and Engel, 2006).

The first cases of cerebral achromatopsia were reported by Verry in 1888. In response to these patients, Verry introduced the concept of a "colour centre" in the brain.

Continued research confirmed the existence of a cortical region devoted to colour processing. Thus, Meadows (1974) demonstrated a correlation between the cortical region sensitive to colour and the damaged cortical regions in achromatopsic patients.

The dorsal stream ("where" path) or occipito-parieto-prefrontal path participates in the appreciation of the spatial relations among objects (spatial vision) as well as for the visual guidance of movements towards objects in visual space (Ungerleider and Haxby, 1994).

The occipitoparietal cortex includes parts of Brodmann's area 19 and area 7 from the superior parietal lobule. The prefrontal part of these paths includes parts of the inferior frontal gyrus corresponding to Brodmann's areas 45 and 47 as well as the dorsal part of premotor area 6.

There seems to be some left hemisphere specialization or dominance for visual form in the ventral stream. Evidence from neuropsychology, electrophysiology, and neuroimaging suggests that there are specialized processing regions for specific categories of visual objects (i.e., faces).

Face recognition is a biological necessity and unique behavioral capacity that requires a dedicated neuronal system that can be selectively damaged (Kanwisher and Yovel, 2006).

Prosopagnosia is a deficit in the general capacity to discriminate between very similar exemplars in a class of objects due to damage to neural representations of objects that are widely distributed and overlapping (Haxby et al., 2001). Prosopagnosia is the result of injury to a specialized neural system that develops with experience and is required when distinguishing between subtle differences within a category of complex visual material (Gauthier et al., 1999; Riesenhuber and Poggio, 2000; Serre et al., 2007). Loss of face recognition and colour vision usually coexist because of the proximity of the areas responsible for them (Gorno-Tempini et al., 2001; Hadjikhani and de Gelder, 2002; Hubel et al., 2003; Schiltz et al., 2006).

The fifth visual area (V5)

Another extrastriate visual area is visual area V5 in the ascending limb of the inferior temporal sulcus. It is found in nonhuman primates towards the posterior end of the superior temporal sulcus. It receives ipsilateral association connections from area V1, V2, V3 and V4, in a topographically organized way.

Other lesser projections are received from widespread visual areas in the temporal and parieto-occipital lobes and from the frontal eye field. This area in nonhuman primates receives input from the magnocellular layers of the lateral geniculate nucleus by way of the primary visual cortex. There may be direct projections from V1 to V5 or indirect to V5 through V2 or V3.

V5 is primarily a movement detection or discrimination area, and contains a high proportion of movement-sensitive, direction-selective cells. This motion pathway likely extends beyond the middle temporal area to the medial superior temporal area, the parietal lobe and the frontal eye fields (Goodale and Milner, 1992; Huck et al., 2002; Schneider et al., 2004; Goodale and Westwood, 2004; Zilles, 2004;).

Feedforward projections of V5 go to surrounding temporal and parietal areas, and to the frontal eye field. Thalamic connections are with the lateral and inferior pulvinar and intralaminar group of nuclei. Other connections follow the general pattern of all neocortical areas (Crossman, 2008).

Patients with lesions in this area may have a selective disturbance of movement vision such as visual tracking. Bilateral lesions of the fifth visual area (V5) are associated with a defect in visual motion perception (**akinetopsia**). This visual area in humans is comparable in many ways to area MT in nonhuman primates.

Preoccipital areas involved in following ocular movements

The posterior parietal eye field corresponds to areas 39, 40, 19 and 18 of Brodmann. This area triggers reflexive, visually guided saccades. It exerts its influence on saccadic eye movements *via* its connections to the frontal eye field or directly to the superior colliculus.

Thus, in the parietal lobe and in part of the occipital lobe, is an area involved in following of the automatic ocular movements (Morrow and Sharpe, 1990; Pierrot-Deseilligny and Gaymard, 1990; Pierrot-Deseilligny et al., 1995; Lekwuw and Barnes, 1996; Afifi and Bergman, 2005).

The posterior parietal cortex (the cortex in the posterior region of the intraparietal sulcus and the adjacent superior parietal lobule) is activated by the primary visual cortex during saccades for which there is a visual goal.

According to Augustine (2008), in the parietal lobe and in part of the occipital lobe, is an area involved in the following of automatic ocular movements.

In the parietal lobe, this area corresponds to Brodmann's area 19, while in the occipital lobe it corresponds to Brodmann's area 18. One is often not aware of these movements as the eyes fix on a moving object. These ocular movements are extrapyramidal in type and obviously significant as emphasized by the presence of two different cortical fields (the frontal eye fields for voluntary ocular movement and preoccipital areas for following movements of the eyes) as well as two separate extrapyramidal paths for their production. (Paus, 1996; Pandya and Yeterian, 1996; Milea et al., 2002).

Cortical stimulation of parietal area 19 and occipital area 18 yields deviation of the eyes upward, downward, or horizontal deviations. If the upper part of area 19, or the lower part of area 18, is stimulated, upward deviation of the eyes will occur. Presumably, there are connections from these two regions of the parietal and occipital lobes, respectively, to the tegmentum of the midbrain by way of the internal corticotectal fibres.

In particular, these fibres pass the rostromedial part of the superior colliculus (Lobel et al., 2001; Schüz and Miller, 2002; Zilles, 2004; Augustine, 2008).

From the rostromedial superior colliculus, tecto-oculomotor fibres pass to the oculomotor and trochlear nuclear complexes of the midbrain. They end on neurons that supply muscles that raise the lids and lift the eyes in an upward direction (Jampel, 1975; King et al., 1976; Bortolami et al., 1977; Augustine et al., 1981; Leigh and Zee, 2006; Augustine, 2008).

If the upper part of area 18, or the lower part of area 19, is stimulated, downward deviation of the eyes will occur. The anatomic basis is by way of internal corticotectal fibres that pass from the parietal and occipital lobes to the caudolateral part of the superior colliculus. From this region, tecto-oculomotor fibres pass to the oculomotor nucleus, particularly to these neurons that supply muscles that lower the eyes (Tijssen et al., 1991; Augustine, 2008).

If the middle part of parietal area 18 and the middle part of occipital area 19 are stimulated, horizontal deviation of the eyes will occur. In this situation, corticotegmental paths pass from the cerebral cortex to the tegmentum of the midbrain. From there, connection fibres project to the contralateral abducens nucleus and the abducens reticular gray matter in order to initiate a horizontal deviation of the eyes (King et al., 1976; Augustine et al., 1981; Leigh and Zee, 2006).

Thus, projections from area 18 and 19 also reach the frontal eye fields (area 8 of Brodmann) in the frontal lobe, as well as the superior colliculus and motor nuclei of the extraocular muscles. These projections play a key role in conjugate eye movement induced by visual stimuli (visual pursuit). However, the connections and functional aspects of ocular movements are exceedingly complex.

Patients with lesions in the posterior parietal eye field lose reflexive visually guided saccades but are able to move their eyes in response to command (intentional saccades).

Saccadic movements are fast eye movements with rapid fixation of vision from point to point with no interest in the points in between. Positron emission tomography (PET) scans and lesion studies indicate that the cerebral areas most important for saccadic control are: (1) the posterior parietal cortex; and (2) the frontal premotor cortex (Pierrot-Deseilligny et al., 1995; Lekwuwa and Barnes, 1996).

Frontal eye field. Three areas in the frontal lobe participate in saccadic processing: (1) the frontal eye field (area 8 of Brodmann); (2) the dorsolateral prefrontal cortex (area

46 of Brodmann); and (3) the supplementary eye field (anterior part of the supplementary motor area). The frontal and supplementary eye fields are activated during all types of saccadic movements. The dorsolateral prefrontal cortex is activated during fixation.

The frontal eye field located in the middle frontal gyrus, anterior to or in the anterior portion of the motor strip, corresponds to area 8 of Brodmann and the immediately adjacent cortex. This field triggers intentional (voluntary) saccades to visible targets in the visual environment, and subserves intentional exploration of the visual environment (Pierrot-Deseilligny et al., 1995; Lekwuwa and Barnes, 1996). The frontal eye field receives multiple cortical inputs, from the parietooccipital cortex, supplementary eye fields, and the prefrontal cortex (Brodmann's area, 46). The frontal eye field elicits intentional (voluntary) saccades through connections to the nuclei of the extraocular muscles in the brain stem.

The pathway from the frontal eye field to the nuclei of extraocular movements is not direct but involves multiple brain stem reticular nuclei, including the superior colliculus, the interstitial nucleus of the longitudinal fasciculus, and the paramedian pontine reticular formation.

This frontal eye field can be functionally subdivided into different sectors depending on the direction of the eye movements that can be elicited from it.

Transcranial magnetic stimulation in humans has permitted the delimitation of the frontal eye field within an area that comprises portions of the dorsolateral prefrontal and premotor cortex (Chouinard et al., 2003; Pierrot-Deseilligny et al., 2004).

Auditory cortex

Primary auditory cortex

The temporal lobe has three parallel gyri on the lateral surface: **superior** (Brodmann's area 22), **middle** (Brodmann's area 21), and **inferior** (Brodmann's area 20). Thus, its lateral surface is divided into three parallel gyri by the superior temporal and inferior temporal sulci (Fig. 21.32). The superior temporal sulcus begins near the temporal pole and slopes slightly up and backwards parallel to the posterior ramus of the lateral sulcus. Its end curves up into the parietal lobe.

The inferior temporal sulcus is subjacent and parallel to the superior one and is often broken into two or three short sulci. Its posterior end also ascends into the parietal lobe, posterior and parallel to the upturned end of the superior sulcus. The temporal lobe is inferior to the lateral fissure.

The cortex of the medial temporal lobe includes major subdivisions of the limbic system, such as the hippocampus and entorhinal cortex. Areas of neocortex adjacent to these limbic regions are grouped together as the medial temporal association cortex. Ferrier (1876; 1878; 1890), a British physician, is credited with localizing the primary auditory cortex of monkeys to the superior temporal gyrus. This localization was not accepted by his contemporaries.

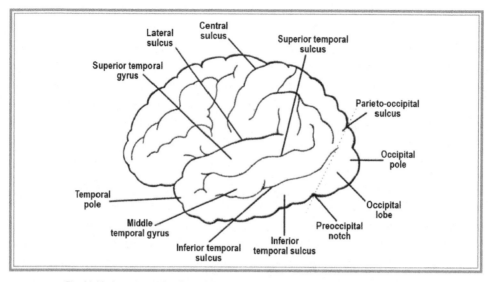

Fig. 21.32. Superolateral surface of the left cerebral hemisphere including the boundaries, major sulci and gyri of the temporal and occipital lobes.

The primary auditory cortex (Brodmann's areas 41 and 42) resides deep in the lateral fissure of Sylvius, in the hidden superior surface of the superior temporal gyrus, containing the transverse temporal gyri of Heschl, and in the floor of the lateral fissure.

Thus, two transversely-oriented gyri, the anterior and posterior transverse temporal gyri are continuous with the superior temporal gyrus but folded and hidden from view when one observes the lateral surface of the cerebral hemisphere. The anterior transverse temporal gyrus (of Heschl), lying in depth of the lateral sulcus and corresponding to Brodmann's area 41 (Fig. 21.33) is **the primary auditory cortex** or **A I.** Recordings of primary evoked responses to auditory stimuli during surgery for epilepsy provide evidence for a restricted portion of Heschl's gyrus as the primary auditory area (Heffner, 1987; Hocherman and Yirimiya, 1990; Liegeois-Chauvel et al., 1994).

However, the two transverse temporal gyri are buried in the lateral sylvian sulcus, covered by parts of the frontal and parietal opercula, and continuous with the superior temporal gyrus. Caudal to the transverse temporal gyri is a smooth area, the **planum temporale**, which is usually larger on the left side than on the right (Fig. 21.34).

The temporal operculum houses the primary auditory cortex. This is coextensive with the granular area 41 in the transverse temporal gyri. Surrounding areas constitute the auditory association cortex (Fig. 21.35).

The length and surface area of the left primary auditory cortex is greater than the right in newborns and adults.

The circular insular sulcus limits area 41 medially while laterally area 43 does not reach the temporal operculum.

Thus, the primary auditory cortex (Brodmann's area 41 or A I) is located in the first (anterior) transverse temporal gyrus but many extend into the second (posterior) gyrus.

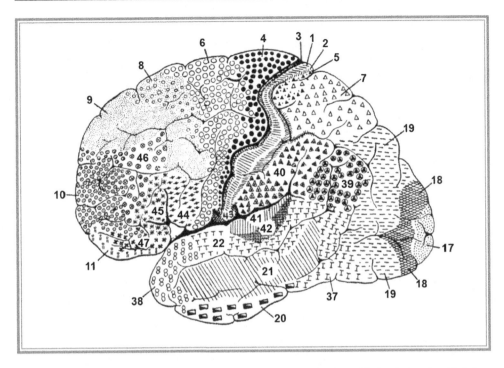

Fig. 21.33. Cytoarchitectural map showing Brodmann areas on the lateral surface of the hemisphere (modified after Brodmann K, from Carpenter MB, Sutin J: Human Neuroanatomy. Baltimore, Williams and Wilkins, 1983).

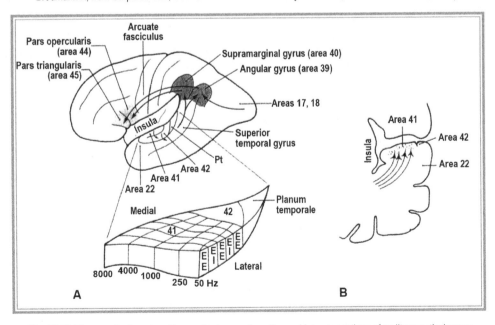

Fig. 21.34. The organization of auditory cortical areas. Location and interconnections of auditory cortical areas (A) and of the granular cortex in area 41 (B), and the orthogonal isofrequency and binaural responses columns in the primary auditory cortex (detail from A) (after Henkel, 2006).

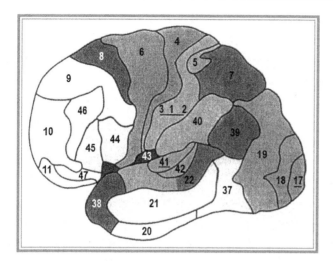

Fig. 21.35. Modern rendition of the cytoarchitectural map showing Brodmann's areas on the lateral surface of the human brain (figure provided by Mark Dubin, University of Colorado, 2006).

Cytoarchitecturally, area 41 encompasses the granular cortex, with its well-developed layer IV containing small granule cells and densely packed small pyramidal cells in layer VI.

Adjacent to the granular cortex in the second transverse gyrus and planum temporale is area 42, which constitutes the secondary auditory cortex (Yost, 1994).

Since studies of the somesthetic and visual cortex indicate that a vertical column of cells constitutes the elementary functional unit, it might be expected that a similar arrangement would exist in the auditory cortex. Thus, a study in anaesthetized cats has indicated that: (1) units responsive to noise bursts are randomly distributed; (2) different regions to a high or low proportion of click stimuli do not follow the direction of vertical columns; and (3) narrowly tuned units aligned with vertical columns tend to occur in clusters (Abeles and Goldstein, 1970).

Microelectrode studies of the auditory cortex in cats and monkeys have revealed a rather precise tonotopic organization (Merzenich and Brugge, 1973; Merzenich et al., 1973). Best frequencies in the full auditory range for monkeys were represented in an orderly fashion in the primary auditory area in a cytoarchitectonic field coextensive with the koniocortex. Lowest frequencies were represented rostrally and laterally, whereas highest frequencies were found caudally and medially.

In monkeys, the primary auditory cortex is surrounded by a belt of auditory cortex which cytoarchitectonically uniform and can be parcelled into several divisions. This cortical belt, which appears to represent the secondary auditory area, has been divided topographically into three main areas designated as the rostrolateral, lateral and caudomedial fields.

Thus, column cells in the auditory cortex share the same functional properties. Columnar organization is thus based on its frequency stripes, each stripe responding to a particular tonal frequency.

The primary auditory cortex is arranged into two dimensional, alternating, vertically oriented columns of neurons. One dimension of the auditory cortex is composed of frequency columns. The cells in each frequency column respond to an auditory stimulus of a particular frequency. So, cells responding to low frequencies reside in the frequency columns located in the rostral extent of the transverse temporal gyri of Heschl, whereas frequency columns containing cells responding to gradually higher frequencies are lined up in sequence towards the caudal extent of the primary auditory cortex.

The other dimension of the auditory cortex is composed of alternating binaural columns. There are two types of binaural columns: summation columns and suppression columns. The neurons residing in the summation columns respond to an auditory stimulus that stimulates both ears simultaneously.

In contrast, the neurons in the suppression columns respond maximally to an auditory stimulus that stimulates only one ear, but respond minimally when the auditory stimulus stimulates both ears (Patestas and Gartner, 2008).

The primary auditory cortex of each side receives information from both ears by way of the medial geniculate body of the thalamus, and then sends projections to the contralateral side *via* the corpus callosum. Area 41 is also reciprocally connected with the anterior division, and area 42 with the posterior division of the medial geniculate body.

The primary auditory cortex receives fibres predominantly from the contralateral side.

Orderly projections from neurons of the medial geniculate body to the primary auditory cortex are termed **thalamotemporal projections** or **acoustic radiations** that reach the temporal lobe through the sublenticular part of the internal capsule. Auditory fibres originate in the peripheral organ of Corti (Fig. 21.36) and establish neural synapses in the neuraxis, both homolateral and contralateral to their side of origin before reaching the medial geniculate nucleus of the thalamus (Altschuler et al., 1986, 1991; Pickles, 1988; Webster et al., 1992).

Physiologic studies of the primary auditory cortex have revealed that it does not play a major role in sound frequency discrimination but rather in the temporal pattern of acoustic stimuli. Sounds are heard in the primary auditory cortex and pattern for tones of different pitch exist here in nonhuman primates and, presumably, also in human.

Frequency discrimination of sound is a function of subcortical acoustic structures. The optimal stimulus that fires auditory cortical units seems to be a changing frequency of sound stimuli rather than a steady-frequency stimulus (Webster et al., 1992; Yost, 1994).

One of the characteristic features of the auditory system is its tonotopic localization. The tonotopic localization present in the cochlea appears to be preserved through all of the relay nuclei of the auditory system to levels of the inferior colliculus (Neff, 1961; Rose et al., 1963; Whitfield, 1977). At higher levels of the auditory system there is an increasing proportion of neural elements not directly concerned with the parameter of stimulus frequency, even though they respond to complex sounds (i.e., noise click) covering broad bands of the audible spectrum (Ades, 1959).

The tonotopic organization of constituent cells of the cortical layers and incoming afferent fibres from a series of orderly isofrequency columns extend through the primary auditory cortex as long stripes. High frequencies are represented medially and low frequencies laterally.

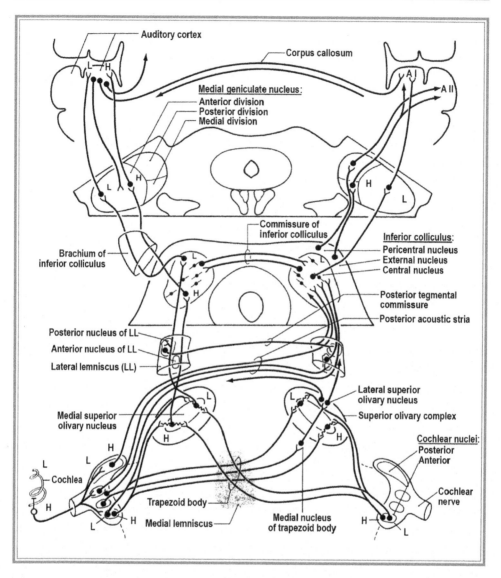

Fig. 21.36. Ascending central auditory pathways. Monoaural pathways , binaural pathways, and other connections. A I and A II, primary and secondary auditory cortices; H, high frequencies; L, low frequencies (after Henkel, 2006).

Single-cell responses are to single tones of a narrow frequency band. Cells in single vertical electrode penetrations share an optimum frequency response.

The series of stripes so formed have one subcomponent composed of cells excited by stimulation of both ears alternating with a subcomponent composed of cells excited by the contralateral ear and inhibited by the ipsilateral ear (Webster et al., 1992; Yost, 1994; Henkel, 2006).

In the cerebral cortex two areas showing tonotopic localization have been defined in cats by determining the loci of potentials evoked in response to stimulation of nerve fibres in the cochlea, or different sound frequencies (Woolsey and Walzl, 1942; Ades, 1943, 1959). In the more dorsal area, referred to as auditory area I (A I), the basal coils of the cochlea (high frequencies) are represented rostrally, and the apical region of the cochlea (low frequencies) caudally. In the more ventral auditory area (A II) the tonotopic localization is reversed. A third cortical zone designated PE (i.e., posterior ectosylvian area) lies posterior to auditory areas I and II and appears to be related functionally to auditory area I.

Anatomical studies of ablations of these auditory areas have provided information concerning the origin of afferent fibres from the medial geniculate body (Rose and Woolsey, 1949, 1958).

Auditory areas I and II have also been identified in monkeys (Ades and Felder, 1942; Pribram et al., 1954). In chimpanzees, tones of low frequency are represented anterolaterally, while tones of high frequency are represented posteromedially (Bailey et al., 1943).

Stimulation of the cortical areas in the temporal lobe near the primary auditory area (i.e., areas 42 and 22), in men, produces sounds described as the noise of a cricket, a bell or a whistle. These sounds are elementary tones which may be high or low pitched, continuous or interrupted, but are always devoid of complicated or changing qualities (Penfiled and Rasmussen, 1950). Most of these auditory responses are referred to the contralateral ear. The largest and most important fibre crossing is in the trapezoid body at the level of the cochlear nuclei, but others also are present, including fibres from auditory cortical areas that cross in the corpus callosum (Mettler, 1932).

Stimulation of the primary auditory cortex produces crude auditory sensations such as buzzing, humming, or knocking. Such sensations are clinically referred to as tinnitus.

Physiological studies (Woolsey and Walzl, 1942; Ades and Brookhart, 1950; Rosenzweig, 1954) indicate that each cochlea is represented bilaterally in the auditory cortex, although some slight differences exist between the two sides. Thus, when the sound is presented on one side, the cortical response is greatest in the contralateral hemisphere. If the sound is presented in a median plane, the cortical activity in the two hemispheres is equal.

Because audition is represented bilaterally at a cortical level, unilateral lesions of the auditory cortex cause impairment in sound localization in space and diminution of hearing bilaterally, but more often contralaterally.

According to Penfield and Evans (1934), the removal of one temporal lobe impairs sound localization on the opposite side, especially judgment of distance of sound.

Clinically, unilateral lesions of the auditory cortex are difficult to recognize.

Experimental studies indicate that bilateral ablations of auditory areas I, II and PE in cats do not abolish auditory localization of sound in space, although discriminations of this kind are impaired (Neff et al., 1956; Neff and Diamond, 1958). Sound localization in space is most critically impaired by bilateral ablations of A I (Strominger, 1969).

Bilateral ablations of the auditory cortical areas have little or no effect on the ability of cats to discriminate changes in frequency (Meyer and Woolsey, 1952; Butler et al., 1957; Neff and Diamond, 1958).

Meyer and Woolsey (1952) reported that following bilateral ablations of auditory areas I, II and PE, and somatic area II, cats could not relearn to discriminate changes in frequency, but could discriminate changes in sound intensity. The ability to localize sound in space is not affected by a section of the corpus callosum, is affected very little by a section of the commissure of the inferior colliculus and is severely affected by a section of the trapezoid body (Neff and Diamond, 1958; Jerger, 1960).

Neurons in each medial geniculate body project fibres to layers IIIb and IV of the auditory cortex. Area 41 in sensorial area of the koniocortex with layers II-IV of densely arranged small neurons surrounded by fields with large and medium-sized IIIc pyramidal neurons.

The primary auditory cortex is connected with the primary (unimodal) association auditory cortex. Other important connections include the auditory cortex of the contralateral hemisphere, the primary somesthetic cortex, frontal eye fields, Broca's area of speech in the frontal lobe, and the medial geniculate nucleus. Thus, the auditory cortex interconnects with the prefrontal cortex, though the projections from A I are small. Generally, posterior parts of the operculum project to areas 8 and 9. Central parts project to areas 8, 9 and 46. More anterior regions project to areas 9 and 46, to area 12 on the orbital surface of the hemisphere, and to the anterior cingulate gyrus on the medial surface. Contralateral corticocortical connections are with the same and adjacent regions in the other hemisphere.

Onward connections of the auditory association pathway converge with those of the other sensory association pathways in cortical regions within the superior temporal sulcus (Pickles, 1988; Webster et al., 1992; Yost, 1994; Crossman, 2008).

Via its projection to the medial geniculate body in the thalamus, the primary auditory cortex controls its own input by changing the excitability of medial geniculate neurons.

Auditory association cortex

Adjacent to the primary auditory cortex is the auditory association cortex (Brodmann's area 22). It is located mainly in the posterior portion of the superior temporal gyrus and is unimodal. It comprises the area adjacent to Heschl's gyri in the superior temporal gyrus, including the posterior portion of the floor of the sylvian fissure (the planum temporale). It is connected to the primary auditory cortex by the arcuate fascicules. Area 22 includes a part of the planum temporale and the posterior portion of the superior temporal gyrus. It receives connections from the primary auditory cortex, as well as visual and somesthetic information. This speech receptive area, known as Wernicke's area, may be as much as seven times larger on the left side then on the right.

Thus, the auditory association cortex is connected *via* the anterior commissure with the prefrontal cortex and *via* the corpus callosum with the prefrontal, premotor, parietal, and cingulate cortices. This area is concerned with the comprehension of spoken sound. Area 22 in the dominant hemisphere is known as Wernicke's area. Lesions in this area are associated with a receptive type of aphasia, a disorder of communication characterized by the inability of the patient to comprehend spoken words. In such cases, comprehension of speech sound is impaired but discrimination of nonverbal sound is largely unaffected. The higher association area of the auditory cortex also extends into the inferior parietal lobule. This lobule is made up of the angular gyrus (area 39) and supramarginal gyrus (area 40). These two areas are important in reading and writing and are sometimes included in the Wernicke area (Webster et al., 1992; Yost, 1994; Afifi and Bergman, 2005).

The auditory association cortex in the nondominant (right) hemisphere is specialised for nonspeech auditory information, such as environmental sounds, musical melodies, and tonal qualities of sound (prosody).

Bilateral lesions in the auditory association cortices result in the inability to recognize sounds (auditory agnosia) in the presence of normal hearing alertness and intelligence (Altschuler et al., 1991; Yost, 1994; Afifi and Bergman, 2005).

Brodmann's areas 44 and 45 are known as the Broca area for expressive speech and language. They are located in the pars opercularis and pars triangularis of the inferior frontal gyrus. The major pathway connecting these areas with the primary and association auditory cortex is the arcuate fasciculus.

If areas 44 and 45 are damaged along with other motor cortices on the left side by a stroke involving branches of the middle cerebral artery, the result is Broca's aphasia. In this disorder, speech is nonfluent, but comprehension of verbal and nonverbal sounds is largely unimpaired (Henkel, 2006).

Disconnection of the auditory association cortex (area 22) from the primary auditory cortex (areas 41 and 42) results in a condition known as **pure word deafness**, characterized by poor comprehension of spoken language and poor repetition with intact comprehension of written language. Thus, Brodmann's area 22, bordering the primary auditory area and presenting typical six-layered isocortex, receives fibres from areas 41 and 42 and has connections with areas of the parietal, occipital, and insular cortex (Bailey et al., 1943; Sugar et al., 1948, 1950).

Lesions of area 22 in the dominant hemisphere, or bilateral lesions, produce word deafness or sensory aphasia. This form of sensory aphasia usually is associated with lesions in the posterior part of area 22. Although patients with these lesions can hear, they cannot interpret the meaning of sounds, especially speech.

Area 21, the middle temporal cortex, is polysensory in men, and it connects with auditory, somatosensory and visual cortical association pathways. The auditory association areas of the superior temporal gyrus project in a complex ordered fashion to the middle temporal gyrus, as does the parietal cortex.

The middle temporal gyrus connects with the frontal lobe: the most posterior parts project to the posterior prefrontal cortex, areas 8 and 9, while intermediate regions connect more interiorly with areas 9 and 46.

The middle temporal region has also connections with the anterior prefrontal areas 10, 11, 12, 14, 46, and with the medial surface of the frontal pole. Further forwards the middle temporal region projects to the temporal pole and the entorhinal cortex.

Thalamic connections are with the pulvinar nuclei and intralaminar group. Physiological convergence of different sensory modalities and many neurons respond to faces (Altschuler et al., 1991; Webster et al., 1992; Yost, 1994; Crossman, 2008). Lesions of area 22 and part of area 21 of Brodmann have no effect on the perception of sound and pure tone.

Area 20 is the higher visual association area. The posterior inferior temporal cortex receives major ipsilateral corticocortical fibres from occipitotemporal visual areas, notably V4.

The anterior inferior temporal cortex projects onto the temporal pole and to paralimbic areas on the medial surface of the temporal pole.

Additional ipsilateral connections of the inferior temporal cortex are with the anterior middle temporal cortex in the walls of the superior temporal gyrus, and with visual areas of the parietotemporal cortex.

Unlike this, these are frontal lobe connections with area 46, with the orbitofrontal cortex, and with the frontal eye field. Reciprocal thalamic connections are with the pulvinar nuclei. Intralaminar connections are with the paracentral and central medial nuclei. Callosal connections are between corresponding areas and the adjacent visual association areas of each hemisphere.

The cortex of the temporal pole receives feedforward projections from widespread areas of the temporal association cortex which are immediately posterior to it. The dorsal part receives predominantly auditory inputs from the anterior part of the superior temporal gyrus. The inferior part receives visual inputs from the anterior area of the inferior temporal cortex (Crossman, 2008).

Other ipsilateral connections are with the anterior insular, the posterior and medial orbitofrontal, and the medial prefrontal cortices.

The temporal pole projects onwards into limbic and paralimbic areas.

Thalamic connections are mainly with the medial pulvinar nucleus, and with intralaminar and midline nuclei.

Physiological responses of cells in this and more medial temporal cortices correspond particularly to behavioral performance and to other recognition of high-level aspects of social stimuli (Crossman, 2008).

Descending auditory pathways. Descending projections make reciprocal connections throughout the auditory pathway. They form feedback loops that provide circuits to modulate information processing from the peripheral level to the cortex (Yost, 1994; Henkel, 2006). Thus, the auditory cortex projects to the medial geniculate nucleus and nuclei of the inferior colliculus. The inferior colliculus projects to the periolivary nuclei, which, in turn, send olivocochlear efferents to the cochlea. There are also descending projections from the periolivary nuclei to the cochlear nuclei (Fig. 21.37).

Acoustic startle reflex, orientation, and attention. Reflexive and learned responses to sound require sensory-motor integration. In addition to corticocortical interconnections for the dissemination of auditory information, there is also an integration of auditory sensory inputs with motor pathways in the brain stem (Henkel, 2006). Reticulospinal neurons in the region of the lateral lemniscus have dendrites that sample lemniscal activity and are involved in rapid acoustic startle reflex pathways (Webster et al., 1992; Henkel, 2006).

Fig. 21.37. Descending auditory pathways that modulate sensory processing at central and peripheral auditory sites. The lateral olivocochlear efferents and the medial olivocochlear efferents A I and A II primary and secondary auditory (cortices) (after Henkel, 2006).

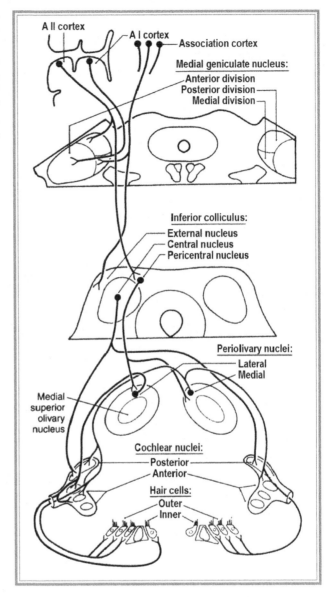

In addition, the deep layers of the superior colliculus receive auditory information from the inferior colliculus and auditory areas (Fig. 21.38). The deep layer of the superior colliculus integrate auditory, visual and somesthetic information and project to the brain stem and cervical spinal cord nuclei *via* tectobulbospinal fibres, which are involved in controlling the orientation of the head, eyes, and body to sound (Altschuler et al., 1986, 1991; Yost, 1994; Henkel, 2006).

In sum, bilateral destructions of the primary auditory cortex, the bordering area 22, or both will result in cortical deafness (bilateral loss of hearing caused by bilateral cerebral injuries).

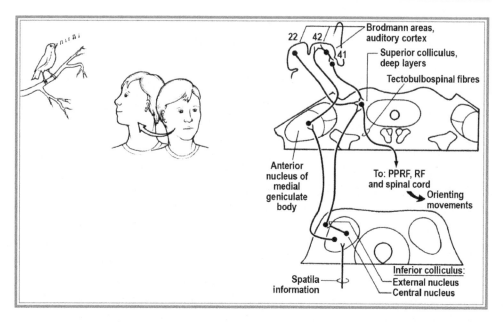

Fig. 21.38. The pathways that subserve auditory-motor integration involved in simple orientation to a novel auditory stimulus. RF, reticular formation; PPRF, paramedian pontine reticular formation (after Henkel, 2006).

Although such patients have bilateral cerebral injury, others often have a reasonably normal audiogram because tones of different pitch came to consciousness at a thalamic level. Destruction of only one primary auditory cortex will lead to subtle auditory deficits. Such patients have difficulty in localizing sounds in the contralateral auditory field and perhaps a loss of discrimination of distorted, interrupted, or accelerated speech (Augustine, 2008).

Destruction of the auditory association cortex (Wernicke's region) in the left cerebral hemisphere often fields a handicapping auditory receptive aphasia. Such patients have normal hearing and a normal production of words (fluent). Yet they are unable to interpret spoken sounds related to language or use words appropriately. Patients with injuries limited to the parietal operculum are often indifferent to loud and unpleasant noise (Eickhoff et al., 2006; Augustine, 2008).

The medial geniculate nucleus forms a small protuberance on the lower caudal surface of the thalamus between the lateral geniculate body and the pulvinar. Low frequencies are represented laterally and higher frequencies are represented medially. Thus, the anterior division of the medial geniculate nucleus receives afferents from the central nucleus of the inferior colliculus and projects to the primary auditory cortex.

The posterior division receives inputs from the pericentral nucleus of the inferior colliculus and projects to secondary auditory cortex. This pathway may convey information about moving or novel stimuli that direct auditory attention.

The medial (magnocellular) division receives afferents from the external nucleus of the inferior colliculus and projects to association areas of the auditory cortex. The medial division projects to temporal and parietal association areas and to the amygdala, putamen and pallidum. So, this pathway may be a part of the reticular activating system (Pickles, 1988; Webster et al., 1992; Henkel, 2006).

INSULA

Vicq d'Azyr was the first, in 1781, to express interest in the insula. He referred to it as the „convolutions" situated between the sylvian fissure and the corpus callosum. In 1809 (a, b), Reil was the first to describe the insula.

In order to view the insula, a highly developed structure in the depth of the sylvian fissure, the frontal, temporal, and parietal opercula have to be pulled apart, since this lobe is submerged within and forms the floor of the lateral sulcus (Eickhoff et al., 2006).

The sulcus separating the insula from the operculae is referred to by different authors as the periinsular sulcus, limiting sulcus, circuminsular sulcus, insular sulcus, or circular sulcus.

The frontal operculum is between the anterior and ascending rami of the lateral fissure, forming a triangular division of the inferior frontal gyrus.

The frontoparietal operculum, between the ascending and posterior rami of the lateral fissure, consists of the posterior part of the inferior frontal gyrus, the lower ends of the precentral and postcentral gyri, and the lower end of the anterior part of the inferior parietal lobule (Varnavas and Grand, 1999).

The temporal operculum (Fig 21.39), below the posterior ramus of the lateral fissure, is formed by the superior temporal and transverse temporal gyri.

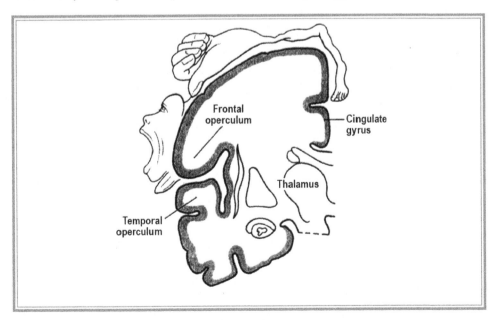

Fig. 21.39 Coronal representation showing the somatotopy of the body in the primary motor cortex, which is located in the precentral and anterior paracentral gyri (adapted from Penfield and Rasmussen, 1968).

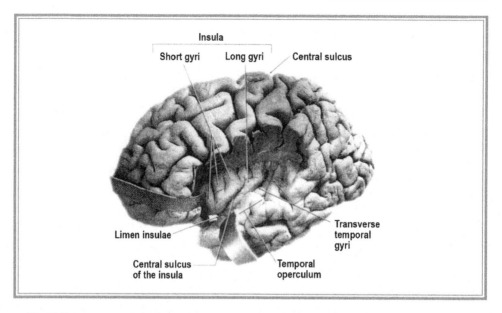

Fig. 21.40. Lateral view of the left cerebral hemisphere. The frontal and parietal opercula are removed, and the temporal operculum is retracted to expose the insula and transverse temporal gyri (after Hains and Mihailoff, 2006).

The term "operculum" (Latin: lid, or covering) refers to the fact that these parts of the respective lobes form a lid or cover for the insular lobe that forms the floor of the lateral sulcus. Anteriorly, the inferior region of the insula adjoins the orbital part of the inferior frontal gyrus. The insula is shaped like a pyramid. The summit of the pyramid is in the insular apex. Its apex is beneath and near the anterior perforated substance where the circular sulcus is deficient. The medial part of the apex is termed the limen insulae (gyrus ambiens). The **limen insulae** (threshold to the insula) is the area in which the inferior surface of the hemisphere is continuous with the insular cortex.

The insula is traversed by an obliquely directed central insular sulcus which divides the insular surface into a large anterior and a small posterior part. The anterior part exhibits transverse and accessory insular gyri and three or four short gyri (anterior, middle, and posterior). The transverse and accessory insular gyri form the insular pole located at the most anterior inferior aspect of the insula (Fig. 21.40).

The posterior part, located caudally to the central insular sulcus, is composed of the anterior and posterior long gyri, separated by the postcentral insular sulcus (Ture et al., 1999). The cortex of the insula is continuous with that of its opercula in the circular sulcus. The insula is approximately coextensive with the subjacent claustrum and putamen.

The insula is surrounded by the arcuate fasciculus which interconnects the frontal and temporal lobes. The superior longitudinal fasciculus, located in the core of the hemisphere, interconnects the frontal, parietal and occipital cortices. In the white matter of the temporal lobe, fibres passing between the frontal and occipital areas make up the inferior fronto-occipital fasciculus.

The insular cortex of the primates shows a sequential transition from allo- to meso- and finally to isocortex (Brackhaus, 1940; Stephan, 1975; Jones and Burton, 1976 b; Mesulam and Mufson, 1982 a, 1985). Its most retro-ventro-mesial portion located right at the limen insulae is allocortical and forms the insular segment of the prepyriform olfactory cortex. Around this allocortical core are arranged three concentric, approximately semicircular belts. The first, the agranular insula, bordering rostroventrally on the allocortical central segment of the prepyriform cortex, is part of the lateral mesocortical belt that runs along the lateral edge of the prepyriform-periamygdaloid allocortex; it is bordered along its dorsal and caudal periphery by the dysgranular insular proisocortex, which at its periphery dorsally and caudally is followed by the isocortical granular insula. Thus, cytoarchitectonically, three zones are recognized within the insula. Anteriorly, and extending caudally into the central insula, the cortex is agranular. It is surrounded by a belt of dysgranular cortex, in which the laminae II and III can be recognized, and this, in turn, is surrounded by an outer zone of homotypical granular cortex which extends to the caudal limit of the insula.

Although the function of the insula is still somewhat unclear, it is known that the insular cortex receives nociceptive and viscerosensory inputs.

Connections. The insula of primates is reciprocally connected to many surrounding and to some more distal cortical areas and to the amygdala (Mesulam and Mufson, 1982 b, 1985; Mufson and Mesulam, 1982; Seleman and Goldman-Rakic, 1988; Cavada and Goldman-Rakic, 1989 a). The connections of the postero-dorsal granular and adjacent portion of the dysagranular insula are part of the transinsular somatosensory association path (Mufson and Mesulam, 1982; Mesulam and Mufson, 1985; Friedman et al., 1986).

This region also seems to receive inputs from the auditory association cortex (Mufson and Mesulam, 1982; Mesulam and Mufson, 1985). It is also connected to a segment of the premotor cortex in area 6 representing the face, to the prefrontal cortex below the principal sulcus (areas 45 and 46), the isocortical portion of the orbitofrontal cortex, the cingulate cortex, and the precentral nucleus of the amygdala (Mesulam and Mufson, 1982 b, 1985; Mufson and Mesulam, 1982).

Rostral to this somatosensory association area in the posterior insula there may be in the dysagranular insula an area of multimodal convergence between gustatory and other afferents emanating from the somatosensory and premotor areas concerned with the representation of the face and mouth region (Sudakov et al., 1871; Mesulam and Mufson, 1971). In monkeys, this dysgranular and agranular area receives afferents from the parvocelullar portion of the ventroposterior medial thalamic nucleus, the thalamic gustatory relay nucleus (Mufson and Mesulam, 1984; Mesulam and Mufson, 1985; Pritchard et al., 1986), and its neurons respond to gustatory stimuli (Sudakov et al., 1971; Yaxley et al., 1990).

The parvocelullar portion of the ventroposterior thalamic nucleus, also receives viscerosensory afferents that, as they ascend from the brain stem through the ventromedial thalamus, are difficult to disentangle from ascending taste pathways (Beckstead et al., 1980).

In rodents, the insula receives afferents from the same thalamic relay nucleus as well as more diverse gustatory and viscerosensory inputs from gustatory-viscerosensory relay nuclei in the brain stem, the parabrachial nuclei (Saper, 1982 a, b; Shipley and Saunders, 1982; Cechetto and Saper, 1987; Krushel and van der Kooy, 1988; Allen et al., 1991).

The rostro-ventral dysgranular-agranular insular cortex of primates is reciprocally connected with the gustatory opercular cortex, the mesocortical orbitofrontal cortex (especially its caudolateral portion), the cingulate cortex, the olfactory prepyriform allcortex, the temporopolar cortex, most of the amygdaloid nuclei, and the peri- and entorhinal cortices (Mesulam and Mufson, 1982 b, 1985; Mufson and Mesulam, 1982; Rolls, 1989 a).

In primates the postero-dorsal granular-dysgranular sector may predominantly function as a unimodal somatosensory association area. This is supported by the fact that this region is reciprocally connected with the somatosensory subdivision (area 7 b) of the parietal association cortex (Cavada and Goldman-Rakic, 1989 a; Neal et al., 1990 b).

Conversely, the anteroventral dysgranular-agranular sector is likely to be multimodal with emphasis on gustatory, viscerosensory, and olfactory modalities together with some visceromotor representations.

Thus, the insular lobe in primates including humans has connection with the cerebral cortex of the frontal lobe (orbital cortex, frontal operculum, lateral premotor cortex, ventral granular cortex and medial area 6) and the parietal lobe (second somatosensory area and retroinsular area of the parietal lobe). Ipsilateral cortical connections of the insula are diverse. Somatosensory connections are with S I, S II and surrounding areas, area 5 of the superior parietal lobe and area 7b of the inferior parietal lobe.

There are also insular connections with the temporal lobe (temporal pole and superior temporal sulcus) and the insular lobe (an abundance of local intra-insular connections) (Augustine, 1985, 1996, 2008).

There are insular projections to subdivisions of the cingulate gyrus and to the lateral, lateral basal, central, cortical and medial amygdaloid nuclei. There are also insular connections with nonamygdaloid areas such as the perirhinal cortex, entorhinal cortex, and the periamygdaloid cortex. The thalamic taste area projects fibres to the ipsilateral insular-opercular cortex (Augustine, 1996; Ture et al., 1999; Augustine, 2008).

The insular cortex projects to almost all the nuclei of the amygdala (Amaral and Insausti, 1992; Carmichael and Price, 1995; Stefanacci and Amaral, 2002).

Most of these projections originate in the rostral insular cortices, specifically the agranular (Ia) and rostral aspects of the dysgranular (Id) division (Amaral and Insausti, 1992; Carmichael and Price, 1995; Mufson et al., 1997; Stefanacci and Amaral, 2000, 2002).

Projections from more caudal division of the insular cortex (caudal divisions of Id and the granular insular cortex Ig) are less dense and less widespread (Amaral and Insausti, 1992; Stefanacci and Amaral, 2000, 2002).

The parainsular cortex sends projections to the lateral nucleus, the basal nucleus, and the accessory basal nucleus (Amaral and Insausti, 1992; Stefanacci and Amaral, 2000).

Most of the insular projections are directed towards the middle to caudal aspects of the amygdala and originate predominantly in layer II and III, with a lesser contribution from layer V (Stefanacci and Amaral, 2002).

The amygdaloidal complex returns projections throughout the insular cortex and to the superficial and deep layers (Carmichael and Price, 1995). These connections are generated by the lateral nucleus, the basal nucleus, the accessory basal nucleus, the medial nucleus, the anterior cortical nucleus, the periamygdaloid cortex, and the anterior amygdaloid area (Amaral and Price, 1984; Carmichael and Price, 1995).

Caudal regions of area Id and area Ig receive fewer projections from the amygdaloid complex (Amaral and Price, 1984).

Thalamic afferents to the insula come from subdivisions of the ventral posterior nucleus and of the medial geniculate body, from the oral and medial parts of the pulvinar, the suprageniculate / nucleus limitans complex, the mediodorsal nucleus and the nuclei of the intralaminar and midline groups. It appears that the anterior (agranular) cortex is connected predominantly with the mediodorsal and ventroposterior nuclei, while the posterior (granular) cortex is connected predominantly with the pulvinar and the ventral posterior nuclei.

The other nuclear groups appear to connect with all areas (Crossman, 2008).

Thus, the anterior insular part connects with the frontal lobe, and the posterior part connects with the parietal and temporal lobes. Lesion-based analysis has shown that distructions of the left anterior part impair coordination of articulation and speech production.

Functional aspects

In rats, single-cell recording in the insular cortex reveals a „viscerotopic" organization. Thus, the taste and gastric representation lies next to the somatosensory representation of the tongue and that for cardiopulmonary receptors next to that of the trunk (Cechetto and Saper, 1987).

In primates and rodents, the anteroventral portion of the insula is concerned with alimentary and related visceral functions (Hoffman and Rasmussen, 1953; Penfield and Faulk, 1955).

There is also a visceromotor representation in the insula. In various animal species including primates, stimulation of the insula affects a number of autonomic functions such as gastric peristalsis, salivation, blood pressure, and heart rate as well as respiration (Kwada, 1951; Hoffman and Rasmussen, 1953; Oppenheimer and Cechetto, 1990).

In humans, insular stimulation affects gastric peristalsis (Penfield and Faulk, 1955), as well as heart rate and blood pressure. Bradycardia and falls in diastolic blood pressure was more often elicited from left insular stimulations whereas tachycardic and pressure responses occured more commonly with stimulation of the right insula (Oppenheimer et al., 1992).

Thus, the insular cortex has been implicated in the mediation of heart rate, in taste, and in gustatory processing. Given the role of the amygdaloid complex in identifying danger in the environment, connections with insular cortex may be a route for gustatory and autonomic information to be processed by the amygdala.

The insular cortex receives nociceptive and viscerosensory inputs. Thus, it has visceral sensory and somatic sensory roles as well as visceral motor and somatic motor roles.

According to Mufson et al. (1997) and Augustine (1996, 2008), the insula participates in the autonomic regulation of the gastrointestinal tract and the heart and is as well functioning as a motor association area. This motor function includes a role in the recovery of motor functions after stroke and in ocular movements.

The insular lobe also serves as a vestibular area and as a language area including memory tasks related to language and auditory processing underlying speech. Other insular functions include a possible role in the verbal component of memory and its role in selective visual attention.

CORTICAL LANGUAGE AREAS

Wernicke's area

Language is an arbitrary and abstract way to represent thought processes by means of sentences and to present concepts or ideas by means of words.

Most components of the language system are located in the left hemisphere, which is the dominant hemisphere for language in approximately 95% of humans.

Nearly all right-handers and about two-thirds of left-handers have such dominance.

Wernicke's area, comprises an extensive region that includes the posterior part of the superior temporal gyrus (Brodmann's area 22) including planum temporale in the floor of the sylvian fissure, and the parietooccipitotemporal junction area including the angular gyrus (Brodmann's area 39).

According to Augustine (2008), those parts of the superior temporal gyrus corresponding to Brodmann's areas 42 and 22 constitute Wernicke's region, an auditory association region.

The upper surface of area 22, the planum temporale, is distinctly longer on the left side (dominant hemisphere for language) in most people. Together, Heschl's gyrus (primary auditory cortex) and the anterior and posterior temporal planes are sometimes referred to as the **planum temporale.**

Brodmann's areas 42 and 22 constitute Wernicke's region, an auditory association region. In this region, sounds are appreciated, they become meaningful for understanding language, and are interpreted as words. Thus, Wernicke's area is concerned with the comprehension of language. The superior temporal gyrus component of Wernicke's area (area 22) is concerned with comprehension of spoken language, whereas the angular gyrus (area 39) and adjacent regions are concerned with comprehension of written language. According to Afifi and Bergman (2005), spoken language is perceived in the primary auditory area (Heschl's gyrus, area 41 and 42) in the superior temporal gyrus and transmitted to the adjacent located Wernicke's area, where it is comprehended.

According to Haines and Mihailoff (2006), the gyri that are part of the Wernicke's area are the supramarginal gyrus – Brodmann's area 40 – and the angular gyrus –

Brodmann's area 39. Clinically, the Wernicke area is regarded as extending into the temporal lobe and encompasses portions of Brodmann's area 22 and some of area 21.

According to Patestas and Gartner (2008), Wernicke's area consists of auditory association cortex (part of Brodmann's area 22), as well as parts of the supramarginal and angular gyri (Brodmann's areas 37, 39, and 40, usually in the left, dominant hemisphere). Wernicke's area is also referred to as the receptive (sensory, language area, general interpretative area, or the gnostic area. It plays an important role in the comprehension and formulation of language. When an individual reads and says the words, the visual pathway relays the sensory visual input to the primary visual cortex where the words are "seen". The primary visual cortex transmits this input to the association visual cortex where the significance of the words is determined. The visual information is then relayed to Wernicke's area where the words are comprehended, and the creation of the words takes place. Wernicke's area then projects to Broca's area, which dictates the motor activity necessary to produce the words.

Reading requires the perception of visual language stimuli by the occipital cortex, followed by correlation with auditory language information, *via* the intermodal association cortex of the angular gyrus. Writing involves the activation of motor neurons projecting to the arm and hand.

In the right cerebral hemisphere this cortical area is an auditory association area that serves to determine the emotional undertones of language. When we hear someone speak, the person's voice often reveals if he / she is happy, upset, angry, etc.

Although several areas in the left hemisphere are dominant in the reception, programming and production of language function, corresponding areas in the right hemisphere are metabolically active during speech. These areas are believed to be concerned with the melodic function of speech (**prosody**). Lesions in such areas of the right hemisphere render speech amelodic (**aprosodic**). Lesions in area 44 on the right side result in a dull monotonic speech. Lesions in area 22 on the right side, on the other hand, may lead to an inability of the patient to detect inflection of speech. Such patients may be unable to differentiate whether a particular remark is intended as a statement or as a question (Afifi and Bergman, 2005).

In right-handed people and in a majority of left-handers as well, clinical syndromes of aphasia result from left hemisphere lesions. Rarely, aphasia may result from a right hemisphere lesion in a right-handed patient, a phenomenon called **crossed aphasia** (Bakar et al., 1996).

Broca's area

Gall and Spurzheim (1809), based on their observations of skull shape, placed the ability to speech and recall words in the inferior aspect of the frontal lobes. Bouillaud (1825) hypothesized that the anterior lobes of the brain contained a centre for speech production. Bouillaud even offered a prize to the first individual who reported a case with loss of speech without lesion to the frontal lobes.

However, there were a number of studies that were real contributions to the knowledge of the clinical phenomenology of aphasia. One is the description by Osborne, in 1833, of a highly educated patient with severe jargon aphasia who understood spoken speech quite well and could read with understanding. His writing was only mildly affected.

Lordat's case, reported in 1843, is of a priest who after a stroke showed an almost complete motor aphasia but steadily improved.

There is also Marcé's paper, in 1856, dealing specifically with impairment in writing. Marcé described a number of cases of agraphia within the setting of oral language disturbances of varying severity and different types, and he postulated the existence of a cerebral centre for writing distinct from the coordinating centre for oral speech.

There is, also, an important reference to receptive aphasia in the 1843 monograph of Lordat.

The association of aphasia with right hemiplegia is usually ascribed by Broca (1861, 1863), but this distinction is often dimmed by the accompanying mention of Marc Dax's earlier contribution in 1836 (1865), a quarter of a century before Broca's first observation. In 1836, Marc Dax presented a work indicating that disturbances in language production were due to lesions of the left hemisphere. Dax's work remained largely unknown until his son, Gustav Dax (1865, 1877), presented and published his deceased father's work in the years after 1863 (see Benton, 2000 and Buckingham, 2006).

Dax's memoir is not only interesting in that it is the first mention of the role of the left hemisphere in the function of speech but also because it raises once again the problem of "priority" in scientific observations (Benton, 2000).

Broca called the inability to produce language in the context of intact comprehension, **"aphenie"**. Trousseau subsequently renamed such disturbances **"aphasia"** in 1864. However, in 1863, Broca published a series of eight cases showing primarily left-frontal lesions with language production deficit. In an 1865 and 1869 manuscript, Broca firmly asserted that the left hemisphere is the dominant seat for language production.

Broca's area is equivalent to areas 45 and 44 located in the opercular and triangular portions of the left inferior frontal gyrus. This area of the cortex not only "programs" the neurons in the adjacent motor cortex subserving the mouth and larynx from which descending axons travel to the brain stem cranial nerve nuclei in the imitation of a sequence of complex movements, but also has expressive language capacities (e.g., grammar).

Within Broca's area, a coordination program for vocalization is formulated. The elements of the program are transmitted to the face, tongue, vocal cords, and pharynx area of the motor cortex for execution of speech.

The supplementary motor area is also necessary in the production of language for the initiation of speech. Broca's area receives input from Wernicke's area *via* the arcuate fasciculus (Wise et al., 1999; Sherwood et al., 2003).

Broca's area is involved in planning the motor activity that is necessary for the word to be produced. Broca's area projects this information to the premotor cortex where motor activity is planned and relayed to the primary motor cortex, which initiated the movements necessary to produce speech. Thus, when a word is heard, the output from the primary auditory area (Heschl's gyrus) is conveyed to the adjacent Wernicke's area, where the word is comprehended. If the word is to be spoken, the comprehended pattern is transmitted *via* the arcuate fasciculus from Wernicke's area to Broca's area in the inferior frontal gyrus. The arcuate fasciculus is a long associated fibre bundle that links Wernicke's and Broca's areas of speech. Damage to the arcuate fasciculus is associated with impairment of repetition of spoken language. If the word is to be read, representations visualized as words or images are conveyed from the visual cortex (areas 17, 18 and 19) to the angular gyrus (area 39), which in turn arouses the corresponding auditory form of the word in Wernicke's area. From Wernicke's area, the information is relayed *via* the arcuate fasciculus to Broca's area (Afifi and Bergman, 2005).

These pathways, and doubtless others, constitute the cortical circuitry for language comprehension and expression. In addition, other cortical centres involved in cognitive processes project into the primary language cortex, influencing the content of language. Finally, subcortical structures play increasingly recognized roles in language function (the thalamus, the reticular activating system, the nuclei of the basal ganglia etc.).

Lesions in Broca's area are associated with a type of aphasia (motor, anterior, expressive, nonfluent) characterized by the inability of a patient to express himself by speech. Such patients are able to comprehend language when Wernicke's area is intact. Autopsy data and neuroimaging studies have shown both the absence of Broca's aphasia in individuals with lesions in this area and also the reverse (Yang et al., 2008).

Depression is a common psychological consequence of aphasia, and is significantly more common after anterior left-hemisphere lesions (including those associated with nonfluent aphasia) than lesions in other areas (Carson et al., 2000).

Cortical localization of music

One should separate musical perception from musical execution by the naive, casual listener and the music professional. Whereas a naive listener perceives music in its overall melodic contour, the professional perceives music as a relation between musical elements and symbols (language).

Thus, a naive listener perceives music in the right hemisphere, whereas the professional perceives music in the left hemisphere.

Musical execution (singing), on the other hand, seems to be a function of the right hemisphere irrespective of musical knowledge and training. The primary auditory cortex of the right temporal lobe appears to make periodicity pitch discrimination (Zatorre, 1984, 2001; Zatorre and Belin, 2001; Zatorre et al., 2002).

Liégeois-Chauval et al. (1998) point out that distinct musical processes may depend on specific cortical sites in the superior temporal gyrus.

Zatorre (2001) suggested that the right temporal lobe has a special function in extracting pitch form sound, regardless of whether the sound is speech of music. In regard to speech, the pitch will contribute to "tone" of voice, which is known as prosody.

The fact that the brain appears to have neural networks dedicated to the processing of language and music leads to the conclusion that both language and music have biological roots. Although this conclusion seems obvious for language, it is less obvious for music, which has often been perceived as an artefact of culture.

Ventral surface and midtemporal cortical areas

The ventral surface of the temporal lobe shows the continuation of the inferior temporal gyrus from the lateral surface. Medial to the inferior temporal gyrus is the occipitotemporal (fusiform) gyrus. The collateral sulcus separates the occipitotemporal gyrus from the more medial parahippocampal gyrus and uncus, which constitute parts of the limbic lobe.

In the middle part of the inferior temporal gyrus, on the lateral and ventral surface, and in the region dorsal to the secondary auditory cortex, are visual and auditory association areas (Schmitt et al., 1981; Schüz and Miller, 2002). These secondary association areas are richly interrelated with occipital, frontal, parietal and insular cortices. Penfield and Evans (1934) and Penfield and Mathieson (1974) suggested these midtemporal areas participate in the recall of past events or so-called remote memory. This appears to be the case especially with events that have visual and auditory components visualized and heard at the same time in the past, and those events accompanied by some emotional stress or intellectual conflict. These areas have connections with the frontal lobe and limbic system including the amygdaloid body and hippocampal formation (Augustine, 2008).

Slight irritation of these midtemporal areas often causes the vague feeling of familiarity that falls under the term *déjà vu*. These seizures usually occur with impairment of consciousness. A distorted memory experience such as the distortion of time sense, a **dreamy state**, a flashback, or a sensation as if a naïve experience had been experienced before, known as *déjà vu*, or as if a previously experienced sensation had not been experienced, known as *jamais-vu,* may occur. When this refers to auditory experiences, these are known as *déjà-entendu* or *jamais-entendu*. Occasionally, seizures manifest as a form of forced thinking, in which the patient may experience a rapid recollection of episodes from his past life, know as **panoramic vision**.

Cognitive disturbances include the dreamy state, distortions of time sense, sensations of unreality, detachment or depersonalization.

Affective symptomatology includes sensations of extreme pleasure or displeasure, as well as fear and intense depression with feelings of unworthiness and rejection.

Anger or rage is occasionally experienced. Fear or terror is the most frequent symptom.

Epileptic or gelastic seizure laughter should not be classified as an affective symptom because the laughter is usually without affect and hollow.

Illusions take the form of distorted perceptions in which objects may appear deformed.

Hallucinations may occur as manifestations or perceptions without corresponding external stimulus and may affect somatosensory, visual, auditory, olfactory, or gustatory sense. Irritation of auditory association areas in these midtemporal regions is likely to produce reminiscent speech or sounds, particularly a piece of music or a sound of someone's voice from our previous experience. The temporal lobe probably plays a vital role in processing olfactory and gustatory information. The human temporal lobe is probably involved in odour detection and is involved in olfactory memory functions, particularly the right temporal lobe. Odour experiences often cause a retrieval of images, an unfolding of past memories, and the imitation of a complex feeling state (Gibbs, 1951; Gastaut, 1970; Geschwind, 1979; Bear, 1979; Mungus, 1982).

Automatisms may occur in both partial and generalized seizures. According to Gastaut (1973), automatisms are described as more or less coordinated adapted (eupractic or dyspractic) involuntary motor activity occurring during the state of clouding of consciousness either in the course of, or after an epileptic seizure, and usually followed by amnesia for the event. They may occur in complex partial seizures as well as in absence of seizures.

Thus, the irritation of the medial or lateral temporal lobe causes temporal lobe epilepsy. Temporal lobe epilepsy is a form of partial epilepsy characterized by recurrent seizures that originate from these regions.

Temporal lobe epilepsy is most commonly associated with complex partial seizures, although a large number of individuals also experience simple partial and / or secondary generalized tonic-clonic seizures.

However, in recent years, most epileptologists distinguish between mesial (amygdalo-hippocampal) and neocortical forms of temporal lobe epilepsy (Williamson et al., 1993; Pacia et al., 1996; Engel and Weiser, 1997; Engel, 2001).

In mesial temporal lobe epilepsy, seizures arise most often in the hippocampus and spread through adjacent cortical region. These seizures begin with an aura consisting of a rising epigastric sensation and progress to an altered state of consciousness with variable types of automatism (French et al., 1993; Williamson et al., 1993; Engel and Weiser, 1997; Engel, 2001). Motor automatism often occurs ipsilateral to the side of seizure, and dystonia of the hand may occur contralateral. The combination of these findings in a simple seizure is very suggestive of mesial temporal lobe epilepsy.

Seizures resulting from neocortical temporal lobe epilepsy can involve the inferior temporal neocortex (excluding the parahippocampal gyrus), the temporal polar region, and the superior plane of the temporal lobe (Pacia et al., 1996). These seizures characteristically begin with an aura, which can include auditory hallucinations, experiential auras, visual misperceptions, or dysphasia when the seizure focus is on the language-dominant hemisphere. Complex partial seizures are evoked if the focus spreads to medial temporal or extratemporal lobe structures (Barr and Karantzoulis, 2011).

The inferior occipital region of the temporal cortex is part of the "what" visual pathway and contributes to the analysis of form.

Specific areas within the occipital temporal cortex are involved in recognition or identification of colour, faces, letters, numbers, or objects. Thus, in the posterior temporal and bordering occipital regions are complex association areas.

Damage can lead to visual agnosia, or the inability to recognize familiar objects, faces, or words. For example, bilateral damage to occipital-temporal regions can result in **prosopagnosia**, the inability to recognize faces (Hadjikhani and Gelder, 2002; Schiltz et al., 2006).

Thus, a severe deficit in discriminating and identifying faces with the inability to recognize one's own pictures or mirror images is likely to occur with injury to both fusiform and lingual gyri. The visual association properties of these regions include the synthesis of specific faces, which requires the complex synthesis of visual input, memory, and other sensory phenomena. Individuals with prosopagnosia or face blindness may learn to recognize people by their clothes, mannerisms, gait, hairstyle or voice. While they connot recognize a person by their face, they are able to recognize facially expressed emotions like happy, sad, and angry (Bodamer, 1947; Damasio et al., 1982; Landis et al., 1986; Schiltz et al., 2006).

Medial regions of the temporal lobe are essential for learning and memory. Bilateral damage results in the inability to learn new information or make new memories (anterograde amnesia). These patients are unable to make new memories, learn new facts, or recall new experiences. Their memory leading up to the surgery is largely intact and general intelligence is also unaffected (French et al., 1993; Engel and Weiser, 1997; Blumer et al., 1998; Engel, 2001).

Anomic aphasia

Anomia can occur in healthy individuals who occasionally experience difficulty in thinking of an intended word during conversation, also known as the tip-of-the-tongue state (Biedermann et al., 2008). It is a frequent occurence in individuals with left hemisphere brain damage and aphasia (Raymer, 2005). Typically associated with difficulties for nouns, anomia also can affect the ability to retrieve other classes of words, such as verbs and adjectives. It is important to note that anomia and the anomic aphasia are not synonymous. **Anomia** is the primary symptom of anomic aphasia and can also be observed in virtually all other forms of aphasia, both as initial and residual signs when other signs and symptoms of aphasia have revolved (Raymer and Rothy, 2008).

Anomia leads to a complete inability to retrieve a word and other times an inappropriate word is retrieved known as a **paraphasia**. In severe forms of anomia, neologisms may occur in which the uttered word may not be recognizable at all.

Anomic aphasia is the language impairment that involves only word finding difficulties or pure anomia in contrast to other forms of aphasia (Goodglass et al., 2001).

In the left temporal / occipital region, particularly in parts of the fusiform and probably the lingual gyrus corresponding to Brodmann's areas 37 and 29, is a region connected by the inferior occipitofrontal fasciculus with the inferior and perhaps midtemporal regions and with other cortical areas along its course.

This region connects with the inferolateral and part of the lateral of the frontal lobe.

Acutely, anomic aphasia has been described following left temporal / occipital lesions (e.g., area 37) and left thalamic lesion (Raymer et al., 1997 a, b).

The grammatical characteristics of the sentence remain intact. Common in anomic aphasia is circumlocution, in which the speaker cannot think of the intended word and instead describes or provides associated information about the word (Laine and Martin, 2006).

Primary gustatory cortex

Clinical and experimental evidence indicates that the cortical area for taste is located in the parietal operculum, ventral to the primary somesthetic area in close proximity to the cortical areas receiving sensory afferents from the tongue and pharynx.

It is represented to Brodmann's area 43 in the parietal operculum and in the adjacent parainsular cortex (Börnstein, 1940; 1940 a; Patton and Ruch, 1946; Penfield and Rasmussen, 1959; Bagshow and Pribram, 1953).

Electrophysiological studies in rats, cats, and squirrel monkeys indicate that afferent taste impulses conveyed by the chorda tympani and glossopharyngeal nerves are projected to the most medial and caudal part of the posteroventral medial nucleus of the thalamus (Landgren, 1961; Emmers et al., 1962; Blomquist et al., 1962; Emmers, 1964). Direct lesions destroying this thalamic region produce gustatory deficits in monkeys (Blum et al., 1943; Patton et al., 1944) and goats (Andersson and Jewell, 1957).

Anatomical studies (Benjamin and Akert, 1959) in rats indicate that unilateral ablations of the cortical area in which potentials could be evoked by stimulating the chorda tympani and glossopharyngeal nerves (i.e., the parietal operculum) did not impair normal taste discrimination.

Bilateral ablation of this area produced a partial loss of taste. Ablation of this cortical taste area produced retrograde degeneration of thalamic neurons confined to the most medial, parvocellular subdivision of the posteroventral medial nucleus.

Ablations of the precentral and postcentral opercula in monkeys and chimpanzees cause a loss of taste.

Similar lesions involving the anterior insular cortex, the postcentral operculum and the anterior supratemporal cortex in monkeys impair taste sensibility (Bagshow and Pribram, 1953). In humans, the gustatory cortex receives fibres from the posteroventral medial nucleus of the thalamus, upon which converge sensory fibres from the face and mouth, including taste fibres. Although crude taste sensation can be perceived at the thalamic level, discrimination among different taste sensations is a cortical function.

Stimulation of the parietal operculum (Penfield and Boldrey, 1937) and adjacent insular cortex (Penfield and Rasmussen, 1950) in conscious patients produce gustatory sensations.

A report of an epileptic patient who experienced a gustatory aura characterized by a sour or bitter taste is cited as providing information concerning localization of taste in the cerebral cortex (Shenkin and Lewey, 1944).

Although this patient could recognize bitter and salty substances bilaterally, he was unable to perceive sweet substances on one side of his tongue. A vascular anomaly was found in the parietal opercular region contralateral to the taste deficit.

In an extensive study of thalamic projections to the insular and opercular cortex in monkeys, it was established that the parvocellular subdivision of the posteroventral medial nucleus projects to the parietal operculum and the insular cortex (Roberts and Akert, 1963).

The gustatory representation in the cerebral cortex is adjacent to the somesthetic area for the tongue (Cohen et al., 1957), suggesting that taste may not have an exclusive primary receiving area.

Different observations in squirrel monkeys suggest cortical areas concerned with taste may be separated from somesthetic areas (Benjamin, 1963).

Irritative lesions in this area in humans have been shown to give rise to hallucinations of taste, usually preceding the onset of an epileptic attack. Such a prodromal symptom preceding an epileptic fit focuses attention on the site of the irritative lesion.

In sum, taste receptors relay gustatory information to the solitary nucleus in the brain stem.

The solitary nucleus then transmits the information *via* the ipsilateral central tegmental tract to the posteroventral medial nucleus of the thalamus.

The thalamus then projects these inputs to the inferior extent of the postcentral gyrus (Brodmann's area 43).

The cortical area where taste information is relayed resides next to the area where the general sensory input from the tongue is transmitted.

The complete loss of taste (**ageusia**) is rarely encountered, in part because of the large numbers of nerves that relay taste information to the central nervous system.

More frequently a patient suffers from **hypogeusia** or **parageusia** (dysgeusia), distorsion in the perception of taste. Foci of seizure activity in central taste processing areas can trigger unpleasant taste sensation (**cacogeusia**).

REFERENCES

Abel LA, Unverzagt F, Yee RD, Effects of stimulus predictability and interstimulus gap on saccades in Alzheimer's disease. Dementia and Geriatric Congnitive Disorders 13; 235-243, 2002.

Abeles M, Goldstein MH, Functional architecture in cat primary auditory cortex: Columnar organization and organization according to depth. J Neurophysiol 33; 172-187, 1970.

Ades HW, A secondary acoustic area in the cerebral cortex of the cat. J Neurophysiol 6; 59-64, 1943.

Ades HW, Central auditory mechanisms. In: J Field (ed.), *Handbook of Physiology*, Section I, Vol I. American Physiological Society, Washington, DC, Ch. 24, 585-613, 1959.

Ades HW, Felder R, The acoustic area of the monkey (Macaca mulatta). J Neurophysiol 5; 49-54, 1942.

Ades HW, Brookhart HM, The central auditory pathway. J Neurophysiol 13; 189-205, 1950.

Adrian ED, Double representation of the feet in the sensory cortex of the cat. J Physiol 98; 16-18, 1940.

Adrian ED, Afferent discharges to the cerebral cortex from peripheral sense organ. J Physiol 100; 159-191, 1941.

Afifi AK, Bergman RA, *Functional Neuroanatomy. Text and atlas.* Lange Medical Books / Mc Graw-Hill. New York, Chicago, San Francisco etc., 246-257, 2005.

Allen GV, Saper CB, Hurley KM, Cechetto DF, Organization of visceral and limbic connections in the insular cortex of the rat. J Comp Neurol 311; 1-16, 1991.

Altman J, Some fiber projections to the superior colliculus in the cat. J Comp Neurol, 119; 77-95, 1962.

Altschuler RA, Bobbin RP, Hoffman DW, Neurobiology of Hearing: the Cochlea. New York. Raven Press, 1986.

Altschuler RA, Bobbin RP, Clapton BM, Hoffman DW, *Neurobiology of Hearing. The Central Auditory System.* New York, Raven Press, 1991.

Amaral DG, Price JL, Amygdala-cortical projections in the monkey (Macaca fascicularis). Journal of Comparative Neurology 230; 465-496, 1984.

Amaral DG and Insausti R, Retrograde transport of D [3H]-aspartate injected into the monkey amygdaloid complex. Experimental Brain Research 88; 375-388, 1992.

Amunts K, Schlaug G, Schleicher A, et al., Asymmetry in the human motor cortex and handedness. NeuroImage 4; 216-222, 1996.

Anderson TJ, Jenkins IH, Brooks DJ et al., Cortical control of saccades fixation in man. A PET study. Brain 117; 1073-1084, 1994.

Andersson B, and Jewell PA, Studies on the thalamic relay for taste in the goat. J Physiol 139; 191-197, 1957.

Ang Jr. ES, Haydar TF, Gluncic V, Rakic P, Four-dimensional migratory coordinates of GABAergic interneurons in the developing mouse cortex. J. Neurosci 23; 5805-5815, 2003.

Arciniegas DB, Beresford TP, *Neuropsychiatry. An introductory approach.* Cambridge: Cambridge University Press, 2001.

Ascoli GA et al., Pelilla terminology: nomenclature of features of GABAergic interneurons of cerebral cortex. Nat. Rev. Neurosci 9; 557-568, 2008.

Augustine JR, *Human Neuroanatomy.* An Introduction. Academic Press. Amsterdam. Boston. Heidelberg etc., 357-371, 2008.

Augustine JR, The insular lobe in primates including humans. Neurol Res 7; 2-10, 1985.

Augustine JR, Circuitry and functional aspects of the insular lobe in primates including humans. Brain Res Rev 22; 229-244, 1996.

Augustine JR, Des Champs EG, Ferguson JG Jr, Functional organization of the oculomotor nucleus in the baboon. Am J Anat 161; 393-404, 1981.

Aziz-Zadeh L, Iacoboni M, Zaidel E et al., Left hemisphere motor facilitation in response to manual action sounds. European Journal of Neuroscience 19; 2609-2612, 2004.

Aziz-Zadeh L, Maeda F, Zaidel E et al., Lateralization in motor facilitation during action observation: A TMS study. Experimental Brain Research 144; 127-131, 2002.

Baars BJ, The brain. In: BJ Baars and NM Gage (eds), *Cognition, Brain and Consciousness. Introduction to Cognitive Neuroscience.* Elsevier, Amsterdam, Boston, Heidelberg. Academic Press, 121-148, 2007.

Baars BJ, The conscious access hypothesis: origins and recent evidence. Trend Cogn Sci 6; 47-52, 2002.

Badamer J, Die Prosopagnosie. Arch Psychiatr Nervenkr 179; 6, 1947.

Bagshaw MH, Pribram KH, Cortical organization in gustation (Macaca mulatta). J Neurophysiol 16; 499-508, 1953.

Bailey P, von Bonin G, *The isocortex of Man.* University of Illinois Press, Urbana, 1951.

Bailey P, van Bonin G, Garol HW, Mc Culloch WS, Functional organization of temporal lobe of monkey (Macaca mulatta) and chimpanzee (Pan satyrus). J Neurophysiol 6; 121-128, 1943.

Bakar M, Kirshner HS, Wertz RT, Crossed aphasia: functioanal brain imaging with PET or SPRECT. Arch Neurol 53; 1026-1032, 1996.

Baloh RW, Honrubia V, *Clinical Neurophysiology of the Vestibular System.* Philadelphia, FA Davis, 1990.

Bartels A, Zeki S, The architecture of the color centre in the human visual brain: New Results and a review. The european Journal of Neuroscience 12; 172-193, 2000.

Barr WB, Karantzoulis S, Temporal lobe epilepsy. In: J Kreutzer, J De Luca, B Caplan (eds.), Encyclopedia of Clinical Neuropsychology. Volume 4, Q-Z, Springer, New York, Dordrecht, Heidelberg, London, 2482-2483, 2011.

Bates JAV, Stimulation of the medial surface of the human cerebral hemisphere after hemispherectomy. Brain 76; 405-447, 1953.

Batista-Brito R, Fishell G, The developmental integration of cortical interneurons into a functional network. Curr Top Dev Biol 87; 81-118, 2009.

Bear D, Temporal lobe epilepsy – a syndrome of sensory-limbic hypoconnection. Cortex 15; 357-384, 1979.

Beck E, Die myeloarchitektonische Felderung des in der Sylcischen Furke gelegenen Tailes des menschlichen Schäfenlappens. J Psychol. u. Neurol 36; 1-21, 1929.

Beckstead RM, Morse JR, and Norgren R, The nucleus of the solitary tract in the monkey: projections to the thalamus and brain stem. J Comp Neurol 190; 259-282, 1980.

Benjamin RM, Some thalamic and cortical mechanisms of taste. In: Y. Zotterman (ed.), *Olfaction and Taste.* Macmillan Company, New York, 309-329, 1963.

Benjamin RM, Akert K, Cortical and thalamic areas involved in taste discrimination in the albino rat. J Comp Neurol 111; 231-260, 1959.

Benton A, *Exploring the History of Neuropsychology* (Selected Papers). Oxford University Press, 2000.

Bertrand G, Spinal efferent pathways from the supplementary motor area. Brain 79; 461-473, 1956.

Biedermann B, Ruh N, Nickels L, Coltheart M, Information retrieval in tip of the tongue: New data and methodological advances. Journal of Psycholinguistic Research 37; 171-198, 2008.

Blakemore C, Cooper GF, Development of the brain depends on visual experience. Nature 228; 478, 1970.

Blakemore SJ, Frith CD, Wolpert DM, The cerebellum is involved in predicting the sensory consequences of action. Neuroreport 12; 1879-1884, 2001.

Blanke O, Seeck M, Direction of saccadic and smooth eye movements induced by electrical stimulation of the human frontal eye field: effect of orbital position. Experimental Brain Research 150; 174-183, 2003.

Blomquist AJ, Benjamin RM, Emmers R, Thalamic localization of afferents from the tongue in squirrel monkey (Saimiri sciureus). J Comp Neurol 118; 77-78, 1962.

Blum M, Walker AE, Ruch TC, Localization of taste in the thalamus of Macaca mulatta. Yale J Biol and Med 16; 175-192, 1943.

Blumer D, Wakhlu S, Davies K, Herman B, Psychiatric outcome of temporal lobectomy for epilepsy: incidence and treatment of psychiatric complications. Epilepsia 39; 478-486, 1998.

Bodegård A, Geyer S, Naito E et al., Somatosensory areas in man activated by moving stimuli: cytoarchitectonic mapping and PET. NeuroReport 11; 187-191, 2000.

Bodegård A, Ledberg A, Geyer S et al., Object shape differences reflected by somatosensory cortical activation, J Neurosci 20; 1-5, 2000.

Bodegård A, Geyer S, Naito E et al., Somatosensory area in man activated by moving stimuli: cytoarchitectonic mapping and PET. NeuroReport 11; 187-191 2000 a.

Bodegård A, Ledberg A, Geyer S et al., Object shape differences reflected by somatosensory cortical activation. J Neurosci 20; 1-5, 2000 b.

Bodegård A, Geyer S, Grefkes C et al., Hierarchical processing of tactile shape in the human brain. Neuron 31; 317-328, 2001.

Börnstein WS, Cortical representation of taste in man and in monkey. II. Localization of cortical taste area in man and method of measuring impairment of taste in man. Yale J Biol and Med 13; 133-156, 1940 a.

Börnstein WS, Cortical representation of taste in man and monkey. I. Functional and anatomical relations of taste, olfaction and somatic sensibility. Yale J Biol and Med 12; 719-736, 1940.

Bortolami R, Veggetti A, Callegari E et al., Afferent fibers and sensory ganglion cells within the oculomotor nerve in some mammals and man. I. Anatomical investigations. Arch Ital Biol 115; 355-385, 1977.

Bouillaud JB, *Traité Clinique et Physiologique de l'Encéphalite*. Paris: Baillière, 1825.

Bouvier SE, Engel SA, Behavioral deficits and cortical damage loci in cerebral achromatopsia. Cerebral Cortex (New York, NY: 1991) 16; 183-191, 2006.

Bowsher D, Some afferent and efferent connections of the parafascicular – center median complex. In: DP Purpura and MD Yahr (eds.), *The Thalamus*. University Press, New York, 99-108, 1966.

Brandt T, Dietrich M, *The vestibular cortex. Its locations, functions, and disorders.* Ann NY Acad Sci 871; 293-312, 1999.

Broca P, Remarques sur le siège de la faculté du langage articulé, suivies d'une observation d'aphémie. Bull Soc Anat (Paris) 6; 330-357, 1861.

Broca P, Localization des fonctions cérébrales. Siège du langage articulé. Bull Soc Anthrop (Paris) 4; 200-203, 1863.

Broca P, Sur la faculté du langage articulé. Bul Soc Antropol 6; 337-393 1865.

Broca P, Sur le siège de la faculté de langage articulé. Tribune Médicale 3; 254-256, 265-269, 1869.

Brockhaus H, Die Cyto- und Myeloarchitektonik des Cortex claustralis und des Claustrums beim Menschen. J Psychol Neurol (Leizig) 49; 248-249, 1940.

Brodal A, *Neurobiological anatomy* (3rd ed) New York, Oxford University Press, 1981.

Brodmann K, *Vergleichende Lokalisationlehr der Grosshirnrinde in ihren Prinzipien dargesteltt auf Grund des Zellenbaues.* Leipzig: JA Barth, 1909.

Brown KN, Chen S, Han Z, et al., Clonal production and organization of inhibitory interneurons in the neocortex. Science 334; 480-486, 2011.

Buccino G, Vogt S, Ritzl A et al., Neural circuits underlying imitation learning of hand actions: An event-related fMRI study. Neuron 42; 323-334, 2004.

Buckingham HW, The Marc Dax (1770-1837) / Paul Broca (1824-1880) controversy over priority in science: Left hemisphere specificity for seat of articulate langage and for lesions that cause aphemia. Clinical Linguistics and Phonetics 20; 613-619, 2006.

Burkhalter A, Bernardo KL, Organization of corticocortical connections in human visual cortex. Proc Natl Acad Sci 80; 1071-1075, 1989.

Butler RA, Diamond IT, Neff WD, Role of auditory cortex in discrimination of changes in frequency. J Neurophysiol 20; 108-120, 1957.

Butt et al., The temporal and spatial origins of cortical interneurons predict their physiological subtype. Neuron 27; 9682-9695, 2005.

Boxer AL, Principles of motor control by the frontal lobes as revealed by the study of voluntary eye movements. In BL Miller and JL Cummings (Eds.), *The Human Frontal Lobe.* Second Edition. The Guilford Press. New York, London, Ch. 17, 262-276, 2007.

Bradley WE, Farrell DF, Ojeman GA, Human cerebrocortical potentials evoked by stimulation of the dorsal nerve of the penis. Somatosens Mot Res 15; 118-127, 1998.

Braitenburg V, Schüz A, *Cortex Statistics and Geometry of Neuronal Connectivity.* 2nd ed, Springer Verlag, Berlin, 1998.

Brodmann K, *Vergleichende localizationslehre der groshirnrinde.* Leipzig: Borth, 1909.

Brouwer B, Ashby P, Altered corticospinal projections to lower limf motoneurons in subjects with cerebral palsy. Brain 114; 1395-1407, 1991.

Bucy PC, Effects of extirpation in man. In: PC Bucy (ed.), *The precentral Motor Cortex,* ed. 2. University of Illinois Press, Urbana, Ch. 14, 353-294, 1949.

Bucy PC, The surgical treatment of abnormal involuntary movements. Neurologia 1; 1-15, 1959.

Burton H, Fabri M, Alloway K, Cortical areas within the lateral sulcus connected to cutaneous representation in area 3b and 1: a revised interpretation of the second somatosensory area in macaque monkeys. J Camp Neurol 355; 539-562, 1995.

Cajal S. Ramón y, Histologie du système nerveux de l'homme et des vertébrés. Norbert Maloine, Paris. 2 vols, 1909, 1911.

Campbell AW, *Histological Studies on the Localization of Cerebral Function.* Cambridge University Press, New York, 360, 1905.

Carmichael ST, Price JL, Limbic connections of the orbital and medial prefrontal cortex in macaque monkeys. Journal of Comparative Neurology 363; 615-641, 1995.

Carpenter MB, *Human Neuroanatomy.* Seventh Edition. The Williams and Wilkins Company, Baltimore, Maryland, USA, 547-599, 1979.

Carpenter MB, Upper and lower motor neurons. In: J.A. Downey, and RC Darling (Eds.), *Physiological Basis of Rehabilitation Medicine*. WB Saunders Company, Philadelphia, Ch. 1; 3-27, 1971.

Carpenter MB, Sutin J, Human Neuroanatomy. Baltimore, Williams and Wilkins, 1983.

Carr L, Iacoboni M, Dubeau MC et al., Neural mechanisms of empathy in humans: A relay from neural systems for imitation to limbic areas. Proceeding of the National Academy of Science of the United States of America 100; 5497-5502, 2003.

Carreras M, Levitt M, Microelectrode analysis of the second somatosensory cortical area in the cat. Fed. Proc, 18; 24, 1959.

Carson AJ, MacHale S, Allen K et al., Depression after stroke and lesion location. A systematic review. Lancet 356; 122-126, 2000.

Casanova Manuel F, *Neocortical Modularity and the Cell Minicolumns*. New York, Nova Science Publisher, 2005.

Cavada C, Goldman-Rakic PS, Posterior parietal cortex in rhesus monkey: I – Parcelation of areas based on distinctive limbic and sensory corticocortical connections. J Comp Neurol 287; 393-421, 1989 a.

Cechetto DF, Saper CB, Evidence for a vinerotropic sensory representation in the cortex and thalamus in the rat. J Comp Neurol 262; 27-45, 1987.

Cerri G, Shimazu H, Maier MA, Lemon RN, Facilitation from ventral premotor cortex of primary motor cortex outputs to macaque hand muscles. Journal of Neurophysiology 90; 832-842, 2003.

Chouinard PA, Van Der Werf YD, Leonard G, Paus T, Modulating neural networks with transcranial magnetic stimulation applied over the dorsal premotor and primary motor cortices. J Neurophysiol 90; 1071-1083, 2003.

Cisek P, Kalaska JF, Neural correlates of mental rehearsal in dorsal premotor cortex. Nature 431; 993-996, 2004.

Cogan DG, *Neurology of the Ocular Muscles,* (Ed. 2), Charles C Thomas, Publisher, Springfield, Ill., 1956.

Cohen MJ, Landgren S, Strom L, Zottermann Y, Cortical reception of touch and taste in the cat. Acta physiol scandinav 40: Suppl 135; 50, 1957.

Collins RC, Cerebral cortex. In: AL Pearlman and RC Collins (eds). *Neurobiology of disease*. New York Oxford University Press, 1990.

Colonnier M, The fine structural arrangement of the cortex. Arch Neurol 16; 651-657, 1967.

Colonnier M, Synaptic patterns and different cells types in the different aminac of the cat visual cortex. An electron microscopic study. Brain Res 9; 268-287, 1968.

Condy C, Rivaud-Pechoux S, Ostendorf F et al. Neural substrate of antisaccades: Role of subcortical structures. Neurology 63; 1571-1578, 2004.

Constantinidis C, Franowicz MN, Goldman-Rakic PS, The sensory nature of mnemonic representation in the primate prefrontal cortex. Nature Neuroscience 4; 311-316, 2001.

Corballis MC, From mouth to hand: Gesture, speech, and the evolution of right-handedness. Behavioral Brain Sciences 26; 199-208, 2003.

Corbetta M, Akbudak E, Cantoro TE et al., A common network of functional areas for attention eye movements. Neuron 21; 761-773, 1998.

Corbin JG, Nery S, Fishell G, Telencephalic cells take a tangent: non-radial migration in the mammalian forebrain. Nat Neurosci 4 (suppl), 1177-1182, 2001.

Coxe WS, Landau WM, Observations upon the effect of supplementary motor cortex ablation in the monkey. Brain 88; 763-772, 1965.

Cramer SC, Finkelstein SP, Schaechter JD, et al., Activation of distinct motor cortex regions during ipsilateral and contralateral finger movements. Journal of Neuropsychology 81; 383-387, 1999.

Crosby EC, Relations of brain centers to normal and abnormal eye movement in the horizontal plane. J Comp Neurol 99; 437-480, 1953.

Crosby EC, Humphrey T, Lauer EW, *Correlative Anatomy of the Nervous System*. Macmillan Company, New York, 731, 1962.

Crossman AR, Cerebral hemisphere. In: bray's Anatomy. First Edition, Chapter 23, Churchill Livingstone. Elsevie, London, 335-359, 2008.

Curtis BA, Jacobson S, Marcus EM, *An Introduction to the Neurosciences*. Philadelphia: Saunders, 1972.

Daffner KR, Scinto LF, Weintraub S et al., Diminished curiosity in patients with probable Alzheimer's disease as measured by exploratory eye movements. Neurology 42; 320-328, 1992.

Damasio AR, Damasio H, van Hoesen GW-Prasopagnosia: Anatomic basis and behavioral mechanisms. Neurology 32; 331, 1982.

Darby DG, Nobre AC, Thangaray V et al., Cortical activation in the human brain during lateral saccades using EPISTAR functional magnetic resonance imaging. Neuroimage 3; 53-62, 1996.

Dax G, Observations tendant á prouver la coincidence constante de dérangements de la parole avec une lésione de l'hémisphere gauche de cerveau. Montpellier Méd. 38; 313-340 and 508-529; 39; 112-130, 226-237, and 413-421, 1877.

Dax M, Lésions de la moitié gauche de l'encephale coincident avec l'oublie de signes de la pensée. Gax. Hbd. Méd. Chir (Paris) 2; 259-262, 1865.

Dănăilă L, Golu M, *Tratat de Neuropsihologie*, Vol 2. Editura Medicală București, 261-319, 2006.

De Felipe J, Jones EC, *Cajal on the cerebral Cortex: An Annotated Translation of the Complete Writings*. New York: Oxford University Press, 1988.

Denny-Brown D, Botterell EH, The motor functions of the agranular frontal cortex. A Rev Nerv and Ment Dis Proc 27; 235-345, 1948.

Denny-Brown D, Motor mechanisms – Introduction: the general principles of motor integration. In: J Field (ed.), *Handbook of Physiology*, Section I. Vol II, American Physiological Society, Washington, DC Ch. 32; 781-796, 1960.

De Renzi E, Disorders of visual recognition. Sem Neurol 20; 479-485, 2000.

De Yoe EA, Felleman DJ, Van Essen DC, McClendon E, Multiple processing streams in occipitotemporal visual cortex. Nature 371; 151-154, 1994.

Déjérine J, Sémiologié du système nerveux. In : C Bouchard (ed), *Traité de Pathologie Générale*. Vol 5. Paris. Masson, 1900.

Desmurget M, Grfton S, Forward modeling allows feedback control for fast reaching movements. Trends Cogn Sci 4; 423, 2000.

Di Pellgrino G, Fadiga L, Fogassi L et al., Understanding motor events: A neurophysiological study. Experimental Brain Research 9; 176-180, 1992.

Dickman JD, The vestibular system. In: DE Haines (ed.), *Fundamental Neuroscience for Basic and Clinical Applications*. Third Edition. Churchill Livingstone. Elsevier. Philadelpia, 351-365, 2006.

Dickman JD, Byer M, Hess BJ, Three-dimensional organization of vestibular related eye movements to rotational motion in pigens. Vision Res 40; 2831-2844, 2000.

Disbrowe-Roberts T, Krubitzer L, Somatotopic organization of cortical field in the lateral sulcus of Human sapiens: evidence for S II and PV. J Comp Neurol 418; 1-21, 2000.

Doerster O, The cerebral cortex in man. Lancet 2; 309-312, 1931.

Dusser de Barenne JG, Mc Culloch WS, Suppression of motor response upon stimulation of areas 4S of the cerebral cortex. Am J Physiol 126; 482, 1939.

Eickhoff SB, Schleicher A, Zilles K, Amunts K, The human parietal operculum. I. Cytoarchitectonic mapping of subdivision. Cereb Cortex 16; 254-267, 2006 a.

Eickhoff SB, Amunts K, Mohlberg H, Zilles K, The human parietal operculum. II. Sterotoxic maps and correlation with functional imaging results. Cereb Cortex 16; 268-279, 2006 b.

Emmers R, Localization of thalamic projection of afferents from the tongue in the cat. Anat Rec 148; 67-74, 1964.

Emmers R, Benjamin RM, Blomquist AJ, Thalamic localization of afferents of the tongue in albino rat. J Comp Neurol 118; 43-48, 1962.

Emery B, Regulation of oligodendrocyte differentiation and myelination. Science 330; 770-782, 2010.

Engel JJ, Mesial temporal lobe epilepsy: What have we learned? The Neuroscientist 7; 340-352, 2001.

Engel JJ, Weiser HG, Mesial temporal lobe epilepsy. In: J Engel and TA Pedley (eds.), Epilepsy: A comprehensive textbook. Philadelphia, PA: Lippincott-Raven, 2417-2426, 1997.

Erickson TC, Woolsey CN, Observations on the supplementary motor area of man. Tr Am Neurol. A. 76; 50-56, 1951.

Ettinger U, Kumari V, Zachariah E et al., Effects of procyclidine on eye movement in schizophrenia. Neuropsychopharmacology 28; 2199-2208, 2003.

Elliott, *Textbook of Neuroanatomy*, Philadelphia: Lippincott, 1969.

Everett NB, *Functional Neuroanatomy*. Philadelphia. Lea and Febiger, 1965.

Fadiga L, Fogassi L, Pavesi G, Rizzolatti G, Motor facilitation during action observation: A magnetic stimulation study. Journal of Neurophysiology 73; 2608-2611, 1995.

Fadiga, Catighero L, Olivier E, Human motor cortex excitability during the perception of others' action. Current Opinion in Neurobiology 15; 213-218, 2005.

Farah MJ, Disorders of visual-spatial perception and cognition. In KM Heilman and E Valenstein (eds). Clinical neuropsychology (4th ed). New York: Oxford University Press, 2003.

Feidel D, Farber RH, Clementz BA et al., Inhibitory deficits in ocular motor behavior in adults with attention-deficit / hyperactivity disorder. Biological Psychiatry 56; 333-339, 2004.

Felleman DJ, van Essen DC, Distributed hierarchical processing in the primate cerebral cortex, Cereb. Cortex 1; 1-47, 1991.

Ferrari PF, Gallese V, Rizzolotti G, Fogassi L, Mirror neurons responding to the observation of ingestive and communicative mouth actions in the monkey ventral premotor cortex. European Journal of Neuroscience 17; 1703-1714, 2003.

Ferrier D, *The Localization of Cerebral Disease*. London: Smith. Elder and Co., 1878.

Ferrier D, *The Cranian Lectures on Cerebral Localization*. London: Smith. Elder and Co., 1890.

Ferrier D, *The Functions of the Brain*. London: Smith, Elder and Co., 1876 (2nd ed., 1886).

Fields RD, Change in the brain's white matter. Science 330; 768-769, 2010.

Fino E, Yuste R, Dense inhibitory conectivity in neocortex. Neuron 69; 1188-1203, 2011.

Flames N, et al., Delineation of multiple subpallidal progenitor domains by the combinatorial expression of transcriptional codes. Neurosci; 9682-9695, 2007.

Flanagan JR, Wing AM, The role of internal models in motion planning and control: evidence from grip force adjustments during movements of hand-held loads. J Neurosci 17; 1519-1528, 1997.

Flechsig P, Anatomie des menschlichen Gehirn and Ruckenmorks. Leipzig: Georg Thieme 1920.

Foerster O, The cerebral cortex in man. Lancet 2; 309-312, 1931.

Fogarty M, et al., Spatial genetic patterning of the embrionic neuroepithelium generates GABAergic interneuron diversity in the adult cortex. J Neurosci 27; 10935-10946, 2007.

Fogassi L, Ferrari PF, Gesierich B et al., Parietal lobe: From action organization to intention understanding. Science 308; 662-667, 2005.

Foerster O, Motor cortex in man in the light of Hughlings Jackson's doctrine. Brain 59; 135-159, 1936 a.

Foerster O, Symptomatologie der Erkrankungen des Grosshirns. Motorische Felder und Bahmen. In: Neurologie. Vol 5. Julius Springer, Berlin, 1-357, 1936 b.

Fox PT, Fox JM, Raichle ME, et al., The role of cerebral cortex in the generation of voluntary saccades: a positron emission tomographic study. J Neurophysiol 54; 348-369, 1985.

Fox PT, Miezin FM, Allman JM et al., Retinotopic organization of human visual cortex mapped with positron-emission tomography. J Neurosci 7; 913-922 1987.

Franckowiak RSJ, Fristan KJ, Frith CD, et al., *Human brain function.* San Diego Academic Press, 1997.

French JA, Williamson PD, Thadani VM et al., Characteristics of medial temporal lobe epilepsy: I. Result of history and physical examination: Annals of Neurology 43; 774-780, 1993.

Friedman DP, Murray EA, O'Neill JB, Mishkin M, Cortical connections of the somatosensory fields of the lateral sulcus of macaques: evidence for a corticolimbic pathway for touch. J Comp Neurol 252; 323-247, 1986.

Fulton JF, Keller AD, *The Sign of Babinski. A study of the Evolution of Cortical Dominance in Primates.* Charles C Thomas, Springfield, Ill., 165, 1932.

Fulton JF, Kennard MA, A study of flaccid and spastic paralysis produced by lesions of the cerebral cortex in primates. A Res Nerv and Ment Dis Proc 13; 158-210, 1934.

Funahashi S, Chafee MV, Goldman-Rakic PS, Prefrontal neuronal activity in rhesus monkeys performing a delayed anti-saccade task. Nature 365; 753-756, 1993.

Fuster JM, *Memory in the cerebral cortex: An empirical approach to neural metworks in the human and nonhuman primate.* Cambridge, MA: MIT Press, 1995.

Fuster JM, The prefrontal cortex – an update: time is of the essence. Neuron 30; 319-333, 2001.

Gabrieli JDE, Poldraqck RA, Desmond JE, The role of left prefrontal cortex in language and memory. Proc Natl Acad Sci USA 95; 906-913, 1998.

Gagnon D, O'Driscoll GA, Petrides M, Pike G, The effect of spatial and temporal information on saccades and neural activity in oculomotor structures. Brain 125; 123-139, 2002.

Gall FJ, Spurzheim G, Recherche sur le système. Nerveux en Général et sur Celui du Cerveau en Particulier. Paris: F Schoell, 1809 (Reprint. Amsterdam: Bonsel, 1967).

Gallese V, Fadiga L, Fogassi L, Rizzolotti G, Action recognition in the premotor cortex. Brain 119; 593-609, 1996.

Gastant H, Clinical and electroencephalographic classification of epileptic seizures. Epilepsia 11; 102, 1970.

Gastant H, Definitions. In: *Dictionary of Epilepsy.* Part I. World Health Organization, Geneva, 1973.

Garey LJ, (Trans), *Brodmann's "Localization in the Cerebral Cortex".* Smith-Gordon, London 1994.

Glimcher PW, *Decisions, Uncertainly and the Brain: The Science of Neuroeconomics*, Cambridge, MA: MIT, Press 2003.

Garey LJ, Jones EG, Powell TPS, Interrelationships of striate and extrastriate cortex with the primary relay sites of the visual pathway. J Neurol Neurosurg and Psychiat 31; 135-157, 1968.

Gauthier I, Tarr MJ, Andersson et al., Activation of the middle fusifom "face area" increases with expertize in recognizing novel objects. Nature Neuroscience 2; 568-573, 1999.

Gazzaniga MS, Cerebral specialization and interhemispheric communication. Does the corpus callosum enable the human condition? Brain 123; 1293-1326, 2000.

Gelman DM, Marin O, Generation of interneuron diversity in the mouse cerebral cortex. Eur. J Neurosci 31; 2136-2141, 2010.

Gelnar PA, Krauss BR, Szeverenyi NM, Apkarian AV, Fingertip representation in the human somatosensory cortex: an fMRI study. NeuroImage 7; 261-283, 1998.

Gennari F, De peculiari structura cerebri, nonnullisque ejus morbis. Parma: ex Regio Typographia, 1782.

Geschwind N, Behavioral changes in temporal lobe epilepsy. Psychological Medicine 9; 217-219, 1979.

Geschwind DH, Iacoboni M, Structural and functional asymmetries of the human frontal lobes. In: BL Miller and JL Cummings (eds.), *The Human Frontal Lobes*. Second Edition. The Guilford Press. New York, London, 68-91, 2007.

Geyer S, Ledberg A, Schleicher A et al., Two different areas within the primary motor cortex of man. Nature 382; 805-807 1996.

Geyer S, Schleicher A, Zilles K, Areas 3a, 3b, and 1 of human primary somatosensory cortex. 1. Microstructural organization and interindividual variability. NeuroImage 10; 63-83, 1999.

Geyer S, Schorman T, Mohlberg H, Zilles K, Areas 3a, 3b, and 1 of human somatosensory cortex. Part 2, Spatial normalization to standard anatomical space. NeuroImage 11; 684-696, 2000.

Gibbs FA, Ictal and non-ictal psychiatric disorders in temporal lobe epilepsy. Journal of Nervous and Mental Disease 113; 522-528, 1951.

Ginhoux F, Greter M, Leboeuf M et al., Fate mapping analysis reveals that adult microglia derive from primitive macrophages. Science 330; 841-845, 2010.

Glickstein M, Whitteridge D, Tatsuji Inoue and the mapping of the visual on the human cerebral cortex. TINS 10; 350-353, 1987.

Godoy J, Lüders H, Dinner DS et al., Versive eye movements elicited by cortical stimulation of the human brain. Neurology 40; 296-299, 1990.

Goldberg E, Gradient approach to neocortical functional organization. Journal of clinical and Experimental Neuropsychology 11; 1489-1517, 1989.

Goldberg E, Higher cortical functions in humans: The gradiental approach. In: E Goldberg (ed). *Contemporary neuropsychology and the legacy of Luria*. Hillsdale, NJ: Erlbaum, 1990.

Goldberg E, Rise and fall of modular orthodoxy. Journal of Clinical and Experimental Neuropsychology 17; 193-2008, 1995.

Goldberg E, Bilder RM, Hughes JE et al., A reticulofrontal disconnection syndrome. Cortex 25; 687-695, 1989.

Goodale MA, Milner AD, Separate visual pathways for perception of action. Trends Neurosci 15; 20-25, 1992.

Goodale MA, Westwood DA, An evolving view of duplex vision: separate but interacting cortical pathways for perception and action. Curr Opin Neurobiol 14; 203-211, 2004.

Gorno-Tempini et al., Explicit and incidental facial expression processing: An fMRI study. NeuroImage 14; 465-473, 2001.

Graeber MB, Changing face of microglia. Science 330; 783, 2010.

Grodzinsky Y, Amunts K, *Broca's Region*. Oxford University Press, New York, 2006.

Guitton D, Buchtel HA, Douglas RM, Frontal lobe lesions in man cause difficulties in suppressing reflexive glances and in generating goal-directed saccades. Experimental Brain Research 58; 455-472, 1985.

Gupta A, Wang Y, Markram H, Organizing principles for a diversity of GABAergic interneurons and synapses in the neocortex. Science 287; 273-278, 2000.

Glickstein M, The discovery of the visual cortex. Sci Am 256; 118-127, 1988.

Gless P, *Experimental Neurology*. Oxford University, Press, London, 1961.

Guldin WO, Grüsser OF, Is there a vestibular cortex? TINS 21; 254-259, 1998.

Hadjikhani N, De Gelder B, Neural basis of prosopagnosia: an fMRI study. Hum Brain Mapp 16; 176-182, 2002.

Häggvist G, Faserabalytische Studien über die Pyramidenbahn. Acta Psychiat et Neurol 12; 457-466, 1937.

Haines DE, Michailoff GA, The telencephalon. In: DE Haines (Ed.), *Fundamental Neuroscience for Basic and Clinical Applications*. Third Edition. Churchill, Livingstone. Elsevier, Philadelphia, 2006.

Hanbery J, Jasper H, Independence of diffuse thalamo-cortical projection system shown by specific nuclear destructions. J Neurophysiol 16; 252-271, 1953.

Happe F, Brownell H, Winner E, Acquired "theory of mind" impairments following stroke. Cognition 70; 211-240, 1999.

Hasegawa RP, Peterson BW, Goldberg ME, Prefrontal neurons coding suppression of specific saccades. Neuron 43; 415-425, 2004.

Haxby JV, Gobbini Mi, Furey ML et al., Distributed and overlapping representation of faces and objects in ventral temporal cortex. Science 293; 2425-2430, 2001.

Heffner HE, Ferrier and the study of auditory cortex. Arch Neurol 44; 218-221, 1987.

Henkel CK, The auditory system. In: DE Haines (ed.), *Fundamental Neuroscience for Basic and Clinical Applications*. Churchill Livingstone Elsevier, Philadelphia, 2006.

Highstein SM, Cohen B, Buttner-Ennerver JA, *New directions in vestibular research.* Ann NY Acad Sci 781; 1-739, 1996.

Hikosaka O, Takikawa Y, Kawagoe R, Role of the basal ganglia in the control of purposive saccadic eye movements. Physiological Reviews 80; 953-978, 2000.

Hillis AE, Language and frontal cortex. In: BL Miller and JL Cummings (eds.), *The Human Frontal Lobes Functions and Disorders,* Second Edition. The Guilford Press, New York, London. Ch. 20; 306-316, 2007.

Hines M, The anterior border of the monkey's (Macaca mulatta) motor cortex and the production of spasticity. Am J Physiol 116; 76, 1936.

Hines M, The "motor" cortex. Bull Johns Hopkins Hosp 60; 313-336, 1937.

Hirsch HVB, Spinelli DN, Visual experience modifies distribution of horizontally and verically oriented receptive fields in cat. Science 168; 869-871, 1970.

Hocherman S, Yirimya R, Neuronal activity in the medial geniculate nucleus and in the auditory cortex of the rhesus monkey reflects signal anticipation. Brain 113; 1707-1720, 1990.

Hoffman BL, Rasmussen T, Stimulation studies of insular cortex of Macaca mulatta. J Neurophysiol 16; 343-351, 1953.

Holmes G, May WP, On the exact origin of the pyramidal tract in man and other mammals. Brain 32; 1-43, 1909.

Huang ZL, Di Cristo G, Ango F, Development of GABA inervation in the cerebral and cerebellar cortices. Nat Rev Neurosci 8; 673-686, 2007.

Hubel DH, Wiesel TN, Receptive fields of single neurons in the cat's striate cortex. J Physiol 148; 547-591, 1959.

Hubel DH, Wiesel TN, Receptive fields, binocular interaction and functional architecture in the cat's visual cortex. J Physiol 160; 106-154, 1962.

Hubel DH, Wiesel TN, Shape and arrangement of columns in cat's striate cortex. J Physiol 165; 559-558, 1963.

Hubel D et al., Functional imbalance of visual pathways indicate alternative face processing strategies in autism. Neurology 61; 1232-1237, 2003.

Huck AC, Dougherty RF, Heeger DJ, Retinotopy and functional subdivision of human areas MT and MST. J Neurosci 22; 7195-7205, 2002.

Hurlbert A, Color vision: primary visual cortex shows its influence. Curr Biol 13; 270-272, 2003.

Hutton S, Kennard C, Oculomotor abnormalities in schizophrenia: A critical review. Neurology 50; 604-609, 1998.

Iacoboni M, Woods RP, Mazziotta JC, Blood flow increases in left dorsal premotor cortex during sensorimotor integration learning. Society for Neuroscience. Abstract 22; 720, 1996.

Iacoboni M, Woods RP, Brass M et al., Cortical mechanisms of human imitation. Science 286; 2526-2528, 1999.

Iacoboni M, Molna-Szakacs I, Gallese I, Gallese V et al., Grasping the intentions of others with one's own mirror neuron system. PloS Biology 3; e79, 2005.

Iamel RS, Ocular torsion and the function of the vertical extraocular muscles. J Comp Ophtalmol 79; 292-304, 1975.

Ishai A, Ungerleider LG, Matin A, Haxby JV, The representation of objects in the human occipital and temporal cortex. J Cogn Neurosci 12 Suppl 2; 35-51, 2000.

Isoda M, Tanji J, Contrasting neuronal activity in the supplementary and frontal eye fields during temporal organization of multiple saccades. Journal of Neurophysiology 90; 3054-3065, 2003.

Ivry RB., Robertson LC, The two sides of perception. MIT Press, Cambridge, MA, 1998.

Iwata M., Modular organization of visual thinking. Behavioral Neurology 2, 153-166, 1989.

Jasper HH, Unspecific thalamocortical relations. In: J Field (ed), *Handbook of Physiology.* Section 1, Vol. II. American Physiological Society. Washington DC. Ch. 53; 1307-1321, 1960.

Jerger JF, Observations on auditory behavior in lesions of the central auditory pathways. AMA Arch Otolaryng 71; 797-806, 1960.

Jerison NJ, *Brain Size and the Evolution of Mind.* New York, American Museum of Natura History, 1991.

Johnston JL, Miller JD, Nath A, Ocular motor dysfunction in HIV-1-infected subjects: A quantitative oculographic analysis. Neurology 46; 451-457, 1996.

Jones EG, Varieties and distribution of non-pyramidal cells in the somatic sensory cortex of the squirrel monkey. J Comp Neurol 160; 205-268, 1975.

Jones EG, Laminar distribution of cortical efferent cells. In: *Cerebral Cortex,* Vol. 1. New York, Plenum Press, 521-553, 1984.

Jones EG, Cortical and subcortical contributions to activity-dependent plasticity in primate somatosensory cortex. Annu Rev Neurosci 23; 1, 2000.

Jones EG, *The thalamus,* Second Edition, Vol. I, Cambridge University Press, Cambridge, 2007.

Jones EG, Leavitt RY, Retrograde axonal transport and the demonstration of non-specific projections to the cerebral cortex and striatum from thalamic intralaminar nuclei in the rat and monkey. J Comp Neurol 154; 349-378, 1974.

Jones EG, Burton H, Areal differences in the laminar distribution of thalamic afferents in cortical fields of the insular parietal and temporal regions of primates. J Comp Neurol 168; 197-247, 1976 b.

Kaada BR, Somato-motor, autonomic and electrocorticographic responses to electrical stimulation of "rhinencephalic" and other structures in primates, cat and dog. Acta physiol Sand 24 (Suppl 83); 285, 1951.

Kaas JH, The transformation of association cortex into sensory cortex. Brain Res Bull 50; 425, 1999.

Kaas JH, Evolution of somatosensory and motor cortex in primates. Anat Rec A Discov Mol Cell Evol Biol 281; 1148-1156, 2004.

Kahane P et al., Reappraisal of the human vestibular cortex by cortical electrical stimulation study. Ann Neurol 54; 615-624, 2003.

Kanwisher N, Dermott J, Chun MM, The fusiform face area: A module in human extrastriate cortex specialized for face perception. Journal of Neuroscience 17; 4302-4311, 1997.

Kätzel D, Zemelman BV, Buetfering C, et al., The columnar and laminar organization of inhibitory connections to neocortical excitatory cells. Nat Neuosci 14; 100-107, 2011.

Kawato Y, Internal models for motor control and trajectory planning. Curr. Opin. Neurobil 9; 718-727, 1999.

Kanwisher N, Yovel G, The fusiform face area: A cortical region specialized for the perception of faces. Philosophical Transactions of the Royal Society of London: Biological Sciences 361; 2109-2128, 2006.

Kennard MA, Somatic functions. In: PC Bucy (ed.), *The Precentral Motor Cortex*. Ed. 2. University of Illinois Press, Urbana, Ch. 9; 243-276, 1949.

Kennard MA, Fulton JF, The localizing significance of spasticity, reflex grasping and the signs of Babinski and Rossolino. Brain 56; 213-225, 1933.

Kennard MA, Viets HR, Fulton JF, The syndrome of the premotor cortex in man: Impairment of skilled movement, forced grasping, spasticity and vasomotor disturbances. Brain 57; 69-84, 1934.

Keubitzer L, Clarey J, Tweedale R et al., Redefinition of somatosensory areas in the lateral sulcus of macaque monkeys. J Neurosci 15; 3821-3839, 1995.

King WN, Lisberger SG, Fuchs AF, Responses of fibers in medial longitudinal fasciculus (MLF) of alert monkeys during horizontal and vertical conjugate eye movements evoked by vestibular or visual stimuli. J Neurophysiol 39; 1135-1149, 1976.

Klein C, Developmental functions for saccadic eye movement parameters derived form pro- and antisaccade tasks. Experimental Brain Research 139; 1-17, 2001.

Klein C, Fischer B, Hartnegg K et al., Optomotor and neuropsychological performance in old age. Experimental Brain Research 135; 141-154, 2000.

Kobayashi Y, Saito Y, Isa T, Facilitation of saccade initiation by brain stem cholinergic system. Brain and Development 23 (Suppl. 1); 24-27, 2001.

Kohler S, Moscovitch M, Unconscious visual processing in neuropsychological syndromes: A survey of the literature and evaluation of models of consciousness. In: MD Rugg (ed). *Cognitive neuroscience*. Cambridge, MA: MIT Press, 1997.

Kohler E, Keysers C, Umiltà MA et al., Hearing sounds, understanding actions: Action representation in mirror neurons. Science 297; 846-848, 2002.

Kolb B, Whishaw QI, *Fundamentals of Human Neuropsychology*. Fifth Edition. World Publishers. New York, 2003.

Kormack DR, Rakic P, Radial and horizontal deployment of clonally related cells in the primate neocortex: relationship to distinct mitotic lineages. Neuron 15; 311-321, 1995.

Krauzlis R and Dill N, Neural correlated of target choice for pursuit and saccades in the primate superior colliculus. Neuron 35; 355-363, 2002.

Krauzlis RJ, Recasting the smooth pursuit eye movement system. Journal of Neurophysiology 91; 591-603, 2004.

Krushel LA, Van Der Kooy D, Visceral cortex: integration of the mucosal senses with limbic information in the rat agranular insular cortex. J Comp Neurol 270; 39-54, 1988.

Küver H, Functional significance of the geniculo-striate system. Biological Sympasia 7; 253-299, 1942.

Kuyspers HGJM, Lawrence DG, Cortical projections to the red nucleus and the brain stem in the rhesus monkey. Brain Res 4; 151-188, 1967.

Laine M, Martin N, *Anomia: Theoretical and clinical aspects.* New York: Psychology Press, 2006

Lanadis T, Cummings JL, Benson F, Palmer EP, Loss of topographic familiarity: An environmental agnosia. Arch Neurol 43; 132, 1986.

Landgren S, The response of thalamic and cortical neurons to electrical and physiological stimulation of the cat's tongue. In: WA Rosenblith (ed.), *Sensory Communication.* Massachusetts Institute of Technology Press, Cambrige, 437-453, 1961.

Lassek AM, The human pyramidal tract. II. A numerical investigation of the Bets cells of the motor area. Arch Neurol and Psychiat 44; 718-724, 1940.

Lassek AM, The pyramidal tract. The effect of pre- and postcentral cortical lesions on the fiber components of the pyramids in monkey. J Nerv and Ment Dis 95; 721-729, 1942 a.

Lassek AM, The human pyramidal tract. IV. A Study of the mature, myelinated fibers of the pyramid. J Comp Neurol 76; 217-225, 1942.

Lassek AM, The pyramidal tract: Basic considerations of corticospinal neurons. A Res Nerv and Ment Dis Proc 27; 106-128, 1947.

Lassek AM, The Pyramidal Tract: Its Status in Medicine. Charles C Thomas, Publisher, Springfield, III, 1-66, 1954.

Lassek AM, Rasmussen GL, The human pyramidal tract. A fiber and numerical analysis. Arch Neurol and Psychiat 42; 872-876,1939.

Lassek AM, Rasmussen GL, A comparative fiber and numerical analysis of the pyramidal tract. J Comp Neurol 72; 417-428, 1940.

Lassek AM, And Evand JP, The human pyramidal tract. XII. The effect of hemispherectomies on the fiber components of the pyramids. J Comp Neurol 83; 113-119, 1945.

Lawrence DG, Kuypers HGJM, The functional organization of the motor system in the monkey. The effects of bilateral pyramidal lesions. Brain 91; 1-14, 1968.

Lee HW et al., Mapping of functional organization in human visual cortex. Electrical cortical stimulation. Neurology 54; 849-854, 2000.

Lee S, Yoon Bo-Eun, Berglund K et al., Channel-mediated tonic GABA release from glia. Science 330; 790-796, 2010.

Leichnetz GR et al., The prefrontal corticotectal projection in the monkey. An anterograde and retrograde horseradish peroxidase study. Neuroscience 6; 1023-1041, 1981.

Leigh RJ, Zee DS, *The neurology of Eye Movements.* Ed 2. Philadelphia: FA Davis, 1991.

Leigh RJ, Human vestibular cortex. Ann Neurol 35; 383-384, 1994.

Leigh RJ, Kennard C, Using saccades as a research tool in the clinical neurosciences. Brain 127; 460-477, 2004.

Leigh RJ, Zee DS, The neurology of eye movements. In: Contemporary Neurology Series. 4th ed. Vol. 70. Oxford University Press, New York, 2006.

Lekwuwa GU, Barnes GR, Cerebral control of eye movements: I. The relationship between cerebral lesion sites and smooth pursuit deficits. Brain 119; 473-490, 1996.

Lemmen LJ, Davis, and Radnor LL, Observation on stimulation of the human frontal eye field. J Comp Neurol 112; 163-168, 1959.

Lennie P, Receptive fields. Curr Biol 13; 216-219, 2003.

Levin PM, Bradford FK, The exact origin of the corticospinal tract in the monkey. J Comp Neurol 68; 411-422, 1939.

Lezak MD, *Neuropsychological Assessment.* 3ʳᵈ Ed. New York: Oxford University Press, 1995.

Lezak MD, Howieson DB, Loring DW, The behavioral geography of the brain. In: MD Lezak, DB Howieson, DW Loring (eds) *Neuropsychological Assessment.* Fourth Edition. Oxford University Press, New York, 39-85, 2004.

Li H, et al. Functional differentiation of a clone resembling embriogenic cortical interneuron progenitors. Neurobiol. 68; 1549-1564, 2008.

Liégeois-Chauvel C et al., Localization of the primary auditory area in man. Brain 114; 139-153, 1994.

Liégeois-Chauvel C, Peretz I, Babai M et al., Contribution of different cortical areas in the temporal lobes to music processing. Brain 121; 1853-1867, 1998.

Livingstone MS, Hubel DH, Specificity of intrinsic connections in primate primary visual cortex. J Neurosci 4; 2830-2835, 1984.

Lloyd D, Virtual lesions and the not-so-modular brain. J. Intern. Neuropsychol. Society 6; 627-635, 2000.

Lobel E, Kahane P, Leonards U et al., Localization of human frontal eye fields: anatomical and functional findings of functional magnetic resonance imaging and intracerebral electrical stimulation. J Neurosurg 95; 804-815, 2001.

Lordat J, Analyse de la Parole pour Servir à la Théorie de Divers Cas d'Alalie et de Paralalie. Paris: JB Baillière. 1843.

Lorente de Nó, The structure of the cerebral cortex. In: JF Dulton (ed.), *Physiology of the Nervous System.* Ed. 3. Oxford University Press, New York, 288-330, 1949.

Lüders H, et al., The second sensory area in humans: Evoked potential and electrical stimulation studies. Ann Neurol 17; 177-184, 1985.

Lüders H, Lesser RP, Dinner DS et al., Localization of cortical function: new information from extraoperative monitoring of patients with epilepsy. Epilepsia 29 (Suppl 2); 56-65, 1988.

Luna B, Thulborn KR, Strojawas MH, et al., Dorsal cortical regions subserving visually guided saccades in humans: a fMRI study. Cereb Cortex 8; 40-47, 1998.

Luria AR, *Higher cortical functions in man.* New York: Basic Book, 1966.

Luria AR, *Working Brain.* Harmondsworth, England, Penguin, 1973.

Lynch JC, The cerebral cortex. In: DE Haines (ed.), *Fundamental Neuroscience for Basic and Clinical Applications.* Churchill Livingstone Elsevier, Philadelphia, 512-526, 2006.

Lynch JC, Tian JR, Corticocortical networks and corticosubcortical loops for the higher control of eye movement. In: Buttner-Ennever JH (ed.): Neuroanatomy of the Oculomotor System. Amsterdam, Elsevier, Vol. 151, 467-508, 2005.

Lynch JC, Columnar organization of the cerebral cortex (cortical columns). In: *Neuroscience Year* (Supplement to Encyclopedia of Neuroscience). Boston, Birkhauser, 37-40, 1989.

Marcé LV, Sur quelques observations de physiologie pathologique tendant à démontrer l'existence d'un principe coordinateur de l'écriture. Mémoires de la Société de Biologie 3; 93-115, 1856.

Marie P, Révision de la question de l'aphasie. Semaine Médicale 26; 241-247, 1906.

Mariss O, Rubenstein JL, Cell migration in the forebrain. Annu Rev Neurosci 26; 441-483, 2003.

Markowitsch H, et al., Cortical afferents to the prefrontal cortex of the cat: A Study with the horseradish peroxidase technique. Neurosci Lett 11; 115-120, 1979.

Markram H, et al. Interneurons of the neocortical inhibitory system. Nat Rev Neurosci 5; 793-807, 2004.

Matelli M, Luppino G, Rizzolatti F, Patterns of cytochrome oxidase activity in the frontal agranular cortex of the macaque monkey. Behavioural Brain Research 18; 125-136, 1985.

Mc Carley RW, Sleep, dreams and states of consciousness. In: PM Conn (ed), *Neuroscience in Medicine*. Philadelphia: JB., Lippincott, 535-554, 1995.

Mc Cormick DA, Neurotransmitter actions in the thalamus and cerebral cortex. J. Clin. Neurophysiol 9; 212-223, 1992.

Meadows JC, Disturbed perception of colors associated with localized cerebral lesions. Brain: A Journal of Neurology 97; 615-632, 1974.

Mesulam MM, Behavioral neuroanatomy. In: MM Mesulam (ed), *Principles of behavioral and cognitive neurology* (2nd ed). New York, Oxford University Press, 2000.

Merzenich MM, Brugge JF, Representation of the cochlear partition on the superior temporal plane of the Macaque monkey. Brain Res. 50; 275-296, 1973.

Merzenich MM, Knight PL, Roth G, Cochleotopic organization of primary auditory cortex in the cat. Brain Res 63; 343-346, 1973.

Mesulam M, Mufson EJ, Insula of old world monkey. 1. Architectonics in the insula-orbito-temporal components of the paralimbic brain. J Comp Neurol 212; 1-22, 1982 a.

Mesulam M, Mufson EJ, Insula of the old world monkey. III. Efferent cortical output and comments on function. J Comp Neurol 212; 38-52, 1982 b.

Mesulam M, Mufson EJ, The insula of Reil in man and monkey. Architectonics, connectivity and function. In: A Peters and EG Jones (eds.), *Cortex*, Vol 4, *Association and Auditory Cortices*. Plenum Press, New York, London, 179-226, 1985.

Mesulam MM, The cholinergic innervations of the human cerebral cortex. Prig Brain Res 145; 67-78, 2004.

Mettler FA, Connections of the auditory cortex of the cat. J Comp Neurol 55; 139-183, 1932.

Mettler FA, On the origin of the fibers in the pyramid of the primate brain. Proc Soc Exper Biol and Med 57; 111-113, 1944 a.

Meyer DR, Woolsey CN, Effects of localized cortical destruction upon auditory discriminative conditioning in the cat. J Neurophysiol 15; 149-162, 1952.

Milea D, Lobel E, Lehéricy S et al., Intraoperative frontal eye field stimulation elicits ocular deviation and saccade suppression. NeuroReport 13; 1359-1364, 2002.

Milner B, Effects of different brain lesions on card sorting. Arch Neural 9; 900-1000, 1963.

Minkowski M, Étude sur les connections anatomiques des circonvolutions rolandiques, pariétales et frontales. Schweiz Arch Neurol in Psychiat 12; 71-104 and 227-268; 14; 255-278; 15; 97-132. 1923-1924.

Miyoshi G, Fishell G, GABAergic interneuron lineage selectively sort into specific cortical layers during early postnatal development. Cereb Cortex 21; 845-852, 2011.

Miyoshi G, Butt SJ, Takebayashi N, Fishell G, Physiologically distinct temporal cohorts of cortical interneurons arise from telencephalic Olig 2 expressing precursors. J. Neurosci 27; 7786-7798, 2007.

Miyoshi et al., Genetic fate mapping reveals that the caudal ganglionic eminence produces a large and diverse population of superficial cortical interneurons. J Neurosci 30; 1582-1594, 2010. 2010,

Molnar-Szakacs I, Iacoboni M, Koski L, Mazziotta JC, Functional segregation within pars opercularis of the inferior frontal gyrus: Evidence from fMRI studies of imitation and action observation. Cerebral cortex 1; 986-994, 2005.

Moore CJ, Stern CE, Corkin S et al., Segregation of somatosensory activation in the human Rolandic cortex using fMRI. J Neurophysiol 84; 558-569, 2000.

Morecraft RJ, Yeterian E, Prefrontal cortex. Enciclopedia of Human brain 4; 11-26, 2000.

Morrow MJ, Sharpe JA, Cerebral hemispheric localization of smooth pursuit asymmetry. Neurology 40; 284-292, 1990.

Mosimann UP, Felblinger J, Bollinari P et al., Visual exploration behavior during clock reading in Alzheimer's disease. Brain 127; 431-438, 2004.

Mosimann UP, Muri RM, Burn DJ et al., Saccadic eye movement changes in Parkinson's disease dementia and dementia with Lewy bodies. Brain 128; 1267-1267, 2005.

Mostofsky SH, Lasker AG, Gutting LE et al., Oculomotor abnormalities in attention deficit hyperactivity disorder: A preliminary study. Neurology 57; 423-450, 2001.

Mountcastle VB, Modality and topographic properties of single neurons of cat's somatic sensory cortex. J Neurophysiol 20; 408-434, 1957.

Mountcastle VB, The cortical organization of the neocortex. Brain 120; 701-722, 1997.

Mountcastle VB, Lynch JC, Georgopoulous A, et al., Posterior parietal association cortex of the monkey. Command function from operations within extrapersonal space. J. Neurophys. 38; 871-908, 1975.

Mufson EJ, Mesulam M, Insula of the old world monkey. II. Afferent cortical input and comments on the claustrum. J Comp Neurol 212; 23-37, 1982.

Mufson EJ, Mesulam M, Thalamic connections of the insula in the rhesus monkey and connects on the paralimbic connectivity of the medial pulvinar nucleus. J Comp Neurol 227; 109-120, 1984.

Mufson EJ, Sobreviela T, Kordower JH, Chemical neuroanatomy of the primate insular cortex: relationship to cytoarchitectonics, connectivity, function and neurodegeneration. In: Björklund T Hökfelt (eds.), *Handbook of Chemical Neuroanatomy. Vol 13: The Primate Nervous System,* Part I, 377-454. Elsevier, Amsterdam, 1997.

Munari C, Kahane P, Tassi L et al., Intracerebral low frequency electrical stimulation: a new tool for the definition of the "epileptogenic area"? Acta Neurochir Suppl 58; 181-185, 1993.

Munari C, Hoffman D, Francione S et al., Stereo-electroencephalography methodology: advantages and limits. Acta Neurol Scand Suppl 152; 56-69, 1994.

Munoz DP, Le Vasseur AL, Flanagan JR, Control of volitional and reflexive saccades in Tourette's syndrome. Progress in Brain Research 140; 467-481, 2002.

Mungus D, Interictal behavior abnormality in temporal lobe epilepsy. Archives of General Psychiatry 39; 108-111, 1982.

Müri R, Iba- Zizen MT, Derosier C et al., Location of the human posterior eye field with functional magnetic resonance imaging. J Comp Neurosurg Psychiatry 60; 445-448, 1996.

Nauta WJH, Whitlock DG, An anatomical analysis of the non-specific thalamic projection system. In: JF Delafresnaye (ed), *Brain Mechanism and Consciousness (Symposium).* Blackwell Scientific Publications, Oxford, 81-98, 1954.

Neal JW, Pearson RCA, Powell TPS, The ipsilateral cortico-cortical connections of area 7b, PF, in the parietal and temporal lobes of the monkey. Brain Res 524; 119-132, 1990 b.

Neff WD, Neural mechanisms of auditory discrimination. In: WA Rosenblith (ed), *Sensory Communications*, Massachusetts Institute of Technology Press and John Wiley and Sons, New York, 1961.

Neff WD, Diamond IT, The neural basis of auditory discrimination. In: HF Harlow and CN Woolsey (eds), *Biological and Biochemical Bases of Behavior.* University of Wisconsin Press, Madison, 101-126, 1958.

Neff WD, Fisher JF, Diamond IT, Yela M, Role of auditory cortex in discrimination requiring localization of sound in space. J Neurophysiol 19; 500-512, 1956.

Nieman DH, Bour LJ, Linszen DH et al., Neuropsychological and clinical correlates of antisaccade task performance in schizophrenia. Neurology 54; 866-871, 2000.

Noctor SC, Flint AC, Weissman TA, et al., Neurons derived from radial units in neocortex. Nature 409; 714-720, 2001.

O'Rourke NA, Sullivan DP, Kaznowski CE et al., Tangential migration of neurons in the developing cerebral cortex. Development 121; 2165-2176, 1995.

O'Sullivan EP, Jenkins IH, Henderson L et al., The functional anatomy of remembered saccades: a PET study. Neuroreport 6; 2141-2144, 1995.

Oppenheimer SM, Cechetto DF, The cardiac chronotopic organization of the rat insular cortex. Brain Res 533; 66-72, 1990.

Oppenheimer SM, Gelb A, Girvin JP, Hachinski VC, Cardiovascular effects of human insular cortex stimulation. Neurology 42; 1727-1732, 1992.

Osborne J, On the loss of the faculty of speech depending on forgetfulness of the art of using the vocal organs, Dublin J Med Chem Sci 4; 157-170, 1833.

Pacia SV, Devinsky O, Perrine K et al., Clinical features of neocortical epilepsy. Annals of Neurology 40; 724-730, 1996.

Pandya DN, Yeterian EH, Architecture and connections of cortical association areas. In: A Peters and EG Jones (eds). *Cerebral Cortex*, Vol. 4, New York: Plenum Press, 1985.

Pandya DN, Yeterian EH, Architecture and connections of cerebral cortex: Implications for brain evolution and function. In: AB Scheibel and AF Wechsler (eds), *Neurobiology of higher cognitive function.* New York: Guilford Press, 1990.

Pandya DN, Yeterian EH, Comparison of prefrontal architecture and connections. Philos Trans R Soc Lond. B Biol Sci 351; 1423-1432, 1996.

Pandya DN, and Yeterian EH, Comparison of prefrontal architecture and connections. In: AC Roberts, TW Robbins and L Weiskrantz (eds), *The prefrontal cortex. Executive and cognitive functions.* New York Oxford University Press, 1998.

Parsons LM, Sergent J, Hodges DA, Fox PT, The brain basis of piano performance. Neuropsychologia 43; 199-215, 2005.

Passingham RE, Brain size and inteligence in man. Brain Behavior and Evolution 16, 253-270, 1979.

Passingham RE, *The Frontal Lobes and voluntary Action.* Oxford: Oxford University Press, 1993.

Passingham R, Functional organization of the motor system. In: RSJ Franckowiak et al., (eds) *Human brain function.* San Diego, Academic Press, 1997.

Patton HD, Ruch TC, The relation of the foot of the pre- and postcentral gyrus to taste in the monkey and chimpanzee. Fed Proc 5; 79, 1946.

Patton HD, Ruch TC, and Walker AE, Experimental hypogeusia from Horsley-Clarke lesions of the thalamus in Macaca mulatta. J Neurophysiol 7; 171-184, 1944.

Paulescu E, Franckowiak RSJ, and Bottini G, Maps of somatosensory system. In: RSJ Franckowiak et al., (eds) *Human brain function.* San Diego, Academic Press, 1997.

Paus T, Location and function of the human frontal eye-field: a selective review. Neuropsychologia 34; 475-483, 1996.

Paxinos G (ed.), The Human Nervous System. San Diego, Academic Press, 439-755, 1990.

Peters A, Jones EG, *Cerebral cortex*. New York, Plenum Press, Vol. 1-14, 1984-1999.

Peele TL, Cytoarchitecture of individual parietal areas in monkey (Macaca mulatta) and distribution of the efferent fibers. J Comp Neurol 77; 693-737, 1942.

Penfield W, Evans J, Functional defects produced by cerebral lobectomies. A Res Nerv and Ment Dis Proc 13; 352-377, 1934.

Penfield W, Boldrey E, Somatic motor and sensory representation in the cerebral cortex of man as studied by electrical stimulation. Brain 60; 389-443, 1937.

Penfield W, Rasmussen T, *The Cerebral Cortex of Man. A clinical Study of Localization of Function*. Macmillan Company. New York, 248, 1950.

Penfield W, Welch K, The supplementary motor area of the cerebral cortex. A clinical and experimental study. A.M.A. Arch. Neurol and Psychiat 66; 289-317, 1951.

Penfield W, Jasper HH, *Epilepsy and the Functional Anatomy of the Human Brain*. Little Brown and Company, Boston, 896, 1954.

Penfield W, Faulk ME, The insula: further observations on its function. Brain 78; 445-470, 1955.

Penfield W, Mathieson G, Memory: autopsy findings and comments on the role of the hippocampus in experimental recall. Arch Neurol 31; 145-154, 1974.

Penfield W, Boldrey E, Somatic motor and sensory representation in the cerebral cortex as studied by electrical stimulation. Brain 60; 389-443, 1958.

Peters A, and Jones EG, *Cerebral Cortex*, Vol. 1-14. New York, Plenum Press, 1984-1999.

Petit L, Orssaud C, Tzourio N et al., PET study of voluntary saccadic eye movements in humans: basal ganglia - thalamocortical system and cingulate cortex involvemenet. J Neurophysiol 69; 1009-1017, 1993.

Petit L, Clark VP, Ingeholm J et al., Dissociation of saccade-related and pursuit-related activation in human frontal eye fields as revealed by fMRI imaging. J Neurophysiol 77; 3386-3390, 1997.

Pettigrew JD, Olson and Hirsch HUB, Cortical effects of selective visual experience: Degeneration or reorganization? Brain Res 51; 354-351, 1973.

Pickles JO, *An introduction to the Physiology of Hearing*, 2nd ed. London. Academic Press, 1988.

Pierrot-Deseilligny C, Gaymard B, Eye movement disorders and ocular motor organization. Curr Opin Neurol Neurosurg 3; 796-801, 1990.

Pierrot-Deseilligny C et al., Cortical control of saccades. And Neurol 37; 557-567, 1995.

Pierrot-Deseilligny C, Muri RM, Rivaud-Pechoux S et al., Cortical control of spatial memory in humans: The visuooculomotor model. Annals of Neurology 52; 10-19, 2002.

Pierrot-Deseilligny C, Muri RM, Ploner CJ et al., Decisional role of the dorsolateral prefrontal cortex in ocular motor behavior. Brain 126; 1460-1473, 2003.

Pierrot-Deseilligny C, Milea D, Muri RM, Eye movement control by the cerebral cortex. Current Opinion in Neurology 17; 17-25, 2004.

Platt ML, and Glimcher PW, Neural correlates of decision variables in parietal cortex. Nature 400; 233-238, 1999.

Polyakov GJ, Modern data on the structural organization of the cerebral cortex. In: AP Luria (ed), *Higher cortical functions in man*. New York: Basic Books, 1966.

Posner MI, Raiche ME, *Images of Mind*. New York: Scientific Library, 1994.

Powell TPS, Mountcastle VB, Some aspects of the functional organization of the cortex of the postcentral gyrus of the monkey: A correlation of findings obtained in a single unit analysis with cytoarchitecture. Bull. Johns Hopkins Hosp 105; 133-162, 1959 a.

Pribram KH, Rosner BS, Rosenblith WA, Electrical response to acoustic clicks in monkey: Extent of neocortex activated. J Neurophysiol 17; 336-344, 1954.

Price J, Thurlow L, Cell lineage in the rat cerebral cortex: a study using retroviral-mediated gene transfer. Development 104, 473-482, 1988.

Pritchard TC, Hamilton RB, Morse JB, Norgren R, Projections of the thalamic gustatory and lingual areas in the monkey. Macaca fascicularis. J Comp Neurol 244; 213-228, 1986.

Provencio I, and 5 others, A novel human opsin in the inner retina. J. Neurosci 20; 600-605, 2000.

Pryse-Phillips W, *Companion to Clinical Neurology*. 2nd ed., Oxford, Oxford University Press, 2003.

Purves D, Riddle DR, La Mantia AS, Iterated patterns of brain circuitry (or how the brain gets its spots). Trends in Neuroscience 15; 362-368, 1992.

Purves D, Augustine GJ, Fitzpatrick D, et al., (eds), The Association Cortices. In: D. *Neuroscience* Third Edition. Sinauer Associates Inc., Publishers Sunderland, Massachusetts USA, 613-636, 2004.

Rakic P, Specification of cerebral cortical areas. Science 241; 170-176, 1988.

Raymer AM, Moberg P, Crosson B et al., Lexical-remantic deficits in two patients with dominant thalamic infarction. Neuropsychologia 35; 211-219, 1997 a.

Raymer AM, Foundas A, Maher L et al., Cognitive neuropsychological analysis and neuro-anatomic correlates in a case of acute anomia. Brain and Language 58; 137-156, 1997 b.

Raymer AM, Naming and word retrieval problems. In: LL La Pointe (ed.), *Aphasia and related neurogenic language disorders*. 3rd ed., New York; Thieme, 72-86, 2005.

Raymer AM, Rothi LJ, Cognitive neuropsychological approaches to assessment and treatment: Impairments of lexical comprehension and production. In: R Chapey (ed). *Language intervention strategies in adult aphasia*. 5th ed., Baltimore: Lippincott, Williams and Wilkins, 607-631, 2008.

Reid CB, Liang I, Walsh C, Sistemic widespread clonal organization in cerebral cortex. Neuron 15; 299-310, 1995.

Reil JC, Das Hirnschenkel-System oder die Hirnschenkel-Organisation im grossen Gehirn. Arch Physiol Halle 9; 147-171, 1809 a.

Reil JC, Die sylvische Grüße Arch Physiol Hall 9; 195-208, 1809 b.

Richter CP, Hines M, Experimental production of the grasp reflex in adult monkeys by lesions of the frontal lobe. Am J Physiol 101; 87-88, 1932.

Riesenhuber M, Poggio T, Models of object recognition. Nature Neuroscience 3 (Suppl.) 1199-1204, 2000.

Rizzolatti G, and Arbib M, Language within our grasp. Trends in Neurosciences 2; 188-194, 1998.

Robert TS and Akert K, Insular and opercular cortex and its thalamic projection in Macaca mulatta. Schweiz Arch Neurol Neurochir Psychiat 92; 1-43, 1963.

Robertson IH, Marshall JC (eds), *Unilateral Neglect: Clinical and Experimental Studies*. Have, UK: Lawrence Erlbaum, 1993.

Roland Ep, Zilles K, Functions and structures of the motor cortices in humans. Curr Opin Neurobiol 6; 773-781, 1996.

Rolls ET, Information processing in the taste system of primates. J EXP Biol 146; 141-164, 1989 a.

Rolls et. al., The orbitofrontal cortex: In AC Roberts et al., *The prefrontal cortex: Executive and cognitive functions*. Oxford University Press, 1998.

Romansky KV et al., Corticosubthalamic projection in the cat: An electron microscopic study. Brain Res 163; 319-322, 1979.

Rosano C, Krisky CM, Velling JS et al., Pursuit and saccadic eye movement subregions in human frontal eye field: A High-Resolution fMRI investigation. Cerebral Cortex 12; 107-115, 2002.

Rose M, Cytoarchitektonic und Myeloarchitektonik der Grosshirnrinde. In: O Bunke and O Foerster (eds.), *Handbuch der Neurologie*. Vol. 1. Springer, Berlin, 588-778, 1935.

Rose JE, Woolsey CN, The relation of thalamic connections, cellular structure and evocable electrical activity in the auditory region of the cat. J Comp. Neurol 91; 441-466, 1949.

Rose JE, Woolsey CN, Cortical connections and functional organization of the thalamic auditory system of the cat. In: HF Harlow and CN Woolsey (eds), *Biological and Biochemical Bases of Behavior*. University of Wisconsin Press, Madison, 127-150, 1958.

Rose JE, Greenwood DB, Goldberg JM, Hind JE, Some discharge characteristics of single neurons in the inferior colliculus of the cat. I. Tonotopical organization, relation of spike-counts to tone intensity, and firing patterns of single elements. J Neurophysiol 26; 294-320, 1963.

Rosenzweig MR, Cortical correlates of auditory localization and of related perceptual phenomena. J Comp Physiol Psychol 47; 269-276, 1954.

Roth G, The evolution and ontogeny of consciousness. In: T Metzinger (ed), *Neural correlates of consciousness*. Cambridge, MA, MIT Press, 2000.

Russell JR, De Myer W, The quantitative cortical origin of pyramidal axons of Macaca rhesus. Neurology 11; 96-108, 1961.

Saper CB, Convergence of anatomic and limbic connections in the insular cortex of the rat. J Comp Neurol 210; 162-173 1982 a.

Saper CB, Reciprocal parabrachial-cortical connections in the rat. Brain Res 242; 33-40, 1982 b.

Scarff JE, Primary cortical centers for movement of upper and lower limbs in man. Arch Neurol and Psychiat 44; 243-299, 1940.

Scarff JE, Unilateral prefrontal lobotomy for relief of intractable pain and termination of narcotic addition. Surg Gynec and Obst 89; 385-392, 1949.

Schall JD, Morel A, King DJ, Bullier J, Topography of visual cortex connections with frontal eye field in macaque: Convergence and segregation of processing streams. Journal of Neuroscience 15; 4464-4487, 1995.

Schall JD, Stuphorn V, Brown JW, Monitoring and control of action by the frontal lobes. Neuron 36; 309-322, 2002.

Scheibel ME, Scheibel AB, Elementary processes in selected thalamic and cortical subsystems – the structural substrates. In: *The Neurosciences*, Second Study Programs, Vol. 2. New York, Rockefeller University Press, 443-457, 1970.

Schiltz C, Sorger B, Caldara R et al., Impaired face discrimination in acquired prosopagnosia is associated with abnormal response to individual faces in the right middle fusiform gyrus. Cereb Cortex 16; 574-586, 2006.

Schmahmann JD, Leifer D, Parietal pseudothalamic pain syndrome: Clinical features and anatomic correlates. Arch Neurol 49; 1032-1037, 1992.

Schlag J, Schlag-Rey M, Evidence for a supplementary eye field. J Neurophysiol 57; 179-200, 1987.

Schmitt FO, Woden FG, Adelman G, Dennis SG, *The Organization of the Cerebral Cortex*. MIT Press, Cambridge, 1981.

Schneider WX, Vam: A neuro-cognitive model for visual attention control of segmentation, object recognition and space-based motor action. Visual Cogn 2; 331, 1995.

Schneider KA, Richter MC, Kastner S, Retinotopic organization and functional subdivision of the human lateral geniculate nucleus: a high-resolution functional magnetic resonance imaging study. J Neurosci 24; 8975-8985, 2004.

Schüz A, Miller R, *Cortical Areas: Unity and Diversity*. Taylor and Francis, London and New York, 2002.

Seleman LD, Goldman-Rakic PS, Common cortical and subcortical targets of the dorsolateral prefrontal and posterior parietal cortices in the Rhesus monkey: evidence for a distributed neural network subserving spatially guided behavior. J Neurosci 8; 4049-4068, 1988.

Serre T, Kreiman G, Kouch M et al., A quantitative theory of immediate visual recognition. In: P Cisek, T Drew and FJ Kalaska (Eds.), *Progress in brain research* (Vol 164), Amsterdam: Elsevier, 33-56, 2007.

Shafiq-Antonacci R, Maruff P, Masters C, Currie J, Spectrum of saccade system function in Alzheimer disease. Archives of Neurology 60; 1272-1278, 2003.

Sharp J, et al., Disturbance of ocular motility. Continuum 1; 41-91, 1995.

Shaywitz SE, Dyslexia. NEJM 338; 307-312, 1998.

Shenkin HA, Lewey FH, Taste area preceding convulsions in a lesion of the parietal operculum. J Nerv. And Ment Dis 100; 352-354, 1944.

Sherwood CC et al., Variability of Broca's area homologue in African great apes: Implications for language evolution. Anat Rec Part A 27; 276-285, 2003.

Shimazu H, Maier MA, Cerri G et al., Macaque ventral premotor cortex exerts powerful facilitation of motor cortex outputs to upper limb motoneurons. Journal of Neuroscience 24; 1200-1211, 2004.

Shipley MT, Saunders MS, Special senses are really special: evidence for a reciprocal bilateral pathway between insular cortex and nucleus parabrachialis. Brain Res Bull 12; 221-226, 1982.

Shmuelof L, Zachary E, A mirror representation of others' actions in the human anterior parietal cortex. J Neurosci 26; 9736-9742, 2006.

Sirigu A et al., The mental representation of hand movements after parietal cortex damage. Science 273; 1564-1568, 1996.

Sirigu A, Daprati E, Ciancia S et al., Altered awareness of voluntary action after damage to the parietal cortex. Nature Neuroscience 7; 80-84, 2004.

Smith WK, The frontal eye fields. In: PC Bucy (ed), *The Precentral Motor Cortex.* Urbana, IL: University of Illinois Press, 308-342, 1944.

Smith EE, and Jonides J, Neuroimaging analysis of human working memory. Proc. Natl. Acad. Sci USA 95; 12061-12068, 1998.

Smutok MA, Grafman J, Salazar AM, et al., The effects of unilateral brain damage on contralateral and ipsilateral upper extremity function in hemiplegia. Physical Therapy 69; 195-203, 1989.

Snyder M, Hall WC, Diamond IT, Vision in tree shrews after removal of striate cortex. Psychoneurol Sc. 6; 243-244, 1966.

Sparks DL, The brain stem control of saccadic eye movements. Nature Reviews: Neuroscience 3; 952-964, 2002.

Spinelli DN, Hirsch HVB, Phelps RW, Metzler J, Visual experience as a determinant of response characteristics of cortical receptive fields in cat. Exper Brain Res 15; 289-304, 1972.

Stefanacci L, Amaral DG, Topographic organization of cortical inputs to the lateral sulcus of the macaque monkey amygdala: A retrograde tracing study. Journal of Comparative Neurology 421; 52-79, 2000.

Stefanacci L, Amaral DG, Some observations on cortical inputs to the macaque monkey amygdala: An anterograde tracing study. Journal of Comparative Neurology 451; 301-323, 2002.

Steinmetz H, Structure, functional and cerebral asymmetry: in vivo morphometry of the planum temporale. Neurosci Biobehav Rev 20; 587-591, 1996.

Sterling P, Retina. In GM Shepherd (ed), The synaptic organization of the brain (4th ed). New York, Oxford University Press, 1998.

Stern P, Introduction. Glee for Glia. Science 330; 473, 2010.

Strominger NL, Subdivisions of auditory cortex and their role in localization of sound in space. Exper Neurol 24; 348-362, 1969.

Stephan H, Allocortex. In: W Bergmann (ed.), *Handbuch der mikroskopischen Anatomie des Menschen*. Vol. 4, Nervensystem, Part 9, Springer Verlag, Berlin, Heidelberg, New York, 998 pp, 1975.

Stuphorn V, Schall JD, Neuronal control and monitoring of initiation of movements. Muscle and Nerve 26; 326-339, 2002.

Sturb RL, Black FW, *Neurobehavioral disorders. A clinical approach*. Philadelphia: Davis, 1988.

Sudokov K, Mac Lean PD, Reeves A, Marino R, Unit study of exteroceptive input to claustrocortex in awake, sitting, squirrel monkey. Brain Res 28; 19-34, 1971.

Sugar O, French JD, Chusid JG, Corticocortical connections of the superior surface of the temporal operculum in the monkey (Macaca mulatta). J Neurophysiol 11; 175-184, 1948.

Sugar O, Amador LV, Griponissiotes B, Corticocortical connections of the walls of the superior temporal sulcus in the monkey (Macaca mulatta). J Neuropath and Exper Neurol 9; 179-185, 1950.

Sutherling WW et al., Cortical sensory representation of the human hand: size of finger regions and nonoverlapping digit somatotopy. Neurology 42; 1020-1028, 1992.

Sweeney JA, Mintun MA, Kwee S, et al., Positron emission tomography study of voluntary saccadic eye movements and spatial working memory. J Neurophysiol 75; 454-468, 1996.

Tanaka DH, et al. Random walk behavior of migrating cortical interneurons in the marginal zone: time lapse analysis in flat-mount cortex. J. Neurosci 29; 1300-1311, 2009.

Tanji J, Shima K, Role of supplementary motor area cells in planning several movements ahead. Nature 371; 413-416, 1994.

Thaker GK, Ross DE, Cassady SL et al., Saccadic eye movement abnormalities in relatives of patients with schizophrenia. Schizophrenia Research 45; 253-264, 2000.

Thompson KG, Bichot NP, A visual salience map in the primate frontal eye field. Progress in Brain Research 147; 251-262, 2005.

Thompson AM, Lamy C, Functional maps of neocortical local circuitry. Front Neurosci 1; 19-42, 2007.

Thompson JM, Woolsey CN, Talbot SA, Visual areas I and II of cerebral cortex of rabbit. J Neurophysiol 13; 277-288, 1950.

Tijssen CC et al., Conjugate eye deviation: Side, site, and size of hemispheric lesion. Neurology 41; 846-850, 1991.

Toga AW, Thompson PM, Mori S et al., Toward multimodal atlases of the human brain. Nature Rev Neurosci 7; 952-966, 2006.

Tonji J, Kurata K, Changing concepts of motor areas of the cerebral cortex Brain Dev 11; 374-377, 1989.

Tower SS, Pyramidal lesion in the monkey. Brain 63; 36-90, 1940.

Tower SS, The pyramidal tract. In: PC Bucy (ed), *The Precentral Motor Cortex,* Ed. 2. University of Illinois Press, Urbana, Ch. 6; 149-172, 1949.

Travis AM, Neurological deficiencies after ablation of the precentral motor area in Macaca mulatta. Brain 78; 155-173, 1955.

Travis AM, Neurological deficiencies following supplementary motor area lesions in Macaca mulatta. Brain 78; 174-198, 1955 a.

Trousseau A, De aphasie, maladie décrite récemment sous le nom impropre d'aphémie. Gazettes des Hopitaux 37; 13-14, 25-26, 37-39, 48-50, 1964.

Truex RC, Carpenter MB, *Human Neuroanatomy*. Baltimore: Williams and Wilkins, 1969.

Ture U et al., Topographic anatomy of the insular region. J Neurosurg 90; 720-733, 1999.

Umiltà MA, Kohler E, Gallese V et al., "I know what you are doing": A neurophysiological study. Neuron 31; 155-165, 2001.

Ungerleider LG, Haxby JV, "What" and "where" in the human brain. Curr Opin Neurobiol 4; 157-165, 1994.

Urasaki E et al., Cortical tongue area studied by chronically implanted subdural electrodes: With special reference to parietal motor and frontal sensory responses. Brain 117; 117-132, 1994.

Van Essen DC, Drury HA, Structural and functional analyses of human cerebral cortex using a surface-based atlas. Journal of Neuroscience 17; 7092-7102, 1997.

Varnas GG, Grand W, The insular cortex: Morphological and vascular anatomic characteristics. Neurosurgery 44; 127-138, 1999.

Verrey D, Hémiachromatopsie Droite Absolue. Conservation Partielle De La Perception Lumineuse Et Des Formes. Ancien Kyste Hémorrhagique De La Partie Inférieure Du Lobe Occipital Gauche. Archives d'Ophtalmologie 8; 289-300, 1888.

Vicq d'Azyr F, Recherches sur la structure du cerveau, du cervelet, du la moelle elongeé, de la moelle épinière; et sur l'origine des nerfs de l'homme et des animaux. Hist Acad Royale Sci: 495-622, 1781.

Vogt C, Vogt O, Allgemeine Ergebnisse Unserer Hirnforschung. Vierte Mitteilung: Die physiologische Bedeutung der architektonischen Rindenreizungen. J Psychol. Neurol 25; 279-462, 1919.

Von Economo CF, *The cytoarchitectonics of the human Cerebral Cortex*. Oxford Medical Publications, London, 1986, 1929.

Walker AE, Fulton JF, Hemidecortication in chimpanzee, baboon, macaque, potto, cat and coati: A study in encephalization. J Nerv and Ment Dis 87; 677-700 1938.

Walker AE, Weaver TA Jr, Ocular movements from the occipital lobe in the monkey. J Neurophysiol 3; 353-357, 1940.

Walsh C, Ccpko CL, Widespread clonal dispersion in proliferative layers of cerebral cortex. Nature 362; 632-635, 1993.

Wanadi J, Adami H, Sherr J et al., Naltrexone treatment of tardive dyskinesia in patients with schizophrenia. Journal of Clinical Psychopharmacology 24; 441-445, 2004.

Webster D, Fay RR, Popper AN, Springer Handbook of Auditory Research, Vol I. *The Auditory Pathway: Neuroanatomy*. New York, Springer-Verlag, 1992.

Weiskrantz L, *Blindsight*. Oxford, UK, Clarendon Press, 1986.

Welch WK, Kennard MA, Relation of cerebral cortex to spasticity and flaccidity. J Neurophysiol 7; 255-268, 1944.

Welker WT, Benjamin RM, Miles RC, Woolsey CN, Motor effects of cortical stimulation in squirrel monkey. (Saimiri sciureus). J Neurophysiol 20; 347-364, 1957.

Williamson PD, French JA, Thadani VM et al., Characteristics of medial temporal lobe epilepsy: II. Interictal and ictal scalp electroencephalography, neuropsychological testing, neuroimaging, surgical results, and pathology. Annals of Neurology 34; 781-787, 1993.

Willie JT and 13 others, Distinct narcolepsy syndromes in orexin receptor-2 and orexin null mice: Molecular genetic dissection of non-REM and REM sleep regulatory processes. Neuron 38; 715-730; 2003.

Winner E, Brownell H, Happe F et al., Distinguishing lies from jokes: Theory of mind deficits and discourse interpretation in right hemisphere brain-damage patients. Brain and Language 62; 89-106, 1998.

Wise SP, The primate premotor cortex: Past, present and preparatory. Ann Rev Neurosci 8; 1-19, 1985.

Wise RJ et al., Brain regions involved in articulation. Lancet 353; 1057-1061, 1999.

Whittfield IC, *The Auditory Pathway.* Williams and Wilkins Company. Baltimore, 1967.

Wolpert DM, Ghahramani Z, Jordan MI, An internal model for sensorimotor integration. Science 269; 1880-1882, 1995.

Wolpert DM, Gharhamani Z, Competitional principles of movement neuroscience. Nat Neurosci 3; 1212-1217, 2000.

Wolpert DM, Gharhamani Z, Flanagan JR, Perspectives and problems in motor learning. Trends Cogn Sci 1; 487-494, 2001.

Wonders CP, Anderson SA, The origin and specification of cortical interneurons. Nat Rev Neurosci 7; 687-696, 2006.

Wonders CP, et al., A spatial bias for the origins of interneuron subgroups within the medial ganglionic eminence. Dev. Biol 314; 127-136, 2008.

Woolsey CN, Walzl EM, Topical projection of nerve fibers from local regions of the cochlea to the cerebral cortex of the cat. Bull. John Hopkins Hosp 71; 315-344, 1942.

Woolsey CN, Fairman D, Contralateral, epsilateral and bilateral representation of cutaneous receptors in somatic area I and II of the cerebral cortex of pigs, sheep and other mammals. Surgery 19; 684-702, 1946.

Woolsey CN, Settlage PH, Meyer DR et al., Patterns of localization in precentral and "suplementary" motor areas and their relation to the concept of a premotor area. A Res Nerv Ment Dis Proc 30; 238-264, 1951.

Woolsey CN, Organization of somatic sensory and motor area of the cerebral cortex. In: HF Harlow and CN Woolsey (eds.) Biological and Biochemical Bases of Behavior. University of Wisconsin, Madison, 63-81, 1958.

Woolsey CN, Erickson TC, Gilson WE, Localization in somatic sensory and motor areas of human cerebral cortex as determined by direct recording of evoked potentials and electrical stimulation. J Neurosurg 51; 476-506, 1979.

Xu Q, et al. Sonic hedgehog signaling confers ventral telencephalic progenitors with distinct cortical interneuron fates. Neuron 65; 240-328, 2010.

Yu YC, Bultje RS, Wang X, Shi SH, Specific synapses develop preferentially among sister excitatory neurons in neocortex. Nature 458, 501-504, 2009.

Zatorre RJ, Musical perception and cerebral functions: A critical review. Music Perception 2; 196-221, 1984.

Zatorre RJ, Neural specializations for tonal processing. Annals of the New York Academy of Sciences 930; 193-210, 2001.

Zatorre RJ, Belin P, Spectral and temporal processing in human auditory cortex. Cerebral Cortex 11; 946-953, 2001.

Zatorre RJ, Belin P, Penhume V, Structure and function of the auditory cortex. Music and speech. Trends in Cognitive Science 6; 37-46, 2002.

Zeki S, Watson JD, Lueck et al., A direct demonstration of functional specialization in human visual cortex. J Neurosci 11; 641-649, 1991.

Zihl J, Von Cramon D, Mai N, Selective disturbance of moment vision after bilateral brain damage. Brain 106; 313-340, 1983.

Zilles K, Werners R, Büsching U, Schleicher A, Ontogenesis of the laminar structure in areas 17 and 18 of the human visual cortex. A quantitative study. Anat Embrieol 174; 339-353, 1986.

Zilles KO, Is the length of the calcarine sulcus associated with the size of the human visual cortex? A Morphometric study with magnetic resonance tomography. J Hirnforsch 36; 451-459, 1995.

Zilles K, Architecture of the human cerebral cortex. Regional and laminar organization. In: Paxinos G, Mai JK (eds.), *The Human Nervous System*. 2nd ed, Chapter 27, 997-1055, Elsevier, Academic Press, Amsterdam, 2004.

Zilles K, Palomero-Gallagher N, Cytomyelo-, and receptor architectonics of the human parietal cortex. NeuroImage 14; 8-20, 2001.

Yang ZH, Zhao XQ, Wang CX et al., Neuroanatomic correlation of the post-stroke aphasias studied with imaging. Neurological Research 30; 356-360, 2008.

Yamamoto J, Ikeda A, Satow T et al., Human eye fields in the frontal lobe as studied by epicortical recording of movement-related cortical potentials. Brain 127; 873-887, 2004.

Yates BJ, Miller AD, *Vestibular Autonomic Regulation*. New York, CRC Press, 1996.

Yaxley S, Rolls ET, Sienkiewicz ZJ, Gustatory responses of single neurons in the insula of the macaque monkey. J Neurophysiol 63; 689-700, 1990.

Yoshimura Y, Callaway EM, Fine-scale specificity of cortical networks depends on inhibitory cell type and conectivity. Nat Neurosci. 8; 1552-1559, 2005.

Yost WA, *Fundamentals of Hearing*: An introduction. San Diego, Academic Press, 1994.

Chapter 22

VENTRICULAR SYSTEM
AND MENINGES

Introduction

The cerebral ventricular system which consists of the four ventricles and the central canal of the spinal cord are the remnants of the lumen of the embryonic neuronal tube.

The cells of the nervous system, both neurons and glia, originated from germinal matrix adjacent to the lining of this tube. The cells multiply and migrate away from the walls of the neural tube, forming the nuclei and cortex. As the nervous system develops, the mass of tissue grows and the size of the tube diminishes, leaving various spaces in different parts of the nervous system.

The parts of the tube that remain in the hemispheres are called the cerebral ventricles, or the lateral ventricles. The ventricles are described in the order in which they are numbered from rostral to caudal.

Thus, each cerebral hemisphere contains a large lateral ventricle that communicates near its rostral end with the third ventricle *via* the interventricular foramen (foramen of Monro) on either side of the median plane.

The third ventricle communicates with the forth ventricle by way of the aqueduct of the midbrain, a wide tent-shaped cavity lying between the brain stem and cerebellum.

The fourth ventricle becomes continuous with the central canal of the medulla oblongata and spinal cord and open by means of apertures into the subarachnoid space.

The ventricular system contains cerebrospinal fluid (CSF), which is mostly secreted by the choroid plexuses located within the lateral, third and fourth ventricle. The total volume of the fluid is about 100 to 140 ml and its pressure is about 150 mm of saline (normal range: 70-180 mm) in the lateral recumbent position. The pressure is several times higher in the lumbar region when sitting, but is about atmospheric at the foramen magnum and is negative in the ventricles.

CSF flows from the lateral to the third ventricle, then through the cerebral aqueduct into the fourth ventricle. It leaves the fourth ventricle through the **foramen of Magendie** and the **foramina of Luschka** to reach the subarachnoid space surrounding the brain.

The neuroglial cells that line the ventricles of the brain and the central canal of the spinal cord are termed **ependymal cells**. The ependyma is nonciliated in adult.

Lateral ventricle

The largest ventricles, the paired ventricles, separated from one another by the **septum pellucidum**, are located in the right and left cerebral hemispheres. Thus, each of the paired lateral ventricle is a C-shaped profile cavity that wraps around the thalamus and is situated deep within the cerebrum. Thus, each lateral ventricle wraps around the superior, inferior, and posterior surface of the thalamus. The superior surface of the thalamus forms the floor of the body, the posterior surface of the thalamus forms the anterior wall of the atrium, and the inferior surface of the thalamus forms the medial part of the roof of the temporal horn.

The caudate nucleus is an arched, C-shaped cellular mass that wraps around the thalamus and constitutes an important part of the wall of the lateral ventricle (Rhoton, 1987).

Each lateral ventricle possesses a body and three horns, the anterior, posterior, and inferior horns. Thus, its various parts are the anterior horn, which lies deep to the frontal lobes; the central portion or body, which lies deep to the parietal lobes; the atrium or trigone where the ventricle widens and curves into the inferior horn, which goes into the temporal lobes. In addition, there may be an extension into the occipital lobes, called the occipital or posterior horn.

The frontal horn of the lateral ventricle has as its inferior boundary the rostrum, its rostral boundary the genu, and its superior boundary the trunk, of the corpus callosum. The anterior horns of the two ventricles are separated by the septum pellucidum.

Laterally the frontal horn of the lateral ventricle is limited by the bulging head of the caudate nucleus. The anterior horn extends back as far as the interventricular foramen. The narrow interventricular foramen is located immediately posterior to the column of the fornix and separates the fornix from the anterior nucleus of the thalamus.

The body or **the central portion** of the lateral ventricle lies within the frontal and parietal lobes and extends from the interventricular foramen to the splenium of the corpus callosum. It is inferior to the trunk of the corpus callosum. The body is also on the medial aspect of the thalamus (inferiorly) and body of the caudate nucleus (superiorly). The bodies of the lateral ventricles are separated by the septum pellucidum, which contains the columns of the fornices in its lower edge (Born et al., 2004). The inferior limit of the body of the ventricle and its medial wall are formed by the body of the fornix. In the central part of the lateral ventricle is the choroid plexus. The body of the lateral ventricle widens posteriorly to become continuous with the posterior and inferior horn at the collateral trigone or atrium (Rhoton, 2002; Born et al., 2004; Kawashima et al., 2006).

The posterior (occipital) horn of the lateral ventricle tapers into the occipital lobe of each cerebral hemispheres. It is usually diamond-shaped or square in outline, and the two sides are often asymmetrical. Fibres of the tapetum of the corpus callosum separate the ventricle from the optic radiation and form the roof and lateral wall of the posterior horn.

Forceps major pass medially as they sweep back into the occipital lobe, and produce a rounded elevation in the upper medial wall of the posterior horn. Lower down, a second elevation, the calcar avis, corresponds to the deeply infolded cortex of the anterior part of the calcarine sulcus (Mc Lone, 2004; Crossman, 2008). The occipital horns are usually asymmetrical – the back part of one horn may appear as a separate entity.

The inferior (temporal) horn of the lateral ventricle extends into the temporal lobe from the fourth part of the central part of the lateral ventricle. This is the largest compartment of the lateral ventricle. It curves round the posterior aspect of the thalamus (pulvinar), passes downwards and posterolaterally and then curves anteriorly to end within 2.5 cm of the temporal pole, near the uncus (Switka et al., 1999; Crossman, 2008).

It corresponds to the superior temporal sulcus. The floor of the ventricle consists of the hippocampus medially and the collateral eminence, formed by the infolding of the collateral sulcus, laterally.

Superiorly, the inferior horn is formed mainly by the tapetum of the corpus callosum, the tail of the caudate nucleus, and the stria terminalis which runs forward to end in the amygdaloid body (Switkaetal, 1999; Mc Lone, 2004).

The temporal extension of the choroid plexus fills this fissure and covers the outer surface of the hippocampus.

The choroid plexus of each lateral ventricle is invaginated along a curve line known as the choroid fissure.

The fissure extends from the interventricular foramen in front and arches over the posterior end of the dorsal thalamus, as far as the end of the temporal horn. The choroid plexus of the lateral ventricle is only in the central part of the lateral ventricle and the temporal horn (Strazielle and Ghersi-Egea, 2000).

At the junction of the central part with the temporal horn it is best developed and is there known as the glomus choroideum.

Calcified areas (corpora amylacea) are frequent in the glomus.

The vessels of the plexus originate from the internal carotid (anterior choroidal artery) and from the posterior cerebral (posterior choroidal arteries).

At the interventricular foramina, the choroid plexuses of both lateral ventricles become continuous and then join that of the third ventricle.

Third ventricle

The third ventricle is a narrow cleft unilocular, located in the center of head, below the corpus callosum and the body of the lateral ventricle; above the sella turcica, pituitary gland, and midbrain; and between the cerebral hemispheres, thalami, and the walls of the hypothalamus (Rhoton, 1987). Over a variable area, the thalami are frequently adherent to each other at the interthalamic adhesion (massa intermedia). This interthalamic adhesion varies in size, and the thalamus and hypothalamus create minor differences in the lateral walls of the third ventricle.

It communicates at its anterosuperior margin with each lateral ventricle through the foramen of Monro and posteriorly with the forth ventricle through the aqueduct of Sylvius. It has an anterior, a roof, a floor, a posterior, and two lateral walls.

Anterior wall

The anterior part of the third ventricle extends from the foramina of Monro, above, to the optic chiasma below, which crosses its floor.

The part of the anterior wall visible on the surface is formed by the optic chiasma and the lamina terminalis. The optic chiasma is a major modifier of the floor of the third ventricle because its size and location affect the size and configuration of the optic and infundibular recesses. The optic recess seems to be a residual space on the floor of the third ventricle of which formation, shape, and size are the result of the varying indentation of the ventricular floor by the chiasma (Yamamoto et al., 1981).

The lamina terminalis is a thin sheet of gray matter and pia mater that attaches to the upper surface of the chiasma, to the anterior commissure and to the rostrum of the corpus callosum.

The lamina terminalis forms the roof of the small virtual cavity lying immediately below the ventricle called the cistern of the lamina terminalis.

Above this, the anterior wall is formed by the diverging columns of the fornices and the anterior commissure.

When viewed from within, the boundaries of the anterior wall from superiorly to inferiorly are formed by the columns of the fornix, foramina of Monro, anterior commissure, lamina terminalis, optic recess, and optic chiasma. The anterior commissure is a compact bundle of myelinated nerve fibres that cross the midline in front of the columns of the fornix. The diameter of the anterior commissure varies from 1.5 to 6.0 mm. The distance from posterior end of the anterior commissure to the anterior border of the foramen of Monro range from 1.0 to 3.5 mm (Yamamoto et al., 1981). The foramen of Monro on each side is located at the junction of the roof and the anterior wall of the third ventricle. The foramen is a ductlike canal that opens between the fornix and the thalamus into the lateral ventricle and extends inferiorly below the fornix into the third ventricle as a single channel. The foramen of Monro is bounded anteriorly by the junction of the body and the columns of the fornix and posteriorly by the anterior pole of the thalamus (Rhoton, 1987). The structures that pass through the foramen are the choroid plexus, the distal branches of the medial posterior choroidal arteries, and the internal cerebral, thalamostriate, superior choroidal, and septal vein.

Roof. A thin layer of ependyma covered by pia mater forms the thin roof of the third ventricle. Above the roof is the body of the fornix. The body forms a gentle arch located between the roof of the third ventricle and the floor of the body of each lateral ventricle.

The upper layer of the anterior part of the roof of the third ventricle is formed by the body of the fornix, and the posterior part of the roof is formed by the crura and the hippocampal commissure. The septum pellucidum is attached to the upper surface of the body of the fornix.

According to Yamamoto et al. (1981), anteroposterior length of the septum pellucidum varied from 28 to 50 mm. The tela choroidea forms two of the three layers in the roof below the layer that is formed by the fornix.

The roof has four layers: one neural layer formed by the fornix, two thin membranous layers of tela choroidea, and a layer of blood vessels between the sheets of the tela choroidea (Rhoton, 1987; Rhoton, 2002).

The final layer in the roof is a vascular layer located between the two layers of tela choroidea. The vascular layer consists of the medial posterior choroidal arteries and their branches and the internal cerebral veins. The internal cerebral veins arise in the anterior part of the velum interpositum, just behind the foramen of Monro, and they exit the velum interpositum above the pineal body to enter the quadrigeminal cistern and join the great vein (Rhoton, 1987).

The velum interpositum is the space between the two layers of the tela choroidea.

The cleft between the lateral edge of the fornix and the superomedial surface of the thalamus is called the choroidal fissure. The choroid plexus of the lateral ventricle is attached along this fissure.

Floor. The floor of the third ventricle extends from the optic chiasma anteriorly, to the orifice of the aqueduct of Sylvius posteriorly.

When viewed from inferiorly, the structures forming the floor from anterior to posterior include the optic chiasma, the infundibulum of the hypothalamus, the tuber cinereum, the mammillary bodies, the posterior perforated substance, and (most posteriorly) the part of the tegmentum of the midbrain located above the medial aspect of the cerebral peduncle (Rhoton, 1987; Rhoton, 2002).

There is a small angular, optic recess at the base of the lamina terminalis, just dorsal to and extending into the optic chiasma. Behind it, the anterior part of the floor of the third ventricle is formed mainly by hypothalamic structures. Immediately behind the optic chiasma lies a thin infundibular recess, which extends into the pituitary stalk. The posterior part of the floor extends posterior and superior to the medial part of the cerebral peduncles and superior to the tegmentum of the midbrain.

Posterior wall. The posterior wall of the third ventricle extends from the suprapineal recess above, to the aqueduct of Sylvius below. Thus, the posterior boundary of the third ventricle is marked by a suprapineal recess above the pineal gland, which extends into the pineal stalk, by the habenular commissure, by the pineal gland, by the posterior commissure, and by the aqueduct of Sylvius. The habenulae are small eminences on the dorsomedial surfaces of the thalamus just in front of the pineal gland. The habenulae are connected across the midline in the rostral half of the stalk of the pineal gland by the habenular commissure (Rhoton, 2002).

The suprapineal recess projects posteriorly between the upper surface of the pineal gland and the lower layer of tela choroidea in the roof.

The shape and size of the suprapineal recess are related to the size of the corpus callosum. The increasing size of the splenium, as seen from the cat and monkey, is associated with a concomitant reduction of the suprapineal recess. The habenular commissure, which interconnects the habenulae, crosses the midline in the cranial lamina, and the posterior commissure crosses in the caudal lamina.

Because of the development of the neocortex and the relative unimportance of olfaction, the habenulae are the smallest.

The position of the anterior and posterior commissures are used as the basic reference points for stereotaxic surgical procedures.

Lateral wall. The walls of the third ventricle are hidden between the cerebral hemispheres. The upper part of the lateral wall is formed by the medial surface of the anterior two-third of the thalamus, and the lower part is formed by the hypothalamus anteriorly and the subthalamus posteriorly.

Hypothalamic sulcus between the interventricular foramen and the cerebral aqueduct marks the boundary between the thalamus and hypothalamus. The superior limit of the thalamic surfaces of the third ventricle is marked by narrow, raised ridges, known as the striae medullaris thalami.

The massa intermedia projects into the upper one-half of the third ventricle and often connects the opposing surfaces of the thalamus. It was present in 76% of the brains examined and was located 2.5 to 6.0 mm posterior to the foramen of Monro (Yamamoto et al., 1981; Rhoton 1987, 2002).

The columns of the fornix form distinct prominences in the lateral walls of the third ventricle just below the foramen of Monro, but inferiorly they sink below the surface.

The third ventricle presents several recesses: (1) the optic recess superior to the chiasma; (2) the infundibular recess in the infundibulum of the neurohypophysis; (3) a less well-defined recess rostral to the mammillary bodies; (4) the pineal recess in the stalk of the pineal body; (5) the suprapineal recess (Augustine, 2008).

Aqueduct of Sylvius

The aqueduct of Sylvius is a small tube in the midbrain, 1-2 mm in diameter and about 1 cm in length. It extends throughout the dorsal quarter of the midbrain in the midline, is widest in its central part, is surrounded by the gray matter and connects the third and fourth ventricle. The superior and inferior colliculi are dorsal to aqueduct and the midbrain tegmentum is ventral. Rostrally it commences immediately behind and below the posterior commissure.

Caudally, it is continuous with the lumen of the fourth ventricle at the junction of the midbrain and pons.

Fourth ventricle

The fourth ventricle is a romboid shaped space in the hindbrain who lies between the brain stem and the cerebellum. Rostrally (superiorly) it is narrow becoming continuous with the cerebral aqueduct (of Sylvius), and caudally (inferiorly), it narrows into the central canal of the medulla oblongata (obex), which, in turn, is continuous with the central canal of the spinal cord (Fig. 22.1). The ventricle is, at its widest, at the level of the pontomedullary junction, where a lateral recess on both sides extends to the lateral border of the brain stem. In the widest part of the ventricle, on either side, it has two openings, the right and left foramina of Luschka and a single median foramen of Magendie.

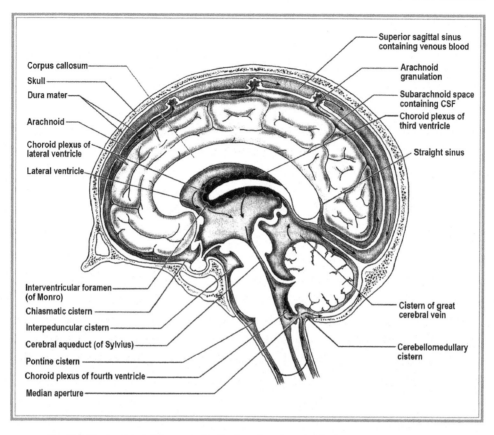

Fig. 21.1. Hemisected skull demonstrating the flow of cerebrospinal fluid in the ventricle of the brain and the subarachnoid spaces (after Patestas and Gartner, 2008).

All three foramina permits cerebrospinal fluid to leave the ventricular system and enter the subarachnoid space. The foramina of Luscha lead to the interpeduncular cistern, whereas the foramen of Magendie delivers the CSF into the cerebellomedullary cistern.

Floor of the fourth ventricle. The floor of the fourth ventricle is a romboid cavity on the dorsal surfaces of the pons and the rostral half of the medulla. It consists largely of grey matter and contains important cranial nerve nuclei.

The superior part of the ventricular floor is triangular in shape and is limited laterally by the superior cerebellar peduncles as they converge toward the cerebral aqueduct.

The inferior part of the ventricular floor is also triangular in shape and is bounded caudally by the gracile and cuneate tubercles, which contain the dorsal column nuclei, and more rostrally, by the diverging inferior cerebellar peduncles (Rhoton, 2010; Crossman, 2008).

A dorsal median sulcus divides the floor into right and left halves. Each half is it-sclf divided, by an often indistinct sulcus limitans, into a medial region known as the medial eminence and a lateral region known as the vestibular area. The vestibular nuclei lie beneath the vestibular area.

The medial eminence, an elevation on the floor of the fourth ventricle, extends the length of the pons and into the open medulla. In the caudal part of the pons, the medial eminence presents a swelling called the facial colliculus, a small elevation produced by an underlying loop of efferent fibres from the facial nucleus which covers the abducens nucleus. Between the facial colliculus and the vestibular area the sulcus limitans widens into a small depression, the superior fovea. In its upper part, a small region of bluish-grey pigmentation denotes the presence of the subjacent locus ceruleus.

Inferior to the facial colliculus, at the level of the lateral recess of the ventricle is the striae medullaris, which runs transversely across the ventricular floor (Rhoton, 2000).

The hypoglossal and vagal trigone are caudal to the facial colliculus and form the caudal part of the medial eminence at medullary levels.

Thus, in the inferior area of the floor of the fourth ventricle, the medial eminence is represented by the hypoglossal triangle (trigone), which lies over the hypoglossal nucleus. Laterally, the sulcus limitans widens to produce an indistinct inferior fovea. Caudal to it, between the hypoglossal triangle and the vestibular area, is the vagal triangle, which covers the dorsal motor nucleus of the vagus. The triangle is crossed below by a narrow translucent ridge, the funiculus separans, which is separated from the gracile tubercle by the small area postrema. They are both covered by ependyma, containing tanycytes and neurons (only area postrema) (Rhoton, 2000; Crossman, 2008).

The lowermost part of the floor of the fourth ventricle has the shape of the point of a pen (calamus scriptorius). Here are nuclei related to respiration, cardiovascular activity and the act of swallowing (deglutition) (Matsushima et al., 1982; Augustine, 2008).

Roof of the fourth ventricle. Sheets of white matter (the superior and inferior medullary vela) which are lined by ependyma and which stretch between both superior and inferior cerebellar peduncles form the roof of the fourth ventricle. The superior medullary velum is continuous with the cerebelar white matter and is covered dorsally by the lingula of the superior vernis (Rhoton, 2000).

The inferior medullary velum formed by ventricular ependyma and the pia mater of the tela choroidea, presents a deficiency, the median aperture (foramen Magendie), just inferior to the nodule of the cerebellum.

CSF flows through this foramen into the *cisterna magna* (Matsushima et al., 1982; Barshes et al., 2005). The ends of the lateral recesses have similar openings, the lateral apertures. These, are not well-defined openings but rather gaps between the cerebellum and medulla oblongata with choroid plexus protruding through them. By turning fila of the glossopharyngeal and vagal nerves medially, one is able to see the choroid plexus projecting through the lateral aperture immediately inferior to the flocculus (Barshes et al., 2005; Augustine, 2008). The choroid plexus of the fourth ventricle invaginates into the roof of the ventricle on either side of the median plane. A prolongation of each plexus protrudes through the corresponding lateral aperture.

The vessels to the plexus arise from cerebellar branches of the vertebral and basilar arteries. The choroid plexus of the fourth ventricle is T-shaped, with vertical and horizontal limbs but the precise form varies widely. The vertical (longitudinal) limb is double, flanks the midline and is adherent to the roof of the ventricle.

The horizontal limbs of the plexus project into the lateral recesses of the ventricle. Small tufts of plexus pass through the foramina of Luschka and emerge, still covered by the ependyma, in the subarachnoid space of the cerebellopontine angle (Rhoton, 2000; Mc Lone, 2004; Crossman, 2008). The blood supply of the fourth ventricular choroid plexus is from the inferior cerebellar arteries.

Capillaries drain into a rich venous plexus served by a single choroidal vein.

The vascular pia mater in the roofs of the third and fourth ventricles and in the medial wall of the lateral ventricle along the line of the choroid fissure, is closely opposed to the ependymal lining of the ventricles, without any intervening brain tissue.

It forms the tela choroidea, which gives rise to the highly vascularized choroid plexuses from which CSF is secreted into the lateral, third and fourth ventricles.

The body or stroma of the choroid plexus consists of many capillaries, separated from the subarachnoid space by the pia mater and choroid ependymal cells (Strazielle and Ghersi-Egea, 2000; Crossman, 2008).

Production of the cerebrospinal fluid (CSF)

A major advance in localizing the site of CSF was made by Dandy in 1918 when he made extirpation of the choroid plexus of the lateral ventricle in communicating hydrocephalus and in 1919 when he completed a crucial experiment by stenosing both foramina of Monroe and performing a unilateral choroid plexectomy in a single dog. After the observing that the ventricle without choroid plexus collapsed, while the opposite ventricle expanded greatly, it was initially thought that the sole source of CSF was localized to the choroid plexus (Du Boulay et al., 1972).

Currently it is believed that while the choroid plexus is an important site of CSF production, other significant sources exist. They include the ependyma and the brain parenchyma (Fishman, 1992). Indeed, it has been estimated that approximately 30% of CSF is produced by the ependyma (Milhorat, 1975).

CSF is secreted at a rate of 0.35-0.40 ml per minute, which means that normally about 50% of the total volume of CSF is replaced every five to six hours (Zakharov et al., 2004).

The total CSF volume is approximately 150 ml, of which 125 ml is intracranial. The ventricles contain about 25 ml, most lying within the lateral ventricles, and the remaining 100 ml is located in the cranial subarachnoid space (Greitz, 2004).

Until Cushing's paper The Third Circulation, in 1925, most had ascribed the idea that CSF moved with an "ebb and flow" movement, an idea begun by Magendie, 100 years before (Milhorat, 1975). Modern radiological technique confirmed the notion that CSF does indeed circulate (Du Boulay et al., 1972; Ohara et al., 1988; Stoodley et al., 1997).

CSF flows from the lateral ventricles to the third ventricle *via* the paired interventricular foramina of Monroe, and then through the cerebral aqueduct to the fourth ventricle. CSF leaves the fourth ventricle through the medial and lateral apertures (foramina of Luschka) to enter the subarachnoid space of the cisterna magna and the subarachnoid cisterns over the front of the pons respectively (Notle, 1993).

Many different routes are possible once the CSF has reached the cisterna magna. The fluid may travel: superiorly toward the cerebellar hemispheres to the ambient cistern; anterosuperiorly toward the interpenduncular and interchiasmatic cistern; anteriorly toward the premedullary, prepontine, and cerebellopontine cistern; or inferiorly toward the spinal subarachnoid space. CSF in the spinal subarachnoid space posterior to the spinal cord and dentate ligaments is directed in the caudal direction. The overall direction of fluid ventral to the spinal cord is in the cephalad direction; therefore, returning the CSF to the basilar cisterns (Milhorat, 1975).

The movement of CSF in the subarachnoid space is complex and is characterized by a fast flow component and a much slower bulk flow component. During systole, the major arteries lying in the basal cisterns and other subarachnoid spaces dilate significantly and exert pressure effects on the CSF, causing rapid CSF flow around the brain and out of the cranial cavity into the upper cervical vertebral canal.

The flow of CSF is propagated by the cardiac cycle. The pulsation of the arterial system transmits pulsation to the brain parenchyma, the choroid plexus, and the large arteries at the skull base (Ohara et al., 1988). The volumetric displacement of the CSF increases with low diastolic pressure and low systolic pressure (Barshes et al., 2005).

Perhaps the smallest contribution is from the outpouring of new CSF and the ciliary beating of the ventricular ependyma. The pressure gradient across the arachnoid villi also contributes to the bulk flow of CSF *via* the creation of a pressure gradient. The mean CSF pressure in the brain is 150 mm saline while the pressure in the superior sagittal sinus in 90 mm saline (Milhorat, 1975).

The amplitude of the CSF pulsations is also affected by the respiratory cycle, the resistance of outflow created by the arachnoid villi, the mean intracranial pressure, and the compliance of the cranial and spinal cord cavities (Fujii et al., 1980; Ohara et al., 1988).

Pulsations of 10-30 mm H_2O and 20-30 mm H_2O in amplitude are seen at particular points in the respiratory and cardiac cycles, respectively, with isovolumetric measurements in the lumbar CSF (Fujii et al., 1980).

The amplitude of pulsations in the cisterna magna is 50 mm H_2O while that of the lumbar fluid is 30 mm H_2O) (Fishman, 1992).

According to Duboulay et al. (1972), an average of 0.1 mL CSF was displaced from the third ventricle during each systole; in comparison to 1.0 mL in the basal cisterns and 0.64 mL in the cisterna magna.

Thus, radiographic studies in humans have shown that pulsations throughout the neuraxis lead to the "pumping" of CSF and that various areas of the brain and spinal cord provide varying contribution to the pumping activity (Ohara et al., 1988; Stoodley et al., 1997).

CSF absorption. CSF is absorbed into the venous system by active diffusion into cerebral capillaries which occurs as a result of the interstitial pressure differential.

Other routes of absorption exist, including the ependyma, the leptomeninges, and the lymphatics of the spine (Milhorat, 1975). The driving forces for absorption of CSF have been attributed to the gradient in both hydrostatic and colloid osmotic pressures between the protein-free CSF in the arachnoid villi and the venous spaces (Barshes et al., 2005).

CSF function. The CSF does act to support as cushion elements in the central nervous system. The CSF acts to lessen the apparent weight of the brain to approximately 4% of this mass (Burt, 1993).

The CSF appears to have a function at least partially analogous to that of lymphatics in other organs – namely, removing fat-soluble and toxic substances from the brain's extracellular fluid. Many fat-insoluble molecules are also removed from the brain extracellular fluid by the circulation of CSF including urea, albumin, homovanillic acid, and norepinephrine (Milhorat, 1975).

The "internal milieu" of the brain may be regulated by exclusion of large and polar molecules from the CSF and also by modification of the CSF by capillary-glial complexes, epithelia, and neurons themselves (Fishman, 1992).

The CSF may also function as a mechanism of intracerebral transport for biogenic amines which initiate the secretion of pituitary hormone release factors. Tanycytes appear to have a role in this function (Milhorat, 1975).

Tanycites are found in clusters in the walls of the third ventricle and cerebral aqueduct, in floor of the fourth ventricle, and in the cervical spinal canal. Clusters of tanycytes are often associated with circumventricular organs, namely the median eminence, the area postrema, the subcommissural organ, and the pineal gland (Peters et al., 1991).

In contrast to the ependymal cells, tanycytes have many microvilli and few cilia. These cells have three portions: a somatic portion, a neck portion, and a tail portion with end-feet which course through the hypothalamus to contact fenestrated blood vessels or pial surfaces (Fishman, 1992).

Fixed macrophages are also present in the arachnoid border layer. These cells are sometimes referred to as Kolmer or epiplexus cells when associated with the choroid plexus. They contain many membrane-bound inclusions and variable vacuoles; they lack cytoplasmic processes (Peters et al., 1991).

Composition of CSF. The fact that the CSF is isosmotic in comparison to the plasma suggests that water freely equilibrates between the two fluid compartments (Fishman, 1992). The composition of CSF compared to that of plasma is presented in Table 22.1.

Thus, CSF is not simply a protein-free dialysate of the plasma but rather a true secretion requiring energy for its production.

According to Barshes et al. (2005), the secretion of CSF is dependent upon the active transport of sodium which is performed by a choroid epithelial sodium-potassium activated ATPase. The in vivo inhibition of choroid plexus fluid formation by ouabain, an inhibitor of this ATPase, support the idea that CSF is a secretion. This ATPase and other transport enzymes are responsible for the transport of other ions and micronutrients into the CSF. Small amounts of protein are transported into CSF mainly by pinocytosis (Barshes et al., 2005).

Table 22.1

**Normal Composition of Cerebrospinal Fluid and Serum
(adapted from Fishman, 1992)**

	CSF	Serum (arterial)
Osmolarity (mOsm/L)	295	295
Water content (%)	99	93
Sodium (mEq/L)	138	138
Potassium (mEq/L)	2.8	4.5
Chloride (mEq/L)	119	102
Bicarbonate	22.0	24.0
Phosphorus (mg/dL)	1.6	4.0
Calcium (mEq/L)	2.1	4.8
Magnesium (mEq/L)	2.3	1.7
Iron (g/dL)	1.5	15.0
Urea (mmol/dL)	4.7	5.4
Creatinine (mg/dL)	1.2	1.8
Uric acid (mg/dL)	0.25	5.50
CO_2 tension (mmHg)	47.0	41.0
*p*H	7.33	7.41
Oxygen (mmHg)	43.0	104.0
Glucose (mg/dL)	60.0	90.0
Lactate (mEq/L)	1.6	1.0
Pyruvate (mEq/L)	0.08	0.11
Lactate: pyruvate ratio	26.0	17.6
Proteins (mg/dL)	0.035	7.0

Meninges

Three connective membranes that envelop the central nervous system are collectively known as the meninges. They provide support and protection for the delicate tissue they surround. Although the dura mater surrounding the brain is continuous with the dura mater surrounding the spinal cord at the level of the foramen magnum, it is customary to discuss the two separately.

Thus, separating the brain and spinal cord from the calcified tissue are three more or less concentric membranes. The outermost, dense, irregular collagenous connective tissue is the dura mater or **pachimeninx.**

The innermost connective tissue membrane is the **pia mater**, the thin translucent membrane, adherent to the surface of the brain and spinal cord, which accurately follows every contour. The middle spiderweb-like is a delicate layer of reticular fibres, the **arachnoid.**

The pia mater and arachnoid collectively are called the **leptomeninges** and are separated from one another by the subarachnoid space.

Cranial dura mater

The cranial dura mater is a thick, dense, opaque, fibrous coat which incompletely divides the cranial cavity into compartments and accommodates the dural venous sinuses. It is predominantly acellular, and consists mainly of densely packed fascicle of collagen fibres arranged in laminae which run in different directions, producing a lattice-like appearance.

The cranial dura mater has two layers, on **outer periosteal dura mater** (endosteal layer) that is attached to the internal table of the diploe and acts as a true periosteum, and an **internal meningeal dura mater** that is in intimate contact with the arachnoid.

There is little histological difference between endosteal and meningeal layers. Both contain fibroblasts, and the endosteal layer also contains osteoblasts. Focal calcification may occur in the falx cerebri.

The periosteal dura mater firmly adheres to the inner aspect of the cranial bones, especially at the sutures and along the base of the skull. The meningeal and periosteal layers serve both meningeal and periosteal function.

Thus, the space external to the cranial dura, the epidural space, is a potential space.

Studies of the fine structure of the dura-arachnoid interface layer in humans reveal that the innermost part of the cranial dura and the outermost part of the arachnoid are intimately fused. However, there is a potential space between the meningeal layer of the cranial dura mater and the cranial arachnoid, known as the subdural space, that, according to some neuroanatomists, is occupied by an extremely thin film of fluid.

The periosteal and meningeal layers of the dura mater are tightly attached to each other throughout much of their extent. The dura mater forms reflections upon itself, some of which contain **dural venous sinuses.**

The periosteal dura mater is a coarse type of connective tissue composed of dense irregular collagenous connective tissue interlaced with some elastic fibres.

It is especially firmly attached at the sutures, cranial base, and around the foramen magnum.

At the foramina of the skull the periosteal dura mater forms a connective tissue sheath around the cranial nerves as they leave the skull and this dural layer is quickly replaced by the epineurium derived from the extracranial connective tissue. The endosteal layer is continuous with the pericranium through the cranial sutures and foramina and with the orbital periosteum through the superior orbital fissure. The dural sheath of the optic nerve is continuous with the ocular sclera. The dura fuses with adventitia of major vessels, such as the internal carotid and vertebral arteries, at sites where they pierce it to enter the cranial cavity (Standring, 2008).

The innermost aspect of the meningeal layer of the dura mater, composed of dense irregular collagenous connective tissue, is lined by a single layer of flattened fibroblasts that form epithelioid sheet that is in direct contact with and separates the arachnoid from, the collagenous connective tissue component of the meningeal dura.

Reflections of the meningeal layer of the dura mater

The meningeal layer of the dura mater give rise to several folds that divide the cranial cavity into compartments, or to separate parts of the brain from one another.

Thus, the meningeal layer of the dura is reflected inwards to form three folds, namely the falx cerebri, falx cerebelli, and tentorium cerebelli that partially divide the cranial cavity into compartments.

Additionally, this meningeal layer forms a diaphragm over the hypophysial fossa, known as the diaphragm sella and Meckel's cave (cavum trigeminale).

Falx cerebri. The largest of these folds is the sickle-shaped fax cerebri which extends in the midline from the crista galli to the internal occipital protuberance. Falx cerebri occupies the longitudinal fissure between the two cerebral hemispheres. The crescent is narrow in front, and broad behind where it is attached to the superiors surface of the tentorium cerebelli. The superior, convex surface of the falx cerebri is attached to the periosteal layer of the dura, leaving only a narrow, endothelial lined channel, the superior sagittal sinus. The inferior border that is free but concave in shape follows the shape of the corpus callosum.

The layers of the falx along the convex border divide to accommodate the superior sagittal sinus whereas those along the concave border divide to accommodate the inferior sagittal sinus.

The superior sagittal sinus begins just behind the crista galli, at the foramen cecum, and terminates posteriorly at the confluence of sinuses. At the junction where the falx cerebri joins and fuses with the tentorium cerebelli is another endothelial lined space, the **straight sinus**, that receives blood from the inferior sagittal sinus and the great cerebral vein. Blood from the straight sinus also enters the confluence of sinuses.

Tentorium cerebelli. The tentorium cerebelli, a horizontal reflection of the meningeal layer of the dura mater, is interposed between the cerebellum and the occipital lobes of the cerebrum. It divides the cranial cavity into supratentorial and infratentorial compartments, which contain the forebrain and hindbrain respectively. Anteriorly, the lateral aspect of the tentorium is attached to the superior surface of the petrous portion of the temporal bone and forms endothelially lined spaces, the right and left superior petrosal sinuses, and continues anteriorly to attach to the posterior clinoid processes of the sphenoid bone. The tentorium forms a large part of the floor of the middle cranial fossa, and fills much of the gap between the ridges of the petrous temporal bones. On both sides, the rim of the tentorial incisures is attached to the apex of the petrous temporal bone and continues forward as a ridge of dura mater to attach to the anterior clinoid process.

This ridge marks the junction of the roof and the lateral part of the cavernous sinus.

The periphery of the tentorium cerebelli (attached to the superior border of the petrous temporal bone), crosses under the free border of the tentorial incisures at the apex of the petrous temporal bone, and continues forward to the posterior clinoid processes as a rounded, indefinite ridge of the dura mater.

The angular depression between the anterior parts of the peripheral attachment of the tentorium and the free border of the tentorial incisure is part of the roof of the cavernous sinus (Standring, 2008).

The free and concave anterior edge of the tentorium forms the **tentorial incisure,** the only opening between the supratentorial and infratentorial components. This tentorial incisure or match is filled by the midbrain and the anterior part of the superior aspect of the cerebellar vermis and permits the ascent of the posterior cerebral arteries to reach the cerebral hemisphere. The convex outer limit of the tentorium is attached posteriorly to the lips of the transverse sulci of the occipital bone and to the posterior-inferior angles of the parietal bones, where it encloses the transverse sinuses.

Laterally, it is attached to the superior borders of the petrous parts of the temporal bones, where it contains the superior petrosal sinuses.

The lateral borders of the tentorium cerebelli extend much further anteriorly than does its midline.

The superior surface of the central region is convex. The layers of the tentorium along the convex border divide to accommodate the transverse sinus.

The compartment inferior to the tentorium contains not only the cerebellum but also the pons and medulla oblongata.

Falx cerebelli. The falx cerebelli, a relatively small reflection of the meningeal layer of the dura lies below the tentorium and attaches to the inferior aspect of the tentorium in the median plane and to the internal occipital crest. This small midsagittal septum partially separates the cerebellar hemispheres.

The posterior margin of the falx cerebelli contains the occipital sinus and is attached to the internal occipital crest. The apex of the falx cerebelli frequently divides into two small folds, which disappear at the sides of the foramen magnum.

Diaphragma sella. The diaphragma sella is a thin reflection of the meningeal layer of the dura mater over the pituitary fossa, which is perforated by the infundibulum (Rhoton, 2002).

This fourth dural projection is circular in shape, forming a roof over the sella turcica and covering its content.

The lateral aspect is attached to the clinoid processes. The anterior and posterior edges of the diaphragma sella house the anterior and posterior intercavernous sinuses. The infundibulum and pituitary stalk pass into the pituitary fossa through a central opening in the diaphragma.

Cavum trigeminale (Meckel's cave). The cavum trigeminale is a narrow, slit-like region interposed between the periosteal and meningeal layers of the dura mater positioned on the trigeminal impression of the petrous portion of the temporal bone. It is occupied by the trigeminal ganglion as well as by the sensory and motor roots of the trigeminal nerve (Patestas and Gartner, 2008).

Vascular and nerve supply. The periosteal layer of the dura mater is richly supplied by blood vessel, whereas the meningeal layer has no vascular supply. The blood vessels of the periosteal layer include the middle meningeal and accessory meningeal arteries of the middle cranial fossa, as well as the meningeal branches of the anterior and posterior etmoidal arteries and meningeal branches of the internal carotid artery of the anterior cranial fossa. Meningeal branches of the vertebral, occipital, middle meningeal, and ascending pharyngeal arteries serve the periosteal dura of the posterior cranial fossa. Blood is drained from the dura by meningeal veins that empty their blood into several of the sinuses as well as into nearby emissary veins and diploic veins. The diploic veins are large, thin-walled vessels that occupy chanels in the diploe of the cranial bones. Four main trunks are usually described; these are the frontal, anterior or posterior temporal, and occipital diploic veins.

Sinus pericranii is a rare condition involving congenital or acquired anomalous connections between an extracranial blood-filled nodule and an intracranial dural venous sinus *via* dilated diploic and / or emissary veins of the skull (Sheu et al., 2002).

Emissary veins traverse cranial apertures and make connections between intra-cranial venous sinuses and extracranial veins. These connections are of clinical significance in determing the spread of injection from extracranial foci to venous sinuses, for example, the spread of infection from the mastoid to the venous sinuses or from the paranasal sinuses to the cavernous sinus (Browder and Kaplan, 1976; Kaplan and Browder, 1976; Ozveren et al., 2002).

Innervation of the cranial dura mater

Sensory nerve supply of the cranial dura mater derived mostly form cranial nerve V (trigeminal nerve) but also from the first three cervical spinal nerves, and the cervical sympathic trunk.

Less well-established meningeal branches have been described arising from the vagus and hypoglossal nerves and possibly from the facial and glossopharyngeal nerves.

In the anterior cranial fossa, the dura is innervated by meningeal branches of the anterior and posterior ethmoidal nerves and anterior filaments of the meningeal rami of the maxillary (nervus meningus medius) and mandibular (nervus spinosus) divisions of the trigeminal nerve. The nervus spinosus re-enters the cranium through the foramen spinosum with the middle meningeal artery. The nervus spinosus contains sympathic postganglionic fibres from the middle meningeal plexus.

Intraoperative mechanical stimulation of the falx may trigger the trigeminocardic reflex (Bauer et al., 2005).

The dura in the posterior cranial fossa is innervated by ascending meningeal branches of the upper cervical nerves which enter through the anterior part of the foramen magnum (second and third cervical nerves) and through the hypoglossal canal and jugular foramen (first and second nerves).

Meningeal branches from the vagus apparently start from the superior vagal ganglion and are distributed to the dura mater in the posterior cranial fossa. Those from the hypoglossal leave the nerve in its canal and supply the diploe of the occipital bone, the dural walls of the occipital and inferior petrosal sinuses, and much of the floor and anterior wall of the posterior cranial fossa. Sensory nerve endings are restricted tot the dura mater and cerebral blood vessels, and are not found in either the brain itself, or in the arachnoid or pia mater. Stimulation of these nerve endings causes pain and is the basis of certain forms of headache (Standring, 2008).

Leptomeninges and CSF space

The term leptomeninges refers to the inner two of the three membranous layers which envelop the brain: the arachnoid membrane and the pia mater.

The prefix **lepto-**, denoting "fine" or "thin" in Greek, contrast of the pachymeningeal layer called the dura mater (Nolte, 1993).

Whereas the dura mater and pia mater have been described since the time of the Egyptians some 3000 years ago, the arachnoid mater was not clearly distinguished as a separate layer until the work of the Dutch anatomist Gerardus Blaes in 1666 (Bakay, 1991).

The term arachnoid was applied by the Dutch anatomist Frederick Ruysch (1638-1731), the name roughly meaning "spider-like" and referring to the web-like structure of these layers (Sanan, van Loveren, 1999).

Key and Retzius (1875) made a landmark contribution to the anatomy of these layers.

Cranial arachnoid

The arachnoid is a delicate nonvascular membrane between the dura and pia mater which passes over the sulci without following their contours. Ultramicroscopic examination of the arachnoid has revealed two components making up this layer: an outer layer, often referred to as the **arachnoid barrier cell layer**; and an inner layer, often referred to as the **arachnoid trabeculae**.

The arachnoid barrier cell layer is a layer of two to three tiers of flattened cells. These cells have a large, oval- to spindle-shaped nucleus, multiple cytoplasmic processes, scant mitochondria, small rough endoplasmic reticulum and a poorly developed Golgi apparatus (Nabeshima et al., 1975; Oba and Nakanishi, 1984; Haines and Frederickson, 1991).

A basement membrane underlies the arachnoid barrier cell layer and separated this layer from the underlying subarachnoid space (Haines and Frederikson, 1991). Numerous zonulae occludens (tight junctions), zonulae adherens and macula adherens (desmosomes) are found interconnecting cells of this layers. These connections function as the meningeal barrier, which excludes proteins and other large molecules from diffusing from the blood to the CSF in the subarachnoid space (Nabeshima et al., 1975; Haines and Frederikson, 1991, Peters et al., 1991).

Thus, the intravascular introduction of dyes will stain the dura but not the underlying meningeal layers, the CSF or the brain parenchyma (Nabeshima et al., 1975).

Occasional intercellular connections (viz. desmosomes) also exist between the cell of the arachnoid barrier cell layer in the cranium and the overlying dura.

From the arachnoid surface trabeculae, known as arachnoid trabeculae, extends toward and attach to the external surface of the pia mater.

Trabeculae, traverse the subarachnoid space from the deep layer of the arachnoid mater to the pia mater, as thin, web-like chordae. Each trabecula has a core of collagen which is coated by leptomeningeal cells. In the meshes of the arachnoid trabeculae (subarachnoid space), cerebrospinal fluid circulates. The cells of the trabecular layer have smaller nuclei, abundant mitochondria, and well-developed Golgi apparatuses and rough endoplasmatic reticulum (Oba and Nakanishi, 1984). Extracellular collagen fibrils are found outside of the cells in this layer (Nabeshima et al., 1975). Gap junctions often connect cells within the arachnoid trabecular layer. The extensive gap junction allow the arachnoid cells to function together to allow the passage of small molecules from cell to cell (Peters et al., 1991).

The trabeculae that cross the subarachnoid space may form compartments, particularly in the perivascular region, which may facilitate directional flow of CSF throughout the subarachnoid space.

The subarachnoid space therefore contains CSF, the larger arteries and veins which traverse the surface of the brain. These arteries and veins in the subarachnoid space are coated by a thin layer of leptomeninges, often one cell thick.

Cranial and spinal nerves that traverse the subarachnoid space, to pass out of cranial or intervertebral foramina, are coated by a thin layer of leptomeninges which fuses with the arachnoid at the exit foramina. Blood vessels from the vascular meninges perforate the arachnoid to reach the pia mater. However, each vessel is completely surrounded by arachnoid fibroblasts and, therefore, the vessels never actually enter the subarachnoid space.

Scanning electron microscopy, however, has revealed that the pia actually surrounds the vessels as it travels through the subarachnoid space but does not accompany the vessel as it descends into the brain parenchyma. Instead, the pia surrounding the vessel spreads out over the pia which is covering the surface of the brain, effectively occluding the perivascular space from the subarachnoid space (Hutchings and Weller, 1985). Thus, the Virchow-Robin space communicates with the brain extracellular space rather than the subarachnoid space.

The subarachnoid space who lies between the arachnoid and pia mater is connected with the fourth ventricle of the brain by the median aperture (foramen of Magendie), and by the paired lateral apertures (foramina of Luschka). Foramen of Magendie provides communication with the cisterna magna, and foramina of Luschka open into the subarachnoid space at the cerebellopontine angle, behind the upper roots of the glossopharyngeal nerves.

Structurally and functionally, arachnoid barrier layer prevents cerebrospinal fluid in the subarachnoid space from reaching the dura.

Arachnoid cisternae

In certain areas of the brain, the arachnoid completely diverges from the pia mater, forming expanded subarachnoid spaces known as subarachnoid cistern. These more expansive spaces identified as subarachnoid cisterns, are continuous with each other through the general subarachnoid space.

As CSF percolates through the subarachnoid spaces it also enters the subarachnoid cisterns, filling them.

The largest cistern, the **cisterna magna** is formed between the caudal aspect of the cerebellum and the dorsal surface of the medulla oblongata, as the arachnoid stretches across these two structures rather than following the contour of the brain. The cistern is continuous above with the lumen of the fourth ventricle through its median aperture, the foramen of Magendie, and below with the subarachnoid space of the spinal cord.

The pontine cistern is a much smaller space than the cisterna magna. It is located along the ventral surface of the pons and communicates with the subarachnoid space of the spinal cord caudally, and rostral to the pons, with the interpeduncular cistern.

The basilar artery runs through the pontine cistern into the interpeduncular cistern.

The interpeduncular cistern is located between the right and left cerebral peduncles and receives CSF by way of the two lateral foramina of Luschka, from fourth ventricle. Anteriorly, the interpeduncular cistern extends to the chiasmatic cistern, frequently, the two are considered to be a single cistern, the cisterna basalis, even though the optic chiasma is interjected between them.

The cistern of the lateral fossa is formed by the arachnoid as it bridges the lateral sulcus between the frontal, parietal, and temporal opercula. It contains the middle cerebral artery.

The cisterna ambiens (superior cistern) or the cistern of the great cerebral vein is located in the vicinity of the superior aspect of the cerebellum, the corpora quadrigemina, and the pineal body. This superior cistern lies posterior to the brain stem and third ventricle, and occupies the interval between the splenium of the corpus callosum and the superior cerebellar surface.

The great cerebral vein traverse the superior cistern, and the pineal gland protrudes into it.

Several smaller cisterns have been described, including the **prechiasmatic** and **postchiasmatic** cistern, which are related to the optic chiasma, and the **cistern of the lamina terminalis** and the **supracallosal cistern,** all of which are extension of the interpeduncular cistern and contain the anterior cerebral arteries.

The subarachnoid space also extends through the optic foramen into orbit where it is bounded by the optic nerve sheath. The latter is formed by fusion of the arachnoid and dura mater, and surrounds the orbital position of each optic nerve as far as the back of the globe, where the dura fuses with the sclera of the eye.

For the carotid bifurcation aneurysms, the entire carotid-ophthalmic and carotid cisterns must be opened, as well as the cisterns surrounding the proximal A1 and M1 arteries.

Arachnoid granulations and villi

Arachnoid granulations were first illustrated by Vesalius in 1543 who observed their imprint on the inner surface of the skull. In 1705, Pacchioni described the structures, but mistakenly thought that they were lymph nodes which irrigated the meninges.

In 1853, Faivre is accredited with correctly proposing that the granulations serve to drain CSF.

Arachnoid granulations are small, but visible mushroom-shaped evagination of the arachnoid protruding into the lumen of the dural sinuses (Fig. 22.2).

Arachnoid villi and arachnoid granulations differ in term of size and complexity. Villi are macroscopic structures that are present in the superior sagittal sinus of the fetus and newborn infant. Granulations are visible to the naked eye by the age of 18 months in the parieto-occipital region of the superior sagittal sinus, and by age of 3 years in the laterally located sinuses of the posterior fossa. They increase in number and size with increasing age, and become more lobulated and complex, and may become calcified, when they are known as Pacchionian bodies. The name Pacchionian granulations has been used to refer to large, elaborate arachnoid granulations in horses and in man (Wolpow and Schaumburg, 1972).

These outpushing of the arachnoid mater and subarachnoid space through the wall of dural venous sinuses, very often are located close to points where veins enter the sinus.

Thus, most of the arachnoid granulations are associated with lacunae lateralis, diverticula of the superior sagittal sinus, although some just into the lumen of the sinus.

At the base of each arachnoid granulation a thin **neck** of arachnoid mater projects through an aperture in the dural lining of the venous sinus and expands to form a core of collagenous trabeculae and interwoven channels.

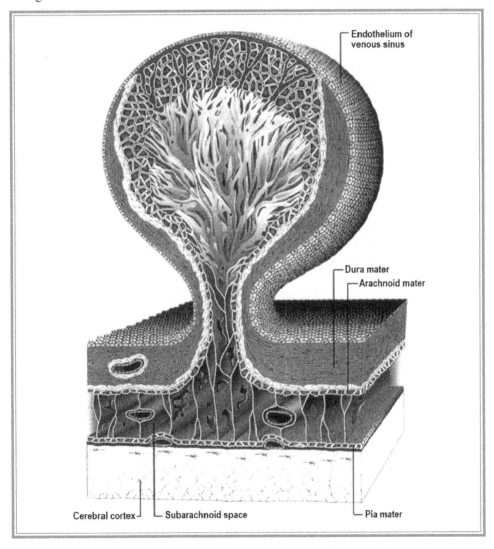

Fig. 22.2. An arachnoid granulation (Modified). Morphology of CSF drainage pathways in man (Raimond, ed, Kida and Weller, 1994).

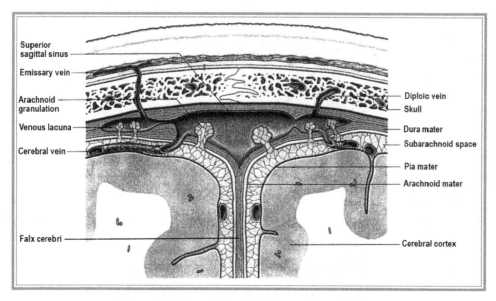

Fig. 22.3. Coronal section through the vertex of the skull to show the relationships between the superior sagittal sinus, meninges and arachnoid granulations (adapted from Drake, Vogl and Mitchell, 2005).

The core of an arachnoid granulation, composed of arachnoid trabeculae, is continuous with the subarachnoid space and is surrounded by the epithelioid layer of the arachnoid and of the dura, forming a membrane that is two cell layer thick.

As the arachnoid granulation evaginates into the lacuna lateralis, it is invested by some cellular and collagenous elements of the meningeal dura mater, which in turn is surrounded by the endothelial lining of the blood vessel (Patestas and Gartner, 2008).

The core is surmounted by an **apical cap** of arachnoid cells, some 150 μm thick (Fig 22.2). Channels extend through the cap to reach the subendothelial regions of granulation. The cap region of each granulation is attached to the endothelium of the sinus over an area some 300 μm diameter, whereas the rest of the core of the granulation is separated from the endothelium by a fibrous dural cupola (Kida and Weller, 1994).

The arachnoid granulation are most prominent along the margins of the great longitudinal fissure, commonly in the lateral lacunae of the superior sagittal sinus, and also protruding directly into the lumen of the sinus (Fig. 22.3).

These leptomeningeal structures are often thought of as one-way valves from the CSF compartment to the venous compartment. They are commonly called arachnoid villi, when microscopic, or arachnoid granulation, when macroscopic.

According to Yamashima (1988), the functional ultrastructure of the human **arachnoid villi** was studied to clarify drainage channels of cerebrospinal fluid. The apical portion of each villus was usually covered by the arachnoid cell layer alone with no endothelial investment, whereas most of the stromal central core was further encompassed by a fibrous capsule with an endothelial investment. According, the CSF-blood interface was assumed to be in both the endothelial cells and the arachnoid cell layer. The former were characterized by abundant micropinocytotic vesicles and occasional intracyto-plasmatic vacuolis, whereas the latter was characterized by numerous extracellular cisterns measuring 10 micron in maximal diameter. There were no free communications such as endothelial open junctions or endothelium-lined tubules. In the villi affected by subarachnoid hemorrhage, endothelial cells were intact and continuous despite the erythrocyte packed subendothelial space, which appeared to be on the verge of rupturing. Intracytoplasmic vacuoles, measuring less than 1 micron diameter, sometimes contained serum protein-like substance. It is conceivable that, in human arachnoid villi, the extracellular cisterns of the arachnoid cell layer contribute to the passive transport of CSF, whereas micropinocytosis and vacuolization mechanisms of the endothelial cells are availed for active transport (Yamashima, 1988).

The function of arachnoid granulation remains controversial. It has long been thought that CSF from the subarachnoid space enters into the core of the arachnoid granulation and from there penetrates, probably by osmosis, the epithelioid layers of the arachnoid granulation and the endothelial lining, to escape into the lacuna lateralis.

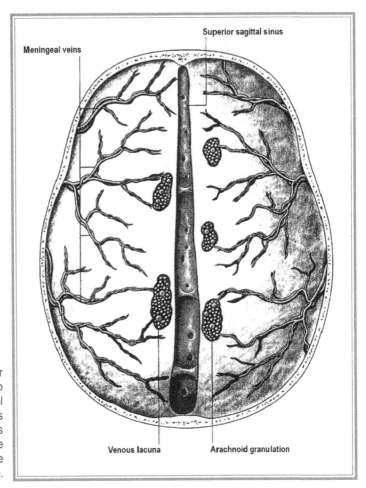

Fig. 22.4. The superior sagittal sinus opened up after removal of the cranial vault. Note the fibrous bands that cross the sinus from two of the venous lacunae (after Standing, 2008).

Meningeal veins

Superior sagittal sinus

Venous lacuna

Arachnoid granulation

Studies of Kida and Weller (1994), Greitz (2004) and Zakharov et al. (2004), have shown that CSF may also be resorbed throughout the ventricles and subarachnoid space, through the walls of pial and subarachnoid vessels. Moreover, there is a growing body of experimental evidence that significant volumes of CSF may be absorbed into extracranial lymphatics in animals. It has been suggested that extracranial lymphatics play a major role in CSF reabsorption at relatively low pressures, but that other routes, including arachnoid granulations, become increasingly important as CSF pressure rises.

A connection between parenchymal interstitial fluid and extracranial lymphatics in humans has yet to be convincingly demonstrated (Crossman, 2008).

Therefore, the function of the arachnoid granulations is transporting CSF manu-factured by the choroid plexuses of the ventricles of the brain into the vascular system.

Cerebrospinal fluid acts as a fluid buffer for the protection of the central nervous system. Cerebrospinal fluid also compensate for changes in blood volume in the cranium, allowing the cranial contents to remain at a constant volume.

No one element of the cranial contents (brain, blood or cerebrospinal fluid) can increase, except at the expense of the other (Monroe-Kellie doctrine).

It is important to note that although the arachnoid granulations protrude into the venous sinuses, they are always separated from the blood by the endothelial lining of the dural sinus / lacuna lateralis (Kida and Weller, 1994) (Fig. 22.4).

Pia mater

This vascular membrane is composed of: (1) an inner membranous layer, the intima pia (Key and Retzius, 1875), and (2) a more superficial epipial layer. The intima pia, adherent to underlying nervous tissue, follows its contours closely and is composed of fine reticular and elastic fibres. Where blood vessels enter and leave the central nervous system, the intima pia is invaginated forming a perivascular space.

The intima pia, like the arachnoid, is avascular and derives its nutrients by diffusion from the cerebrospinal fluid and the underlying nervous tissue (Millen and Woollam, 1961, 1962). The epipial layer is formed by a meshwork of collagenous fibre bundles continuous the arachnoid trabeculae. Cerebral vessels lie on the surface of the intima pia within the subarachnoid space.

However, the cranial pia mater is the most delicate layer of the cranial meninges, which closely invests the surface of the brain, from which it is separated by a microscopic subpial space. It follows the contours of the brain into concavities and the depths of fissures and sulci. The cranial pia also lines the basal cistern.

The cranial pia mater is composed of a single layer (or, occasionally, two layers) of attenuated fibroblasts that form a transparent epithelioid membrane that closely invests the contours of the brain (Patestas and Gartner, 2008).

Since the pia mater is vascular, it has numerous blood vessels associated with it; however, because this is so, thin vessels are in part surrounded by cells derived from the arachnoid trabecular and, in part, by cells of the pia mater. Deep to the epithelioid sheath is a thin, discontinuous layer of collagen and elastic fibres. The end-feet of the astrocytes form a protective layer that underlies this subpial extracellular matrix, separating it from the neural tissue (Kida and Weller, 1994; Patestas and Gartner, 2008). The cell of the pia mater are modified fibroblasts similar to the cells of arachnoid membrane. Their morphology is often undistinguishable from that of the arachnoid cells (Cloyd and Low, 1974; Peters et al., 1991).

According to Kida and Weller (1994) and Crossman (2008), pia mater is formed from a layer of leptomeningeal cells, often only 1 to 2 cells thick, in which the cells are joined by desmosomes and gap junctions but few, if any, tight junctions. The cells are continuous with the coating of the subarachnoid trabeculae and separated from the basal lamina of the glia limitans by bundles of collagen and fibroblasts-like cells, and the arteries and vein that lie in the subpial space (Fig. 22.5).

The intimal layer of pia is an avascular layer. In contrast to the overlying epipial layer, it is adherent to the brain throughout all its contours. It has been proposed that the vascular epipial layer represents the contribution of mesenchyme to the pia, while the avascular intimal layer represents the contribution of the neural crest (Millen and Woollam, 1961).

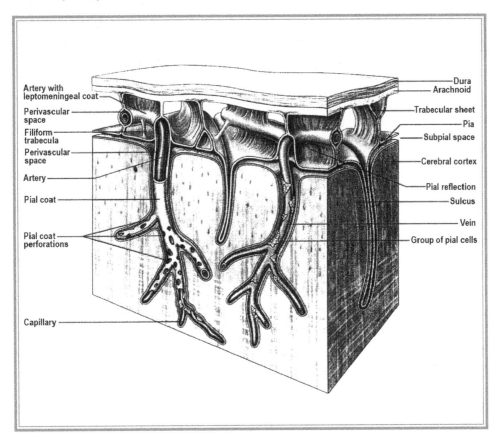

Fig. 22.5 The relationships between the dura, the leptomeninges and the blood vessels that enter and leave the cerebral cortex. The subarachnoid space is divided by trabeculae (after Crossman, 2008).

The cranial arachnoid trabeculae join the pia to the arachnoid mater. Although very thin and apparently fragile, cranial pia nonetheless exhibits a high level of stiffness, thus influencing the mechanical properties of the brain. The cerebral vessels that are in the subarachnoid space have a superficial covering of the cranial pia. Smaller vessels ramify on the pia before penetrating the brain (Barshes et al., 2005). Thus, pia mater is reflected from the surface of the brain onto the surface of the blood vessels in the subarachnoid space, which means that the subarachnoid space is separated by a layer of pia from the subpial and perivascular space of the brain (Nicholas and Weller, 1988).

Interrelationships of the pia mater and the perivascular (Virchow-Robin) spaces in the human cerebrum was studied by Zhang et al. (1990).

In addition to separating the subarachnoid space from the brain tissue, the pia mater also serves to degrade neurotransmitter substances and to prevent material in the subarachnoid space from entering the nervous tissue, as evidenced by the inability of erythrocytes to cross the pia mater in case of subarachnoid hemorrhage (Barshes et al., 2005; Patestas and Gartner, 2008).

Thus, despite its delicate nature, the pia mater appears to form a regulatory interface between the subarachnoid space and the brain. Pial cells contain enzymes such as catechol -O- methyltransferaze and glutamine synthetaze (which degrade neurotransmitters), they also exhibit pinocytotic activity and ingest particles up to 1 in diameter.

A subpial space of variable thickness exists between the pia and the basement membrane of the glial limitans (outer glial layer of the brain and spinal cord). This space contains collagen fibrils (Cloyd and Low, 1974). Pial cells are often joined to arachnoid trabecular cells with desmosomes (Haines and Frederikson, 1991).

REFERENCES

Augustine JR, *Human Neuroanatomy. An introduction*. Academic Press. Amsterdam. Boston. Heidelberg etc., 393-404, 2008.

Bakay L, Discovery of the arachnoid membrane. Surg Neurol 36; 63-68, 1991.

Barshes N, Demopoulos A, Engelhard HH, Anatomy and physiology of the leptomeninges and CSF space. Cancer Treat Res 125; 1-16, 2005.

Bauer DF, Youkilis A, Schenck C et al., The falcine trigeminocardiac reflex: case report and review of the literature. Surg Neurol 63; 143-148, 2005.

Born CM, Meisenzahl EM, Frodl T et al., The septum pellucidum and its variants. A MRI study. Eur Arch Psychiatry Clin Neurosci 254; 295-302, 2004.

Browder J, Kaplan HA, *Cerebral Dural Sinuses and their Tributaries*. Springfield, Illinois: Thomas, 1976.

Burt AM, Textbook of Neuroanatomy. Philadelphia: WB. Saunders Co, 1993.

Cloyd MW, Low FN, Scanning electron microscopy of the subarachnoid space in the dog. J Comp Neurol 153; 325-368, 1974.

Crossman AR, Neuroanatomy, In: S Standring (ed), *Gray's Anatomy*. Fortieth Edition. UK. Churchill Livingstone Elsevier, 223-394, 2008.

Cushing H, Discussion. AJR 13; 10-11, 1925.

Dandy WE, Extirpation of the choroid plexus of the lateral ventricles in communicating hydrocephalus. Ann Surg 68; 569-579, 1918.

De Boulay G, O'Connel J, Currie J et al., Further investigating on the pulsatile movements in the cerebrospinal fluid pathway. Acta Radial 13; 496-523, 1972.

Faivre E, Observations sur les granulations méningiennes ou glandes de Pacchioni. Ann Sci Natl (Zool) 3rd ser; 20: 321-333, 1853.

Fishman RA, *Cerebrospinal Fluid in Diseases of the Nervous System*. Philadelphia: WB. Saunders Co, 1992

Fujii K, Lenkey C, Rhoton AL Jr, Microsurgical anatomy of the choroid arteries: Lateral and third ventricles. J Neurosurg 52; 165-188, 1980.

Greitz D, Radiological assessment of hydrocephalus: new theories and implications for therapy. Neurosurg Rev 27; 145-165, 2004.

Haines DE, Frederikson RG, The Meninges. In Al-Mefty O. Meningiomas. New York, Raven Press, 9-25, 1991.

Hutchins M, Weller RO, Anatomical relationships of the pia mater to cerebral blood vessels in man. J Neurosurg 65; 316-325, 1985.

Kaplan HA, Browder J, Neurosurgical consideration of some features of the cerebral dural sinuses and their tributaries. Clin Neurosurg 23; 155-169, 1976.

Kawashima M, Li X, Rhoton AL Jr et al., Surgical approaches to the atrium of the lateral ventricle: microsurgical anatomy. Surg Neurol 65; 436-445, 2006.

Key A, Retzius G, Studien in der Anatomie des Nervensystems und des Bindegewebes. Samson und Wallin, Stockholm, 1875.

Kida S, Weller RO, Morphology of CSF drainage pathways in man. In: A Raimondi (ed), *Principles of Pediatric Neurosurgery*. Vol 4. Berlin: Springer, 1994.

Matsushima T, Rhoton AL Jr, Lenkey C, Microsurgery of the fourth ventricle: Part 1. Microsurgical anatomy. Neurosurgery 11; 631-667, 1982.

Mc Lone DG, The anatomy of the ventricular system. Neurosurg Clin N Am 15; 33-38, 2004.

Millen JW, Woollam DHM, Observations on the nature of the pia mater. Brain 84; 514-520, 1961.

Millen J, Woollam DHM, *The Anatomy of the Cerebrospinal Fluid*. Oxford University Press, New York, 90-102, 1962.

Milhorat TH, The third circulation revisited. J Neurosurg 42; 628-645, 1975.

Nabeshima S, Reese TS, Landis DM, Brightman MW, Junctions in the meninges and marginal glia. J Comp Neur 164; 127-134, 1975.

Nicholas DS, Weller RO, The fine anatomy of the human spinal meninges. J Neurosurg 69; 276-282, 1988.

Nolte J, *The Human Brain: An introduction to its functional anatomy*. St. Louis: Mosby Year Book 33-47, 1993.

Oba Y, Nakanishi J, Ultrastructure of the mouse leptomeninx. J Comp Neur 225; 448-457, 1984.

Ohara S, Nagain H, Matsumoto T, Banno T, MR imaging of the CSF pulsatory flow and its relation to intracranial pressure. J Neurosurg 69; 675-682, 1988.

Ozveren MF, Uchida K, Aiso S, Kawase T, Meningovenous structures of the petroclival region: clinical importance for surgery and intravascular surgery. Neurosurgery 50; 829-836, 2002.

Pacchioni A, Dissertatio epistolaris de glandulis conglobatis durae meningis humanae, indeque ortis lymphaticis ad piam meningem productis Romae: typis Io. Francisci Buagni, Dissertatio 1705.

Patestas MA, Gartner LP, *A text book of Neuroanatomy*. Blackwell Publishing USA, 84-98, 2008.

Peters A, Palay SL, Webster H, *The Fine Structure of the Nervous System*. New York: Oxford University Press, 1991.

Rhoton AL Jr, The sellar region. Neurosurgery 51 (Suppl 1); 335-374, 2002.

Rhoton AL Jr, Microsurgical anatomy of the third ventricular region. In: MLJ Apuzzo (ed), *Surgery of the Third Ventricle*. Williams and Wilkins, Baltimore. London. Los Angeles. Sydney, 92-166, 1987.

Rhoton AL Jr, Cerebellum and fourth ventricle. Neurosurgery 17 (Suppl 3); 7-27, 2000.

Rhoton AL Jr, The foramen magnum. Neurosurgery 47 (Suppl 3); 155-193, 2000.

Rhoton AL Jr, The lateral and third ventricles. Neurosurgery 51 (Suppl 1); 207-271, 2002.

Sanan A, van Loveren HR, The arachnoid and the myth of Arachne. Neurosurgery 45; 152, 1999.

Sheu M, Fauteux G, Chang H et al., Sinus pericranii: dermatologic considerations and literature review. J Am Acad Dermatol 46; 934-941, 2002.

Standring S, Head and Neck. In S Standring (ed.), Gray's Anatomy. Fortieth Edition, Section 4. London UK, Churchill Livingstone Elsevier, 423-434, 2008.

Stoodley MA, Brown SA, Brown CJ, Jones NR, Arterial pulsation-dependent perivascular cerebrospinal fluid flow into the central canal in sheep spinal cord. J Neurosurg 86; 689-693, 1997.

Strazielle N, Gherzi-Egea JF, Choroid plexus in the central nervous system: biology and physiopathology. J Neuropathol Exp Neurol 59; 561-574, 2000.

Switka A, Narkiewicz O, Dziewiatkowski J, Morys J, The shape of the inferior horn of the lateral ventricle in relation to collateral and occipitotemporal sulci. Folia Morphol (Warsz) 58; 69-80, 1999.

Vesalius A, De humani corporis fabrica libri septem. Basel: Johannes Oporinus, 1543.

Wolpow ER, Schaumburg HH, Structure of the human arachnoid granulation. J Neurosurg 37; 724-727, 1972.

Yamamoto I, Rhoton AL Jr, Peace DA, Microsurgery of the third ventricle: Part I. Microsurgical anatomy. Neurosurgery 8, 334-356, 1981.

Yamashima T, Functional ultrastructure of cerebrospinal fluid drainage channel in human arachnoid villi. Neurosurgery 22; 633-641, 1988.

Zakharov A, Papaiconomou C, Koh L, et al., Integrating the roles of extracranial lymphatics and intracranial veins in cerebrospinal fluid absorption in sheep. Microvasc Res 67; 96-104, 2004.

Zhang ET, Inman CBE, Weller RO, Interrelationships of the pia mater and the perivascular (Virchow-Robin) spaces in human cerebrum. J Anat 170; 111-123, 1990.

Chapter 23

CEREBRAL ASYMMETRY
in nonhumans

Introduction

For many years it has been generally believed that lateralization of cerebral function was uniquely human characteristic and in fact arose on response to specifically human selective processes (Levy, 1969).

However, evidence of lateralization of functions has been documented in the brain of several animal species (Le May, 1977; Webster and Thurber, 1978; Nottebohm, 1981; Glick et al., 1982), and some studies (Denenberg, 1981; Glick et al., 1982) have brought into question the view (Warren, 1977) that the human pattern of cerebral laterality is "species unique".

In 1885, Ernest Mach postulated a mechanism of spatial behavior that applied to both man and beast. He recounted: "The idea that the distinction between right and left depends upon an asymmetry, and possibly in the last resort upon a chemical difference, is one which has been present to me from my earliest years". It was not until about nine decades later that the implications of Mach's idea were investigated. In 1873, Nothnagel found that injections of chromic acid into the striatum caused a bending of the trunk to the side of lesion (Wilson, 1914).

Ferrier (1876) stated that "irritation of the corpus striatum causes general muscular contraction on the opposite side of the body. The head and body are strongly flexed to the opposite side, so that the head and tail become approximated.

In 1921, Lashley described a rotation syndrome after combined unilateral destruction of caudate nucleus and the motor cortex above it.

"Circus" movements after "parietal and unsymmetrical injuries to the striatum" in rats were reported by Herrick in 1926.

Thus, when subjected to repeated testing with the same dose of a given drug, some animals rotate consistently to the left whereas others rotate to the right. It was further shown that nonlesioned, untreated rats also rotate at night (the more active half of their circadian cycle) and that this rotation is in the same direction as that induced by amphetamine (Glick and Cox, 1978).

Mach (1885) noted that "human being and animals that have lost their direction move, almost without exception, nearly in circle".

Behavioral and biological laterality is also ubiquitous in many nonhuman species, with many instances of asymmetry being at least analogous to asymmetries found in humans. At least some may also be homologous, in the sense of sharing common structures and developmental origins.

Motor asymmetries have been discovered for a number of species, with individuals sometimes showing very strong left-right preference. Furthermore, preference seems to depend on variables such as age and sex and on specific task demands. Despite these caveats, in several species of primates there tends to be left-hand preference for reaching and maintaining postural control but a right hand preference for manipulation and other skilled activities (Hellige, 2002).

According to Corballis (1997), in freely moving animals, there is strong evolutionary pressure for bilateral symmetry, in the placement of sense organs and limbs and those parts of the brain that are associated to them. This is so because such animals must be equally attentive to both sides of space and be able to move in a straight line.

For other systems, asymmetry may be favored in such cases as a way of packaging organs more efficiently into the body cavity or of packaging cognitive functions more efficiently into a brain whose size is limited.

Once an organism's brain becomes functionally asymmetric, additional asymmetries are likely to arise *via* the same kind of snow ball mechanism (Christman, 1997; Banich and Heller, 1998).

That is, some of the additional evolutionary adaptations are favored by the environment, with the result that those adaptations also become asymmetric.

This would occur regardless of whether the environment favored hemispheric asymmetry for a new adaptation. As this process is repeated, the extent of functional brain asymmetry increases (Hellige, 1993, 2002).

One of the most fundamental divisions of the human brain is that of the left and right cerebral hemispheres.

Numerous studies have revealed the consistent presence of both behavioral and anatomical asymmetries that reflect the specialized capacities of each hemisphere (Gazzaniga, 1970; Geschwind and Galaburda, 1985; Annett, 1985; Galaburda, 1991; Bogen, 1993). Apparently, the left and right hemisphere appear to be anatomically and biologically identical, leading one to wonder why there are so many functional asymmetries.

However, postmortem studies of anatomy and structural imaging studies of the living brain have documented a number of consistent physical asymmetries.

The ability to measure structure within the normal, living brain has made it possible to search for relationships between structural asymmetry and a variety of other nonmotoric behavioral and perceptual asymmetries, but no clear-cut picture has emerged.

Perhaps those structural characteristics revealed by contemporary imaging techniques are still relatively gross.

However, it should be noted that attempts to relate structural asymmetries to other dimensions, such as sex, psychopathology, and cognitive deficit, have produced mixed results.

Among other things, laterality in other species indicates that the emergence of language is not a prerequisite for the emergence of other behavioral and biological asymmetries. However, the various functional aspects of asymmetry correlate with each other weakly or not at all. The relative independence of different manifestations of asymmetry indicates that there are probably several different environmental influences to determine an individual's pattern of asymmetry. Thus, the asymmetry patterns that are characteristic of mature individuals are likely to be rooted in early stage of ontogenetic development.

Rogers (1997) has shown that it is possible to eliminate these population-level asymmetries by including the eggs in darkness and to reverse them by experimentally manipulating the embryo. Similar developmental scenarios might exist for humans.

Various possibilities have been suggested in humans, in which certain functional asymmetries could arise from the interaction of maturational asymmetries and changes in the nature of environmental stimulation.

By being more responsive to early environmental influences, the right hemisphere may become dominant for perceiving various nonphonetic sounds, for processing global properties of visual stimuli and for maintaining postural control.

In contrast, by being on a later developmental trajectory, the left hemisphere may be saved for complementary specialization that involves processing of more detailed or finer-grained information and sensorimotor feedback and control. In addition, other asymmetric growth spurts during childhood may provide a mechanism for the continuing unfolding of functional hemispheric asymmetry (Hellige, 2002).

Thus, there are indications that even in newborns there is a kind of left hemisphere dominance for speech perception and that activation of the left and right hemispheres is associated with positive and negative emotions, respectively.

According to Heilman (1997), the existence of hemispheric asymmetry for emotion has led to consideration of the possible relationship of laterality to psychopathology.

Among the more promising hypotheses is the idea that schizophrenia is related to dysfunction of an anterior region within the left hemisphere, an area that is believed to be important for language and for controlling parietal areas involved in attention. In a complementary way, depression has been linked to disturbances of the right hemisphere.

At the other end of the life span, it has been hypothesized that performance of the right hemisphere declines more rapidly in old age than does performance of the left hemisphere (Corballis, 1997; Christman, 1997; Beeman and Chiarello, 1998; Banich and Heller, 1998).

The seeds of laterality may be related to asymmetry in the molecules and particles of which all living things are constructed.

The existence of the left hand preference for visual guided reaching in present-day prosimians suggests that at least some type of motor asymmetry was present in our ancestral line by the time of our line branched from the prosimian line, nearly 60 million years ago (mya). This left-hand advantage extends to some species of Old World monkeys. In addition, some species of Old World monkeys show right hemisphere dominance for processing monkey faces and left hemisphere dominance for processing communicatively relevant vocalizations (Corballis, 1997; Christman, 1997; Banich and Heller, 1998; Hellige, 2002).

The similarity of these asymmetries to those of humans suggests that their precursors were present in our last common ancestors, approximately 40 mya (Corballis, 1997).

Asymmetry in rats

The phenomenon of rotation in normal rats was one of the first indications that normal animals may have an intrinsic asymmetry in nigrostriatal function that is accentuated by some drugs. Several experiments have been concerned with the general functional significance of nigrostriatal asymmetry revealed by the rotation studies. All results suggested that rotation is a stereotyped form of spatial behavior and that spatial tendencies are derived, at least in part, from a nigrostriatal asymmetry.

Comparison of rats having stronger or weaker directional biases showed that the strength of the biases was related generally to overall learning ability, as well as specifically to the ability to discriminate between left and right (Zimmerberg et al., 1978). Rats lacking clear spatial biases were hyperactive, had difficulty in learning a variety of tasks, and were unable to distinguish left from right.

Cerebral lateralization in the rat is clearly present at birth, changes during development, and is sexually dimorphic.

However, it is apparent that left- and right-sided rats differ behaviorally as well as neurochemically (Valdes et al., 1981). Behavioral and cerebral differences between left- and right-handed human beings are well documented. Whereas right-handed individuals almost always have left cerebral dominance, left-handed individuals have either right cerebral dominance, left cerebral dominance, or ambivalent dominance (Kolb et al., 1982).

It was generally observed that approximately 50% of rats rotated to the right and 50% to the left.

Because left frontal cortex was usually more active than right frontal cortex, the implication was that, in a large population, more rats should have right side preferences than left side preferences and right preferences should be greater than left preferences (Glick and Ross, 1981). These scientists reexamined the data accumulated for the past several years and determined that, in a group of 602 rats, there was small (54.8%) but significant ($p < 0.025$) right population bias; right-sided rats were also found to be both more active and have greater side preferences than left-sided rats (Glick and Ross, 1981).

Research with rats and chicks has also demonstrated asymmetry for emotional behaviors. For example, in both handled rats and chicks the right hemisphere tends to produce emotional activity, whereas the left hemisphere tends to inhibit emotional activity. In addition to providing interesting instances of laterality, effects such as these also illustrate the importance of reciprocal activity between the left and right sides of the brain (Rogers, 1997; Vallortigara, 2000).

Ross and Glick (1981) speculated that the increase in population bias in human being as compared with rodents is perhaps related to the evolution and growth of the cortex in relation to subcortical structures. The population bias would be expected to increase in parallel with phylogeny if the left - right asymmetry in cortex increased as the cortex became more convoluted in conjunction with an enhanced modulation of subcortical structures (e.g., striatum).

Differences in the neurotransmitters found in each hemisphere have also been associated with differences in hemisphere function (Glick et al., 1982; Direnfeld et al., 1984; Robinson and Starkstein, 2002; Berridge et al., 2003) and sex (Arato et al., 1991).

It has been hypothesized that the distribution of two important neurotransmitters is asymmetric in the human brain, with dopamine being more prevalent in the left hemisphere and norepinephrine being more prevalent in the right hemisphere.

These differences may have an evolutionary foundation, for they have been found in primates and other animals (Nottebohm, 1979; Geschwind and Galaburda, 1985; Corballis, 1991).

The lateralized size differential in primates is paralleled in some species by left lateralization for vocal communication (Mac Neilage, 1987).

Rossor et al. (1980) investigated directly the possibility of neurochemical symmetry in postmortem human brain. They measured concentration of three to five neurotransmitters in nine structures, both left and right sides, of normal brain; their primary goal was to learn whether left - right differences need consideration in comparisons of abnormal and normal brain. Because only one substance (GABA-gamma-aminobutyric acid) in one structure (substantia nigra) showed a left - right difference by a t test, it was concluded that neurochemical laterality, although still possibly a substrate for functional asymmetry, was unlikely to be an important consideration in such comparisons. Afterwards, data were eventually subjected to correlational analysis.

The results showed that human brain indeed has lateral asymmetries in several structures and transmitter systems (Glick et al., 1982).

There were several similarities between the human data and those previously reported in rats.

Thus, even though information on cerebral dominance was lacking in human beings it was clearly demonstrated that levels of ChAT (choline acetyltransferaze) and DA (dopamine) were higher in the left globus pallidus than in the right globus pallidus. Since most of the patients (N = 14) should have been right-handed pallidal ChAT and DA levels were obviously higher on the side contralateral to hand preference (Glick et al., 1982). Similarly, in rats striatal DA levels were higher on the side contralateral to side preferences (Zimmerberg et al., 1974).

The similarities between rat and human brains demonstrated that studies in the rat may reveal mechanisms and functions of brain asymmetry that are relevant to human beings.

In sum, studies in rats and mice focus on two rather different types of asymmetry.

The first emphasizes postural and motor asymmetries such as paw preference and direction of movement. Unlike handedness in humans, most postural asymmetries in rodents are random across the population.

The second type of lateralization in rodents is more interesting in the current context because it is seen in the population, much as we saw in birds.

As in humans, there is an asymmetry in the anatomy of the two cerebral hemispheres, with the right hemisphere being larger. In addition, the cortex of the right hemisphere is thicker, especially in the visual and posterior parietal regions, and this difference is modulated by hormones.

Male rodents have a greater difference than females.

Both prenatal stress and postnatal castration were shown to abolish the anatomical asymmetry in males, presumably owing to alterations in the normal hormonal environment (Stewart and Kolb, 1988, 1994).

Evidence is accumulating to support the conclusion that the hemisphere is specialized for the processing of species-specific calls.

The auditory asymmetry may represent a left-hemisphere advantage in the processing of rapidly changing acoustic stimuli. Claims that the right hemisphere is specialized for controlling emotional and spatial behavior remain speculative (Kolb and Whishaw, 2003).

The results of studies on nonhuman primates and rodents show that the increased aggression in males is probably a result of the male hormone testosterone both pre- and postnatally. Castrating infant male rats or monkeys decreases aggression and treating female with testosterone increases aggression (Kolb and Whishaw, 2003). Generally, men are physically more aggressive than women.

An intriguing asymmetry in rodents is an apparent lateralization of immune responses. So, lesions in the left hemisphere of mice, but not in the right, suppress T-cell function. The T-cell suppression may be due to lateralized control of the secretion of the specific hormones, such as prolactin. Whether similar asymmetries exist in the control of immune functions in humans is not yet known, although such asymmetry has been hypothesized by Kang et al. (1991).

Stress may alter anatomical asymmetries in the rat cortex, and many researchers have suggested that stress may also alter functional asymmetries.

Thus, Denenberg (1981) hypothesized that specific experiences might alter the two hemispheres differentially during development. So, Denenberg's results could be explained by the lateralized responses to various stress-related hormones, such as glucocorticoids.

Asymmetry in birds

In 1981, Nottebohm severed the hypoglossal nerve in canaries and found a severe disruption in the bird's song after left lesions but not after right ones. Subsequent work showed anatomical differences in the structure controlling birdsong in the two avian hemispheres and identified many song-related regions as sexually dimorphic.

Although a left hemisphere dominance for song has been shown in many species of songbirds (and even in chickens), it is not characteristic of all songbirds. Apparently, the zebra finch has little anatomical and functional asymmetry, even though it sings. It may be that the lateralization is not for singing itself but for some other still-unrecognized feature of bird vocalizations (Kolb and Whishaw, 2003).

Nottebohm's discovery led to interest in the possibility of asymmetry in the visual system of birds because the optic nerve of the most birds cross over almost completely at the optic chiasma. Thus, each hemisphere receives most input from a single eye. Furthermore, birds have no corpus callosum and, although other small commissures connect the hemisphere, there is less interhemispheric transfer in birds than in mammals.

According to Bradshaw and Rogers (1993), the right-eye system is specialized for categorizing objects, such as food *versus* nonfood items, whereas the left-eye system is specialized for responding to the unique properties of each stimulus (color, size, shape, and so forth), including topographical information. Thus, the left hemisphere of birds appears to be specialized for categorizing objects and the right for processing topographical information.

The result of research by Horn (1990) showed an asymmetry for memory formation in the chicken brain.

One curious asymmetry is in sleep. Birds spend much of their sleep time with only one hemisphere asleep, which presumably allows them to monitor the environment. On the other hand, it also means that there is a transient asymmetry in sensory processing, which might have significant implications for the animals. Kolb and Whishaw (2003) note parenthetically that unilateral sleep is also characteristic of cetaceans (whales, dolphins) and seals, a sensible adaptation in mammals that can drown.

In sum, lateralization takes many forms in the brain and is not a unique property of mammals.

Asymmetry in nonhuman primates

A trend in primate brain evolution is the shift of the Sylvian fissure from an almost vertical orientation to a more horizontal orientation. This shift implies an expansion of the parietal lobe, which pushes the Sylvian fissure low, usually in the left hemisphere. Thus, there is a greater upward slope in the Sylvian fissure in the right hemisphere in apes and Old-World monkeys. In addition, the right frontal lobe and left occipital lobe extend farther in the same species, again as in humans. So, there is an asymmetry in the Sylvian fissure (Mac Neilage et al., 1988; Kolb and Whishaw, 2003).

Bradshaw and Rogers (1993) concluded that the asymmetries in the language-related parietal and temporal lobe structure were not fully developed until the arrival of hominids. Contemporary chimpanzees show right-hand dominance for certain high-level tasks as well as left and right hemisphere dominance for processing communicatively relevant symbols and certain visuospatial tasks, respectively. Thus, it is possible that these asymmetries were present in the last common ancestors we shared with chimpanzees, appropriately 5 mya (Corballis, 1997). So, it is sufficiently plausible to suggest that some forms of hemispheric asymmetry were already present in our ancestral line before the first hominids emerged approximately 4 mya (Hellige, 2002).

Tool making and language are both forms of praxis and involve properties such as recursion, embeddedness, and generativity. Both gestural communication and vocalization also require sequences of precisely time movements. So, there may have been pressure for the same brain hemisphere to become dominant for those aspects of vocalization and language that are shared with tool making and gestural communication. Thus, the increased development of language-related structures in the posterior part of the brain is suggested to have occurred after the advent of hominids.

Studies in the 1977 by Warren unequivocally failed to find any systematic hand preference in rhesus monkeys, and he concluded that observed preferences are task dependent and are strongly affected by learning.

Afterwards, Mac Neilage et al. (1987) argued that, because earlier studies concentrated on particular types of movements, a hand preference in monkeys has been overlooked. Their basic premise is that primates evolved a preference for reaching with one limb (the left) while supporting the body with the other (the right). As the prehensile hand developed and primates began to adopt a more upright posture, the need for a hand used primarily for postural support diminished and, because this hand was free, it became specialized for manipulating objects. They later proposed that the hand specialization was accompanied by hemispheric specializations: a right-hemisphere (left-hand) perceptuomotor specialization for unimanual predation (grasping fast-moving insects or small animals) and a left-hemisphere specialization for whole-body movements.

A significant difficulty of this hypothesis is that studies of limb use in primates are hampered by poor control of myriad confounding factors including species, age, sex, task difficulty, learning, and sample size (Kolb and Whishaw, 2003). One objection to the theory is that cerebral asymmetry must precede handedness, and whether this asymmetry did indeed precede handedness and why it might have done so is not clear.

Hoster and Ettlinger (1985) trained 155 rhesus monkeys to make a tactile response in a task in which the subjects had to discriminate a cylinder from a sphere. The results showed that the 78 monkeys spontaneously using the left hand outperformed the 77 using the right hand. Thus, as in the humans, the right hemisphere outperformed the left one, suggesting an asymmetry.

Hamilton and Vermeire (1988) took a different approach. They taught 25 split-brain monkeys to discriminate two types of visual stimuli that have shown lateralization in humans. In one task, the animals had to discriminate between pairs of lines differing in slope by 15° (15° *versus* 30°, for example, or 105° *versus* 120°). For each pair, the more vertical line was designated as positive, and the monkey received a food reward for choosing it.

Most monkeys learned the line-orientation discriminations faster with the left hemisphere.

The second task required the animals to discriminate different monkey faces. The right hemisphere of most animals showed better discrimination and memory of the faces.

There was no hemispheric difference in making a simple discrimination of black-and-white patterns.

However, the line-orientation task appears to be one in which humans would show a right-hemisphere bias, rather than the left-hemisphere bias shown by the monkeys. At any rate, it is safe to conclude that there appears to be evidence in nonhuman primates of hemispheric specialization for the processing of different types of visual information. There is also evidence from primates that the two hemispheres may differ in their production of facial expressions. The number of facial expressions elicited from the right hemisphere was greater than the number made when using the left hemisphere, which is what one would predict from studies of humans.

In another study, Hauser (1993) found that the left side of the monkey's face began to display facial expression before the right, and it was more expressive. A similar result was reported for humans. Many studies look asymmetries in auditory perception.

Thus, Dewson (1977) removed the superior temporal gyrus (roughly equivalent to Wernicke's area in humans) in four rhesus monkeys, producing a lasting deficit on an auditory-visual task if the lesion was in the left hemisphere but not if it was in the right. The monkeys were required to press a panel that activated one of two acoustical stimuli, either a 1-kilohertz (kHz) tone or white noise. They were then presented with two panels, one green and one red. If the tone was heard, the monkeys pressed the red panel; if the white noise was heard, they pressed the green panel to receive the reward. Lesions on the left impaired performance of this task, but lesions on the analogous area on the right did not.

Petersen et al. (1978) compared the ability of Japanese macaques to discriminate between communicatively relevant sounds and irrelevant sounds. The animals could discriminate relevant sounds presented to the right ear better than those presented to the left. The researchers suggested that the Japanese macaques engage in the left-hemisphere processing in a way that is analogous to that in humans.

The results of a further study by Heffner and Heffner (1984) support this conclusion. However, with training, the animals with left temporal lesions were able to relearn the task. When the remaining side was later removed, the animal had a permanent deficit in the task and were unable to relearn it.

There are certain parallels between left hemisphere language dominance in human and asymmetries in other species for the production and perception of vocalization.

In Japanese macaque, the left hemisphere is dominant for the discrimination of species-specific vocalization that is relevant for communication but not for discrimination of other vocalization (Petersen et al., 1978; Rogers, 1997; Springer and Deutsch, 1998; Vallortigara, 2000). Also, chimpanzees that have been trained to use certain visual symbols to communicate, there is evidence of left hemisphere dominance for processing those symbols but not for processing other nonmeaningful symbols. There is evidence that the ultrasonic calls emitted by rat pups are processed preferentially by the left hemisphere of their mother and it is well-known that there is left-brain dominance for the control of song in some species of song birds (Hellige, 2000, 2002).

In language-trained chimpanzees, there is a right hemisphere advantage for processing the location of a line within a geometric figure and for identifying complex visual patterns that are not relevant for communication. In addition, rhesus monkeys have been reported to have right hemisphere superiority for recognizing monkey faces.

In rats, there is evidence that the right hemisphere may be more involved than the left hemisphere in spatial exploration, although the asymmetry emerges only in rats that have been handled during the course of their early development.

Pigeons and newly hatched chicks exhibit left hemisphere dominance for visual pattern discrimination. In chicks, this population-level bias occurs because light strikes only the right eye during a critical period of incubation during which the visual system is developing rapidly (Hellige, 1993; Provins, 1997; Rogers, 1997; Springer and Deutsch, 1998; Ivry and Robertson, 1998; Hellige, 2002).

Some biological asymmetries found in the human brain characterize the brain of certain primates, although the nonhuman asymmetries are smaller and less frequent than those of humans. For example, the brain of both humans and apes shows the kind of counterclockwise torque described earlier, and in chimpanzees as well as in humans, the Sylvian fissure tends to be longer on the left side than on the right side (Kosslyn, 1996; Hellige, 2002).

However, it is difficult to know which laterality effects in other species are truly homologous to the effects found in humans. Nevertheless, the presence of so many asymmetries in other species provides a useful range of animal models that can be used to learn about the development of laterality across the life span of an individual and across evolutionary time (Corballis, 1997; Provins, 1997; Rogers, 1997; Vallortigara, 2000; Hellige, 2002).

Handedness and functional asymmetry

People use the word sinister as a synonym for wicked or evil.

Originally a Latin word, meaning "left-hand side", the contemporary English meaning implies that left-handedness has been historically viewed at best as strange or unusual.

Thus, handedness refers to the fact that most people consistently use the same hand for task in which skill and dexterity are required and only one hand can be used.

Thus, a person who almost always uses his or her right hand when writing, throwing a ball, cutting with a knife, or using a hammer would be defined as being right-handed. Estimates of number of right-handers in the population are between 88 and 92% (Coren, 2002).

However, the handedness is only one aspect of a group of lateral biases.

In footedness, humans also show a right-sided bias, with approximately 80-82% of the population being right footed (Bishop, 1990; Springer and Deutsch, 1995).

Coren (1990, 2002) demonstrates eyedness by consistently choosing the same eye to right down a telescope or to peep through a small hole. They would be showing earedness by usually choosing the same ear to listen to the faint ticking of a clock or to press against a door to hear noises on the other side.

Thus, approximately 66-71% of the population is right-eyed, and 58-60% are right-eared.

Today, terms such as southpaw in baseball suggest an evolution of tolerance toward left-handers and in professional sports, even admiration (Kolb and Whishaw, 2003).

The most common cited statistics for left handedness in the general population is 10%, referring to the percentage of people who write with the left hand. But, when broader criteria are used, estimates range from 10% to 30%. The problem is that handedness is not absolute; some people are nearly totally left- or right-handed, whereas others are ambidextrous (that is, they use either hand with equal facility) (Annett, 1970). The evidence of left handedness on Annett's task varies from a low of about 6% when cutting with scissors to a high of about 17% when dealing cards.

The evolution of handedness

Some animals must manipulate something with only one paw, but the nature of human handedness is unique among mammallian species. Thus, most cats, rats, and monkeys are right- or left-pawed. Although individual animals show behaviors analogous to handedness, there is one major difference between these animals and humans. Whereas 9 of 10 humans are right-handed, in other species the proportion of right- and left-sided individuals is approximately 50%. In other words, there is no right-sided bias to the animal population (Coren, 1990, 2002).

It is possible to estimate the handedness of humans over history to determine if we were always right-handed.

Coren's study shows that examined paintings and drawings, reasoning that if artists were drawing from life, then they would draw the tools and weapons held by their models in the hand that they saw the person using (Coren, 2002). Analysis of more than 50 centuries of such drawings found that the proportion of right-handedness remained at approximately 90% from the Paleolithic Era (the Old Stone Age) until the present (Corballis, 1991; Coren, 2002). The date when right-handedness became dominant in our species can be pushed further back in time.

Language and tool use are among the critical milestones that set us apart from other species, and along with other milestone, such as walking upright, they are likely to have played an important role in the continued evolution of brain laterality (Corballis, 1991). An upright stance freed the hands from the need to provide postural support and minimized their use in locomotion. As a result, the hands were under less environmental pressure to be controlled in a symmetrical fashion.

The precursors of handedness in other primate species suggest that sufficient asymmetry already existed to produce a bias toward right-handedness for the more skilled aspects of movement. In fact, an analysis of the flaking patterns on stone tools manufactured by *Homo habilis* suggests that the majority of the population was already right-handed as far back as 1.5-2 mya.

Certain structural asymmetries, as longer left hemisphere Sylvian fissure, were also characteristic of the brains of *H. habilis* (Corballis, 1997; Hellige, 2002).

Thus, tool use and language seem to have interacted in a synergistic fashion to produce dramatic changes in human skull in the period from 10,000 to 30,000 years ago (Hellige, 2002).

Paleontologists have examined the wear patterns on stone tools and the grinding marks on devices used to grind grains.

These tools and implements date back between 8 000 and 35 000 BC and involve the early humanoid *Homo habilis*, one of the earliest tool makers. The wear patterns of these artefacts confirm that, even at that early date, there appeared to be a consistent predominance of right-handers. Perhaps the most astounding evidence derives from more than 1.5 million years ago, involving one of our very early hominid ancestors, Australopithecus (Corballis, 1991; Coren, 2002).

Although Australopitheciens were not tool makers, they were tool users and would pick up an appropriately sized and shaped rock or stick and use it for a weapon.

Examination of the skulls of baboons hunted by this early precursor to humans shows that the vast majority of these hominids were already right-handed (Corballis, 1991; Iacoboni and Zaidel, 2002; Coren, 2002).

Theories of hand preference

Environmental theories

Behavioral utility. Sometimes called the theory of the Peloponnesian Wars, or the sword-and-shield hypothesis, the behavioral theory proposes that a soldier who held his shield in his left hand better protected his heart and improved his chances of survival. Because the left hand was holding the shield, the right hand became more skilled at various offensive and defensive movements, and it was eventually used for most tasks. The mother, like soldier, used the free right hand for executing skilled movements (Kolb and Whishaw, 2003).

Environmental reinforcement. The child's world is right-handed in many ways, which reinforces the use of that hand. In addition, children in many countries, including the United Sates, have been forced to write with their right hands (Kolb and Whishaw, 2003). However, reinforcement theory also seems to be contradicted by what happened when children were given their choice of hand in learning to write: the incidence of left-hand writing rose to only 10%, which is the norm in most societies that have been studied (Kolb and Whishaw, 2003).

It should not be surprising that a technological and constructed environment created by a species in which 9 of 10 individuals are right-handed should have a bias toward use of the right hand.

Most tools, equipment, furniture and everyday implements such as scissors, gear shifts, in cream scoops, pencil, sharpeners, are biased toward right-handed usage.

Given this right bias to the environment, it is apparent that left-handers are forced to learn to do many things with their right hand that a right-hander would never be expected to do with his or her left hand. If there is a learned component to handedness, this should serve to greatly reduce the number of left-handers in the world (Coren, 2002).

The presence of approximately 10% of left-handers among humans is even more surprising due to direct cultural pressures to make the whole world right-handed. At some level, our society seems to intensely dislike left-handers and for proof one need go no further than our own language (Coren, 2002).

The very word "left" in English comes from the Anglo-Saxon word "lyft", which means "weak" or "broken".

Many common phrases in the English language demonstrate their culture's negative view of left-handedness.

For instance, a left handed compliment is actually an insult. In general, there is not one positive phrase to be found in the language regarding "left" or "left-handed" (Coren, 2002).

In French, the word for left is gauche, which also conveys the meanings "crooked", "ugly", "clumsy", "awkward", "uncouth", and "bashful". The German word for left-hand is links. The dictionary definition of the term linkisch is "akward, clumsy, and maladroit". Even in early Latin, in which the word for left was sinister, it had already taken on its alternate contemporary meaning of evil (Coren, 2002).

Culture and language

In many societies, use of the left hand for activities as eating or writing is considered impolite, insulting, or the sign of ill breeding. It is therefore not surprising that perhaps between 70% and 80% of the population of left-handers report that parents or teachers made over attempts to change them to right-handers. Some of these attempts could be quite brutal, involving punishment for using the left hand or even strapping or tying the left hand down to force right hand use (Coren, 1993; Springer and Deutsch, 1995; Coren, 2002).

What is most surprising about cultural pressure on handedness is that it has such a poor success rate. For female, 4 of 10 left-handers fail to change their handedness, whereas 3 of 4 males do not shift their handedness. Even for those who do change, the change appears to be only for selected actions, which society puts direct pressure on. Thus, a left-handed child may learn to eat or write with his or her right hand, but he or she will still throw a ball or brush his or her teeth with the left hand (Coren, 2002). Thus, handedness is not a causal learned set of behaviors. Handedness is determined early and is quite intractable to change.

Those who speak two or more languages may develop a different pattern of language organization from that of those who speak only one.

Uyehara and Cooper (1980) and Obler et al. (1982) support the idea that Asian and Native American languages may be represented more bilaterally in the brain than, for example, Spanish. Thus, inferring cultural differences in brain organization from the results of these studies should be done with caution.

Rapport et al. (1983) evaluate the language function of seven Chinese-English polyglots whose mother tongue was Malay, Cantonese or Hokkien. Their methods included the use of carotid sodium amobarbital, cortical stimulation, and clinical examination. They found that all these patients were left-hemisphere dominant for both Chinese and English languages: this was no consistent evidence of increased participation by the right hemisphere for language functions.

All language is probably located in the left hemisphere of bilingual people, but the possibility that their left-hemisphere language zones are enlarged or slightly different in microorganization from those who speak only a single language cannot be ruled out (Kolb and Whishaw, 2003).

However, the major effects of language and environment on the brain heavily depend on culture rather than on changes in cerebral asymmetry.

Exposure to multiple languages does not change the normal pattern of brain organization.

The results of PET studies by Klein et al. (1995, 1999) showed that no difference appears in the cerebral activation for various language tasks performed in English and French or English and Chinese by bilingual subjects. In particular, no activation of the right hemisphere was recorded for any task in either language. There may, however, be subtle differences in the cerebral representation of different languages within the left hemisphere.

Using fMRI, Kim et al. (1997) showed that languages acquired later in life may activate different, although adjacent, frontal regions from those activated by first languages or second languages acquired early in life.

Sensory or environmental deficits

Brain organization in nonhearing people. Educational and congenital deafness are alleged to alter hemispheric specialization. As for hearing people, left hemisphere damage produces aphasia in people who converse by using American Sign Language, possibly because of the praxic requirements. However, the congenitally deaf may have atypical patterns of cerebral organization (Kolb and Whishaw, 2003).

Several laboratories report independently that congenitally deaf persons fail to show the usual right-visual-field superiority in tasks of linguistic processing. These data could result from strategy differences due to absence of auditory experience (Kolb and Whishaw, 2003).

Neville (1977) reported that, during the perception of line drawing, visual evoked potential was significantly larger on the right in children with normal hearing and significantly larger on the left in deaf children who used American Sign Language to communicate.

There was no asymmetry at all in deaf children who could not sign but merely used pantomime to communicate. Neville (1977) inferred that the deaf signers acquire their visual signing symbols, much as hearing children acquire auditory verbal symbols, with the left hemisphere.

Thus, visuospatial functions may have developed in the left hemisphere of people who sign, producing an unexpected left-hemisphere effect.

So, absence of language experience somehow abolished certain aspects on cerebral asymmetry or that the expression of cerebral asymmetry depends on language experience.

Although congenital deafness may be suspected to affect the development of certain aspects of cerebral lateralization, the results of studies of brain-injured patients show little difference between hearing and nonhearing subjects.

Hickock et al. (2001) studied 34 congenitally deaf patients who had unilateral brain injury. Left-hemisphere patients performed poorly on all measures of language use, whereas right-hemisphere patients performed poorly on visuospatial tasks, exactly what would be expected in hearing people.

Environmental deprivation. According to Kolb and Whishaw (2003), an adolescent girl endured nearly 12 years of extreme social and experimental deprivation and malnutrition. She was discovered at the age of 13½ , after having spent most of her life isolated in a small closed room during which time she was punished for making any noise. After her rescue, Genie's cognitive development was rapid, although her language lagged behind other abilities.

Results of her dichotic listening tests showed a strong left-ear (hence right-hemisphere) effect for both verbal and nonverbal environmental sounds. The right ear was nearly totally suppressed. Genie's right hemisphere appeared to be processing both verbal and nonverbal acoustical stimuli, as would be the case in people with a left hemispherectomy in childhood (Kolb and Whishaw, 2003).

Probably, in the absence of appropriate auditory stimulation, the left hemisphere lost the ability to process linguistic stimuli. Another explanation is that Genie's left hemisphere was either being inhibited by the right hemisphere or by some other structure or it was performing other functions (Kolb and Whishaw, 2003).

Environmental accident. This theory postulates a genetically determined bias toward being right handed.

Left-handedness develops through a cerebral deficit caused by accident. This idea comes from correlating statistics on the incidence of the left-handedness and neurological disorders in twins. About 18% of twins are left handed, close to twice the occurrence in the population at large. Twins also show a higher incidence of neurological disorders, which are suspected to result overwhelmingly from intrauterine crowding during fetal development and stress during delivery (Kolb and Whishaw, 2003).

Bakan et al. (1973) argued for a high probability of stressful birth among left-handers, which increases the risk of brain damage to the infant and so maintains the statistical incidence of left handedness.

So, most deviation from the expected pattern of fetal development occurs because something has gone wrong during pregnancy or the birth process. For this reason, researchers began to focus on the handedness and birth stressors or pregnancy complications. Such pathological factors are associated with an increased likelihood of left-handedness.

These factors are premature birth, prolonged labor, Rh incompatibility, breech delivery, multiple birth, anoxia, cesarian delivery, and forceps or other instruments to assist the delivery. Thus, it is not surprising that older mothers (aged 40 and older), who are prime candidates for pregnancy and birth complications, are more than twice as likely to produce left-handed children (Bishop, 1990; Corballis, 1991; Springer and Deutsch, 1995).

Functional cerebral organization of left-handers

Left-handers can be subdivided into two genetic populations differing in cerebral organization: familial left-handers, who have a family history of left-handedness, and nonfamilial left-handers, who have no such family history. According to Hécaen and Sauguet (1971), the performance of nonfamilial left-handed patients with unilateral lesions is like that of right-handed patients on neuropsychological tests. In contrast, familial left-handers perform much differently, suggesting to Hécaen and Sauguet that they have a different pattern of cerebral organization.

Rasmussen and Milner (1977) found that, in left-handers, language is represented in the left hemisphere in 70%, in the right hemisphere in 15%, and bilaterally in 15%. Kimura (1999) reported the incidence of aphasia and apraxia in a constitutive series of 520 patients selected for unilateral brain damage only. The frequency of left-handedness in this population was within the expected range, and these patients did not have a higher incidence of either aphasia or apraxia than right-handers did. In fact, the incidence of aphasia in left-handed patients was approximately 70% of the incidence in right-handers, exactly what would be predicted from the sodium amobarbital studies. Thus, although a small proportion of left-handers have bilateral speech or right-hemisphere speech, the majority of left-handers do not (Kolb and Whishaw, 2003).

However, there is larger incidence of left-handedness among mentally defective children and children with various neurological disorders than it is found in the general population. Thus, it can be excepted by probability alone that right-handed children with left-hemisphere damage would switch to right-hemisphere dominance than in the reverse direction.

Anatomical theories

One anatomical theory attributes right-handedness to enhanced maturation and ultimately greater development of the left hemisphere.

Generalizing from assumption, the theory predicts that nonfamilial left-handers will show an asymmetry mirroring the right-handers, whereas familial left-handers will show no anatomical asymmetry (Kolb et al., 1982; Kolb and Whishaw, 2003).

However, no study has specifically considered anatomical asymmetry with respect to handedness or to familial history and handedness (Kolb and Whishaw, 2003).

Another theory have emphasized that many animals have a left-sided developmental advantage that is not genetically coded (Morgan, 1977).

For example, there is a left-sided bias for location of the heart, the size of the ovaries in birds, the control of birdsong, the size of left temporal cortex in humans, the size of the left side of the skull in the great apes, and so on (Morgan, 1977; Moscovitch, 1977). This predominance of left-favoring asymmetries puts the celebrated left-hemisphere speech dominance in the more general, structural perspective of all anatomical asymmetries (Moscovitch, 1977).

Because neither genetic evidence nor genetic theory accurately predicts these human asymmetries, Morgan (1977) assumes that they all result from some fundamental asymmetries in human body chemistry. Thus, Morgan's theory fails to explain left-handedness in the presence of other normal asymmetries such as the location of the heart (Kolb and Whishaw, 2003).

Hormonal theories

Geschwind and Galaburda (1987) proposed that brain plasticity can modify cerebral asymmetry significantly during early life, leading to anomalous patterns of hemispheric organization. A central factor in their theory is the action of the sex linked male hormone testosterone in altering cerebral organization during development.

Testosterone does affect cerebral organization; so it is reasonable to suggest that differences in testosterone level might influence cerebral asymmetry (Mc Glone, 1977, 1980).

Thus, while in the uterus, if the fetus is exposed to an elevated concentration of the hormone testosterone, this fact could produce left-handedness by altering the relative rate at which the two hemispheres of the brain develop. Since testosterone is also the male hormone, this could also explain the observation that men are more likely to become left-handed than are women (approximately 12% left-handedness for men *versus* 8% for women).

Geschwind and Galaburda (1987) suggested that testosterone's effect is largely inhibitory, meaning that higher-than-normal levels of testosterone will slow development, possibly acting directly on the brain or indirectly through an action on genes. Thus, testosterone's inhibitory action is largely in the left hemisphere, allowing the right hemisphere to grow more rapidly, which leads to altered cerebral organization and, in some people, to left-handedness.

Testosterone also affects the immune system, leading to more diseases related to a malfunctioning immune system (Gualtieri and Hicks, 1985).

Unfortunately, the bulk of available evidence does not support the model of Geschwind-Galaburda theory (Grimshaw et al., 1993; Bryden et al., 1994).

Although there is sufficient homogeneity there is also sufficiently reliable heterogeneity to warrant consideration of individual variation. Of particular interest has been the possible relationship of functional hemispheric asymmetry to a number of other between-subject factors including handedness, sex, intellectual ability and psychopathology.

Thus, hand dominance is determined by a variety of genetic and environmental factors, both before and after birth.

Environmental influences include pre- and postnatal trauma, prenatal levels of testosterone and other hormones (higher prenatal levels of testosterone are associated with greater incidence of left-handedness), asymmetric positioning of the fetus in the utero, as well as the biases of the postnatal world.

There are many effects of fetal hormone levels on brain development in other species and in humans there are clear relationships between biological sex and cognitive ability. For example, women tend to outscore men on tests of verbal fluency, and men tend to outscore women on tests of spatial ability. Thus, the incidence of left-handedness is slightly higher in men than in women, consistent with the hypothesis that higher levels of fetal testosterone promote development of the right hemisphere relative to the left hemisphere (Corballis, 1997; Halpen, 2000), so, deficits in patients with unilateral brain damage, finding evidence of greater functional hemispheric asymmetry in men than in women.

Behavioral laterality studies using neurologically intact men and women provide, at best, weak support for the hypothesis of greater functional laterality in men because the results have been quite variable.

There are indications that individual variations in brain laterality may be related to individual differences in cognitive ability. Relative performance on tests of verbal and visuospatial ability are related to handedness. There is also evidence that extreme intellectual precocity, especially for mathematical reasoning, is related to advanced development of the right hemisphere relative to the left, perhaps as a result of increased levels during fetal development (Hellige, 2000, 2002).

Genetic theories

Given the evidence that handedness pattern in humans extends far back into evolutionary history it is not surprising that the vast majority of theories of handedness have included the suggestion of a genetic factor.

Most genetic models for handedness postulate a dominant gene or genes for right-handedness and a recessive gene or genes for left-handedness (Hardyck and Petrovich 1977). Annett (1970) rejects this idea in favor of a dominant gene (rs$^+$) responsible for the development of speech in the left hemisphere.

Annett (1970) hypothesizes further that the processes necessary for left-hemisphere speech also confer advantage on motor control in the right hand. The recessive form of the gene (rs$^-$) result in no systematic bias either for speech or for handedness. If both alleles occurred equally often statistically, then 50% of the population would be (rs^{+-}) and the rest would be equally divided, 25% (rs^{++}) and 25% (rs^{--}). People in the rs^{+-} and rs^{++} groups, constituting 75% of the population, would show a left-for-speech and right-handedness shift. The remaining 25%, people in the rs^{--} group, would show no bias; so half would, by chance, be left-handed (Annett, 1970).

Thus, Annett's model predicts about 12.5% left-handers, which is pretty close to what we see in the population. Unfortunately, her theory neither predicts the number of left-handers with right-hemisphere speech nor attempts to differentiate between familial and nonfamilial left-handers (Kolb and Whishaw, 2003).

Unfortunately, the empirical evidence on handedness does not strongly support genetic theories. Some theorists are still trying to work out more sophisticated mathematical descriptions that might show that handedness is inherited; however, there still is a strong element of doubt in the data (Coren, 2002).

One way to investigate the contributions of genes and experience to cerebral organization is to analyze MRIs from normal brain and to vary the genetic relationships among the subjects.

Thompson et al. (2001) varied genetic relatedness by comparing the MRIs of unrelated people, dizygotic twins, and monozygotic twins. The results were striking, because the quantity of gray matter, especially in frontal, sensorimotor, and posterior language cortex was dissimilar in unrelated people but almost identical in monozygotic twins.

Because monozygotic twins are genetically identical, we can presume that any differences must be attributable to environmental effects. Curiously, there was an

1793

asymmetry in the degree of similarity, the left-hemisphere language zones being significantly more similar than the right in the monozygotic twins. The high similarities among monozygotic twins likely accounts for their highly similar cognitive abilities.

Thus, perhaps the most compelling evidence against a simple, strong genetic determinant for handedness comes from the results of studies that compared the handedness of monozygotic or identical twins with those of dizygotic or fraternal twins. Twin studies are usually considered as providing the clearest indication of the presence or absence of inherited components for most behavioral traits. Monozygotic twins have an identical set of genes they come from a single egg fertilized by a single sperm, that later split into two individuals in the early stages of cell division.

Dizygotic twins come from two eggs cells fertilized by different sperm; hence, they share only the level of genetic similarity that we would find between any pair of brothers or sisters. This means that, at a minimum, if there is a genetic component in handedness, one would at least expect that pairs of monozygotic twin would be more likely to have same handedness than dizygotic twins.

According to Coren (2002), there is no difference between monozygotic twins and dizygotic twins with regard to the likelihood that they will share the same handedness. Even more striking is that the likelihood that any form of twins will have the same handedness is no greater than if we randomly chose pairs of unrelated individuals and determined whether or not they had the same handedness (Coren, 2002).

Although there is a genetically fixed bias toward right-handedness, and this implies some set of genes that determine handedness, in specific situations there might be partial penetrance (which simply means that the gene does not express its full set of characteristics). If the right-handed gene does not express itself, then handedness becomes a matter of chance, and a left-hander could be the result.

Natural left-handedness could occur due to nonpathological differences in the uterus during pregnancy, such as the position in which the fetus lies. If the fetus comes out with the head directed to the back of the mother's right side (right occiput anterior position), the child is more likely to be left-handed than if it were born from the more common left occiput anterior position (with the head directed toward the back of the mother's left side) (Coren, 2002).

More recently, social analysis of gene expression was performed by Sun et al. (2005). They were able to show clear asymmetric gene expression in human brain for the first time. The asymmetry was variable between individuals, and quite regional, being most marked in perisylvian regions for the genes studied in most details.

Striking, the pattern of asymmetry in mouse was random for the cause of one gene, LM04, whereas it was clearly enriched in right perisylvian cortex in majority of humans. They have yet to identify any genes with a predominantly frontal asymmetry, although several genes they identified using microarrays in their such screen have frontal lobe enrichment. Such genes are candidates for patterning of frontal lobe structures and can be used to probe evolutionary conservation of frontal lobe regions across primate species and lower mammals (Preuss et al., 2004).

This raises one very important issue – the relevance of animal models to human development and function. Thus, what happens in the mouse is relevant to humans, but many human diseases have proven hard to model in the mouse.

According to Abu-Khalil et al. (2003), there are few human studies of important patterning molecules or signaling centers involved in mouse brain patterning.

Similarly, given those various diseases, such as schizophrenia and some dementias, witch affect the integrity of the cortex, the high correlation between the brain structures of identical twins could account for the strong genetic component of these diseases (Thompson et al., 2001; Kolb and Whishaw, 2003).

Sex differences in cerebral organization

Generally, men and women behave differently. On average, women tend to be more fluent than men in using language, and men tend to perform better than women in spatial analysis. But sex, like handedness, is not absolute (Kolb and Whishaw, 2003).

Sex differences in behavior

In her book, *Sex and Cognition*, Kimura (1999) examines five cognitive behaviors and finds compelling sex differences in all – namely, motor skills, spatial analysis, mathematical aptitude, perception, and verbal abilities. Table 23.1 summarizing her major conclusion, shows that the verbal-spatial dichotomy is a gross oversimplification.

Table 23.1

Summary of sex differences in cognitive behavior (after Kimura, 1999)

Behavior	Sex difference	Basic reference
Motor Skills		
Target throwing and catching	M > F	Hall and Kimura, 1995
Fine motor skills	F > M	Nicholson and Kimura, 1996
Spatial Analysis		
Mental rotation	M > F	Collins and Kimura, 1997
Spatial navigation	M > F	Astur et al., 2002
Geographical knowledge	M > F	Beatty and Troster, 1987
Spatial memory	F > M	McBurney et al., 1997
Mathematical Aptitude		
Computation	F > M	Hyde et al., 1990
Mathematical reasoning	M > F	Benbow, 1988
Perception		
Sensitivity to sensory stimuli	F > M	Velle, 1987
Perceptual speed	F > M	Majeres, 1983
Sensitivity to facial and body expression	F > M	Hall, 1984
Visual recognition memory	F > M	McGivern et al., 1998
Verbal Abilities		
Fluency	F > M	Hyde and Linn, 1988
Verbal memory	F > M	McGuinness et al., 1990

Motor skills

One obvious difference in motor skills is that, on average, men are superior in throwing objects, such as balls or darts at targets, and are superior at intercepting objects thrown toward them. These differences are present in children as young as 3 years of age (Kimura, 1999). In contrast, women have superior fine motor control and surpass men in executing sequential and intricate hand movement. However, young girls are superior to young boys at each of these skills (Mc Coby and Jacklin, 1974; Majeres, 1983; Hall, 1984; Hall and Kimura, 1995).

Spatial analysis

According to Kimura (1999), although men are generally believed to be superior to women at spatial analysis, this belief applies to only some types of spatial behaviors. Men are superior at tasks requiring the mental rotation of objects, and they are superior at spatial navigation tasks (Collins and Kimura, 1997).

Subjects are given a tabletop map on which they must learn a designated route. On average, men learn such tasks faster and with fewer errors than women do (Kimura, 1999). Although this map test is not a real-world test of spatial navigation, the findings are consistent with those of studies showing that the men have better overall map knowledge than women (Corsi-Cabrera et al., 1997).

Male superiority in spatial-navigation tasks contrasts with female superiority on test of spatial memory. Women are better than men at identifying which objects have been moved. In the map test women have better recall for landmarks along the route. Thus, the spatial information itself is not the critical factor in this sex difference; rather the critical factor is required behavior, that is the way in which the spatial information is to be used (Kimura, 1999; Kolb and Whishaw, 2003).

In accounting for findings that the spatial performance of right hemisphere damaged patients is adversely affected by lesions occurring anywhere in a fairly wide area while only those left hemisphere damaged patients with relatively severe damage to a well defined area show impaired performance on spatial tasks, De Renzi and Faglioni (1967), too, hypothesized more diffuse representation of functions in the right hemisphere and more focal representation in the left.

Mathematical aptitude

Stanley founded **The Study of Mathematically Precocious Youth** (SMPY) in 1971. The project primarily included holding talent search with the intent of identifying gifted youth, particularly in the area of mathematics.

Within a 15-year period, thousands of 12-year-old children were given the Scholastic Aptitude Test Mathematics exam. Stanley was particularly interested in the children with the highest scores because they might be assumed to be least affected by extraneous environmental factors such as social pressures. Benbow and Stanley (1980) and Benbow (1988) have shown that the sex difference increased as the scores increased: 12 times as many "gifted" boys than girls at the top. Furthermore, this ratio was found worldwise across different cultures, although the absolute scores varied with the educational system.

Benbow and Stanley (1980) have searched for support for a primarily environmental explanation of their data but they have not found it.

On average, men get better scores on tests of mathematical reasoning, whereas women do better at tests of computation.

Perception

According to Kimura (1999), perception refers to the recognition and interpretation of the sensory information that we take in from the external world (Kolb and Whishaw, 2003).

There would appear to be no a priory reason to expect a sex difference, but the evidence suggests that women are more sensitive to all forms of sensory stimulation, except for vision. However, women are more sensitive than men to facial expressions and body postures. They also detect sensory stimuli faster.

Males may have one perceptual advantage, however, in that their drawing of mechanical things such as bicycles are superior (Kolb and Whishaw, 2003).

Verbal ability

According to Kimura (1999), women are superior to men on tests of verbal fluency, on average, and they have superior verbal memory. The sex differences in verbal ability have long been known, in part because girls begin talking before boys and appear to be more fluent throughout life.

For example, the **Chicago Word-Fluency Test** asks subjects to write as many words beginning with "s" as possible in 5 minutes and as many four-letter words beginning with "c" as possible in 4 minutes. Girls performed better – at some ages, by as many as 10 words – in a broad study that Kolb and Whishaw (2003) did with children.

It is often argued that sex-related differences are related to life experience, but Kimura (1999) argues compellingly that this relation is unlikely for the cognitive behaviors. In particular, most if not all these differences, as well as differences in aggression are found in both children and adults, and the differences are largely unaffected by training. There are certainly training effects on most tests, but the effects tend to be of similar magnitude in both sexes (Kolb and Whishaw, 2003).

The same sex differences seem unrelated to life experience.

Sex differences in the brain structure

In one study, Ankney (1992) compared the brain of men and women of the same body size and found that men's brains are about 100 g heavier than women's throughout the range of body sizes.

In another study, Pakkenberg and Gundersen (1997) found that the male brains in their sample had about 4 billion more neurons than female brains, and body size did not more account for this difference.

Lynn (1994) and Alexopoulos (1996) have concluded that men have small (4 point) advantage in IQ scores, on average.

When different cerebral regions are examined separately, with results being correlated for relative size of the cerebrum of different brains, the findings of many studies show areal-dependent sex differences, as summarized in Table 23.2.

Table 23.2

Summary of sex differences in gross brain anatomy
(after Kolb and Whishaw, 2003)

Sex difference	Basic reference
Differences Favoring Female Brains	
Larger language areas	Harasty et al., 1997
Larger medial paralimbic areas	Filipek et al., 1994
Larger lateral frontal areas	Schlaepfer et al., 1995
Greater relative amount of gray matter	Gur et al., 1999
More densely packed neurons in temporal lobe	Witelson et al., 1995
Differences Favoring Male Brains	
Larger medial frontal areas	Goldstein et al., 2001
Larger cingulate areas	Paus et al., 1996
Larger amygdala and hypothalamus	Swaab et al., 1985
Larger overall white matter volume	Gur et al., 1999
Larger cerebral ventricles	Murphy et al., 1996
Larger right planum parietale	Jänke et al., 1994
More neurons overall	Pakkenberg and Guderson, 1997

Sex-related differences in brain volume are not diffusely spread across the cerebral hemispheres. Generally, female brain appear to have larger volumes in region associated with language functions, in medial paralimbic regions, and in lateral frontal areas (Filipek et al., 1994; Schlaepfer et al., 1995; Harasty et al., 1997). In addition, women have a greater relative amount of matter and in the temporal lobe, they have more densely packed neurons (Witelson et al., 1995; Gur et al., 1999).

Conversely, men have a larger medial frontal (Goldstein et al., 2001), and cingulate areas (Paus et al., 1996), a larger amygdala and hypothalamus (Swaab and Fliers, 1995), a larger overall white matter volume (Gur et al., 1999), a large cerebral ventricle (Murphy et al., 1996), and a larger right planum parietale (Jäncke et al., 1994).

However, male brains tend to have more neurons (Pakkenberg and Gundersen, 1997) and female brain more neuropils (that is dendrites and axons) per neuron (Kolb and Whishaw, 2003).

The influence of sex hormones

Goldstein et al. (2001) did a large MRI study of sexual dimorphism in the male and female brain, and have documented that sex differences were largest in regions of the human brain in which the results of studies of nonhumans have shown that there are sex differences in the developmental expression of estrogen or androgen receptors. Thus, Goldstein team proposed that a large part of the observed sex differences in cerebral organization is related to differences in the distribution of receptors for gonadal hormones during development.

However, their conclusions have limitations, because they do not consider differences in cerebral organization that might be related to circulating hormones in adulthood. Furthermore, the findings in many studies suggest that the rate of cell death during aging may be higher in men than in women, especially in the frontal lobe (Kolb and Whishaw, 2003).

The presence of sex differences in overall size and in relative size of different regions does not speak directly to the question of whether there are sex differences in the degree of cerebral asymmetry (Kolb and Whishaw, 2003).

However, there are several reliable sex differences in anatomical asymmetry:

Left larger than right in the planum temporale is seen more often in men than in women. An MRI study by Kulynych et al. (1994) found a large asymmetry in males (left, 38% larger) but no asymmetry in females. Because Aboitiz et al. (1992) obtained different results, this result must be interpreted with caution.

Witelson and Kigar (1992) quantified the slope of the Sylvian fissure with reference to various cortical landmarks. This quantification led to separate measure of the horizontal and vertical components of the Sylvian fissure. They found that, although the horizontal component was larger in the left hemisphere of both sexes, men had a larger horizontal component in the left hemisphere than women had.

Thus, male brain has a larger asymmetry in the Sylvian fissure than had female brain. These sex differences are important in the organization of language-related functions.

Jäncke et al. (1994) found that the planum parietale, which favor right hemisphere, is about twice as large in men as in women.

The callosal studies have proved controversial, but consensus appears to be that the posterior part of the callosum (the splenium) is significantly larger in women than in men (Witelson, 1985).

Allen and Gorski (1991) found that women have a larger anterior commissure than men have. This difference is likely due to a difference in the number of neural fibres in the two sexes, a difference presumably due to some difference in the way in which the two hemispheres interact.

Kimura (1983) found that the ridges in our fingerprints, which are established early in fetal life, are asymmetrical, with the finger on the right hand having more ridges. Given that this pattern is visible in utero, it could not be influenced by environmental factors such as differences in limb use. Kimura (1983) found that most people have the asymmetry, but women are far more likely to show an optical pattern, much as we saw for brain asymmetries. The cortical part of Kimura studies and others is that the pattern of ridges is correlated with performance on certain cognitive tests (Kolb and Whishaw, 2003).

Generally, EEG (Corsi-Cabrera et al., 1997), MEG (Reite et al., 1995), blood flow (Gur et al., 1982; Esposito et al., 1996), PET (Haverkort et al., 1999), and fMRI (Pugh et al., 1996; Frost et al., 1999) studies show more asymmetrical activity in men than in women, particularly in language-related activities (Table 23.3).

Table 23.3

Sex differences in imaging studies
(after Kolb and Whishaw, 2003)

Measure	Result	Representative references
EEG	Males more asymmetrical	Corsi-Cabrera et al., 1997
MEG	Males more asymmetrical	Reite et al., 1995
Blood flow	Females > males	Gur et al., 1982
	Females > males in frontal lobe tests	Esposito et al., 1996
PET	Males > females in anterior blood flow	Haverkort et al., 1999
	Females > males in posterior blood flow	
fMRI	More left-hemisphere activity in language-related tasks (but see Frost et al., 1999) in males	Pugh et al., 1996

Measures of the blood flow, including those obtained with the use of PET, show that women have more rapid overall blood exchange than men have, possibly due to the difference in the density of neurons or the distribution of gray matter and white matter (Kolb and Whishaw, 2003).

From these results there are differences in anatomical organization and functional activity of the male and female brain. Presumably, the anatomical differences correspond to the functional differences that researchers have found (Kolb and Whishaw, 2003).

Because of these anatomical and functional differences, two types of lesion-related differences are possible in the neurological patients.

Such difference might exist if the two hemispheres were more similar functionally in one sex than in the other sex. Indeed, the greater asymmetry observed in EEG (Corsi-Cabrera et al., 1997), MEG (Reite et al., 1995) and fMRI (Pugh et al., 1996, Frost et al., 1999) studies in men suggests that men might show more asymmetry effects of unilateral lesions than women.

Injury to the frontal lobe might have greater effects in one sex than in the other, a difference that would be consistent with a greater relative volume of much of the frontal lobes in women (Kolb and Whishaw, 2003).

One way to assess the asymmetry of left- or right-hemisphere lesions is to look at the effects of lesions on general tests of verbal and nonverbal abilities.

So, Inglis and Lawson (1982) showed that, although left- and right-hemisphere lesions in men affected the verbal and performance subscales of the WAIS (Wechsler Adult Intelligence Scale) differently, left-hemisphere lesions in women depressed both

IQ scores equally, and right-hemisphere lesions in women failed to depress either score. A clear sex difference emerged in which males with left-hemisphere lesions exhibited a depression in verbal IQ, whereas males with right-hemisphere exhibited a complementary deficit in performance IQ. In contrast, females with right-hemisphere lesions showed no significant depression in either IQ scale.

Thus, Inglis and Lawson (1982) found an equivalent effect of left-hemisphere lesions on verbal IQ in both sexes, but men with right-hemisphere lesions were more disrupted than woman were.

Work of Kimura (1999) shows that the pattern of cerebral organization within each hemisphere also differs between the sexes. Men and women are almost equally likely to be aphasic subsequent to left-hemisphere lesion. But apraxia is associated with frontal damage to the left-hemisphere in women and with posterior damage in men. Aphasia develops most often when damage in to the front of the brain in women but to the rear of the brain in men (Kimura, 1999).

Thus, men are likely to be aphasic and apraxic after damage to the left posterior cortex, whereas women are far more likely to experience speech disorders and apraxia after anterior lesion.

Kimura (1999) also suggests an analogous sex-related difference subsequent to right-hemisphere lesions.

Anterior, but not posterior lesions in women impaired their performance of the block-design and object-assembly subtests of WAIS, whereas men were equally affected on these tests by either anterior or posterior lesions.

Kolb and Stewart (1991) have found parallel results in their studies of rats with prefrontal lesions: male rats with these lesions have much smaller deficits in various tests of spatial navigation than do female rats with similar lesions. This finding may suggest a fundamental difference between the sexes in the intracerebral organization in mammals.

Kolb and Stewart (1991), in an anatomical study, show a large difference between male and female rats in the dendritic organization of neurons in the prefrontal cortex. This sex difference was affected by treatment that either increased or decreased testosterone levels during development (Kolb and Stewart, 1991).

Strauss et al. (1992) gave sodium amobarbital to 94 epileptic patients who were being considered for elective surgery after infant brain damage. Left-hemisphere injury in infancy leads to the shifting of language to the right hemisphere: so Strauss expected this shift in those patients with left-hemisphere injury. The unexpected result was a sex difference in the likelihood of cerebral reorganization subsequent to left-hemisphere injury after one year of age: girls were unlikely to show reorganization, whereas boys appeared likely to shift language, perhaps as late as puberty. This suggests that the male brain may be more plastic after cortical injury.

According to Kolb and Stewart (1991), males showed a better recovery and more synaptic changes than females did.

Thus, unilateral cortical lesions have different effects on male and female brain.

Explanation of sex differences

Kolb and Whishaw (2003) identified five explanations for sex differences: (1) hormonal effects on cerebral function; (2) genetic sex linkage; (3) maturation rate; (4) environment; and (5) preferred cognitive mode.

Hormonal effects. In birds and mammals, the presence of testosterone at critical times in the course of development has unequivocal effects on the organization of both hypothalamic and forebrain structures, and the observed morphological effects are believed to be responsible for the behavioral dimorphism (Kolb and Whishaw, 2003).

However, the hormones may have an organizing effect on the brains of mammals only during development, although they can still influence neuronal function later in life. Regions of the human brain that have clear sex-related differences in adulthood are the same ones that have a high density of estrogen receptors during development. Women have significantly higher volumes in the major frontal and medial paralimbic regions than those of men, whereas men have larger relative volumes in the medial frontal cortex and the angular gyrus. These areas correspond to region in which there are higher levels of estrogen receptors and to regions high in androgen receptors during development (Goldstein et al., 2001).

Androgens appear to be converted into estradiol (female hormones) in the brain, and the binding of this estradiol to receptors leads to masculinization of the brain. Estradiol receptors have been found in the cortexes of developing rodents and nonhuman primates, but they are not found in the adults.

However, there is a relation between behavior and the level of hormones observed at different times in adult of each sex. Hampson (1990) and Hampson and Kimura (1992) showed that the performance of women on certain tasks changes throughout the menstrual cycle as estrogen levels rise and fall. High estrogen levels are associated with relatively depressed spatial ability as well as enhanced articulatory and motor capability.

Woolley et al. (1990) showed that, during the female rat's estrous cycle, there are large changes in the number of dendritic spines on hippocampal neurons. Thus, the number of synapses in the female rat's hippocampus goes up and down in 4-days cycles. Similarly, female rats that have their ovaries removed in middle age show a dramatic increase in dendrites and spines of cortical neurons (Stewart and Kolb, 1988). Thus, estrogen has direct effects on cerebral neurons in the adult animal.

On the other hand, testosterone affects cognition in men. Kimura (1999) showed that men's spatial scores fluctuate with testosterone levels: men with lower testosterone levels get the highest scores. Testosterone levels in men are higher in the autumn than in the spring, and they are higher in the morning than in the evening. Thus, men do better at the spatial tests in the spring and in the evening. Furthermore, men with lower average levels of testosterone do better on both spatial tests and on mathematical reasoning tests than do those with higher levels.

In the early part of the twentieth century, testosterone was believed to be able to reverse senescence, but there is little evidence that the hundreds of given testicular implants actually benefited from this treatment (Hamilton, 1986).

Nonetheless, some evidence suggests that testosterone treatments may influence spatial cognition in older men. Janowsky et al. (1994) gave retired men testosterone (or placebo) in scrotal patches and found a significant improvement in the performance of spatial tasks but not in verbal or other cognitive measures.

When the researchers measured blood-hormone levels, they found a decrease in estradiol as well as an increase in testosterone. Hampson (1990) found that the low estradiol levels correlated with the improved spatial performance. Thus, the suppression of estrogen is more beneficial than the presence of testosterone.

However, the estrogen treatment in postmenopausal women improves verbal memory.

In sum, gonadal hormones alter the brain and make male and female brains more or less responsive in different environments. Thus, Juraska (1986) has demonstrated that exposure to gonadal hormones perinatally determines the later ability of environmental stimulation to alter the synaptic organization of the cerebrum. On the other hand, she showed that environmentally induced changes in the hippocampus and neocortex are affected differently by gonadal hormones. Thus, the female hippocampus is far more plastic in new environments than the male hippocampus, and this plasticity depends on estrogen.

This type of hormonally mediated selective effect of experience on the brain is important because experimental factors (including social factors) could influence the male and female brain differently, leading to sex-related various in brain and behavior. So, the cognitive functions of the two sexes may diverge functionally at puberty and begin to converge again after menopause (Kolb and Whishaw, 2003).

Genetic sex linkage. If a gene for particular trait, such as spatial analysis, is recessive, the trait will not be expressed in a girl unless the recessive gene is present on both X chromosomes. However, the recessive gene need to be present only on one chromosome if the child is a boy. Thus, if a mother carries the gene on both X chromosomes, all her sons will have the trait, but her daughters will possess it only if their father also carries the recessive gene on his chromosome. However, a thorough review by Boles (1980) concludes that it has yet to be proved.

Maturation rate. It has long been known that girls begin to speak sooner than the boys, develop larger vocabularies in childhood, and, as children, use more complex linguistic construction than the boys do (Kolb and Whishaw, 2003).

Findings from dichotic and tachistoscopic studies often indicate an earlier evolution of cerebral asymmetry in girls than in boys. Because girls attain physical maturity at an earlier age than boys do, it is responsible to propose that the male brain matures more slowly than the female brain and that maturation rate is a critical determinant of brain asymmetry.

That is, the more slowly a child matures, the greater is the observed cerebral asymmetry (Weber, 1976; Kolb and Whishaw, 2003).

Weber (1976) found that, regardless of sex, early-maturing adolescents performed better on tests of verbal abilities than on tests of spatial ones, whereas late-maturing adolescents did the opposite.

Because the girls mature faster than boys, superior spatial abilities in boys may be directly related to their relatively slow development (Weber, 1976).

Environment. In regard to spatial ability, boys are expected to exhibit greater independence than girls and thus to engage in activities such as exploring and manipulating the environment.

Harris (1978) concluded that, although a few studies can be found to support the environmental view, the bulk of the evidence fails to do so.

In the study, by Thomas et al. (1973), on the horizontality of a liquid, women who failed the task were repeatedly shown a bottle half-filled with red water that was tilted at various angles. Women stated that "water is level when the bottle is upright but inclined when the bottle is tilted".

Men and women who performed correctly stated that "water is always level".

Thus, although environmental theories may be appealing, there is no evidence that environmental or social factors can solely account for the observed sex differences in verbal and spatial behaviors (Kolb and Whishaw, 2003).

Preferred cognitive mode. According to Kolb and Whishaw (2003), the difference in strategies used by men and women to solve problems may be at least partly responsible for the observed sex differences in behavior.

Genetic maturational and environmental factors may predispose men and women to prefer different modes of cognitive analysis.

Women solve problems primarily by using a verbal mode. Because this cognitive mode is less efficient in solving spatial problems, women exhibit an apparent deficit (Kolb and Whishaw, 2003).

In sum, at least six significant behavioral differences are related: verbal ability, visuospatial analysis, mathematical ability, perception, motor skills, and aggression (Kolb and Whishaw, 2003).

Harshman et al. (1983), in a very ambitious study of the interaction of sex and handedness in cognitive abilities, found a significant interaction between sex and handedness; that is, sex-related differences in verbal and visuospatial behavior vary as a function of handedness.

Witelson (1985, 1989) found that callosal size also varies by sex and handedness.

Anatomical studies

Generally, the left-hemisphere of the brain controls the right side of the body and the right hemisphere of the brain controls the left side of the body.

Broca (1861) discovered that the major language production center in the brain is located in the left hemisphere of the brain. Another speech center called Wernicke's area (Wernicke, 1874), that is associated with speech comprehension, is also located in the left hemisphere of the brain.

The fact that the right-hand and primary speech functions are controlled by the same half of the brain has fuelled speculations attempting to link brain organization language functions, and handedness. Thus, Broca introduced the notion of the "dominant hemisphere", by which he meant the hemisphere that directs not only the movements of writing, drawing, and other fine movements but also language and perhaps even major aspects of logical thought. He then suggested that left-handers might: have a brain that is organized in a mirror image to that of right-handers, with language control on the right side of the brain.

The data, however, suggest that this relationship is unfounded. So, acquired a pathology that damages the left side of the brain, or an injection of sodium amytal into the left side of the brain results in the development of aphasia.

Although virtually all right-handers have language area in their left hemisphere, Coren (2002) did not find the mirror imaged brain that we expected in left-handers.

The data show that the vast majority of left-handers have the same brain organization as right-handers, with their language control exclusively confined to the left hemisphere. According to Coren (2002), only about 2 of 10 left-handers have language exclusively in the right hemisphere, as had been predicted by Broca.

There is also a small group of individuals who seem to have their language control split between both sides of the brain or duplicated on both sides of the brain (Springer and Deutsch, 1995; Coren, 2002).

The overwhelming number of studies with the new technology (positron emission tomography, functional magnetic resonance imaging, magnetoencephalography) have found that there is a remarkable similarity between brains, regardless of handedness, with the only major difference being that hand control regions are somewhat larger and more active on the side opposite to the dominant hand.

However, right-handers seem to have brains that are slightly more asymmetrical, in terms of both their structure and their functional specialization.

A larger proportion of left-handers seem to have more symmetrical brains and are more likely to have functions equally represented in both hemispheres (Corballis, 1991; Springer and Deutsch, 1995; Toga et al., 2006).

Certain cerebral anatomical asymmetries are apparent at both the macroscopic and histological levels.

Hand preference is correlated with differential patterns of right - left asymmetry in the parietal operculum, frontal cortex, occipital region, vascular patterns, and cerebral blood flow (Carmon et al., 1972; Hochberg and Le May, 1975; Le May, 1977).

Thus, in comparison with right-handers, a higher proportion of left-handers show no asymmetry.

Ratcliffe et al. (1980) correlates the asymmetry in the course of the sylvian (lateral) fissure, as revealed by carotid angiography, and with the results of carotid sodium amobarbital speech testing. They found that left- and right-handers with speech in the left hemisphere had a mean right - left difference of 27° in the angle formed by the vessels leaving the posterior end of sylvian fissure. In the left- and right-handers with speech in the right hemisphere or with bilaterally represented speech, the mean difference shrank to 0°. Thus, the anatomical asymmetry in their population was related to speech representation and not necessarily to handedness.

The location of speech proved a better predictor of individual variation in cerebral organization than handedness.

Asymmetries in areal size, cytoarchitecture or neurocytology occur elsewhere in the cerebral cortex as well as subcortically.

For example, many brains have a wider right frontal pole and a wider left occipital pole. Brodmann's area 45 in the inferior frontal lobe, corresponding to Broca's area, contains a population of large pyramidal neurons that are found only on the left side. The cortical surface surrounding the central sulcus is larger in the left hemisphere, especially in the areas containing the primary somatosensory and motor maps of the arm, suggesting that one cerebral manifestation of hand preference is a larger amount of neural circuitry in the relevant parts of the cortex. Histological asymmetries are also found in areas that are not usually considered to be closely related either to language or handedness.

The left entorhinal cortex has significantly more neurons than the right one (Toga et al., 2006; Crossman, 2008).

Handedness may appear to be more closely related to anatomical anomalies because left-handers display more variation in lateralization of speech.

In a study of more than 300 cases, Yakovlev and Rakic (1966) found that, in 80%, the pyramidal tract that is descending to the right hand contains more fibres than does the same tract going to the left hand. Apparently, more fibres descend to the right hand both from the contralateral left hemisphere and from the ipsilateral right hemisphere than to the left hand. In addition, the contralateral tract from the left hemisphere crosses at a higher level in the medulla than does the contralateral tract from the right hemisphere.

Thus, lateralized central differences may also occur at the level of cellular organization (Pelet et al., 1998; Anderson et al., 1999; Galuske et al., 2000; Gazzaniga, 2000 b).

As early as 1963, Hécaen and Angelergues, on careful review of the neuropsychological symptoms associated with lesions of the right or left hemisphere, speculated that neural organization might be more closely knit and integrated on the left, more diffuse on the right.

For example, the extent of higher order dendritic branching seems to be greater in certain speech areas of the left hemisphere (e.g., Broca's area) than in the corresponding regions of the right hemisphere. Conversely, lower order dendritic branches seem to be longer in the right hemisphere than in the left hemisphere (Hellige, 1993, 2000; Zaidel and Iacobini, 2002).

A difficulty in accounting for variations in anatomical asymmetries is that some left- and right-handers show a marked dissociation between morphological (structural) and functional asymmetry. Kolb and Whishaw (2003) suggest that other variables, still unknown, may also account for individual differences in both left and right-handers.

Witelson (1977, 1985, 1989), Witelson and Goldsmith (1991), Witelson and Kigar (1992), and Witelson et al. (1995) studied the hand preference of terminally ill subjects on a variety of unimanual tasks. She later did postmortem studies of their brains, paying particular attention to the size of the corpus callosum.

She found that the cross-sectional area was 11% greater in left-handed and ambidextrous people than in the right-handed people.

Although no two human brains are exactly alike in their structure, in most people the right frontal area is wider than the left and the right frontal pole protrudes beyond the left, while the reverse is true of the occipital pole: the left occipital pole is frequently wider and protrudes further posteriorly than the right but the central portion of the right hemisphere is frequently wider than the left (Damasio and Geschwind, 1984; Jäncke and Steinmetz, 2003).

Men show greater degree of frontal and occipital asymmetry than women (Bear et al., 1986). These asymmetries exist in fetal brains (de Lacoste et al., 1991; Witelson, 1995).

The left sylvian fissure, the fold between the temporal and frontal lobes, is larger than the right in most people (Witelson, 1995), even in newborns (Seidenwurm et al., 1985). Most attention has focused on asymmetry of the posterior portion of the superior surface of the temporal lobe, the planum temporale.

This region, which is involved in auditory processing, is larger on the left side in most right-handers (Strauss et al., 1985; Beaton 1997).

Thus, for the right-handed individuals the planum temporale is larger in the left hemisphere in approximately 65% of the cases, larger in the right hemisphere in approximately 10% of the cases and approximately equal in 25% of the cases. The corresponding percentages for non-right-handers are approximately 25, 10, and 65% respectively. Similar distributions characterize asymmetry of the sylvian fissure (Hellige, 2000; Zaidel and Iacobini, 2002).

In sum, one of the most notable anatomical asymmetries is in the planum temporale, which is usually larger on the left than on the right side.

Subtle asymmetries in the superior temporal lobe have been demonstrated in terms of overall size and shape, sulcal pattern, cytoarchitecture, and at the neuronal level.

It seems reasonable to assume that these differences underlie some of the functional asymmetries for language representation (Toga et al., 2006).

Handedness and the longevity

A significant number of left-handers arrived at their left-handedness through some form of pathological event during their fetal development or associated with their birth, and this same pathology also resulted in other physical or pathological problems (Coren, 2002).

A number of studies have examined handedness as a function of demographic factors, such as age, sex, and race. These studies found a diminishing percentage of left-handers in older age groups (Bishop, 1990; Springer and Deutsch, 1995). Forced switching of left-handers to right-handedness in older age groups could explain this age-related decline in the number of left-handers.

The alternative explanation for failing to find older left-handers might be that they are simply no longer in the population. That is, left-handers have a shorter life span, and the reason that we fail to find many older left-handers is because a large proportion of them have died early (Coren, 2002).

Although many left-handers were dying of factors traceable to the problems in Table 23.4, there was a surprise in the data: left-handers were five times more likely to die of accident-related injuries (Coren, 2002).

Table 23.4

Conditions That Two or More Research Reports Have Shown to Be Associated with a Disproportionately High Number of Left-Handers

Negative conditions associated with left-handedness

Alcoholism	Hashimoto's thyroiditis	Poor spatial ability
Allergies	Hayfever	Poor verbal ability
Asthma	High and low extremes in numerical ability	Predispositions toward aggression
Attempted suicide	Homosexuality	Psychosis
Autism	Hypopigmentation	Reading disability
Bed-wetting	Immune disorders	Reduced adult height
Brain damage	Impulsive aggression	Reduced adult weight
Chromosomal damage	Infection susceptibility	Regional ileitis
Celiac disease	Juvenile delinquency	Schizophrenia or schizotypal thinking
Crohn's disease	Juvenile-onset diabetes	School failure
Clinical depression	Language problems	Sleep difficulty
Criminality	Learning disabilities	Slow maturation
Deafness	Lower intelligence scores	Slow physical development
Depression	Maniac-depressive phychosis	Strabismus
Drug abuse	Mental retardation	Stuttering
Drug hypersensitivity	Migraine headaches	Sudden heart attack death
Emotionality	Myasthenia gravis	Transsexuality
Epilepsy	Neural tube defects	Ulcerative colitis
Excessive smoking	Neuroticism	Urticaria
Eczema	Poor school performance	

Positive conditions associated with left-handedness

Extremely high intelligence	Good divergent thinking ability	High spatial ability
	High musical ability	

Thus, the left-handers suffer injuries while playing sports, during the traffic, working with tools and motorized equipment, working with kitchen and home implements and devices, and even while engaged in military activities (Coren, 2002).

Left-handedness might be a marker (at least, statistically) for the possible existence of some form of neural pathology, psychological deviance, or developmental abnormality. Thus, the same pathology that caused the left-handedness might have also caused some form of collateral damage that can reduce the individual's physiological or psychological fitness through direct or secondary mechanisms (Coren, 1993, 2002). So, a substantial body of research found that left-handedness is frequently associated with a variety of symptoms or syndromes. However, the number of findings in which left-handedness is associated with positive outcomes in the research literature is much rarer.

A review of the literature indicated at least 60 negative pathological or undesirable conditions associated with left-handedness as opposed to only 4 positive or desirable conditions. Table 23.4 provides an idea of the positive and negative conditions related to an increased proportion of left-handers (Coren, 2002).

The research literature is repleted with suggestions that left-handedness is predominantly associated with negative conditions, and with a range of pathological antecedents. Example of rare traits include animals that are colored differently from the vast majority of their species. For instance, a "blue-marl" collie, a white dog, or an albino human often have major sensory deficits affecting their vision or hearing. These rare traits could include rare palm crease patterns, rare fingerprint patterns, or rare distribution of toe lengths, and even unusual ear shapes are often found to be associated with cognitive or physical deficits.

Left-handedness, which affects only about 10% of the population, would also be qualified as a rare trait (Coren, 2002).

Thus, the rare *versus* the common trait can be influenced by pathological factors. According to Coren (2002), half of the resulting population of left-handers are pathological, whereas only 1.2% of the right-handers are pathological. This means that the relative risk of left-hander being pathological is approximately 41% greater than that of right-hander being pathological.

Left-handedness might be seen as a soft sign indicating increased risk for many problems: however, which specific problems an individual might suffer from, or which neural loci are involved, is not determinable (Coren, 2002).

From the standpoint of behavioral medicine, we may view left handedness as a risk factor that may well predict susceptibility to illness, physiological deficits, psychological problems, and perhaps even a shortened life span (Coren, 2002).

Effects of hemispherectomy

The catastrophic epilepsies, in which panhemispheric syndromes are associated with intractable seizures, include Rasmussen's encephalitis, developmental syndromes (i.e., hemimegaencephaly, tuberous sclerosis, hamartomas, Sturge-Weber syndrome), and congenital hemiplegia or porencephaly (Carson et al., 1996).

Although the original surgical approach of anatomic complete, en bloc hemispherectomy with spearing of basal ganglia, hypothalamus, and diencephalon (Krynaw, 1950; Rasmussen, 1975) was successful from the standpoint of seizure control, the immediate and delayed complications were daunting (Pilcher and Ojeman, 1993).

Postoperative complications were significantly reduced with the introduction, by Rasmussen (1975), of the technique of modified or functional hemispherectomy, in which a generous central and temporal resection is juxtaposed with deafferentation of the frontal and occipital lobes (Rasmussen, 1987). With deafferentation rather than removal of the frontal and occipital lobes, the volume of intracranial dead space is reduced, and in 7.3-year follow-up study of 14 patients, no hemosiderosis or hydrocephalus occurred, and 10 of 14 patients were seizure free. Villemure and Mascott (1995) introduced the peri-insular hemispherectomy, in which a smaller craniotomy and a much reduced peri-insular (i.e., opercular frontal, parietal, and temporal) resection are combined with deafferentation of frontal, parietal, occipital and temporal lobes. In addition, to a favorable seizure outcome (i.e., 9 of 11 patients were seizure free, and 1 of 11 improved 95%), reduced operative time and preoperative and delayed complications were documented.

The trans-sylvian keyhole functional hemispherectomy advanced by Schramm et al. (1995, 2001) represents a true minimalist approach to hemispheric deafferentation. A linear scalp incision and 4 × 4 cm craniotomy provide the limited exposure required for a trans-sylvian approach to the circular sulcus, through which access to the entire ventricular system is gained. Transventricular hemispheric deafferentation and amygdalo-hippocampectomy are performed, with significantly reduced blood loss and a mean operating time of 3.6 hours.

For 20 patients, 88% were seizure free, and seizure improved for 6%.

Although most hemispherectomies are performed in the patient's early adolescence, the surgery is sometimes done in the first year of life, before the speech has developed.

If the hemispheres vary functionally at birth, then the left and right hemispherectomies would be expected to produce different effects on cognitive abilities. If they do not vary at birth, then no cognitive differences would result from left or right hemispherectomies (Kolb and Whishaw, 2003).

Generally, results of studies of linguistic and visuospatial abilities in patients with unilateral hemidecortications support the conclusion that both hemispheres are functionally specialized at birth, although both hemispheres appear capable of assuming some functions usually performed by the missing hemisphere (Kolb and Whishaw, 2003). Thus, hemidecortication produces no severe deficit in visuospatial abilities. The left hemisphere cannot completely compensate the right hemisphere.

Dennis and Whitaker (1976) found that both hemispheres understand the meaning of words and both can spontaneously produce lists of names of things. However, the left hemisphere has an advantage over the right.

In an analysis of reading skills, Dennis et al. (1981) found that both hemispheres had almost equal ability in higher-order reading comprehension; however, the left hemisphere is superior to the right in reading and spelling unfamiliar words and in using sentence structure to achieve fluent reading. The left hemisphere also reads prose passages with greater decoding accuracy, more fluency and fewer errors that violate the semantic and syntactic structure of sentence, performances better with the right hemisphere in a task that requires learning and association between nonsense words and symbols.

So, Dennis (1980) suggests that, if written language structure is thought as a combination of meaning cues (morphology), sound cues (phonology), and picture cues (logography), then the isolated left hemisphere will show superior performance with morphology and phonology and inferior performance with logographic cues.

The isolated right hemisphere will show superior performance with logographic cues and inferior performance with morphological and phonological cues (Dennis, 1980).

Kohn and Dennis (1974) found an almost analogous pattern of results on test of visuospatial function.

Thus, although patients with right hemispherectomies performed normally on simple tests of visuospatial functions such as drawing, they were significantly impaired in complex tests such as negotiating a maze and reading a map (Kohn and Dennis, 1974; Kolb and Whishaw, 2003).

In sum, each hemisphere can assume some of its opposite's functions if the opposite hemisphere is removed in the course of development, but neither hemisphere is totally capable of mediating all of the missing hemisphere's function (Kolb and Whishaw, 2003). There is convincing evidence against equipotentiality: both hemisphere appear to have a processing capacity that probably has an innate structural basis (Kolb and Whishaw, 2003).

With few exception, patients undergoing hemispherectomy are of below-average or, at least, average intelligence, and their proficiency at tests of the intact hemisphere's function is often less than normal (Dennis, 1980; Dennis et al., 1981; Kolb and Whishaw, 2003).

Although such children have severe behavioral difficulties after hemispherectomy, they often compensate remarkably, communicating freely and, in some cases, showing considerable motor control over the limbs opposite the excised hemisphere.

Using both fMRI and SEPs (somatosensory evoked potentials), Holloway et al. (2000) investigated the sensorimotor functions of 17 hemispherectomy patients.

Ten patients showed SEPs in the normal hemisphere when the nerves of the limb opposite the excised hemisphere were stimulated. Similarly, fMRI shows that, for at least some of the patients, passive movement of the same limb produced activation in a region of somatosensory cortex that normally responds to the opposite hand.

The Holloway's team concluded that the responses to the hand ipsilateral to the normal hemisphere must occur because direct ipsilateral pathways run from the normal hemisphere to the affected limb.

However, the novel ipsilateral responses were found in patients with both congenital and acquired disease, suggesting that although age at injury may be important, the ability of nervous system to alter its organization to compensate for injury may influence the cerebral reorganization.

Ontogeny of asymmetry

Generally, adultlike cerebral asymmetries are present before birth, a result that supports an innate predisposition for cerebral asymmetry in humans.

In a MRI study, Sowell et al. (2002 a and b) confirm this general impression.

Thus, a basic template for cortical development appears to lay down an asymmetrical organization prenatally, and the pattern progresses after birth.

The results of ERP studies by Dennis (1980), and Molfese and Molfese (1988) confirm a functional asymmetry in which the left hemisphere showed a greater response to speech stimuli as early as one week of age. There is apparently little change in this difference during development.

However, initially it permits some flexibility or equipotentiality. The cognitive functions of each hemisphere can be conceived as hierarchical. Simple, lower-level functions are represented at the base of the hierarchy, corresponding to functions in the primary sensor, motor, language, or visuospatial areas. More complex, higher-level functions ascend the hierarchy, the most complex being at the top. These advanced functions are the most lateralized (Kolb and Whishaw, 2003).

At birth, the two hemispheres overlap functionally because each is processing low-level behaviors.

By age of 5, the newly developing higher-order cognitive processes have very little overlap, and each hemisphere becomes increasingly specialized. By puberty, each hemisphere has developed its own unique functions (Kolb and Whishaw, 2003).

Thus, Moscovitch (1977) emphasized the possibility that one hemisphere actively inhibits the other, thus preventing the contralateral hemisphere from developing similar functions. This active inhibition presumably develops at about age of 5, as the corpus callosum becomes functional. According to Moscovitch (1977), this inhibitory process not only prevents the subsequent development of language processes in the right hemisphere but also inhibits the expression of the language processes already in the right hemisphere.

The right hemisphere of commissurotomy patients appears to have greater language abilities than expected from the study of normal patients, presumably because the right hemisphere is no longer subject to inhibition by the left. Netley (1977) showed that people born with no corpus callosum demonstrate little or no functional asymmetry as inferred from dichotic listening, suggesting that the absence of interhemispheric connection results in attenuated hemispheric asymmetry.

Popularized accounts of laterality have suggested that people can be classified as "right-brained" or left-brained", depending on whether they prefer to use strategies and models of cognition associated with one hemisphere or another.

Thus, left-brained people are said to be rational and analytic, whereas right-brained people are said to be intuitive, artistic, and creative.

However, there is individual variation on the various dimensions of laterality, but there is no evidence that any neurologically intact individuals are functionally half-brained in the manner referred to as hemisphericity. Individuals do differ reliably in cognitive style, personality, creativity and so forth (Hellige, 2002).

However, hemispheric asymmetries are subtle, with no indication that aspects such as rationality and creativity are the exclusive product of one brain hemisphere. Instead, both hemispheres contribute to virtually everything we do (Hellige, 2000, 2002).

The discovery that both of disconnected hemispheres of split-brain patients have a good deal of competence with respect to perception and motor control has led to speculation about whether or not the surgery has produced a doubling of consciousness or resulted in people with two minds.

Sperry (1986) believed that this was the case. In part, he based his conclusion on the fact that the disconnected right hemisphere has its own perceptions, cognitions, and memories of which the disconnected left hemisphere is completely unaware.

Others, however, have questioned whether the right hemisphere can truly think and whether its limited abilities include the same level of awareness and consciousness that seems typical on the left hemisphere.

Certainly, the disconnected right hemisphere is usually incapable of speech and other forms of verbal communication that are uniquely human and that some have argued, are essential for the concept of "mind". There is much debate among philosophers and cognitive scientists about the extent to which language is essential for thinking, conscious reflection, or mental life.

Le Doux and Gazzaniga (1978) hypothesized that an important function of an individual's verbal left hemisphere is the construction of internal, subjective reality or ongoing narrative based on its observations of his or her own overt behavior.

In this view, observation of one's own behavior is necessary because many processes that influence behavior are not open to conscious experience. Le Doux and Gazzaniga (1978) emphasize this with respect to behavior and bodily sensations produced by the right hemisphere, of which the left hemisphere would have no direct knowledge.

However, even within the left hemisphere there appear to be a great many modules whose processes may influence behavior but that are not themselves open to conscious awareness.

Thus, the need to create an ongoing personal narrative by making inferences about one's own behavior is likely to extend to covert processes performed by both hemispheres. Although, neither hemisphere is uniformly superior for processing nonverbal perceptual information. Instead, both hemispheres contribute to perceptual processing and do so in ways that could be described as complementary.

This chapter is not meant to solve all of the mysteries of lateralized functions, but merely to highlight anatomical and functional asymmetries as they relate to language, complex motor behaviors, and sensorimotor integration.

It is often assumed that anatomical asymmetries invariably reflect functional asymmetries. However, physiological asymmetries, asymmetries in gene expression, or subtle differences in neuronal cytoskeletal architecture may play a more significant role in hemispheric specialization than gross anatomical or cytoarchitectonic asymmetries (Geschwind and Iacoboni, 2007).

The intensification of morphological asymmetries associated with language is important because of a wealth of evidence that these asymmetries are functionally relevant (Witelson, 1977, 1992; Galaburda et al., 1978; Geschwind and Galaburda, 1985).

Furthermore, a number of studies support the general notion that the amount of cerebral cortex dedicated to a particular function may reflect the brain capabilities in that area (Eccles, 1977; Jerison, 1977; Garraghty and Kaas, 1992).

However, the size of a brain region is not always positively correlated with its capabilities. Often, a larger cerebral hemisphere can be observed due to neuronal migration abnormalities or other cortical malformations. In the domain of language more specifically, the brains of individuals with dyslexia appear to be more symmetrical, with a larger than usual planum temporale on the right, rather than a smaller planum temporale on the left (Galaburda, 1993; Kushch et al., 1993).

Thus, anatomical asymmetries, whether gross or fine, cannot be viewed in isolation and must eventually be considered in the context of physiology of the neuronal systems to which they contribute (Geschwind and Iacoboni, 2007).

Handedness is of particular interest because it is a behavioral manifestation of brain laterality for certain manual activities and it is also related to other, more cognitive aspects of laterality.

Direction and magnitude of hand dominance may even be determined by different factors, with the magnitude being more heritable and with the direction being more subject to environmental influence.

Handedness is at least moderately related to other form of laterality. Thus, there is a greater proportion of left-handed individuals who show a laterality effect in a direction opposite to that which is considered prototypical.

ASYMMETRY BETWEEN THE HEMISPHERES
in humans
Introduction

For more than a century, studies of behavioral defects produced by unilateral cerebral lesions had focused on motor planning, language, perceptual analysis, and afterwards on emotions and affects.

In reality, the emotional behavior of some patients affected by extensive lesions of the right hemisphere is so striking that it had attracted the attention of such important neurologists and psychiatrists as such Babinski (1914), Schilder (1935), and Critchley (1955, 1957).

However, much current theorizing about the nature of cerebral asymmetry is based on laterality research. The noninvasive studies are indirect measures of brain function and are far less precise than anatomical measures.

Behavioral measures of laterality do not correlate perfectly with invasive measures of cerebral asymmetry. However, laboratory studies of normal subjects and "split brain" patients have shown which hemisphere processes are dependent on relative weighting of many variables (Beaumont, 1997). In addition to underlying hemispheric organization, these include the nature of the task (e.g., modality, speed factors, complexity), the subject's set of expectancies with the task, previously developed perceptual or response strategies, and inherent subject variable such as sex and handedness (Bryden, 1978; Bouma, 1990; Levine, 1995; Kuhl, 2000). Thus, in these subjects the degree to which hemispheric specialization occurs at any given time is a relative phenomenon rather than an absolute one (Hellige, 1995).

Before summarizing a number of the most well-established asymmetries, it is useful to consider three general characteristics of laterality effects: ubiquity, subtlety, and complementarity (Hellige, 2000 and 2001).

Ubiquitary refers to the fact that the two cerebral hemispheres have different levels of ability and different processing propensities in a great many domains (motor activity, language, perception, emotion, etc.).

Subtlety refers to the fact that it is rarely the case that one hemisphere can perform a task or accomplish a specific process quite well, whereas the other hemisphere cannot perform the task or process at all. Instead, both hemispheres typically have some ability, though they may go about a task in different ways and one hemisphere may do a better job than the other. A notable exception to this is speech production, which tends to be controlled exclusively by a single hemisphere (usually the left).

1814

Complementarity refers to the fact that, in many domains, the role for which each hemisphere is dominant can be described as complementary. Consequently, both hemispheres normally play a role in virtually all complex activities, such as understanding language or identifying faces, with their contributions fitting together like two pieces of a puzzle (Hellige, 2000).

Individual differences in the behavior of normal subjects result, at least in part, from individual differences in how the cerebral hemispheres are organized and how functions are lateralized.

At one extreme, people who are logical, analytical, verbal, and meticulous are assumed to rely more on their left hemispheres to solve problems in everyday life, whereas people who are visual, intuitive and synthesizer are more concerned with organizing concepts and visualizing meaningful wholes are assumed to rely more on their right hemisphere.

Anyhow, factors other than brain organization probably contribute to preferred cognitive mode.

On the one hand, strategies used by subjects can significantly influence tests of lateralization, and, on the other hand, cognitive mode may be due to biases in socialization or environmental factors in addition to neuronal, genetic, or constitutional biases.

Nevertheless, the idea that individual differences in behavior and cognition result in part from individual differences in brain organization is a provocative assumption worthy of serious study.

Clinical and neuroimaging studies, including PET, fMRI, ERP, and MEG, allowed researchers to map cerebral activity as it takes place in normal subjects, and performances related to left and right hemisphere functions.

Because both hemispheres are scanned, however, it is possible to assess left - right differences in cerebral activation during a large range of behavioral measures.

Anyhow, clinical study has limitations of functional localization because "symptoms must be viewed as expressions of disturbances in a system, not as direct expressions of focal loss of neuronal tissue" (Benton, 1981).

Aphasics with similar symptoms may present lesions which vary in site or size. On the other hand, cortical mapping by electrode stimulation (Ojemann, 1979) and neuro-imaging techniques (Mazziota et al., 1997) demonstrates a great deal of interindividual variability in cortical patterning. Examples from functional imaging studies show that many different areas of the brain may be engaged during a cognitive task (Franckowiak et al., 1997; Gazzaniga, 2000). For even the relatively simple task of telling whether words represent a pleasant or unpleasant concept, the following areas of the brain showed increased activation: left superior temporal cortex, posterior cingulate, left para-hippocampal gyrus, and left inferior frontal gyrus (McDermott et al., 1999).

It is important to recognize that normal behaviors are functions of the whole brain with important contributions from both hemispheres entering into every activity and emotional state. Only laboratory studies on intact or split brain subjects or studies of persons with lateralized brain damage demonstrate the differences in hemisphere function.

Tradition and common sense favor verbal (left hemisphere) *versus* nonverbal (right hemisphere) dichotomy. However, some theories see this dichotomy as unsatisfactory because a number of facts have been brought forth to support their position. There is the centuries-old observation that some aphasic patients, if primed, can recite familiar prayers faultlessly (Benton and Joynt, 1960).

Some aphasic patients can sing a song (with its words) while some nonaphasic right hemisphere-damaged patients cannot (Benton, 1977; Burkland and Smith, 1977). An aphasic patient who does not understand the propositional content of an utterance may appreciate the import of its prosodic component, i.e., he will know whether the examiner is making a statement, asking a question, or issuing a command.

Conversely, the verbal functions of many right hemisphere-damaged patients are not fully intact, with examination disclosing and at least modest decline in performance level as measured by controlled word association and taken tests.

Another point that is brought up is the sizable number of subjects who show a left ear (i.e., right hemisphere) superiority when processing verbal information in dichotic listening studies.

Observations such as these have impelled some theories to look for a more basic dichotomy. The leading candidates are the "serial-parallel" and "analytic-holistic" pairs.

The two human cerebral hemispheres are not simply mirror images of each other.

Much information on the lateralization of cerebral function has come from studying patients in whom the corpus callosum had been divided (commissurotomy) as a treatment for intractable epilepsy, and from those rare individuals who lack part, or all, of their corpus callosum.

Commissurotomy produces the "split-brain" syndrome, which has provided evidence supporting the notion that abilities or functions are predominantly associated with one or another hemisphere.

Thus, patients with chrome epilepsy, who have undergone surgical section of the corpus callosum in order to relieve their seizures, portray few difficulties under normal circumstances. However, when these "split brain" patients undergo psychological testing, the two halves of the brain appear to behave relatively autonomously, e.g., visual information directed to the right cerebral hemisphere alone does not evoke verbal response, and consequently individuals cannot name objects or real words solely presented to the left visual field. Destruction of the splenium of the corpus callosum and its connections to the left occipital cortex, either by stroke or tumor, leads to the posterior disconnection syndrome of "alexia without agraphia". Such individuals speak and write without difficulty but cannot understand written material (alexia). Disconnection of visual processes in the right hemisphere from the verbal processes of the dominant left cerebral hemisphere is thought to explain the syndrome.

Knowledge of such lateralization of function has been advanced more recently by functional brain imaging techniques.

In sum, in the human brain, the left cerebral hemisphere is usually the dominant hemisphere (in absolute 95% of the population), whereas the right hemisphere is the nondominant hemisphere.

The left hemisphere usually prevails for verbal and linguistic function, for problem solving, for mathematical skills, and for analytical thinking.

The right hemisphere is mostly non-verbal. It is more involved in spatial and holistic or "Gestalt" thinking, in recognition of faces, and in many aspects of musical and poetry skills, and in some emotions (Table 23.5).

Table 23.5

Summary of data on cerebral lateralization (after Kolb and Whishaw, 2003)

Function	Left hemisphere	Right hemisphere
Visual system	Letters, words	Complex geometric patterns Faces
Auditory system sound	Language / related	Nonlanguage environmental sounds Music
Somatosensory system	?	Tactile recognition of complex patterns Braille
Movement	Complex voluntary movement	Movements in spatial patterns
Memory	Verbal memory	Nonverbal memory
Language	Speech Reading Writing Arithmetic	Prosody?
Spatial processes		Geometry Sense of direction Mental rotation of shapes

Note: Functions of the respective hemispheres that are predominantly mediated by one hemisphere in right-handed people.

Memory also shows lateralization. Thus, verbal memory is primarily of left hemisphere function, while non-verbal memory is represented in the right hemisphere. These asymmetries are relative, not absolute, and vary in degree according to the function and individual concern. Moreover, they apply primarily to right-handed men. Those men with left-hand preference, or mixed handedness, make up a heterogeneous group, which (as an approximation) shows reduced or anomalous lateralization, rather than a simple reversal of the situation in right-handers. For example, speech representation can occur in either or both hemispheres. Women show less functional asymmetry, on average, than men (Crossman, 2008).

Historical aspects

Bouillaud

Jean Baptiste Bouillaud (1796-1881) read a paper before the Royal Academy of Medicine in France in which he argued from clinical studies that certain functions are localized in the neocortex and, specifically, that speech is localized in the frontal lobes, in accordance with Gall's beliefs and opposed to Flourens's beliefs. Beginning in 1825 and for a half-century thereafter, Bouillaud was the great champion of Gall's localization of the centers of speech and language in the frontal lobes and he argued repeatedly, vigorously and, at times, rancorously that aphasic disorders resulted only from lesions in this territory. In his *Traité ... de l'encephalite* (1825), he presented 29 cases with and without aphasia and with and without lesions in the anterior, middle, and posterior lobes. All of the aphasic patients had lesions that were in, or close to the anterior lobes. Inspection of Bouillaud's 29 cases shows that 25 had lesions confined to a single hemisphere, 11 in the left hemisphere and 14 in the right. Eight (73%) of the 11 left hemisphere cases were aphasic. Four (29%) of the right hemisphere cases were aphasic. Reviewing his own autopsied cases as well as those in the literature, he typically presented just a few words on the loci of the lesions and sometimes these few words were very imprecise indeed. In some cases, the flat statement that the lesion was in one or the other anterior lobes (or both) is made. However, in other cases, the locus of the lesions is described as being in the "anterior" part of the hemispheres.

Perhaps one reason why Bouillaud did not perceive this trend toward a higher frequency of aphasic disorder in his left hemisphere patients is that not only he was obsessed with the frontal lobe localization of aphasic disorder but he also accepted Gall's dual localization of the centers of speech and language in both hemispheres.

Observing that acts such as writing, drawing, painting, and fencing are carried out with the right hand, Bouillaud also suggested that a part of the brain that controls them might possibly be the left hemisphere.

Marc Dax

Marc Dax was born in 1770 and died in 1837. He studied medicine in Montpellier, his graduate thesis being an interesting survey of the incidence and nature of the diseases occurring over a 5-year period in the small town of Aigues-Mortes. As Gibson (1962) has pointed out, in this thesis Dax called attention to the occasional occurrence of post-seizure focal paralysis in some children. This observation preceded by many years, those of Bravais and Todd, who are usually credited with the first descriptions of the phenomenon.

Dax had a keen interest in the study of language, and this may account for the special attention which he paid to language disturbances. In 1836, 1 year before his death, he wrote a paper (Dax, 1836, 1865) on the association between aphasic disorders and lesions of the left hemisphere for presentation at a regional medical congress at Montpellier. He was, thus, about 66 year old when he wrote his famous mémoire. It is a remarkable document. Dax describes successive observations that led him gradually to the conviction that aphasia was a product of left hemisphere disease. He collected cases over the ensuing 20 years, so that at the time of writing his paper he reported having a series of over 40 cases in which the diagnosis of left hemisphere disease had been made, primarily on clinical ground, without pathological confirmation.

The paper was not published and, as it will be seen, there is no evidence that Marc Dax actually presented it at the congress. When it was, belatedly, submitted for publication, in 1865, by his physician-son, Gustav Dax, 4 years after Broca's initial observation (Broca, 1865), it initiated a controversy about priority which has persisted up to the present day. At the same time, together with his father's memoir, Gustav Dax (Dax, 1865) published a summary of his own observations and views on aphasia (Joynt and Benton, 2000).

From a scientific standpoint, Marc Dax's generalization on the role of the left hemisphere in speech was hardly derived from well documented observations. The clinical descriptions were scanty, and the pathological confirmation was entirely lacking. Dax made no mention of handedness nor did he, in any way, link hand preference to hemispheric localization of speech function. Nonetheless, Marc Dax did make, and for the first time, a clinical observation of the highest importance.

Gustav Dax

Dax's paper (M. Dax, 1865) was published in 1865 by his son, Gustav Dax (G. Dax, 1865), who stated that it had been read at a regional medical meeting in Montpellier in 1836. In fact, there is no evidence that he did present the paper on that occasion (Joynt and Benton, 1964). It is not mentioned in account of the meeting, nor could anyone be found who remembered having heard it. It seems almost certain that, if the paper had been presented, it would not have been totally neglected and would have had some repercussions (Benton, 2000).

The tone of Dax's paper is personally modest but firm in conviction. Its style indicates that it was meant to be a communication to his peer. He was quite aware of the importance of his discovery and he made one or two copies which he sent to professional friends. Why he did not make his discovery known at the time through publication or oral presentation is not clear (Benton, 2000).

Anyhow, there is suggestive evidence that Gustav Dax, the son, did know of the preferential involvement of the left hemisphere in aphasia prior Broca's 1863 report. Presumably, this knowledge was gained from his father – for Gustav Dax had prepared an extensive treatise of his own on aphasia (Dax, 1877) entitled: "Observations intended to prove the constant coincidence of the derangements of speech with a lesion of the left cerebral hemisphere". In the introduction, Gustav Dax pays respect to his father's memory and mentions his father's views on the localization of lesions responsible for the loss of speech. This work of Gustav Dax was received by the Academy of Medicine of Paris on March 24, 1863. Broca's statement on the eight cases of aphasia with left hemisphere lesions was delivered on April 2, 1863. Unfortunately, the commission appointed by the Academy to examine Gustav Dax's essay did not publish a report on it until 2 years later. Additional support for Dax's claim was provided in 1879 by Caizergues, who reported he had discovered a copy of Marc Dax's memoir when classifying the papers of his grandfather who had been dean of the faculty of Montpellier (Caizergues, 1879). There is, therefore, excellent evidence that Marc Dax did make his observation prior to Broca.

In short, Marc Dax had made an observation for which he was unwilling to take public responsibility, and hence he recorded it in the form of an essentially private communication (Benton, 2000).

Broca

In 1861, Pierre Paul Broca (1824-1880) reported two instances of aphasia with lesions in the left third frontal convolution (Broca, 1861).

He made no mention at that time of the significance of both these lesions occurring on the left side. Later, at a meeting of the Anthropological Society of Paris on April 2, 1863, Broca reported on eight autopsies (Broca, 1863) of patients with aphasia and noted that they all had lesions in the third frontal convolution. In 1865, Broca expanded his views of the special role of the left hemisphere in speech and also discussed his priority in making these observations (Broca, 1865).

In consequence Broca located speech in the third convolution of the frontal lobe on the left side of the brain. Thus, he discovered that functions could be localized to a side of the brain, a property that is referred to as lateralization. Because speech is thought to be central in human consciousness, the left hemisphere is frequently referred to as the dominant hemisphere, to recognize its special role in language. Thus, the concept of hemispheric cerebral dominance was born when Broca (1865) was led to conclude from his observations that "we speak with the left hemisphere". He had read Marc Dax's paper as published by his son in 1865 and, naturally, wished to read the original presentation along with any discussion. He searched in vain throughout the medical literature for the original report or even for a reference to the 1836 paper. He then asked the librarian of the Montpellier Faculty of Medicine to make personal inquiries regarding the 1836 presentation. The librarian reported that he had interviewed 20 physicians who had attended the 1836 congress at Montpellier, and none could recall such a presentation. Hence Broca was, with good reason, quite skeptical that Marc Dax had actually presented his paper at the congress.

The discussion on priority was reopened by Broca in 1877 (Broca, 1877). He stated that he had obtained a manuscript of the Marc Dax paper, purportedly presented in 1836, and compared it with the Gustav Dax manuscript on aphasia. Broca admits that the style, the mode of expression and the discussion all demonstrated no difference in origin. Therefore, he did not doubt that the paper was written in 1836 by Marc Dax for presentation, but he did not believe that it was ever presented. Broca speculated that Marc Dax probably felt ensure of his ground and did not have the courage to face a discussion as there was no confirmation of his cases by autopsy findings (Benton, 2000).

However, Broca's anatomical analysis was criticized by French anatomist Pierre Marie, who reexamined the brains of Broca's first two patients, Tan, and a Monsieur Lelong, 25 years after Broca's death. Marie pointed out in his article titled "The Third Left Frontal Convolution Plays No Particular Role in the Function of Language" that Lelong's brain showed general nonspecific atrophy, common in senility, and that Tan had additional extensive damage in his posterior cortex that may have accounted for his aphasia. Broca had been aware of Tan's posterior damage but concluded that, whereas the posterior damage contributed to his death, the anterior damage had occurred earlier, producing aphasia.

Anyhow, a lesion in Broca's area resulted in a loss of motor memory-images and hence produced a primarily expressive aphasia with preservation of the capacity to understand speech. The speech pattern is nonfluent: on beside examination, the patient speaks hesitantly, after producing the principal, meaning-containing nouns and verbs but omitting small grammatical words and morphemes. This pattern is called agrammatism or telegraphic speech. Patients with acute Broca's aphasia may be mute or may produce single words, often with dysarthria and apraxia of speech, naming is deficient, but the patient often manifests a "tip of the tongue" phenomenon, getting out the first letter or phoneme of the correct name.

Paraphasic errors in naming are more frequently of literal than verbal type (Kirshner, 2000).

Auditory comprehension seems intact, but detailed testing usually reveals some deficiency, particularly in the comprehension of complex syntax. Repetition is hesitant in these patients, resembling their spontaneous speech. Reading is often impaired. Broca's aphasics may have difficulty with syntax in reading, just as in auditory comprehension and speech. Writing is virtually always deficient in Broca's aphasias. Most patients have a right hemiparesis necessitating use of nondominant, left hand for writing. Many patients can scrawl only a few letters.

Associated neurological deficits of Broca's aphasics include right hemiparesis, hemisensory loss, and apraxia of the oral apparatus and the nonparalyzed left limbs.

An important clinical feature of Broca's aphasia is its frequent association with depression (Robinson, 1997).

The lesions responsible for Broca's aphasia usually include the traditional Broca's area in the posterior part of the inferior frontal gyrus, along with damage to adjacent cortex and subcortical white matter.

Lesions involving the traditional Broca's area (Brodmann's areas 44 and 45) resulted in difficulty initiating speech, and lesions combining Broca's area, the lower precentral gyrus, and subcortical white matter yielded the full syndrome of Broca's aphasia.

Aphemia, a rare variant of Broca's aphasia, is a nonfluent syndrome in which the patient is initially mute and then able to speak with phoneme substitutions and pauses. Aphemia may be equivalent to pure apraxia of speech (Kirshner, 2000).

Wernicke

Broca himself was not greatly concerned with the neurological mechanisms underlying speech and its disturbance. It was left to a younger physician, German anatomist Carl Wernicke (1848-1904), to develop a mature theory of the nature of aphasic disorders. In a monograph appeared in 1874, Wernicke demonstrated that a fluent aphasic disorder, characterized by impaired understanding of speech and disordered expressive speech, was specifically associated with disease in the territory of the posterior temporal lobe of the left hemisphere (Wernicke, 1874). Wernicke was aware that the part of the cortex that receives the sensory pathway, or projection, from the ear – and this is called the auditory cortex – is located in the temporal lobe, behind Broca's area. He, therefore, suspected a relation between the functioning of hearing and speech, and he described cases of aphasic patients with lesions in this auditory projection area that differed from those described by Broca. Like Broca, he conceived aphasia as a disorder of the sign function of language. He denied that aphasic patients were necessarily impaired in intellect even though, as a clinician, he knew that many aphasics, perhaps a majority, did in fact show cognitive defects that extended beyond the realm of language. But he insisted that "nothing could be worse for the study of aphasia than to consider the intellectual disturbance associated with aphasia as an essential part of the disease picture".

However, Wernicke went beyond his empirical discovery and his restriction of aphasia to a disorder of the sign function of language to create a model of the neurological mechanisms, derangements of which produced aphasic disorder. His model, and the revision of it, developed by other neurologists, postulated the existence of interconnected cerebral centers of speech in which memory-images of the different modalities of speech were stored. A center for memory-images of the movement patterns of expressive speech was located in Broca's area in the posterior frontal region. A center for auditory memory-images of words was located in Wernicke's area in the posterior temporal lobe. A center for visual memory-images of words was located further back in the angular gyrus. Whether or not there was a specific center for memory-images of the movements patterns of writing was a subject of debate. Those who believed in the existence of such a center placed it either in the second frontal gyrus above Broca's area or in the supramarginal gyrus close to the center for visual memory-images of words (Benton, 2000).

In any case, Wernicke provided the first model for how language is organized in the left hemisphere. It hypothesizes a programmed sequence of activities in Wernicke's and Broca's language areas. Wernicke proposed that auditory information is sent to the temporal lobes from the ear. In Wernicke's area, sounds are turned into sound images or ideas of objects and stored. From Wernicke's area, the ideas can be sent through a pathway called the arcuate fasciculus to Broca's area, where the representations of speech movements are retained. From Broca's area, instructions are sent to muscles that control movements of the mouth to produce the appropriate sound.

If the temporal lobe were damaged, speech movements could still be mediated by Broca's area, but the speech would make no sense, because the person would be unable to monitor the words.

Because damage to Broca's area produces loss of speech movements without the loss of sound images, Broca's aphasia is not accompanied by a loss of understanding (Kolb and Whishaw, 2003).

Wernicke's aphasia may be considered a syndrome opposite to Broca's aphasia, in that expressive speech is fluent but comprehension is impaired. The speech pattern is effortless and sometimes even excessively fluent (logorrhea). A speaker of a foreign language would notice nothing amiss, but a listener who shares the patient's language detects speech empty of meaning, containing verbal paraphasias, neologisms, and jargon productions. Neurologists refer to this pattern as paragrammatism. In milder cases, the intended meaning of an utterance may be discerned, but the sentence goes away with paraphasic substitutions (Kirshner, 2000). Naming in Wernicke's aphasia is deficient, often bizarre with paraphasic substitutions for the correct name. Auditory comprehension is impaired, sometimes even for the simple nonsense questions. Auditory perception of phonemes is deficient in Wernicke's aphasia, but deficient semantics is the major cause of the comprehension disturbance; disturbed access to semantics and to the internal lexicon is central to the deficit of Wernicke's aphasia. Although the patients were able to hear, they could not understand or repeat what was said to them. Reading comprehension is usually affected, but occasional patients show greater deficit in one modality. Writing is also impaired, but in a manner quite different from that of Broca's aphasia (Kirshner, 2000).

The diverse symptom-pictures of aphasia encountered in clinical practice were explained in terms of either a lesion in one or more centers (i.e., the "central" aphasia) or a lesion in the connections between them (i.e., the "conduction" aphasia). Temporal lobe aphasia is sometimes called fluent aphasia, to emphasize that the person can say words. It is more frequently called Wernicke's aphasia, however, in honor of Wernicke's description. The region of the temporal lobe associated with the aphasia is called Wernicke's area.

Most patients have no elementary motor or sensory deficits, although a partial or complete right homonymous hemianopsia may be present.

The psychiatric manifestations of Wernicke's aphasia are quite different from those of Broca's aphasia.

Depression is less common; many Wernicke's aphasics seem unaware of, or unconcerned about their communicative deficits. With time, some patients become angry or paranoid about the inability of family members and medical staff to understand them.

The lesions of patients with Wernicke's aphasia are usually in the posterior portion of the superior temporal gyrus, sometimes extending into the inferior parietal lobe.

Damage to Wernicke's area (Brodmann's area 22) has been reported to correlate most closely with persistent loss of comprehension of single words, although others (Kertesz et al., 1993) have found only larger temporoparietal lesions in patients with lasting Wernicke's aphasia.

A receptive speech area in the left inferior temporal gyrus has been suggested by electrical stimulation studies and by a few descriptions of patients with seizures involving this area (Kirshner et al., 1995), but aphasia has not been recognized with destructive lesions of this area.

Extension of the lesion into the inferior parietal region may predict greater involvement of reading comprehension.

Wernicke also predicted a new language disorder although he never saw such a case. He suggested that, if the arcuate fibres connecting the two speech areas (Wernicke's and Broca's area) were cut, disconnecting the areas but without inflicting damage on either one, a speech deficit that Wernicke described as conduction aphasia would result. Conductive aphasia has been advanced as a classical disconnection syndrome. Geschwind later pointed to the arcuate fasciculus, a white matter tract traveling from the deep temporal lobe, around the sylvian fissure to the frontal lobe, as the site of disconnection (Geschwind, 1965). Conduction aphasia is an uncommon but theoretically important syndrome that can be remembered by its striking deficit of repetition. Most patients have relatively normal spontaneous speech, although some make literal paraphasic errors and hesitate frequently for self-correction. Naming may be impaired, but auditory comprehension is preserved. A patient who can express himself at a sentence level and comprehend conversation may be unable to repeat even single words. Reading and writing are somewhat variable, but reading aloud may share some of the same difficulty as repeating.

Associated deficits include hemianopsia in some patients; right-sided sensory loss may be present, but right hemiparesis is usually mild or absent (Kirshner, 2000).

The lesions of conduction aphasia are usually in either the superior temporal or inferior parietal regions. Patients with limb apraxia have parietal lesions (supramarginal gyrus). The supramarginal gyrus appears to be involved in auditory immediate memory and in phoneme generation. Lesions in this area are associated with conduction aphasia and phonemic paraphasic errors.

Wernicke proposed that, although different regions of the brain have different function they are interdependent in that to work, because they must receive information from one another. Using this same reasoning, French neurologist Joseph Déjérine (1849-1917), in 1892, described a case in which the loss of the ability to read (alexia, meaning "word blindness", from Greek lexia, for "word") resulted from a disconnection between the visual area of the brain and Wernicke's area. So, Déjérine (1892) elucidated the neuroanatomic substrate of pure alexia on the basis of autopsy study of a patient with this disorder. His patient, an educated man and an accomplished musician, suddenly lost the ability to read musical scores as well as conventional written material. Yet he could write, perform music from memory, and showed no difficulty in the expression or understanding of oral speech. He had a right visual field defect – in all probability a hemiachromatopsia, not a hemianopsia. Autopsy study disclosed infarctions in the territory of the left posterior cerebral artery, specifically, the mesial occipital area and the splenium of the corpus callosum. Déjérine inferred that the lesions had the effects of preventing the transmission of visual information to the language centers of the left hemisphere, thus making reading impossible while leaving the interpretation of nonverbal visual stimuli intact.

Déjérine and others accept the proposition that aphasia involves a defect in intelligence.

Neurolinguists and cognitive psychologists have divided alexias according to breakdowns in specific stages of the reading process. The linguistic concepts of surface structure *versus* the deep meanings of words have been instrumental in these new classifications. Four patterns of alexia (or dyslexia, in British usage) have been recognized: letter-by-letter, deep, phonological, and surface dyslexia.

Like reading, writing may be affected either in isolation (pure agraphia) or in association with aphasia (aphasic agraphia). In addition, writing can be impaired by motor disorders, by apraxia, and by visuospatial deficits. Isolated agraphia has been described with left frontal or parietal lesions.

Disconnection is an important idea because it predicts that complex behaviors are built up in assembly-line fashion as information collected by sensory systems enters the brain and travels through different structures before resulting in an overt response of some kind. Furthermore, the disconnection of structures by cutting connecting pathways can result in impairments that resemble those produced by damaging the structures themselves (Kolb and Whishaw, 2003).

The conflict between the "noetic" and "connectionist" school on the issues of the nature of aphasic disorder and its underlying neural substrate continued through the early decades of the twentieth century.

The decades since World War II have witnessed a tremendous surge of interest in the aphasic disorders.

Pitres and amnesic aphasia

Clinicians such as Batteman (1870), Kussmaul (1876) and Banti (1886) identified patients whose most prominent (and, sometimes, only) disability was their incapacity to produce the names of objects and persons. Applying the old term "amnesic aphasia" to this symptom-picture, they regarded it as a distinctive type of speech impairment and included it as such in their classification of the aphasic disorders.

Broadbend (1878) proposed that amnesic aphasia resulted from destruction or dysfunction of a "naming centre" in the posterior region of the left hemisphere, and Milles and McConnell (1895) localized this centre in the third and second temporal gyri.

In 1898, Pitres began by describing what he considered to be a case of pure amnesic aphasia. He distinguished between three forms of amnesic aphasia. The first is antonomasia (word substitution) in which the patient fails to recall and produce substantives within setting of adequate conversational speech and understanding. The second is agrammatism, i.e., inability to formulate acceptable sentences. The third is differential loss of language in polyglots. The anomic patient is less severely impaired than the agrammatic patient who has difficulty in recalling verbs and connectives as well as substantives. The differential loss in polyglots is attributable to differences in the depth of a patient's knowledge of the languages. Thus, Pitres' concept of amnesic aphasia was fairly broad, extending beyond anomia to encompass the lexical and syntactical impoverishment of agrammatism.

Pitres indicated that the causative lesion is most frequently found to be in the inferior parietal lobule, sometimes with extension into the angular gyrus. Amnesic aphasia is produced by breaks in the outflow from psychosensory centers to the whole cortex and hence there cannot be an absolutely constant localization of the responsible lesion. The patient with amnesic aphasia should not only experience difficulty in producing words corresponding to his ideas but also be unable to grasp the ideas represented by words said to him. Anyhow, pure amnesic aphasia is rare. The disorder in naming is usually accompanied by other disabilities.

"The existence of a clinical form of aphasia, uniquely determined by the loss of the evocation of words", cannot be questioned. The syndrome cannot be identified with any major category in current classifications and its autonomy should be recognized. It is an associative aphasia that may be placed between the motor or emissive and sensory or receptive aphasias.

Amnesic or anomic aphasia has figured prominently in modern classifications of the aphasic disorders (Albert et al., 1981). However, reservations about its neuropathologic significance are often expressed and not uncommonly it is described as being merely a symptom-complex that appears in the course of recovery from a more pervasive fluent, non-fluent or transcortical aphasic disorder. Finally, modern neurodiagnostic techniques have yet to be brought to bear on the question of lesional localization and underlying neurological mechanisms. Thus, whether or not Pitres's amnesic aphasia is a useful and meaningful neuropsychological concept remains to be determined.

In summary, anomic aphasia refers to aphasic syndromes in which naming, or access to the internal lexicon, is the principal deficit.

Isolated, severe anomia may indicate focal left hemisphere pathology. Alexander and Benson (1991) refer to the angular gyrus as the site of lesions producing anomic aphasia, but lesions there usually produce other deficits as well, including alexia and the four elements of Gerstmann's syndrome: agraphia, right - left disorientation, acalculia, and finger agnosia, or inability to identify fingers. Isolated lesions of the temporal lobe can produce pure anomia, and positron emission tomography studies of naming in normal subjects have also shown consistent activation of the superior temporal lobe.

Anomic aphasia thus serves as an indicator of left hemisphere or diffuse brain disease (mass lesions elsewhere in the brain, and diffuse degenerative disorders), but it has only limited localization value.

Geschwind

Norman Geschwind (1926-1984) presented his ideas in a now classic paper, "Disconnexion Syndromes in Animals and Man", which was published in 1965. This comprehensive analysis, some 100 pages in length, presented the concept of discon-nection and illustrated its far-reaching implications. Its impact was immediate and far-reaching. In a real sense, it brought neuroanatomy back into the field of aphasia, apraxia, and agnosia, and it provided a fruitful approach to the understanding of these types of disorders, as well as other behavioral manifestations of brain disease.

Today, when we undertake to analyze the mechanisms underlying aphasic disorders, amnesic syndromes, perceptual defects, and visuomotor disabilities, we think in terms of disconnection – not simple disconnection, to be sure, but rather of disturbances of progression and interaction in information processing that are based on the destruction of specific pathways (Benton, 2000).

Wernicke's speech model was updated by American neurologist Norman Geschwind in the 1960s and is now sometimes referred to as the Wernicke-Geschwind model.

Aphasia and thought

A majority of aphasic patients do show impairment on one or another measure of cognitive functions and their defects are by no means restricted to tests of abstract reasoning or symbolic thinking. They are generally more impaired than are nonaphasic patients with left-hemisphere disease.

Among aphasic patients, those with significant defects in oral verbal comprehension are most likely to show defective nonverbal test performance.

Moreover, certain nonverbal tasks, such as the identification of environmental sounds and pantomime recognition, are failed only by aphasics (and perhaps severely demented patients) but not nonaphasics with brain disease (Vignolo, 1969; Duffy et al., 1975; Varney, 1978; Varney and Benton, 1982; Dănăilă and Golu, 2006).

However, the overriding finding (often overlooked in intergroup comparisons) is one of extreme interindividual variability among aphasic patients, even among those with severe disturbances in comprehension. This variability indicates that in virtually every sample of aphasics some will perform normally, a fact which has been convincingly documented in case reports (Alajouanine and Lhermitte, 1964; Zangwill, 1964).

In addition, there is no evidence for a significant relationship between the degree of deficit in nonverbal task performance and the severity of aphasic disorder (Basso et al., 1973), in part because stroke-produced aphasia is such an important cause of socio-economic disability. At the same time, neurodiagnostic procedures, such as CT, magnetic resonance imaging, functional magnetic resonance imaging, magnetoencephalography, and positron-emission tomography, permit investigators to collect a substantial amount of clinicopathologic data fairly quickly and new discoveries have modified concepts about classification and lesional localization.

ASYMMETRIES OF THE HUMAN FRONTAL LOBES

In the course of the brain evolution, the frontal lobes developed most recently to become its largest structures. It was natural to conclude that the frontal lobes must therefore be the seat of the highest cognitive functions. Thus, when Hebb reported in 1939 that a small series of patients who had undergone surgical removal of frontal lobe tissue showed no loss in IQ score on a standard intelligence test, he provoked a controversy. Afterwards, Klebanoff (1945) noted the seemingly unresolvable discrepancies between studies reporting on the cognitive status of patients with frontal lobe lesions. He found that since Fritsch and Hitzig (1870) first reported mental deterioration in patients with traumatic frontal lesions, more authors had described cognitive deficits in patients with frontal lobe damage than denied the presence of such deficits in their patients. The large number of World War II missile wound survivors and the popularity of psychosurgery on the frontal lobes for treatment of psychiatric disorders in the 1940s and 1950s ultimately provided enough cases of frontal brain damage to eliminate speculative misconceptions about frontal lobe functions (Dănăilă and Golu, 1988; Lezak et al., 2004). The frontal lobes are the closest neural representation of popular notions of "intelligence" or Spearman's g factor because of their important role in contributing to success on diverse cognitive tasks (Duncan et al., 2000). Thus, we know now that many cognitive and social behaviors may be disrupted by frontal lobe damage. The three major divisions of the frontal lobes (precentral division, premotor division, and prefrontal division) differ functionally, although each is involved more or less directly with behavior output (Stuss and Benson, 1986; Pandya and Barnes, 1987; Goldberg, 1990; Damasio, 1991; Stuss et al., 1994; Pandya and Yeterian, 1998).

Asymmetries in language

In the last two decades, functional imaging has provided a revealing view of areas involved in healthy and neurologically impaired subjects (Roland, 1984; Petersen et al., 1988; Binder et al., 1995; Klein et al., 1995; Warburton et al., 1996). Most observant clinicians have remarked on the variability and overlap of aphasic syndromes, especially in the immediate period following brain injury, as well as the individual differences in symptoms between patients with apparently similar lesions (Benson, 1986; Galaburda et al., 1990). In light of the individual variability in gross morphology in humans (Andrianov, 1979; Rajkowska and Goldman-Rakic, 1995) there is a left-hemisphere superiority and proficiency for the majority of vocal, motor, and language function (Geschwind, 1970; Benson, 1986).

However, some language capacity exists in most right hemispheres (Dănăilă and Golu, 1987; Iacoboni and Zaidel, 1996). Especially, is the predominance of the right frontal lobe in the production of the melodic components that contribute to prosody, as well as the expression of the emotional content of language.

Because spoken and written language are human specializations, detailed animal models of the role of different frontal subregions serving language are not available (Geschwind and Iacoboni, 2007).

This is in contrast to frontal lobe participation in other cognitive functions, such as working memory and sensorimotor integration, in which studies in primates have vastly accelerated our knowledge of regional subspecializations and provided models that can be tested in humans (Goldman-Rakic, 1987; Funahashi et al., 1989; Wilson et al., 1993; Petrides, 1994).

Broca's original belief that lesions confine to the posterior portion of the third left frontal gyrus caused loss of articulatory function (aphémie) occurred on the background of conviction (Broca, 1861 a, b, c; 1864 a, b; 1865), shared by his contemporaries, that the left and right frontal lobes were identical in size and anatomy (Flourens, 1824; Broca, 1865; Berker et al., 1986).

The recovery of language function occurred through the compensatory effort of homologous, essentially equipotential regions in the right frontal lobe (Geschwind and Iacoboni, 2007). Following Broca, numerous cases supported the left hemispheric localization of language in right-handers, while expanding the cerebral territory responsible for language functions (Wernicke, 1874; Jackson, 1880, 1915; Broca, 1888).

Jackson (1868) presented the first case of the left-handed man with aphasia and right-sided lesions, further supporting between hand dominance and language lateralization. Afterwards studies have confirmed the functional localization of language to the left hemisphere in 99% of right-handers (Hécaen et al., 1981; Annett, 1985; Benson, 1986). However, this relationship is less certain in left-handers, with most demonstrating either left-hemisphere or bilateral language, and, less frequently, right-hemisphere language (Geschwind, 1970; Hécaen et al., 1981; Geschwind and Galaburda, 1985).

Anyhow, removal of the first two to three gyri of the left frontal operculum pars opercularis (area 44) and triangularis (area 45) anterior to Brodmann's area 4 on the left in epilepsy surgery resulted in nonfluent aphasia in every case except one (Penfield and Roberts, 1959).

Cortical stimulation studies by these same investigators demonstrated speech arrest from stimulation of the first two opercular gyri on the left, but never on the right.

Stimulation of the left supplementary motor area (SMA), and not of the right, produced speech arrest (Penfield and Roberts, 1959). Lesions of the SMA can produce transcortical motor aphasia, whereas similar lesions on the right do not, consistent with the proposed role of the SMA in speech initiation (Masdeu, 1978; Freedman et al., 1984).

Thus, in the left hemisphere, lesions in the portion of the motor association area that mediates the motor organization and patterning of speech may result in speech disturbances that have as their common feature disruption of speech production with intact comprehension. These deficits may range in severity from total suppression of speech (Caplan, 1987; Jonas, 1987; Eslinger and Reichwein, 2001) to mild slowing and reduced spontaneously of speech production (Stuss and Benson, 1990). Other alterations in speech production may include stuttering, poor or monotonous tonal quality, or diminished control of the rate of speech production.

Luria (1970) and Dronkers et al. (2000) demonstrated a motor pattern apraxia of speech (oral apraxia) which may include difficulty imitating simple oral gestures in connection with lesions in this area, although this condition can also occur with somewhat more posterior lesions (Tognola and Vignola, 1980).

Lesion studies support the presence of an anterior frontal lobe language area that encompasses Broca's area and additional perisylvian areas more posteriorly. In a series of patients there are lateralized left-sided lesions of the posterior part of the inferior gyrus, 17 out of 19 patients had difficulties in language fluency (Hécaen and Consoli, 1973). Patients with lesions largely confined to the cortical surface corresponding to Broca's region did not have significant agrammatism, or writing difficulties, whereas those with deeper lesions tended to have more profound language impairment. None of 15 patients with a homologous right-sided lesion demonstrated any language or articulatory deficits, confirming the relative specialization of the left inferior frontal gyrus for language output (Geschwind and Iacoboni, 2007).

Numerous case studies have underscored the relationship between the extension of lesion into cortical regions adjacent to the third frontal gyrus and the severity of the Broca's aphasia (Tonkonogy and Goodglass, 1981). Articulatory disturbances (dysarthria and dysprosody) are typically associated with lesions that extend into the opercular precentral gyrus (Alexander et al., 1990).

A combination of word-finding difficulties, paraphasias, and slowness in speech is observed with lesions of the pars triangularis and pars opercularis. Involvement of both regions typically leads to a more severe and lasting nonfluent aphasia. Mohr et al. (1978)

1829

have also demonstrated that lesions localized to Broca's area lead to nonfluent aphasia or nonmotor articulatory disturbance, as well as persistent apraxia and dysprosody, but not frank agrammatism, as is paradigmatic in many current formulations of nonfluent (Broca's) aphasia. Those with typical Broca's aphasia have larger lesions that encompassed deeper white matter structures, anterior insula, and adjacent perisylvian regions (Mohr et al., 1978; Alexander et al., 1990).

Morphological asymmetries. Comparison of the weights of both hemispheres yielded variable and inconclusive results (Thurman, 1866; Broca, 1875; Aresu, 1914; Von Bonin, 1962). However, the left hemisphere is greater than the right, suggesting more cortical surface area overall on the left (Von Bonin, 1962). Indirect measurements taken of indentations in the skull, called petalias, reflect outgrowth of the adjacent cerebral hemisphere. Thus, the presence of marked left occipital petalia, the nature of frontal lobe asymmetries has been less obvious (Tinley, 1927; Hadziselmovic and Cus, 1966). However, most careful quantitative studies in adequate numbers of cases show a predominance of the right frontal petalia (Hadziselmovic and Cus, 1966; Geschwind and Galaburda, 1985).

Le May and Kido (1978) made direct measurements of the frontal lobes and demonstrated that the width of the right frontal region was greater in 58% of right-handed patients and extended further in 31%, as opposed to only 14% that extend further forward on the left. This gross structural asymmetry has been consistently observed in more recent studies (Geschwind and Galaburda, 1985; Bear et al., 1986; Glickson and Myslobodsky, 1993).

However, the meaning of these observations is unclear, because they do not reflect the total extent of cortical surface area because much of cortical surface area is contained in the sulcal folds. This explanation is likely to hold for the studies of Wada et al. (1975), that demonstrated a right-side size advantage when only the lateral cortical surfaces of areas 44 and 45 were measured (Fig. 23.1).

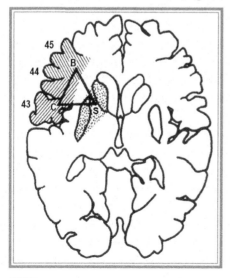

Fig. 23.1. Cerebral structures concerned with language output and articulation.
B = Broca's area; C = pre- and postcentral gyri; S = striatum. Areas 43, 44, and 45 are Brodmann's cytoarchitectonic areas. A lesion in any of the components of this output network (B, C, or S) can produce a mild and transient Broca's aphasia.
Large lesions, damaging all three components, produce severe persistent Broca's aphasia with sparse, labored, agrammatic speech but
well-preserved comprehension. (Illustration by courtesy of Dr. Andrew Kertesz).

One of the first detailed measurements based on cytoarchitectonic divisions of the frontal lobes were carried out by Kononova (1935, 1949).

This work on five right-handed subjects not only showed that the total area of the left frontal lobe was larger than the right by 16%, but also that Brodmann's areas 45 and 47 were larger on the left by a margin of 30% and 45% respectively.

Kononova also observed a larger amount of individual variation in these and other regions of frontal lobe, highlighting the difficulty in drawing firm conclusions from this study of only six cases.

Galaburda's (1980) detailed study of the magnocellular region of the pars opercularis, which largely coincides with area 44, demonstrated the left side to be larger than the right, in the majority of 10 cases.

Hayes and Lewis (1993) have demonstrated a population of magnopyramidal neurons that are 15% larger in left Brodmann's area 45 than in the right.

No difference was seen between similar large pyramidal neurons in area 4 (Hayes and Lewis, 1995). However, in area 46 of the dorsolateral prefrontal cortex, the magnopyramidal neurons were about 10% smaller on the left. These differences are not large. Other investigators have demonstrated consistent morphological asymmetries in more extensive regions of the third or inferior frontal gyrus using autopsy material and MRI in living patients (Falzi et al., 1982; Albanese et al., 1989; Foundas et al., 1995, 1996).

Foundas et al. (1996) demonstrated a striking correlation between the direction of pars triangularis (area 45) asymmetry and hemispheric language lateralization, providing the most convincing evidence to date of the correspondence between language and anatomical asymmetries in the frontal lobe. Nine of 10 patients with Wada test-proven lateralization of language to the left hemisphere displayed asymmetry in favor of the left pars triangularis.

Although it is most likely that an increased neuron number underlies the larger areas 44 and 45 of the left hemisphere (Galaburda, 1993), an increase in neuropil size could also account for the left-hemispheric predominance.

Scheibel et al. (1985) and Simonds and Scheibel (1989) emphasize that pars triangularis and pars opercularis have been shown to have increased complexity of higher-order dendritic branching on the left relative to the primary motor cortex in both hemispheres, and pars triangularis and pars opercularis on the right. However, significance of dendritic branching is uncertain.

Functional imaging

Positron emission tomography (PET) and functional magnetic resonance imaging (fMRI) have supported the functional specialization of the left frontal cortex in language and language-related tasks (Frith et al., 1991; Mc Carthy et al., 1993; Binder et al., 1995; Klein et al., 1995; Just et al., 1996). Indeed, widespread areas of lateral frontal hypometabolism are even seen in patients with aphasia and lesions in parietal and temporal cortex, further implicating the lateral left frontal cortex in language function and recovery (Metter, 1991).

Even simple language tasks, although highly lateralized, activate a network of widely distributed left-hemisphere cortical areas (Petersen et al., 1988; Binder et al., 1995; Just et al., 1996). In most careful PET of fMRI studies of language, homologous regions are often activated on the right side, although typically at far lower levels than those on the left (Habib et al., 1996; Just et al. 1996; Warburton et al., 1996). The left-hemisphere activations are highly variable and extend beyond Broca's region, including the supplementary motor area, and cingulate medially, and the dorsolateral prefrontal cortex and the premotor area laterally.

One of the factors confounding the interpretation of PET language data is the variability in activated areas across different studies. In spite of this variability, left perisylvian regions in general, and Broca's area in particular show consistent activation in language tasks. So, the Broca's area is a critical structure dedicated solely to language output. Since Broca's region comprises cytoarchitectonically and physiologically diverse areas, it may serve several language-related functions (Poppel 1996).

Thus, lesions studies, intraoperative electrical stimulation, and PET imaging studies confirm its role in phonological process (Lecours and Lhermitte, 1970; Denny-Brown 1975; Ojemann and Mateer, 1979; Demonet et al., 1994; Zatorre et al., 1996).

PET data indicate that Broca's region is activated in a wide variety of non-output-related language tasks, including listening tasks (Roland, 1984).

Phonological discrimination tasks often engage verbal working memory functions, which are typically associated with left frontal lobe predominance as well (Milner and Petrides, 1984; Paulescu et al., 1993; Petrides et al., 1993).

Thus, Broca's region comprises contiguous area serving separate functions that can be simultaneously engaged in the same task.

Denny-Brown (1965, 1975) emphasize the importance of visual input in language acquisition and visual influences on aphasia caused by lesions of Broca's area.

Thus, disruption of the integration of these visual inputs is a component of the lateral alexia that can sometimes be observed in patients with Broca's area lesions (Benson, 1977; Boccardi et al., 1984).

In sum, the functional supremacy of one cerebral hemisphere is crucial to language function. There are many ways of determining that the left side of the brain is dominant: (1) by the loss of speech that occurs with disease in certain parts of the left hemisphere and its preservation with lesions involving corresponding parts of the right hemisphere; (2) by preference, for greater facility in the use of the right hand, foot, and eye; (3) by the arrest of speech with magnetic cortical stimulation or a focal seizure or with electrical stimulation of the anterior language area during surgical procedure; (4) by the injection of sodium amytal into the left internal carotid artery (Wada test – a procedure that produces mutism for a minute or two, followed by misnaming, including preservation and substitution; misreading; and paraphasic speech – effects lasting 8 to 9 min in all); (5) by the dichotic listening test, in which different words or phonemes are presented simultaneously to two ears (yielding a right ear – left hemisphere advantage); (6) by observing increases in cerebral blood flow during language processing: (7) by lateralization of speech and language function following commissurotomy (Adams et al., 1997); and (8) by studies with PET, fMRI and magnetoencephalography.

Asymmetry of prosody and emotion

Despite its minimal contribution to the purely linguistic as well as propositional aspects of language, the right hemisphere does have an important role in the communication of feelings and emotion. It has long been known that globally aphasic patients can shout a curse, when angered. These aspects of language are subsumed under the term prosody, by which is meant the melody of speech, its rhythm, intonation, inflection, and pauses that transmit emotional overtones. The prosodic components, and gestures that accompany them, enhance the meaning of the spoken word and endow language with its richness and vitality (Adams et al., 1997).

Thus, speech involves not only the communication of vocabulary and grammatical content, but also social and emotional content.

The critical role of the right hemisphere in the melodic and musical aspects of speech and language output is supported by the observation of preservation of simple singing ability in many patients with nonfluent aphasia (Yamadori et al., 1977).

Syndromes of loss of emotional aspects of speech are termed **aprosodias**. Motor aprosodia involves loss of expressive emotion with preservation of emotional comprehension; sensory aprosodia involves loss of comprehension; sensory aprosodia involves loss of comprehension of affective language, also called affective agnosia.

Several studies show that patients with right-hemisphere lesions can demonstrate deficiency in interpreting and expressing the emotional content of speech (Ross and Mesulam, 1979).

The lesions described in loss of expressive prosody mostly involve large portions of the frontal lobe and often extend into the parietal lobe, hindering precise anatomical localization (Dordain et al., 1971; Ross and Mesulam, 1979).

The involvement of the basal ganglia in prosody is demonstrated by lesion studies (Cancelliere and Kertesz, 1990; Starkstein et al., 1994).

A PET study supports the role of the right lateral prefrontal cortex in simple pitch discrimination, analogous to the role of Broca's area in phoneme perception (Zatore et al., 1994). Another PET study of emotional prosody comprehension also suggests that right prefrontal cortex is preferentially active in tasks requiring perception and interpretation of emotional prosody, and is not simply dedicated to prosodic expression (George et al., 1996).

The deficit in prosody observed after right frontal lesions is not entirely limited to the expression of emotional and melodic content, however, and can extend into nonemotional semantic aspects, such as syllable stress (Weintraub et al., 1981; Dănăilă and Golu, 1987).

In addition, prosodic elements of speech comprehension and expression can also be impaired in anterior left-hemisphere lesions resulting in Broca's aphasia (Danny and Shapiro, 1982; Benson, 1986).

In the foreign accent syndrome, which can result from left frontal lesions involving Broca's area, and neighboring cortical and subcortical regions, inappropriate syllable stress, phoneme misproduction, rhythm, and pauses occur, changing a patient's accent often without chronically altering other aspects of language (Monrad-Krohn, 1947).

Exaggerated prosody, sometimes observed in nonfluent aphasia, reflects the speaker's attempts to communicate using retained right frontal abilities in the face of minimal linguistic capabilities (Geschwind and Iacoboni, 2007).

The role of orbital frontal lobes in the regulation of emotion and mood has been well established in studies of patients with brain injury (Benson and Stuss, 1986) and tumors.

The orbitofrontal cortex is the cortex of the ventral aspect of the frontal lobe. It comprises mainly areas 11 and 13. The orbital prefrontal syndrome can ensue from a variety of disease processes, including tumors (Fig. 23.2), and aneurisms of the anterior communicating artery (Fig. 23.3).

Attention is disturbed mainly in its exclusionary aspect. The patient is unable to suppress interference from external stimuli or internal tendencies.

Imitation of other and utilization behavior – the compulsion to utilize objects or tools prompted simply by their presence – may be symptoms related to that lack of interference control (Lhermitte et al., 1986)

Orbitofrontal hypermotility is the opposite of the hypomotility and aspontaneity of the apathetic syndrome from lateral and medial lesions. In a substantial number of patients the prevalent effect is euphoria, often accompanied by irritability and a contentious, paranoid stance (Cummings, 1985).

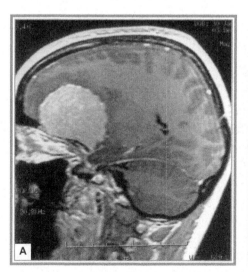 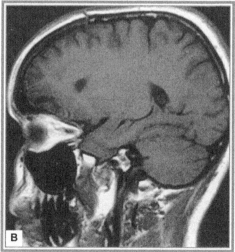

Fig. 23.2. A preoperative contrast enhanced computed tomographic (CT) scan of a 56-year-old man shows a giant size olfactory grove meningioma and displacement of anterior and fronto-basal frontal lobes (A). The patient presents an orbitofrontal syndrome. Postoperative contrast-enhanced CT-scan showing no residual tumor (B) and orbitofrontal syndrome disappeared.

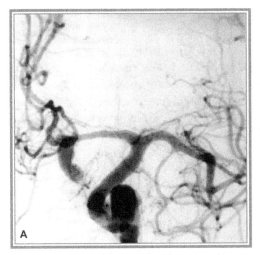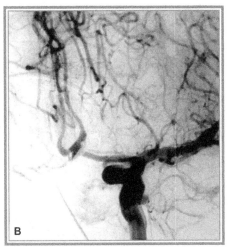

Fig. 23.3 (A) The left carotid angiogram demonstrates an ACoA aneurysm which projects inferiorly. (B) Postoperative angiography demonstrated complete obliteration of the aneurysm with a clip.

Instincts are disinhibited and normal judgement impaired. These patients may show by their behavior a blatant disregard for even the most elementary ethical principles. Thus, orbitofrontal syndrome is oftentimes undistinguishable from mania.

Criminal sociopathy is another psychiatric condition analogous in some respect to the orbitofrontal syndrome (Gorenstein, 1982; Lapierre et al., 1995).

Left frontal damage, especially damage to the anterior frontal lobes, is far more likely to cause depression than similar lesions on the right (Gainotti, 1972; Sackeim et al., 1982; Robinson et al., 1984; Starkstein et al., 1991). Lesions on the right more frequently lead to mania (Jorge et al., 1993), especially regions of the orbitofrontal cortex (Starkstein et al., 1987, 1989). In healthy subjects, left prefrontal cortex cerebral blood flow increases when patients induce a state of dysphoria by thinking sad thoughts (Pardo et al., 1993; George et al., 1995).

A transcranial magnetic stimulation (causing transient hypofunctioning) of the left, but not right prefrontal cortex, resulted in decreased self-report of happiness and a significant increase in sadness rating (Pascual-Leone et al., 1996).

Electrophysiological evidence suggests that the left frontal lobe is more specialized for positive emotions related to approach and exploratory mechanisms and the right for negative avoidance-related reactions (Davidson, 1992; Davidson and Sutton, 1995).

Lateral wall (prefrontal, premotor and primary motor cortex)

The lateral wall of frontal lobe can be subdivided in three main sectors along the anterior-posterior axis: **prefrontal, premotor,** and **primary motor.**

Each of these sectors can be further subdivided in subsectors that are anatomically and functionally differentiated (Matelli et al., 1985; Cavada and Goldman-Rakic, 1989; Stepniewska et al., 1993; Petrides, 1994; Fogassi et al., 1996; Fujii et al., 1996; Geyer et al., 1996; Rizzolatti et al., 1996 a, b).

Prefrontal cortex

The lateral prefrontal cortex is the prefrontal cortex of the lateral convexity of frontal lobe. It comprises part or entirely of areas 8, 9, 10 and 46. It is known to be primarily involved in working memory processes (Goldman-Rakic, 1987). Working memory is the ability to retain an item of information for the prospective execution of an action that is dependent on that information. It is an essential cognitive function for the mediation of cross-temporal contingencies in the temporal integration of reasoning, speech, and goal-directed behavior (Fuster, 2009). Working memory, however, can fail in many patho-logical conditions of the brain. The reason why is failure especially evident and consistently found in the frontal patient is because that kind of memory is necessary for prospective action, whether the action is a motor act, a mental operation, or a piece of spoken language (Fuster, 2009).

Judging from the effects of a prefrontal lesion, working-memory of all modalities seems distributed through lateral cortex, without anatomical compartmentalization for spatial working memory (Müller et al., 2002; Müller and Knight, 2006).

However, the reversible transient lesions by transcranial magnetic stimulation (TMS) have been reported to segregate spatial and non-spatial deficits to the dorsal and ventral lateral cortex, respectively (Mottaghy et al., 2002).

A frontal eye-field (area 8) lesion leads to deficit of working memory for ocular saccades (Ploner et al. 1999). Left-frontal patients have the most difficulty with working memory of verbal items, and right-frontal patients with non-verbal areas.

Right-visuospatial specialization, in patients with right frontal lesions is more likely to demonstrate poor use and representation of visuospatial data in a variety of tasks that require working memory, and those with left frontal lesions are more likely to have disordered memory for episodic information (Kolb and Whishaw, 1985; Milner, 1995). Of patients with unilateral frontal damage, those with right frontal damage show the poorest performance in design fluency tasks (Benson and Stuss, 1986).

Frontal patients, unlike temporal patients, have been noted to perform poorly in spatial as well as nonspatial conditional association tests probably because of the working memory component that those tests contain (Petrides, 1985).

Interference and the failure to control interference clearly play a role in the memory deficit of the frontal patients.

This has been demonstrated by use of memory tasks with proper control of interference factor (Oscar-Berman et al., 1991; Stuss, 1991; Chao and Knight, 1995; Ptito et al., 1995).

So, in patients with brain injury, left frontal lobe damage typically leads to more profound verbal recall deficits than right-sided damage, whereas right frontal damage causes deficits primarily in categorization (Milner and Petrides, 1984; Incisa della Rocchetta, 1986; Incisa della Rocchetta and Milner, 1993).

Deficits in the retrieval of verbal material in patients with left frontal damage may be specific to certain lexical categories, in that injury to the left, but not to the right, premotor areas produced a specific deficit in verb, but not noun retrieval (Damasio and Tranel, 1993).

However, left-hemisphere deficits in short-term or working memory are not limited to the sphere of language and suggest the importance of the left prefrontal cortex in programming strategies, control of executive function, and motor responses (Milner and Petrides, 1984).

Patients with frontal lesions that spare the dorsolateral prefrontal cortex do not exhibit these deficits (Goldman-Rakic, 1987). So, specialization of the left hemisphere is for language and of the right for visuospatial information.

Thus, according to Fuster (2009), frontal patients show deficits in working memory, especially if their lesions include lateral prefrontal cortex. The magnitude and qualities of one such deficit depend on the context of testing, and most important, on the degree to which the test requires the suppression of interference.

A specific framework of the neural substrates of human planning and executive functions comprising working memory suggests that the dorsolateral prefrontal cortex serves mechanisms of active manipulation and monitoring of sensorimotor information within working memory. In this model, the ventrolateral prefrontal cortex serves only working memory mechanisms that support simple retrieval of information for sensory-guided sequential behavior (Petrides, 1994).

The lateral prefrontal cortex receives strong input from extrastriate cortical areas of visual significance (Milner and Goodale, 1995).

The occipitofugal corticocortical pathways consists of a dorsal occipitoparietal stream concerned with the processing of spatial relationships, and a ventral occipito-temporal stream mainly concerned with the processing of object identity (Ungerleider and Mishkin, 1982). This view has been refined, in that the dorsal stream is thought to be primarily related to pragmatic aspects of spatial behavior, whereas the ventral stream is primarily related to semantic aspects of spatial behavior (Goodale and Milner, 1992, Jeannerot et al., 1995).

Thus, working memory for spatial locations is served by the dorsolateral prefrontal cortex, whereas working memory for object identity is served by the ventrolateral prefrontal cortex (Funahashi et al., 1993; Wilson et al., 1993).

Spatial information, for instance, can be readily coded with language. It is probably for such reasons (Milner and Teuber, 1968) that early studies of frontal patients in spatial delay tasks yielded negative results (Ghent et al., 1962; Chorover and Cole, 1966).

Other early studies, using delay task with complex spatial or nonspatial cues and appropriate delays, clearly demonstrated that frontal patients, unlike patients with posterior cortical lesions, have trouble with performance of delay tasks (Konorski, 1959; Milner, 1964). Delays were of up to 60 seconds, and stimuli were such that verbal rehearsal was extremely difficult.

In that nonspatial working memory task, patients with unilateral frontal damage made significantly more errors than normal subjects or than patients with temporal lobe damage.

Lewinsohn et al. (1972) demonstrated similar deficits with visual, auditory, and kinesthetic stimuli. Thus, frontal patients with unilateral right or left lesions showed poorer performance than normal subjects. The authors concluded that the frontal deficit was supramodal, and reflected both faulty registration and faulty retention.

Later, even conventional delay tasks were shown to be impaired after a frontal lesion (Milner et al., 1985; Freedman and Oscar-Berman, 1986; Oscar-Berman et al., 1991; Pierrot-Deseilligny et al., 1991; Verin et al., 1993; Dubois et al., 1995).

Other neuropsychological studies, further substrate the prefrontal working-memory deficits in digit span tests (Vidor, 1951; Hamlin, 1970, Janowsky et al. 1989 a; Stuss, 1991), in certain recognition tests (Milner and Teuber, 1968), and in temporal order and recency tests (Milner, 1971, 1982; Milner et al., 1985; Shimamura et al., 1990; Kesner et al., 1994; Jurado et al., 1997, 1998; Marshuetz, 2005).

PET studies have shown that listening to digits activates the left dorsolateral prefrontal cortex in normal subjects when active monitoring and manipulation of external information held in memory are required only to make judgements about the same stimuli, and no active manipulation is required (Petrides et al., 1993). Similarly, visuospatial information activates the right dorsolateral prefrontal cortex in normal subjects when active manipulation and monitoring of information are required.

The same visuospatial information activates only the right ventrolateral prefrontal cortex when only "reproduction" of information without active manipulation and monitoring is demanded by the task (Owen et al., 1996).

The general patterns of lateralization of verbal working memory function to the left frontal lobe and of visuospatial working memory function to the right frontal lobe, are consistent with the clinical lesion data (Smith et al., 1996).

The dorsolateral prefrontal cortex seems to be a critical structure in a number of delayed response and conditional sensorimotor learning tasks in nonhuman primates (Goldman-Rakic, 1987).

Neurophysiological evidence showed that the neuronal discharge in dorsolateral prefrontal neurons of monkeys performing conditional sensorimotor tasks is dependent upon the learning component of the task (Fuster, 1995).

Learning related rCBF (regional cerebral blood flow) increases seem to be lateralized to the left dorsolateral prefrontal cortex even when learning effects in conditional motor tasks are largely parallel in both hands (Iacoboni et al., 1996 b). This suggests that transfer of learning might occur through the anterior regions of the corpus callosum, interconnecting the prefrontal cortex of the two cerebral hemispheres (Iacoboni and Zaidel, 1995).

Working memory can be characterized as sustained attention to an internal representation (Fuster, 2009).

Working memory is subject to destructibility and interference, which are likely after prefrontal damage.

In a "rich" environment, with plentiful stimuli and distractors the frontal patient's memory is more likely to fail than in a quiet and simple environment. Just as critically, interference may come from whithin – that is from the reservoir of memories and alternatives that the subject has experienced or is likely to experience in that particular context.

The greater the similarity between these and the memory currently "on line", the greater is the probability that they will interfere with it (Fuster, 2009).

Callosal lesion in primates interfere with transfer of visuomotor conditional learning (Eacott and Gaffan, 1990). The lateralization of conditional sensorimotor learning to the left prefrontal cortex may not be specific to the human brain. Indeed, a lateralized left prefrontal-dependent activity during sensorimotor learning has been reported in a nonhuman primate (Gemba et al., 1995). Different from the frontal lobe receive segregated cortical inputs from a variety of cortical areas of sensory significance. In addition, the frontal lobe controls voluntary actions through planning of movements in prefrontal areas, preparation of movements in premotor areas and execution of movements in primary motor areas (Fuster, 1995).

However, little relevant data on structural asymmetries relate to functional asymmetries in sensory motor integration, first in the lateral wall, and then in the medial wall of the frontal lobe.

Premotor cortex

Situated just anterior to the precentral area, the premotor (area 6) and supplementary motor areas have been identified as the site in which the integration of motor skills and learned action sequences takes place (Kolb and Whishaw, 1996; Nilson et al., 2000; Eslinger and Geddes, 2001; Damasio and Anderson, 2003). The concept of a premotor cortex was first proposed in 1905 by Campbell, who called it the intermediate precentral cortex. The term premotor cortex was first used by Hines in 1949.

Independent anatomical and physiological evidence in nonhuman primates (Matelli et al., 1985; Fogassi et al., 1996; Fujii et al., 1996; Rizzolatti et al., 1996) and PET data in humans (Iacoboni et al., 1996 a; Rizzolatti et al., 1996) support the division of premotor cortex into four fields: a rostral (PMdr) and a caudal (PMdc) field in the dorsal premotor cortex, and a rostral (PMvr) and a caudal (PMvc) field in the ventral premotor cortex.

Neurophysiological evidence from studies of nonhuman primates suggests that PMdr is associated with saccade-, arm-, and eye-, eye position-, and stimulus-related activity, whereas PMdc is associated with arm motor preparation- and arm movement-related activity (Fujii et al., 1996). The ventral premotor cortex seems to be associated with grasp representations and action recognition in PMvr (Rizzolatti et al., 1996), and with peripersonal space coding of somatosensory and visual stimuli in PMvc (Fogassi et al., 1996).

The medial premotor cortex is the so-called supplementary motor area (SMA) of Woolsey et al. (1952). In both premotor areas, arcuate (prearcuate area 8 and postarcuate area 6) and SMA, there is a degree of somatotopical organization – that is, differential representation of the body (Woolsey et al., 1952; Muakkassa and Strick ,1979). Premotor areas participate in afferent / efferent loop with the basal ganglia and the thalamus: the looped interconnections are probably targeted to specific sites on both cortical and subcortical structures (Passingham, 1997; Middleton and Strick, 2000).

The dorsal premotor cortex is traditionally associated with neglect in extrapersonal space with selection and preparation of movements guided by external sensory stimuli, and with the retrieval of responses associated with specific sensory stimuli (Halsband and Freund, 1990; Passingham, 1993).

The ventral premotor cortex is associated with neglect in peripersonal space (Rizzolatti et al., 1983).

PET evidence seems to suggest a left-hemisphere lateralization in the human PMvr (inferior frontal gyrus, Brodmann's area 45) for the observation / execution matching system of grasping action (Grafton et al., 1996; Rizzolatti et al., 1996). This functional lateralization seems consistent with the hypothesis that primate communicative gestures could be the precursors of human language and that the "grammar of communicative gestures" could be represented in nonhuman primate PMvr, considered as the anatomical homologue of human Broca's area (Rizzolatti et al., 1996).

However, in these PET studies the subjects were required to grasp objects or to imagine grasping objects, or to observe other grasping objects, only with the dominant right hand.

Also, it has been shown with PET that the left PMvr (Brodmann's area 45) is activated in normal subjects while observing other making silent monosyllable mouth movements ("lip reading"), whereas no acoustic or language receptive areas were activated (Grafton et al., 1996). This would be consistent with the hypothesis that visual information feeds forward directly to Broca's area in the left hemisphere, as emphasized by Denny-Brown (1975).

PET studies of dorsal premotor cortex in humans showed that left PMdr superiority in establishing explicit stimulus - response association, and the left PMdc superiority in implicit sensorimotor learning (Iacoboni et al., 1996 a). This would suggest a functional rostrocaudal fractionation of human dorsal premotor cortex similar to the one observed in nonhuman primates.

The lateralization to the left dorsal premotor cortex, suggested by chronometric investigations, showed that the human left hemisphere is superior in tasks in which stimulus - response associations and response selection are required (Anzola et al., 1977).

In the dorsolateral prefrontal cortex, sensorimotor learning seems to be associated only with blood flow increase in PMdc. This suggests that, in contrast with other types of learning that may be associated with blood flow decreases, frontal lobe mechanisms of sensorimotor learning are generally associated with blood flow increases that correspond to an increase in neural activity (Raichle et al., 1994).

Primary motor cortex

Motor cortex is located in the posterior part of the frontal lobe or frontal cortex, just anterior to somatosensory cortex. Motor cortex includes a primary area, M1, where electrical stimulation of neurons evokes muscle contraction at low levels of current (Jinnai and Matsuda, 1979). M1 is characterized by large pyramidal or Betz cells and the lack of an obvious layer 4 of granular cells.

Thus, M1 is referred to as agranular cortex and as area 4 of Brodmann's classical terminology. The pyramidal cells in M1 project *via* the pyramidal tract to motor neurons pools in the contralateral brain stem and spinal cord (Brodal, 1978; Iwatsubo et al., 1990; Kaas and Stepniewska, 2002).

The primary motor cortex is the site of origin of about 30% to 40% of the fibres in the pyramidal tract.

Furthermore, all the large-diameter axons (approximately 3% of pyramidal fibres) originate from the giant motor neurons (of Betz) in the primary motor cortex.

Most of the neurons contributing fibres to corticospinal tract have glutamate or aspartate as their excitatory neurotransmitter (Holmes and May, 1909; Levin and Bradford, 1938; Lassek, 1940, 1954).

Stimulation of the motor cortex in conscious humans gives rise to discrete and isolated contralateral movement limited to a single joint or a single muscle.

Bilateral responses are seen in extraocular muscles and muscles of the face, tongue, jaw, larynx, and pharynx.

Thus, the primary motor area corresponds to the precentral gyrus (area 4 of Brodmann). On the medial surface of the hemisphere, the primary motor area comprises the anterior part of the paracentral lobule.

The contralateral half of the body is represented in the primary motor area in a precise but disproportionate manner, giving rise to the motor homunculus in the same way as that described for the primary somesthetic cortex.

The primary motor cortex functions in the initiation of highly skilled fine movements.

The motor area receives fibres from the ventrolateral nucleus of the thalamus, the main projection area of the cerebellum. The motor area also receives fibres from the somesthetic cortex (areas 1, 2 and 5) and the supplementary motor cortex.

The connections between the primary motor and somesthetic cortices are reciprocal.

Although the primary motor cortex is not the sole area from which movement can be elicited, it is nevertheless characterized by initiating highly skilled movement at a lower threshold of stimulation than the other motor areas.

One of the most striking lateralized behaviors in humans is hand preference, which is typically associated with manual skill (Annett, 1985). Fine manual coordination is lateralized to the left motor cortex in most right-handed individuals (Liepmann and Mass, 1907; Annett, 1985; Goldberg, 1985).

Some fMRI studies in human demonstrate asymmetric activation of primary motor cortex during volitional fine movements of the hand (Kawashima et al., 1993; Kim et al., 1993).

Stepniewska et al. (1993) and Geyer et al. (1996) demonstrated that the primary motor cortex in human and nonhuman primates is divided functionally into a rostral sector and a caudal sector. However, the functional asymmetries of the primary motor cortex do not differentiate between rostral and caudal sectors (Fuster, 2007).

Hemispatial neglect is typically associated with right temporal-parietal lesions, but it is observed with right frontal lobe lesions as well (Heilman and Valenstein, 1972; Heilman et al., 1993).

Patients with right pre-Rolandic lesions, often encompassing primary motor areas, tend not to move the hand ipsilateral to the lesion in the contralateral hemispace (Bisiach et al., 1990) and exhibit motor impersistences well, which is thought to reflect an attentional deficit (Benson and Stuss, 1986). Paradoxically, these patients tend to neglect lines seen on the left under free vision, and lines seen on the right under mirror-reversed vision (Bisiach et al., 1995). Furthermore, a double dissociation in patients with unilateral neglect is often seen.

Some patients have unilateral neglect only for near space; others have unilateral neglect only for far space (Halligan and Marshall, 1991). This double dissociation suggests that the representations of extrapersonal and personal space are differentiated and segregated in the human brain.

In the nonhuman primate, there is evidence for two parietal-frontal circuits sub-serving extrapersonal and personal space. **A dorsal** parietal-frontal circuit comprises area 7a, lateral intraparietal area, and dorsal premotor cortex, and codes extrapersonal space.

A ventral parietal-frontal circuit comprises area 7b, anterior intraparietal area, and ventral premotor cortex, and codes personal space.

These two circuits are anatomically largely independent, but both input to primary motor cortex (Passingham, 1993).

A PET observation has suggested that the right motor cortex is a critical structure in mapping extrapersonal onto personal space (Iacoboni et al., 1997).

A number of fMRI studies have suggested a major role for the primary motor cortex in motor learning (Grafton, 1995). Most of these studies have resulted in lateralized activation of the left primary motor cortex. The only fMRI studies of which Iacoboni et al. (1996) are aware that have used an unbiased learning paradigm in which left- and right-hand motor activity was completely counterbalanced (Iacoboni et al., 1996 a, b; Iacoboni et al., 1997) have resulted in blood flow increases consistently lateralized to the left frontal lobe. These blood flow increases occurred mainly in dorsal premotor cortex and in dorsolateral prefrontal cortex and only sporadically in primary motor cortex (Iacoboni et al., 1996 b).

Medial wall (anterior cingulate cortex and SMA)

The medial prefrontal cortex comprises parts of the areas 8 through 10, and areas 12, 24 and 32. The latter two areas constitute the anterior cingulate cortex (Fig. 23.4).

It has important influences on attention, response selection, and emotional behavior (Rolls, 1999; Brunia and Van Boxtel, 2000; Chelazzi and Corbetta, 2000).

Anterior and posterior portions have different projections and roles.

In general, the disorders due to medial lesions are poorly defined except for the case of large lesions (Cummings, 1985, 1993).

Anterior cingulate cortex. Together with the lateral prefrontal cortex, the anterior cingulate cortex controls behavior by detecting errors and signaling the occurrence of conflicts during information processing. These functions are critical for the regulation of behavior according to self-determined intention. The relative contribution of the two structures is a matter of debate (Cohen et al., 2000; Gehring and Knight, 2000).

Fig. 23.4. Modern rendition of the cytoarchitectural map showing Brodmann's areas on the medial surface of the human brain (figure provided by Mark Dubin, University of Colorado, 2006).

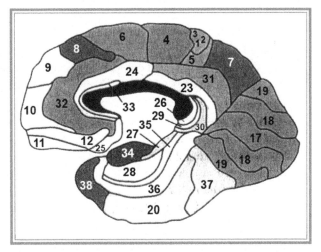

In the macaque, three areas, buried in the cingulate sulcus, seem to have significance in sensorimotor processes: the **rostral** cingulate motor area, located anterior to the genu of the arcuate sulcus, and the **dorsal** and the **ventral** cingulate motor areas, located caudal to the genu of the arcuate sulcus (Picard and Strick, 1996).

PET findings have suggested at least two cortical fields in the human anterior cingulate cortex: **a large rostral** one, anterior to the anterior commissure, associated with complex sensorimotor tasks and with a somatotopic arrangement; and **a small caudate** one, posterior to the anterior commissure, associated with simple tasks and not showing a clear somatotopy (Picard and Strick, 1996).

Area 24 is at the crossroads of pathways linking the limbic system with the frontal lobe, and, at the same time, is one of the so-called "suppressor areas", which upon stimulation induce general muscular hypotonia (Smith, 1945).

The anterior cingulate has been associated with attentional functions (Bench et al., 1993; Posner and Dehaene, 1994). However, asymmetries in the anterior cingulate in attentional mechanisms have not been systematically described (Pardo et al., 1991). Furthermore, widespread areas of right dorsolateral prefrontal cortex are preferentially activated during a variety of attentional tasks (Bench et al., 1993; Vendrell et al., 1995; Lewin et al., 1996).

Picard and Strick (1996) observed a slower learning in right hand in subjects practicing in a random fashion, associated with blood flow increases in the left SMA-proper and the left rostral anterior cingulate area, in a region overlapping with the arm representation in the human anterior cingulate cortex. Thus, behavioral data and rCBF findings suggest a greater sensitivity of the left rostral cingulate region to contextual cues. This is in line with a general role of the cingulate cortex in context-specific learning in other mammals (Freeman et al., 1996).

The most striking asymmetry in the anterior cingulate region is at morphological level. In the left hemisphere, there are often two cerebral sulci in the cingulate region, the cingulate sulcus and the paracingulate sulcus, whereas in the right hemisphere, there is generally only one sulcus, the cingulate sulcus. It has been speculated that this asymmetry might be related to certain aspects of effortful *versus* automatic vocalization (Paus et al., 1996).

Indeed, the PET study that compared reversed speech (effortful) with overpracticed speech, foci of activation were largely observed overlapping with the paracingulate sulcus in the left hemisphere (Paus et al., 1993).

Lesions of the anterior cingulate region generally lead to hypokinesia or akinesia, depending on their size (Kreindler, Macovei, Cardas and Dănăilă, 1966; Meador et al., 1986; Verfaellie and Heilman, 1987). They are also frequently accompanied by defective self-monitoring of behavior and of the ability to correct errors.

Akinetic mutism often results from massive bilateral lesions (Kreindler, Macovei Cardas and Dănăilă, 1966). It is usually accompanied by severe neurovegetative deterioration (Fuster, 2009). Some patients with lesions of the anterior cingulate region have been noted to suffer from cataplexy (Ethelberg, 1950) – that is the paroxysmal and general loss of muscle tonus commonly induced by strong emotion (Levin, 1953).

Once, the global adynamia results from irritation of area 24 (Fuster, 1955).

Mutism and apathy are the most prevalent disorders of medial frontal damage, especially if that damage is large. Thus, subjects with a large medial lesion appear characteristically unaware of their own condition (Nielsen and Jacobs, 1951; Barris and Schuman, 1953).

Supplementary motor area. The supplementary motor area (SMA) is located on the medial surface of the frontal lobe, anterior to the medial extension of the primary motor cortex (area 4). It corresponds roughly to the medial extension of area 6 of Brodmann. Although the existence of a motor area in the medial aspect of the frontal cortex rostral to the precentral area of primates has long been known.

Penfield and Welch (1951) were the first to call this portion of the cortex the supplementary motor area.

A homunculus has been defined for the supplementary motor area in which face and upper limbs are represented rostral to the lower limb and trunk. Stimulation in humans give risk to complex movement in preparation for the assumption of characteristic postures (Brinkman and Porter, 1979; Tanji, 1994).

Two distinct areas can be differentiated in SMA: a rostral area called pre-SMA and a caudal area called SMA-proper. In macaques, the pre-SMA is located mainly anterior to the genu of the arcuate sulcus, whereas SMA-proper is located posterior to the genu of the arcuate sulcus. In the human brain, the pre-SMA is located rostral to the level of the anterior commissure, and the SMA-proper is located caudal to the level of the anterior commissure. Anatomical and neurophysiological evidence suggest that the pre-SMA is related to selection and preparation of movements, whereas the SMA-proper is more related to aspects of motor execution (Picard and Strick, 1996). Although simple motor tasks are elicited from stimulation of the supplementary motor area, the role of this area in simple motor tasks is much less significant and is likely to be subsidiary to that of the primary motor area. On the other hand, the supplementary motor area assumes more significance in executing simple motor tasks as a compensatory mechanism when the primary motor area is destroyed (Tanji, 1994).

The supplementary motor area seems crucial in the temporal organization of movement, especially in sequential performance of multiple movements, and in motor tasks that demand retrieval of motor memory.

When subjects perform sensorimotor tasks, practice in blocked fashion (where each task pattern is practiced separately from the others) produces a faster learning slope than practice in random fashion (where each practiced task pattern is mixed with the others; Stelmach, 1996).

In a PET experiment on sensorimotor conditional learning, Iacoboni (2000) has observed that contextual interference affects learning in the right hand more than in the left hand. This was associated with blood flow increases in the left SMA-proper (Iacoboni, 2000). Thus, the left SMA-proper seems to be more sensitive to contextual interference than the right SMA-proper, which might suggest that the differential contextual effect observed in patients with left and right SMA lesions occurs more specifically at the level of the SMA-proper (Geschwind and Iacoboni, 2007).

Lesions in the medial aspects of area 6 (SMA), and 8, frequency lead to difficulties in initiation and performance of limb, eye, or speech movements.

Patients with long-term unilateral medial frontal lobe lesions in the left hemisphere benefit from preparatory information regarding a motor response and can inhibit inappropriate responses.

In contrast, patients with similar long-term lesions in the right hemisphere cannot benefit from preparatory information regarding a motor response and cannot inhibit an inappropriate motor response (Verfaellie and Heilman, 1987).

Thus, it seems there is a differential effect of contextual cues on motor performance in the left and right SMA. On the other hand, in right-handed neurological patients with unilateral SMA lesions, functional asymmetry is related to the temporal control of movement sequences.

This function is generally subserved by the SMA (Tanji and Shima, 1994).

Patients with left SMA lesions are much more impaired in reproducing rhythm patterns using the left hand, the right hand, or both hands in an alternating manner, than patients with right SMA lesions (Halsband et al., 1993). Furthermore, patients with left SMA lesions are more disturbed in the chronology of memory-guided saccade sequences than patients with right SMA lesions (Gaymard et al., 1993).

This differential role of the left and right SMA in sequential control of movements, at least in right-handers, explains why strategically placed callosal lesions producing motor disconnection tend to be associated with alien syndrome in the nondominant hand, but not the dominant hand in right-handers (Geschwind et al., 1995).

If the motor areas of the right hemisphere that control the left hand do not receive inputs on sequential control of movements from the right SMA because of callosal disconnection, then motor control disturbances in the left hand are likely to appear (Geschwind et al., 1995). They propose that this pathophysiological mechanism might be a unitary mechanism of praxis disturbances following callosal lesions (Gonzales-Rothi et al., 1994).

In sum, one model of frontal specialization proposes a dichotomy in which the right frontal lobe is specialized for novelty and the left frontal lobe for the routine (Goldberg and Podell, 1995). That the right frontal lobe is predominant in novelty processing fits with its role in attentional mechanism (Heilman et al., 1993).

PET studies in healthy volunteers demonstrate strikingly increased blood flow and metabolic activity in the right prefrontal cortex, including Brodmann's areas 8, 9, 44, and 46 during selective attention tasks in different sensory modalities (Roland, 1984; Pardo et al., 1991; Bench et al., 1993; Lewin et al., 1996).

According to Geschwind and Iacoboni (2007), the specialization of one hemisphere for a given function does not require that the contralateral hemisphere be involved in that function. Thus, any attempt to unify lateralized frontal lobe functions under one model is simplistic and likely to be flawed (Geschwind and Iacoboni, 2007).

The only functional asymmetry for which a corresponding structural asymmetry is that of language and Broca's area.

Asymmetry in the motor system

The most obvious behavioral asymmetry in humans is handedness, with approximately 92% of woman and 88% of men favoring and being more proficient with the right hand for performing a variety of skilled activities, such as writing, drawing, eating, and using a needle to sew.

Of the remaining non-right-handed individuals a few exhibit strong and consistent left-handedness, a few are truly ambidextrous, and others show hand preferences that vary from one skilled activity to another (Vallortigara, 2000).

In general, for both right-handed and left-handed individuals, hand differences are weaker for unskilled activities as picking up a small object.

Furthermore, for tasks that require the coordinated activity of both hands, their roles are often complementary (Corballis, 1997).

Generally, for right-handed individuals the left hand (controlled by the right hemisphere) performs movements of relatively low spatial and temporal frequency, whereas the right hand (controlled by the left hemisphere) performs movements of relatively high spatial and temporal frequency.

An example of this complementary arrangement is handwriting, during which the left hand arranges and steadies the paper while the right hand makes more frequent and smaller movements with the writing instruments.

Though handedness is the most obvious example, there are also other motoric asymmetries.

For example, for right-handed individuals the left side of the body is frequently preferred for postural support. In addition, the right side of the face (controlled by the left hemisphere) is superior for making certain oral movements associated with language and other precisely sequenced activities, whereas the left side of the face (controlled by the right hemisphere) is more emotionally expressive (Provins, 1997).

Anyhow, two different types of experiments have been devised to assess motor asymmetries: 1) direct observation of motor asymmetry; and 2) interference tasks (Kolb and Whishaw, 2003).

1) Direct observation

If asymmetry in the control of movement is inherent, this asymmetry might be observable when people are engaged in other behavior.

For example, perhaps the right hand is more active during the performance of verbal tasks, which do not require a manual response, and the left hand is more active during the performance of nonverbal tasks, such as listening to music, which also do not require a manual response. To examine this possibility, Kimura (1964 and 1973) videotaped subjects talking or humming. They found that right-handed people tend to gesture with their right hands when talking but are equally likely to scratch, rub their noses, or touch their bodies with either hand. Kimura interpreted the observed gesturing with the limb contralateral to the speaking hemisphere to indicate a relation between speech and certain manual activities.

Differences in gesturing, which favor the right hand in right-handed subjects, could simply be due to a difference in preferred hand rather than to functional asymmetry in motor control.

A second observed motor asymmetry was reported in the performance of complex movements of the mouth. Wolf and Goodale (1987) did single-frame analyses of videotaped mouth movements produced when people make verbal or nonverbal sounds. These observations support the idea that the left hemisphere has a special role in the selection, programming, and production of verbal and nonverbal oral movements.

Considerable evidence shows that the left side of the face displays emotions more strongly than the right side, and Wolf and Goodale (1987) showed that the onset facial expressions occur sooner on the left side of the face. Thus, it is not the control of movement itself that is asymmetrical but rather movement for a particular purpose.

2) Interference tasks

A variety of interference tasks examine a well-known phenomenon that most people manifest: the difficulty of doing two complex tasks at the same time. Perhaps the most interesting interference study known to us is an unpublished experiment by Robert Hicks and Marcel Kinsbourne (Kolb and Whishaw, 2003). They persuaded several unemployed musicians to come to their laboratory daily to play the piano. The task was to learn a different piece of music with each hand so that the two pieces could be played simultaneously. When the musicians had mastered this very difficult task, the experimenters then asked them to speak or to hum while playing.

Speaking disrupted playing with the right hand, and humming disrupted playing with the left.

Interference studies provide a useful way to study the roles of two hemispheres in controlling movement, but much more work is needed before researchers can identify the complementary roles of the two hemispheres (see reviews by Murphy and Peters, 1994, and by Carosseli et al., 1997). It will be necessary to identify which types of movements each hemisphere is especially good at controlling, because these movements will probably be resilient to interference effects.

Studies of interference effects are intriguing because they may be sources of fresh insights into the cortical organization of the motor system, but interference effects are poorly understood and appear to be capricious. In addition, as we become proficient at motor tasks, we are less prone to interference effects (Kolb and Whishaw, 2003).

The left hemisphere as interpreter

The left hemisphere is considered to be the "dominant" hemisphere in most right-handed people. The term dominant is usually taken to mean language-dominant, but Gazzaniga (1995) has suggested that the left hemisphere is not only superior in terms of language function, but also in the ability to make simple inferences and to interpret its own behavior and emotions (Gazzaniga and Smylie, 1984).

Such observations strongly suggest that the left hemisphere is not only more able than the right to express itself verbally but that it plays a dominant role in interpreting behavior and providing a rationale for events in the world.

These observations can also yield insight regarding the confabulatory behavior seen in some amnesic patients who are unable to encode new information.

Finding themselves in situations for which they cannot remember the antecedents, they may be compelled to explain them in the same way that the left hemisphere explains behavior motivated by right hemisphere (Baynes and Gazzaniga, 1997).

Asymmetries for the language in humans

Introduction

The most obvious functional difference between the hemispheres is that, for most people, the left hemisphere is the primary mediator of verbal function, including reading and writing, understanding and speaking, verbal ideation, verbal memory, numerical symbol system, and even comprehension of verbal symbols traced on the skin. Processing the linear and rapidly changing acoustic information needed for speech comprehension is better with the left than with the right hemisphere (Schwartz and Tallal, 1980; Haward 1997; Beeman and Chiarello, 1998).

Males show a stronger left hemisphere lateralization for phenological processing than females (Shaywitz et al., 1995; Zaidel et al., 1995).

So, left hemisphere dominance for many aspects of language is the most obvious and cited asymmetry outside of the motor domain. From clinical neurological data as well as other sources, it is estimated that speech production is limited to the left hemisphere in approximately 95% of right-handed individuals. Left hemisphere is also dominant for many aspects of language perception and for the verbal processing of stimulus material.

Moreover, left hemisphere lateralization extends to control of posturing and of sequencing hand and arm movements, and of the musculature of speech, although bilateral structures are involved (Lezak et al., 2004).

One of the most obvious cognitive aspect associated with left hemisphere damage is aphasia. This complex of disorders reflects a very basic underlying capacity of the left hemisphere that is not dependent on hearing, as deaf persons who sign can develop an aphasia for their nonauditory language in the areas associated with aphasia in hearing persons (Bellugi et al., 1983; Posner et al., 1990).

Other left hemisphere disorders include verbal memory or verbal fluency deficits, concrete thinking, specific impairments in reading or writing, and impaired arithmetic ability characterized by defects or loss of basic mathematical concepts of operations and even of numbers (Grafman and Rickard, 1997; Delazer and Bartha, 2001; Dănăilă and Golu, 2006).

Right hemisphere language capacities have been demonstrated for comprehension of speech and written material. One significant contribution is the appreciation and integration of relationships in verbal discourse and narrative materials (Delis et al., 1983, Beeman and Chiarello, 1998; Kiehl et al., 1999), which is a capacity necessary for enjoying a good joke (Beeman, 1998; Gardner, 1994). The right hemisphere also appears to provide the possibility of alternative meaning, getting away from purely literal interpretations of verbal material (Bottini et al., 1994; Brownell and Martino, 1998; Fiore and Schooler, 1998).

The right hemisphere appears to have a reading lexicon (Bogen, 1997; Coslett and Saffran, 1998), but the more verbally adept left hemisphere normally blocks access to it so that the right hemisphere's knowledge of words becomes evident only in laboratory manipulations or left hemisphere damage (Landis et al., 1983; Landis and Regard, 1988).

The right hemisphere seems to be sensitive to speech intonations (Borod et al., 1998, Ivry and Lebby, 1998) and is necessary for voice recognition (Van Lancker et al., 1989).

Following commissurotomy, when speech is directed to the right hemisphere, much of what is heard is comprehended so long as it remains simple (Searleman, 1977; Bayness and Eliassen, 1998). Although functional imaging studies show a preponderance of left cerebral activity in reading (Price, 1997), not surprisingly, given its visuospatial components, reading also engages the right hemisphere, activating specific areas (Ornstein et al., 1979; Gaillard and Converso, 1988; Huettner et al., 1989; Banich and Nicholas, 1998; Indefrey and Levelt, 2000). In contrast to the ability for rapid, automatic processing of printed words by the intact left hemisphere, the healthy right hemisphere takes a slower and generally inefficient letter by letter approach (Chiarello, 1988; Burgess and Lund, 1998), which may be useful when word shapes have unfamiliar forms (Banich and Nicholas, 1998).

Less can be said fore the verbal expressive capacities of the right hemisphere since they are quite limited, as displayed – or rather, not displayed – by split brain patients who make few utterance in response to right brain stimulation (Zaidel, 1978; Baynes and Gazzaniga, 2000).

The right hemisphere appears to play a role in organizing verbal production conceptually (Joanette et al., 1990; Browell and Martino, 1998), with specific temporal and prefrontal involvement in comprehending story meanings (Nichelli et al. 1995).

It may be necessary for meaningfully expressive speech intonation (prosody) (Filley, 1995; Borod et al., 1998; Ross, 2000). The right hemisphere contributes to the maintenance of context-appropriate and emotionally appropriate verbal behavior (Joanette et al., 1990; Brownell and Martino, 1998), although this contribution is not limited communication but extends to all behavior domains (Lezak, 1994).

That the right hemisphere has a language capacity can also be inferred in aphasic patients with left-side lesions who showed improvement from their immediate post-stroke deficits accompanied by measurably heightened right hemisphere activity (Papanicolaou et al., 1988; Murdoch, 1990; Dănăilă et al., 1990; Franckowiak, 1997; Heiss et al., 1999; Gold and Kertesz, 2000).

Based on the data obtained following the investigation of patients with organic pathological foci in the right hemisphere, Dănăilă et al., (1990) demonstrate the thesis of bilateral integration of the language system by the interaction of the two cerebral hemispheres.

The study of aphasic patients showed that the dominance of the left hemisphere for language was of a relative rather than an absolute nature.

It had been noted that, although the aphasic patients were incapable of truly proportional language, they did produce automatic, interjectional, and emotional speech; these positive features of an aphasic's language behavior were interpreted as reflecting the operation of mechanisms in his unaffected minor hemisphere (Benton, 2000).

In a stressful situation, an aphasic patient might produce perfectly intelligible propositional speech which he could not utter under ordinary circumstances. It was presumed that this speech was produced by the minor hemisphere. This meant that in the course of language learning, verbal engrams were laid down in the right hemisphere as well as in the left. These minor hemisphere engrams remained inactive because of the specialization of the major hemisphere for language (Benton, 2000).

The same explanation was applied for recovery from aphasic disorder. It seemed clear that the minor hemisphere must have participated in the original learning of language.

So, the right hemisphere has been erroneously called the "minor" or "nondominant" hemisphere because the often subtle character of right hemisphere disorders led early observers to believe that it played no specialized role in behavior. However, although limited linguistically, the right hemisphere is "fully human with respect to its cognitive depth and complexity" (Levy, 1983).

When we consider understanding language for the purpose of communication, this is growing evidence that both hemispheres make important contributions. Whereas the left hemisphere is dominant for the perception of phonetic information, for the use of syntax and for certain aspects of semantic processing, the right hemisphere is dominant for processing the sort of information cues and prosody that communicate such things as emotional tone. So, the right hemisphere is superior to the left in using the intonation cues of speech to identify emotional tone of voice. The right hemisphere is also involved in processing narrative-level linguistic information (Hellige, 2001). Some of these complementary language-related asymmetries may be related to hemispheric difference in the efficiency of processing different aspects of acoustic signals.

For example, identification of many spoken phonemes requires efficient processing of rapid changes in the acoustic signal over brief periods of time, a type of processing for which the left hemisphere is hypothesized to be superior.

In contrast, identification of the emotional tone of voice requires efficient processing of much slower modulations of the acoustic signal over longer periods of time, a type of processing for which the right hemisphere is hypothesized to be superior (Heilman, 1997; Christman, 1997; Hellige, 2000).

So, patients with right hemisphere damage may be quite fluent, even verbose (Brookshire, 1978; Rivers and Love, 1980; Cutting, 1990), but illogical and given to lose generalization and bad judgment (Stemmer and Joanette, 1998). They have difficulty in ordering, organizing and making sense out of complex stimuli or situations, and thus many display planning defects (Lezak et al., 2004). Verbal comprehension may be compromised by confusion of the elements of what is heard by personalized intrusions, by literal interpretations, and by generalized loss of gist in a morass of details (Beeman and Chiarello, 1998). Their speech may be uninflected and aprosodic, paralleling their difficulty in comprehending speech intonations (Ross, 2003).

These patients are vulnerable to difficulty in maintaining a high level of alertness (Ladavas et al., 1989), which may be akin to the association of right hemisphere lesions with impersistence – the inability to sustain facial or limb posture (Pimental and Kingsbury, 1989).

Dănăilă et al. (1990) evaluated speech disorders at 15 patients with tumors and strokes localized in the right hemisphere. They noted there main categories of speech impairments: disturbances of contents of "semantic structure", disturbances of forms of the logical-grammatical structure, and disturbances of dynamics – volume, output, fluency, rhythm, intonation and writing.

The two hemispheres also appear to access word meanings in complementary ways.

When a word is present, the left hemisphere restricts processing very quickly to one possible meaning, usually the dominant meaning or the meaning most consistent with the present context, whereas the right hemisphere maintains activation of multiple meanings and remote associated words for a more expended period of time (Springer and Deutsch, 1998).

Anyhow, viewed in retrospect and taken in their totality these clinical contributions would seem to have produced at least suggestive evidence for the view that the right hemisphere should not be considered simply as a minor hemisphere with no distinctive functional properties (Benton, 2000).

Asymmetry in visuospatial functions

The expected right hemispheric superiority in visuospatial function has been demonstrated in callosotomy patients (Bogen and Gazzaniga, 1965; Milner and Taylor, 1972).

In contrast, superior use of visual imagery has been demonstrated in the left hemisphere, using a letter-based task (Farah et al., 1985).

The use of tactile information to build spatial representations of abstract shapes also appears to be better developed in the right hemisphere (Milner and Taylor, 1972).

Tasks such as Block Design from the Wechsler Adult Intelligence Scale (WAIS), however, which are typically associated with the right parietal lobe, appear to require integration between the hemispheres in some patients (Gazzaniga, 1989). Furthermore, while the right hemisphere is better able to analyze unfamiliar facial information than the left hemisphere (Levy et al., 1972; Gazzaniga and Smylie, 1983) and the left is better able to generate voluntary expressions (Gazzaniga and Smylie, 1990), both hemispheres share in the management of facial expression when spontaneous emotions are expressed.

Although the right hemisphere demonstrates superior levels of performance on a variety of perceptual and spatial tasks, the left hemisphere appears to have at least some competence in most areas and some cases are essential for the solution of complex visual problems.

The left hemisphere is superior at all language tasks and in a variety of tasks that require interferences (Baynes and Gazzaniga, 1997).

Moreover, verbal IQ appears to be stable following callosotomy, although performance IQ may decline (Zaidel, 1990).

Gazzaniga (1995) suggests that the hemisphere is also dominant for intelligent behavior, although that conclusion assumes a contemporary concept of intelligence that rests heavily on verbal abilities.

Hemispheric isolation of visual and tactile information

Subjects can independently report visual material that has been isolated to one hemisphere or other, but they cannot make comparison between the two hemifields.

Performance is at or near chance levels in simple same / different comparison when items are presented in different visual fields (Holtzman et al., 1981; Seymour et al., 1994; Baynes and Gazzaniga, 1997).

Despite reports of integration of higher-order information following callosotomy (Sergent, 1983, 1990), such results have not always been replicated or have proved explicable through the patient's strategic maneuvers (Seymour et al., 1994; Corballis, 1994; Kingstone and Gazzaniga, 1995).

At present, it appears that if visual or tactile information is presented so that it is initially perceived by only one hemisphere, the perception remains isolated within that hemisphere.

The animal literature, however, has documented that information from areas close to the visual midline is shared by both hemispheres (Stone, 1966; Fukuda et al., 1989).

It appears that this observation is also true for the human species in an area no more than 2° from the vertical meridian (Fendrich and Gazzaniga, 1989).

Although represented the visual information in this area has little utility, as neither detailed shape comparisons nor brief displays could be reliably compared across the meridian (Fendrich and Gazzaniga, 1989).

Sharing of attention control

Although both higher cognitive function and basic perceptual information appear to be isolated within each hemisphere, there is some evidence for sharing the control of visual attention. The hemispheres appear to share control of the "attentional spotlight" *via* their subcortical connections (Baynes and Gazzaniga, 1997). That is, if attention is directed to particular position in the visual field a cue in one field, that information can be used by both hemispheres (Holtzman et al., 1981, 1984). Nonetheless, explicit inter-field comparisons of spatial location cannot be made accurately (Holtzman et al., 1981), nor can attention be simultaneously directed to different points in each visual field (Holtzman et al., 1984).

It also appears that attentional resources are limited despite the "splitting" of conscious. Holtzman and Gazzaniga (1982) demonstrated that increasing processing demands in one hemisphere had a deleterious effect on performance in the other hemisphere. Nonetheless, in comparison with normal subjects, there was less decrement in a dual-task condition for callosotomized subjects (Holtzman and Gazzaniga, 1985).

Thus, although the two hemispheres may compete for cognitive resources, there is evidence for independence of function. This latter finding is consistent with the observation of Luck et al. (1989) that visual search is independently mediated by both hemispheres.

Mangun et al. (1994) demonstrated differential processing of spatial cues, with only the left visual field (right-hand) trials yielding an advantage for validly cued trials.

According to Baynes and Gazzaniga (1997), although the behaving is remarkably intact following callosotomy, investigation reveals hemispheric capacities that refine and confirm hypotheses based on normal subjects and patients with focal lesions.

The isolated right hemisphere usually cannot read, write, or speak, despite displaying a variety of conscious behaviors. Dissociation like left-handed tactile anomia or agraphia may be an indication of less language-competent right hemispheres.

However, the ability to comprehended auditory and visual language may be present and can contribute to the presentation of aphasic and alexic patients. Observations indicate that the right hemisphere may participate in long-term recovery from aphasia (Baynes and Gazzaniga, 1997).

Independent function of the hemispheres was demonstrated as a result of which the important role played by the verbal left hemisphere in allowing the organism to observe and interpret its own actions and emotional states was recognized. Insights regarding the components of perception, memory, attention, and language continue to arise from this population and to inform models of normal perceptual and cognitive processing (Baynes and Gazzaniga, 1997).

Asymmetries in processing spatial informations

Tradition and common sense favor the verbal (left hemisphere) *vs.* nonverbal (right hemisphere) dichotomy.

Speech expression and comprehension, as well as reading text and writing, take place serially in a fixed temporal order. In contrast, the appreciation of a spatial display, whether it is a form, an object, or face, permits parallel information processing and hence an almost instantaneous grasp of the complex stimulus (Benton, 2000).

Matching of unfamiliar face is regarded as a configurational task par excellence. In accord with expectation, one finds a right frequency of failure in patients with right hemisphere disease, particularly those with posterior temporo-occipital lesions where the frequency of failure is about 50%. However, there is a subgroup of patients with posterior left hemisphere lesions and impaired understanding of speech who also show a notable frequency of failure, in this instance, 35% to 40% (Hamsher et al., 1979). Similarly, tachitoscopic visual field studies of facial recognition in normal subjects find a highly significant left field advantage, indicating a major participation of the right hemisphere in the performance. But again, there is a substantial minority of normal right, handed subjects who exhibit a left field advantage, the proportion being 20-25% (Helliard, 1973; St. John, 1981).

Anyhow, the right hemisphere dominates the processing of information that does not readily lend itself to verbalization. This includes the reception and storage of visual data, tactile and visual recognition of shapes and forms, perception of spatial orientation and perspective, and copying and drawing geometric and representational designs and pictures. The left hemisphere seems to predominate in metric distance judgments (Hellige, 1988; Mc Carthy and Warrington, 1990), while the right hemisphere has superiority in metric angle judgments (Benton et al., 1994; Mehta and Newcombe, 1996).

Thus, both hemispheres contribute to processing spatial information, with some differences in what they process most efficiently (Sergent, 1991; Banich, 1995).

In the spatial domain, the brain computes at least two kinds of a spatial relation representation – a categorical representation used to assign a spatial relation to a category such as "connected to" or "above" and a coordinate representation used to represent precise distances and locations. The right hemisphere makes more effective use of this latter coordinate system, whereas there is either no hemispheric difference or a left hemisphere advantage for processing categorical spatial relationships. Neural network simulation suggests that hemispheric asymmetry for making categorical *versus* coordinate judgments may be related to the nature of visual information that is most useful for processing categorical *versus* coordinate properties.

It is interesting that categorical spatial processing is disrupted by manipulations (blurring of stimuli) that selectively interfere with information carried by channels with small, discrete receptive fields, whereas coordinate spatial processing is disrupted by manipulations (use of a diffuse red background) that selectively interfere with information carried by channels with large overlapping receptive fields (Beeman and Chiarello, 1998; Hellige, 2001).

The same networks that favored coordinate spatial processing also favored coding the identify of specific shapes, whereas the same networks that favored categorical spatial processing also favored the assignment of shapes to categories. Interestingly, there is evidence of right hemisphere superiority for processing the sort of specific shape information that would be needed to distinguish among the exemplars of single category, but left hemisphere superiority for classifying the prototypes used to define different categories.

Arithmetic calculations (involving spatial organization of the problem elements or distinct from left hemisphere – mediated linear arithmetic problems involving) have a significant right hemisphere component (Grafman and Rickard, 1997; Dehaene, 2000).

Arithmetic failures are most likely to appear in written calculations that require spatial organization of the problems' elements (Grafman and Rickard, 1997; Dănăilă and Golu, 2006).

Visuospatial and other perceptual deficits show up in these patients' difficulty copying designs, making constructions, and matching or discriminating patterns or faces. Prosopagnosia (inability to recognize faces) occurs only when the cortex on the undersides of the occipital and temporal lobes is damaged bilaterally (Mesulam, 2000; Dănăilă and Golu, 2006). Patients with right hemisphere damage may have particular problems with spatial orientation and visuospatial memory such that they get lost, even in familiar surroundings, and can be slow to learn their way around a new area. Visual functions have to do with dorsal-ventral distinction. Two now well-identified visual systems have separate pathways with different cortical loci (Mesulam, 2000; Goodale, 2000; Dănăilă and Golu, 2006).

Their constructional disabilities may reflect both their spatial disorientation and defective capacity for perceptual or conceptual organization. Stereoscopic vision may be affected (Benton and Hécaen, 1970).

The distinctive processing qualities of each hemisphere become evident in the mediation of spatial relations. In the right hemisphere the tendency is to deal with the same visual stimuli as a spatially related whole.

Patients with left hemisphere damage may make defective constructions largely because of tendencies toward simplification and difficulties in drawing angles, but they also may display deficits in visuospatial orientation and short-term recall (Mehta et al., 1989).

The ability to perform complex manual – as well as oral – motor sequences may be impaired (Harrington and Haaland, 1992; Meador et al., 1999; Schluter et al., 2001).

The distinctive processing qualities of each hemisphere became evident in the mediation of spatial relations. Left hemisphere processing tends to break the visual percept into details that can be identified and conceptualized verbally in terms of number or length of lines, size and direction of angles, etc. Together, the two processing systems of the left and the right hemisphere provide recognition, storage and comprehension of discrete and continuous, serial and simultaneous, detailed and holistic aspects of experience across at least the major sensory modalities of vision, audition and touch (Lezak et al., 2004).

Thus, model has clinical value, because loss of tissue in a hemisphere tends to impair its particular processing capacity. A diminished contribution from one hemisphere may be accompanied by augmented or exaggerated activity of the other when released from the inhibitory or competitive constraints of normal hemispheric interactions (Novelly et al., 1984; Lezak, 1994; Starkstein and Robinson, 1997; Shimizu et al., 2000). This phenomenon appears in the verbosity and overwriting of many right hemisphere damaged patients (Lezak and Newman, 1979; Yamadori et al., 1986; Cutting, 1990).

The functional difference between hemispheres also appears in the tendency for patients with left-sided damage to be more accurate in remembering large visually presented forms than the small details making up those forms; but when the lesion is on the right, recall of details is more accurate than recall of the whole composed figure (Delis et al., 1986). These examples suggest that one hemisphere's function is enhanced when the other hemisphere is impaired. In an analogous manner, patients with left hemisphere disease tend to reproduce the essential configuration but leave out details when copying, drawing, and they may perform some visuo-perceptual tasks better, intact subjects (Kim et al., 1984; Wasserstein et al., 1987).

Perceptual deficits, particularly left-sided inattention phenomena and those involving degraded stimuli or unusual presentation, are not uncommon (McCarthy and Warrington, 1990).

Asymmetry in memory and learning

Along with the limbic system, many regions of the temporal lobes are critical for normal learning and retention. Anyhow, memory and learning show hemispheric differences.

Awake patients undergoing brain surgery report vivid auditory and visual recall of previously experienced scenes and episodes upon electrical stimulation of the exposed temporal lobe cortex (Penfield, 1958; Gloor et al., 1982). Nauta (1964) speculated that these memories involve widespread neural mechanisms and that the temporal cortex and, to a lesser extent, the occipital cortex play roles in organizing the discrete components of memory for orderly and complete recall.

Thus, retrieval of visual information is impaired by lesions of the visual association cortex of the occipital lobe, impaired retrieval of auditory information follows lesions of the auditory association of the temporal lobe, and so on.

Anyhow, memory and learning show hemispheric differences. So, loss of the left hippocampus and nearly cortical areas impairs verbal memory, and destruction of the right hippocampus results in defective recognition and recall of "complex visual and auditory patterns to which a name cannot readily be assigned" (Milner, 1970, Morris et al., 1995; Sass et al., 1995; Abrahams et al., 1997; Pillon et al., 1999). In some cases, lesions of the temporal neocortex may impair retention and learning by disconnecting the hippocampus from cortical input (Jones-Gotman et al., 1997). Cortical regions appear to be organized for long-term storage of memories (Fuster, 1999).

The subjects for most studies of memory and the temporal lobe are patients who have had portions of one or both temporal lobes excised, usually for seizure control. These studies show that memory deficits with temporal lobe lesions also differ according to the side of the lesion (Milner, 1972; Lee et al., 1989; Smith, 1989; Morris et al., 1995, Pillon et al., 1999).

Impaired verbal memory appears with surgical resection of the left temporal lobe (Seidenberg et al., 1998), and nonverbal (auditory, tactile, visual) memory disturbances accompany right temporal lobe resection (Lezak et al., 2004). With left temporal lobectomies, deficits have been found for different kinds of verbal memory, including episodic (both short-term and learning), semantic and remote memory (Smith, 1989; Frisk and Milner, 1990; Loring and Meador, 2003).

These patients also lag behind normal controls in learning designs, although once learned their retention is good unlike patients with right temporal lesions who fail both aspects of this memory task (Jones-Gotman, 1986).

Same patients with cortical lesions have shown selective deficits in retrieving highly specific types of information, such as items in certain categories, but not others (Martin et al., 1997; Gabrieli, 1998). This finding suggests that cortical representation of knowledge is highly organized.

Reduced access to verbal labeling may explain the left temporal patients' slowed learning. Learning manual sequences becomes more difficult following left but not right lobectomy (Jason, 1987).

Cortical stimulation of the anterior left temporal cortex interferes with verbal learning without affecting speech, while stimulation of the posterior left temporal cortex is more likely to result in retrieval (word finding) problems and anomia (literally, no words) (Fedio and Van Buren, 1974; Ojemann, 1978).

Lesions in different areas of the left temporal lobe differentially affect the degree and nature of impairment in immediate auditory recall of tones or digits (Gordon, 1983).

Memory deficits documented for patients with right temporal lobectomies and other temporal lobe lesions involve designs, faces, melodies, and spatial formats such as those used in maze learning (Abrahams et al., 1997).

In short, these patients display memory impairments when perceptions or knowledge cannot be readily put into words (Shapiro et al., 1981; Smith, 1989). This left - right difference has been found in brain activation studies comparing the effect of stimulus material on temporal lobes (Ojemann, 1978; Dolan et al., 1997), and on the prefrontal cortex's role in memory (Wagner et al., 1998; Mc Dermott et al., 1999; Lee et al., 2000).

However, current evidence suggests that the relationship between the type of material (verbal *vs.* nonverbalizable) to be learned or modality of stimulus input and hemisphere involvement is not simple. Functional neuroimaging data demonstrate that both hemispheres may be activated by a verbal memory task (Buckner et al., 1998; Johanson et al., 2001).

This finding suggests that cortical representation of knowledge is highly organized. Loss of facts, knowledge of objects, and meaning of words have been reported with selective damage to the inferolateral temporal gyri of one or both temporal lobes, with sparing of the hippocampal and parahippocampal gyri (Graham and Hodges, 1997).

Thus, while the hippocampus and medial limbic structures are involved in the processing of newly learned information that has not been consolidated yet, the temporal cortex appears to house old learned information.

Asymmetry in the information process

The supramodal nature of hemisphere specialization shows up in a number of ways: one is the organization of the left hemisphere for "linear" processing of sequentially presenting stimuli such as verbal statements, mathematical proposition, and the programming of rapid motor sequences. The right hemisphere is superior for "configurational" processing required by material that cannot be described adequately in words or strings of symbol, such as the appearance of a face or three-dimensional spatial relationship (Bogen, 1969 a and b; Lezak, 1994, Carlesimo and Caltagirone, 1995; Swithenby et al., 1998). The two hemispheres process global / local or whole / detail information differently (Robertson and Rafael, 2000; Rossion et al., 2000), what Delis et al. (1988) refer to as the level or hierarchical analysis. When asked to copy or read a large-scale stimulus such as the shape of a letter or other common symbol composed of many different symbols in a small scale, patients with left hemisphere disease will tend to ignore the small bits and interpret the large-scale figure; those whose lesions are on the right are more likely to overlook the big symbol but respond to the small ones. This can be interpreted as indicating a left hemisphere superiority in processing detailed information, a right hemisphere predilection for large-scale or global percepts (Fig. 23.5) (Lezak et al., 2004).

Yet another processing difference between the hemisphere has to do with stimulus familiarity, as the right hemisphere appears to be best suited to handle novel information while the left tends to be more adept with familiar material such as "well-routinized codes" (Goldberg and Costa, 1981; Goldberg, 1990).

Other studies have associated the right hemisphere with early less detailed stages of processing, which may also be those that emerge first in the course of development, leaving the left hemisphere to perform later stage operations on more detailed features (Sergent, 1984, 1988; Bouma, 1990).

Asymmetry in the attention

Data from a variety of sources suggests right hemisphere dominance for spatial attention specially, if not attention generally: patients with compromised right hemisphere functioning tend to have diminished awareness of or responsiveness to stimuli presented to their left side; reaction times mediated by the right hemisphere are faster than those mediated by the left; and the right hemisphere is activated equally by stimuli from either side in contrast to more exclusively contralateral left hemisphere activation (Heilman and Van Den Abell, 1980; Meador et al., 1988; Mesulam, 2000; Heilman and Rothi 2003).

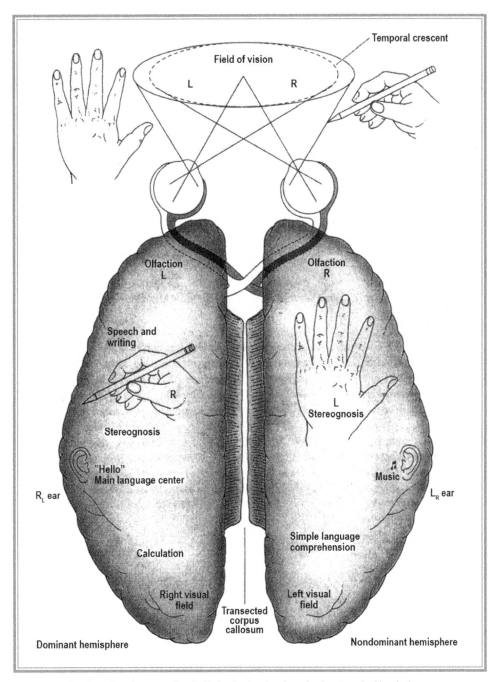

Fig. 23.5. Functions associated with the dominant and nondominant cerebral hemispheres.
(Modified from Noback CR et al. (1996), *The Human Nervous System*, 5ᵗʰ edn., Williams and Wilkins, Baltimore).

However, other studies suggest that neither hemisphere has an attentional advantage, but rather each hemisphere directs attention contralaterally (Mirsky, 1989; Posner, 1990), and that they are equally capable of detecting stimuli (Prather et al., 1992). The right hemisphere directs attention to far space while the left hemisphere directs attention to near space (Heilman et al., 1995). The appearance of right hemisphere superiority for attention in some situations may stem from its ability to integrate complex, nonlinear information rapidly.

Asymmetry in the music

Musical perception may be considered in terms of the reception of those perceptual-acoustic characteristics that define the basic elements of musical sounds, such as frequency, pitch, consonance, timbre, duration, intensity, and spatial location.

The sparing of musical abilities in patients with congenital, acquired language defects or aphasic was noted by Dalin (1745), Bouillaud (1865), Proust, 1866 and 1872), Finkelnburg (1870).

Conversely, instance of loss of musical skills were also described in patients who showed left hemiparesis and without aphasia (Mann, 1898; Jossmann, 1926, 1927). Loss of the capacity to sing hum or whistle a tune is one of the more frequently described forms of amusia. Anyhow, neural mechanism underlying disorders of receptive functions and those of expressive functions of music, and the nature of their relationship to cognitive and linguistic activity remains obscure.

Nevertheless, despite the close qualitative and quantitative association between disorders of music and language, there is incontrovertible evidence that the two spheres of activity are mediated by distinctive neurobehavioral systems.

The long-standing observation that patients with severe expressive language disorder are able to sing is in itself sufficient proof of this. The same dissociation may be observed in patients with receptive language disorder.

The fact that disturbances in musical function can occur in patients who are free of any aphasic disorder is equally cogent evidence for the independence of a two "language" system (Benton, 2000).

Patients with purely or predominantly oral-expressive impairment are about as likely to be nonaphasic as aphasic. However, it must be remarked that most of them do in fact show dysprosodic speech which might be interpreted as another expression of a general defect in the oral production of sounds, rhythms, and melodic intonations.

Clinopathological correlations with respect to disturbances in musical function are much less abundant than for the aphasic disorders and only a limited amount of information about the site of lesions associated with the amusias has been amassed.

Lesions in either hemisphere can produce both expressive and receptive disorders of musical function in a right-handed patient while aphasia in such a patient is almost invariably an expression of left hemisphere disease.

Analysis of the clinical literature suggests that "pure" expressive amusia (vocal or instrumental) with preservation of receptive function and without aphasia is most likely to be associated with anterior lesions of the right hemisphere. The case reports of Mann (1898), Jossmann (1926, 1927), and Botez and Wertheim (1959) illustrate this relationship.

A predominantly expressive amusia in combination with a predominantly expressive aphasic disorder is associated with anterior lesion of the left hemisphere, as illustrated by the inability of many Broca aphasics to reproduce a heard tone or sing a tune. Here appears to be no hemispheric bias in respect to the lesions that may produce a disorder of expressive musical function (Benton, 2000).

Anyhow, the most fundamental musical motor activity is singing. Perry et al. (1999), measured increased cerebral blood flow (CBF) during simple singing using positron emission tomography (PET). Repetitive singing of a single pitch was contrasted with listening to complex tones at the same pitch rate. The set of regions activated overlapped those previously observed during speech (SMA, anterior cingulate, insula / frontal operculum, and precentral gyrus). The main differences were in the direction of hemisphere asymmetry within a subset of these regions. First, the CBF increase was much greater in the right primary auditory region, a result that Zatorre and Binder (2000) and Zatorre and Peretz (2001) later replicated for singing a single pitch continuously on each breath in contrast to listening to playback of that singing.

They hypothesized that this asymmetry may be related to deriving the fundamental frequency of one's own voice for feedback guidance of vocal motor production (given a right auditory cortex preference for spectral analysis).

The fundamental frequency of subjects' vocalization was measured. When the total amount of pitch excursion within each continuously sung note was quantified and covaried against CBF in the whole brain, a region of positive covariation was observed in the right primary auditory region.

Second, though less striking, an asymmetry favoring the right hemisphere was also observed within the right ventral precentral gyrus or the orofacial region. The classsic correspondence between the region activated by singing and speaking suggests that both may have evolved from a complex system for the voluntary control of vocalization. Their divergences suggest the lateral evolution of complementary hemispheric specialization for both the perception and production of singing and speech (Perry et al., 1999).

The simple acts of motor production require the execution of learned motor program or an integrated sequence of movements. More complex sequences that follow a precise temporal plan and involve multiple vocal instrumental pitches and variable timing and intensity are integrated to musical expression. Such sequential movements performed as a unit require advance programming prior to their execution (Pascual-Leone et al., 1995; Blood and Zatorre, 2001). The cortical areas involved in the control of manual motor output in a quasi-musical context, is consistent with what would be expected for timed manual movements in general.

In an experiment, Perry et al. (1999), asked their subjects to listen to a two-note sequence drawn from a major scale and either imagine it in their heads, or hum it out loud. When they hummed out loud, in contrast to just listening to the sequences, activation was seen not only in motor cortex, SMA, and the right putamen as seen during imaging but also in the left putamen, cerebelum, right primary auditory region, and more extensively in motor cortex bilaterally. Thus, this simple act of musical motor programming activated the same areas through to be involved in the execution of movement sequences generally (i.e., primary and premotor cortex, SMA, basal ganglia, and the cerebellum).

Musical perception

Musical perception may be considered in terms of the reception of those perceptual-acoustic characteristics that define the basic elements of musical sounds, such as frequency, pitch, consonance, timbre, duration, intensity and spatial localization.

Disturbance in receptive musical capacities in combination with aphasic disorder have been found to be associated with lesions involving the middle and posterior parts of the first and second temporal gyri, the transverse temporal gyri, and the anterior temporal region of the left hemisphere.

The three surgically explored cases of Dorgeuille (1966) may be cited to illustrate this point.

They showed a fluent aphasia, impairment in the discrimination of tones, expressive musical defects, defective reproduction of sounds and rhythmic patterns and defects in singing melodies with which thay had been quite familiar.

Receptive amusia without concomitant aphasic disorder has been found to be associated with temporal lobe disease of either hemisphere or of both hemispheres (Schuster and Taterka, 1926; Pötzl and Uiberall, 1937; Pötzl, 1939, 1943; Spreen et al., 1965).

A plausible interpretation is that some individuals show dissociated dominance, i.e., thay are left hemisphere dominant for language but right hemisphere dominant for music. Henschen (1920) localized a center for singing in the upper part of the third frontal gyrus, a venter for oral musical comprehension in the left temporal pole and a center for reading music in the angular gyrus.

The idea that each hemisphere makes a distinctive contribution to receptive and expressive musical performance has been proposed. For example, Barbizet et al. (1969) and Barbizet (1972) have advanced the concept that the right hemisphere participates primarily on the perceptual and executive levels of musical activity while the left hemisphere mediates the recognition and memory of musical structures, the symbolic processes in reading and writing music, and the higher level integrative functions involved in musical composition. It is clear that there can be a dissociation between expressive and receptive functions.

But why one aphasic patient with focal lesion will show concomitant disturbances in musical function while another patient with a similar type of disorder and lesion will show no musical disabilities is a complete mystery (Benton, 2000). It is possible that the contribution which each hemisphere makes to the mediation of musical function varies quantitatively from one individual to another.

Reliable knowledge about interhemispheric relations in this respect no doubt would go far toward helping us understand a cognitive problem, namely, why some patients are rendered amusic as a consequence of disease of the right hemisphere while the majority of patients in this category are not affected (Benton, 2000).

A number of questions remain unanswered. Investigation in the field of the aphasic disorders has generated findings that have given much insight into the relations between handedness and hemispheric cerebral dominance for the language functions (Benton, 1965; Subirana, 1969; Hécaen, 1972).

Asymmetry in the visual perception and language of temporal-lobe lesions

TH and TF at the posterior end of temporal lobe are often referred to as the parahippocampal cortex. The fusiform gyrus and inferior temporal gyrus are functionally part of the temporal cortex.

Functionally, mesial structures of the temporal lobe (amygdala, hippocampus, and rhinal cortex) all have demonstrated role in some aspects of the establishment of new memories.

The amygdala, in particular, has been seen as contributing to normal and abnormal emotional responses and experiences. Bilateral amygdaloid destruction causes a severe disturbance of normal affective behavior (Kluver-Bucy syndrome, schizophrenia, and bipolar disorder).

The contribution of the temporal lobe to visual perception has been clarified by the division of visual projection from the occipital lobe in two directions or "streams": a dorsal route into parietal lobe that is involved in spatial localization and a ventral route into the temporal lobe that is involved in the appreciation of the qualities of objects (and their identification) in visual scene.

Damage to posterior inferior temporal lobe, especially when bilateral, and when portions of inferior areas 18 and 19 are involved, can lead to a condition called prosopagnosia.

Patients with this disorder can see a face but do not recognize the person from the face alone.

Prosopagnosia can usually recognize and correctly interpret facial expressions, and they may be able to recognize a person from other visual but nonfacial cues, such as gait or posture. It is clear that the disorder caused by IT (inferior temporal) lesions has to do with conscious recognition.

The disorder may be accompanied by difficulty in recognizing (naming) famous buildings, and such individuals may also have difficulty with texture discriminations and color perception.

When the damage is on the left posterior inferior temporal lobe, the person may identify the face incorrectly but still give an answer in the correct category (e.g., naming a different figure in politics or entertainment). This is called "deep" prosopagnosia in analogy with "deep" dyslexia in which the person reads a word semantically related to a word on the page.

Milner (1968) found that her patients with right temporal lobectomies were impaired in the interpretation of cartoon drawings in the Mc Gill Picture – Anomalies Test. But, although patients with right temporal lesions can describe the contents of the cartoon accurately, they are impaired at recognizing the anomalous aspects of this picture and others. So, when the damage is on the right, the person may be slow and erratic at recognizing faces but not profoundly prosopagnosic.

Language. Electrical stimulation of the superior temporal sulcus (especially in the posterior half) in the left hemisphere of typical right-handers often causes speech arrest or other alterations of language abilities. PET findings show bilateral activation of Heschel's gyrus and unilateral activation of Wernicke's area (left hemisphere only) when typical right-handed subjects listen to a verbal material such as a narrative.

Speech-related areas are occasionally found in the middle temporal gyrus, although it is possible that such unusual patterns of speech representation might be found predominantly in patients with preexisting brain damage.

Damage to the anterior parts of the inferior and lateral portions of the temporal lobe of the speech hemisphere causes problems with confrontational naming, but repetition and grammar are usually unaffected.

An inferior speech area has been seen in some patients (speech arrest following electrical stimulation) and surgeons have usually assumed that these areas can be removed without significant loss of language ability.

Some patients have isolated naming deficits (e.g., proper names) with unilateral lesions of the anterior and lateral tip of the temporal lobe.

Damage to the anterior parts of the inferior and lateral portions of the temporal lobe of the right hemisphere has been associated with memory deficits for autobiographical episodes, although other retrograde memory functions may remain intact.

Using functional activation with PET or fMRI has confirmed the hypothesis that visual analysis extends into the inferior portions of the temporal lobes. The activation appears to be bilateral in most cases, but there is a predominance of left-sided activation if the object's name is being sought.

Anyhow, it is worth mentioning that one of the disadvantages of functional brain scans is that patterns of activation reveal what is activated not what must be activated for successful completion of the task.

The following symptoms are associated with disease of temporal lobes: disturbance of auditory sensation and perception; impaired long-term memory; altered personality and affective behavior: disorders of music perception; disorders of visual perception; disturbance in the selection of visual and auditory input; inability to use contextual information; impaired organization and categorization of sensory input; and altered sexual behavior (Kolb and Whishaw, 2003).

Asymmetry in the auditory system

The temporal lobes comprise all the tissue that lies below the sylvian sulcus and anterior to the occipital cortex. They share borders with the occipital and parietal lobes, but the precise boundaries are not clearly defined by landmarks.

Subcortical temporal-lobe structures include the limbic cortex, the amygdala, and the hippocampal formation. Connection to and from the temporal lobe extents throughout the brain.

We can divide the temporal regions on the lateral surface into those that are auditory (Brodmann's areas 41, 42, and 22) and those that form the ventral visual stream on the lateral temporal lobe (areas 20, 21, 37 and 38). The visual regions are often referred to as inferotemporal cortex.

The medial temporal region (limbic cortex) includes the amygdala and adjacent cortex (uncus), the hippocampus and surrounding cortex (subiculum, entorhinal cortex, perirhinal cortex), and the fusiform gyrus. The entorhinal cortex is Brodmann's area 28, and the perirhinal cortex comprises Brodmann' areas 35 and 36.

In contrast with the visual-system, pathways, the projections of the auditory system provide both ipsilateral and contralateral inputs to the cortex; so there is bilateral representation of each cochlear nucleus in both hemispheres.

In the early 1960s, Doreen Kimura (1961 and 1967) studied neurological patients while they performed dichotic listening tasks. Pairs of spoken digits (say, "two" and "six") were presented simultaneously through headphones, but one digit only was heard in each ear. The subjects heard three pairs of digits and then were asked to recall as many of the six digits as possible, in any order. Kimura and Folb (1968) noticed that subjects recalled more digits that had been presented to the right ear than had been presented to the left.

This result led Kimura to propose that, when different stimuli are presented simultaneously to each ear, the pathway from the right ear to the speaking hemisphere has preferred access and the ipsilateral pathway from the left ear is relatively suppressed.

Thus, during a dichotic task, the stimulus to the left ear must travel to the right hemisphere and then across the cerebral commissures to the left hemisphere. This longer route puts the left ear at a disadvantage, and words played to the right ear are recalled more accurately.

Having found a right ear advantage for the perception of dichotically presented speech stimuli, an obvious next step was to search for tasks that gave a left-ear superiority. In 1964, Kimura reported just such an effect in the perception of melodies. Two excerpts of instrumental chamber music were played simultaneously through headphone, one to each ear. After each pair, four excerpts (including the two that had been played dichotically) were presented binaurally (to both ear), and the subject's task was to identify the two that had been heard previously. Amazingly, Kimura (1964) found a left ear advantage on this task.

Not all normal subjects show the expected ear advantages in dichotic studies, the effects are not large when they occur (seldom exceeding a twofold difference in accuracy in the two ears), and dichotic results are apparently affected by various contextual and practice effects.

Patients with damage to the corpus callosum exhibit an almost complete inhibition of words presented to the left ear, even though they can recall words presented to this ear if there is no competing stimulus to the right ear.

The Kimura's experiments imply that the left hemisphere is specialized for processing language related sounds, whereas the right hemisphere processes music-related sounds.

Papcun et al. (1974) showed that Morse-code operators have a right-ear superiority for the perception of the code, even though the sounds are distinguished only by their temporal structure. Thus, the results of this study might be taken as evidence that the left hemisphere is not specialized for language so much as for "something else".

Asymmetry in the somatosensory system of parietal-lobe lesions

The postcentral gyrus, at the most forward part of the parietal lobe, contains the primary sensory (somatosensory) projection area. Kinesthetic and vestibular functions are mediated by areas low on the parietal lobe near the occipital and temporal lobe boundary regions. Anyhow, the parietal lobe can be divided into three functional zones for somatosensory processes, movement, and spatial cognition. The most anterior zones take part in somatosensory functions.

Sensory information undergoes extensive associative elaboration through reciprocal connections with other cortical and subcortical areas (Kolb and Whishaw, 1996; Mesulam 1998; Dănăilă and Golu, 2006). The superior parietal region primarily controls the visual guidance of movements of the hands and fingers, limbs, head, eyes. The region has expanded in humans to include regions controlling not only the actual manipulation of objects, but also the mental manipulation of objects. Movements around the body, or in the imagination, necessarily include the space around the body and the object. Thus, the posterior parietal region can be conceived of as having a "spatial" function, although the precise nature of this spatial function is far from clear.

The inferior parietal region has a role in processes related to spatial cognition and in what have been described as quasi-spatial processes, such as are used in arithmetic and reading.

Thus, the posterior parietal region can be conceived of having a "spatial" function but no clear-cut demarcation exists among any of the functions localized on the posterior cortex.

Rather, although the primary centers of the major functions served by the posterior cerebral regions are relatively distant from one another, secondary association areas gradually fade into tertiary overlap, or heteromodal, zones in which auditory, visual, and body-sensing components commingle (Lezak et al., 2004).

Anyhow, the parietal cortex processes and integrates somatosensory and visual information, especially with regard to the control of movement.

The anterior parietal zone processes somatic sensations and perceptions; the posterior parietal zone is specialized primarily for integrating sensory input from the somatic and visual regions and, to a lesser extent, from other sensory regions, mostly for the control of movement.

Somatosensory system, like the others, is not a single sensory system, but a multiple one composed of several submodalities. Three major submodalities are: pain and temperature; the perception of objects using fine touch and pressure receptors, or hapsis; and the perception of body awareness, called proprioception.

Somatosensory cortex is composed of a primary area S I (somatosensory area I, or Brodmann's area 3-1-2) and a number of secondary areas (somatosensory area II or S II) areas 5 and 7. Area SI also sends projections into the adjacent motor cortex, area 4.

Penfield and Boldrey (1958) created a map that topographically represented the body surface on the primary somatosensory cortex. The regions representing feeling in the mouth and eyes were in the ventral part of S I, the regions representing hand and finger sensation were in the middle, and the regions corresponding to feet were in the dorsal area. The map is called homunculus. In humans, the areas representing the hands and tongue are extremely large, whereas the areas representing the trunk and legs are small.

The results of subsequent studies, mainly using monkeys and making use of smaller recording electrodes, suggest that the primary somatosensory cortex contains a number of homunculi, one for each of its four known subregions, 3a, 3b, 1, and 2.

Each of these areas is dominated by responses to one type of body receptor, although there is overlap. Area 3a represents muscle sense (position and movement of muscle), area 3b represents both slowly and rapidly adapting skin receptors, area 1 represents rapidly adapting skin receptors, and area 2 represents deep pressure and joint sense. Thus, the body is represented at least four times in S I (Kolb and Whishaw, 2003).

The primary somatosensory system is almost completely crossed, which allow an easy behavioral comparison of the two sides testing the right and left limb separately.

One line of somatosensory research compares the performance on the left and right hands in the recognition of shapes, angles and patterns. The left hand of right-handed subjects is superior at nearly all tasks of this type (Kolb and Whishaw, 2003).

Rudel et al. (1974) found that both blind and sighted subjects read Braille more rapidly with the left hand. Some children are actually fluent readers with the left hand but are totally unable to read with the right. Because Braille patterns are spatial configurations of dots, this observation is congruent with the proposal that the right hemisphere has a role in processing spatial information that is not shared by the left.

Another type of somatosensory test which employs an analogue of the dichotic listening procedure, is the dichaptic test. Subjects feel objects and then look at an array of objects and select those that they had previously touched. Using this, Gibson and Bryden (1983) presented subjects with cutouts of irregular shapes or letters made of sandpaper, which were moved slowly across the fingertips. Their subjects showed a right-hand advantage for identifying letters and a left-hand advantage for identifyng other shapes.

Milner et al. (1994), suggest that the brain operates on a "need to know" basis. Having too much information may be counterproductive for any given system.

Somatosensory symptoms associated with damage to the postcentral gyrus and the adjacent cortex are very different. Within the brain, no other territory supposes the parietal lobes in the rich variety of clinical phenomena that are exposed under conditions of disease.

However, the clinical manifestations of parietal lobe disease may be subtle, requiring special techniques for their elicitation.

Somatosensory symptoms of parietal-lobe lesions

Semmes et al. (1960 and 1963), Semmes and Turner (1977) and Corkin et al. (1970), found that lesions of the postcentral gyrus produced abnormally high sensory thresholds, impaired position sense, and deficits in stereognosis (tactile perception). In Corkin study, patients performed poorly at detecting a light touch to the skin (pressure, sensibility), at determining if they were touched by one or two sharp points (two point threshold), and at localizing points of touch on the skin on the side of the body contralateral to the lesion.

Anyhow, the classical doctrine that somatic sensation is represented only in the contralateral parietal lobe is not absolute.

Beginning with Oppenheim (1898), there have been sporadic reports of patients who showed bilateral astereognosis or loss of tactile sensation as a result of an apparently unilateral cerebral lesion. Semmes et al. (1960 and 1963) found that the impairment of sensation (particularly, discriminative sensation) following right and left-sided lesions was not strictly comparable: the left hand as will as the right tended to be impaired by injury to the left sensorimotor region, whereas only the left hand tended to be affected by injury to the right sensorimotor region.

These observations with minor qualifications were confirmed by Carmon (1971) and also by Corkin et al. (1970), who investigated the sensory effects of cortical excision in patients with focal epilepsy. More recently, Caselli (1991) has described six patients with extensive right-sided cerebral infarction, associated in each case with bilateral impairment of tactile object recognition but without impairment of primary sense modalities in the right hand. In each of these patients, there was also a profound hemineglect, which confounded the interpretation of left side sensory signs.

Thus, it appears that certain somatic sensory functions are mediated not only by the contralateral hemisphere, but also by the ipsilateral one, although the contribution of the former is undoubtedly the more significant.

The traditional concept of the left hemispheric dominance in respect to tactile perception has been questioned by Carmon and Benton (1969), who found that the right hemisphere is particularly important in perceiving the direction of tactile stimuli. Also, Corkin et al. (1964) and Corkin (1965) observed that patients with right-hemisphere lesions show a consistently greater failure of tactile-maze learning than those with left-sided lesions, pointing to a relative dominance of the right hemisphere in the mediation of tactile performance involving a spatial component. Noteworthy in this respect is that the phenomenon of sensory inattention or extinction is more prominent with the right than with the left parietal lobe lesions and is most informative if the primary and secondary sensory cortical areas are spared.

Lesion of the postcentral gyrus may also produce a symptom that Luria (1973) called afferent paresis.

Movements of the finger are clumsy because the person has lost the necessary feedback about their exact position.

Head and Holmes (1911) drew attention to a number of the interesting points about patients with parietal sensory deficits – the easy fatigability of their sensory perception;

the inconsistency of responses to painful and tactile stimuli; the difficulty in distinguishing more than one contact at a time; disregard of stimuli on the affected side when the healthy side is stimulated simultaneously (tactile inattention or extinction); the tendency of superficial pain sensation to outlast the stimulus and to be hyperpathic; and the occurrence of hallucinations of touch.

More precise testing is possible by using a von Frey hair. By this method, a stimulus of constant strength can be applied and the threshold for tactile sensation determined by measuring the force required to bend a hair of known length.

Thus, the defect is essentially one of sensory discrimination, i.e., an impairment or loss of the sense of position and passive movement and the ability to localize tactile, thermal and noxious stimuli applied to the body surface; to recognize figures written on the skin; to distinguish between single and double contacts (two point discrimination); and to detect the direction of movement of a tactile stimulus. In contrast, the perception of pain, touch, pressure, vibratory, and thermal stimuli is relatively intact. This type of sensory defect is sometimes referred to as "cortical", although it can be produced just as well by lesions of the subcortical connections.

In tests of pressure sensibility, two points discrimination, point localization, position of sense, and tactile object recognition, Semmes and Turner (1977) and Corkin et al. (1970) found bilateral disturbance in nearly half of their patients with unilateral lesions, but the deficits were always more severe contralaterally and mainly in the hand.

A pseudothalamic pain syndrome on the side deprived of sensation has also been described by Biemond (1956). The discomfort (burning or constrictive pain, identical to the thalamic pain syndrome) resulted from vascular lesions restricted to the cortex.

Another somatosensory symptom is simultaneous extinction that can be demonstrated only by special testing procedures. The logic of this test is that a person is ordinarily confronted by an environment in which many sensory stimuli impinge simultaneously, yet the person is able to distinguish and perceive each of these individual sensory impressions.

To offer more-complicated sensory stimulation, two tactile stimuli are presented simultaneously to the same or different body parts. The objective of such a double simultaneous stimulation is to uncover those situations in which both stimuli would be reported if applied single, but only one would be reported if both were applied together. A failure to report one stimulus is usually called extinction and is most commonly associated with damage to the somatic secondary cortex, especially in the right parietal lobe.

Blind touch

Paillard et al. (1983), reported the case of a woman who appears to have a tactile analogue of blindsight. This woman had a large lesion of areas PF, PE (area PE is equivalent to area 5 and PF to area 7b in Felleman and van Essen's flat map of cortical areas in the macaque) and some of PG (area PG in the monkey includes areas 7a, VIP, LIP, IPJ, PP, MSTc, and MSTp), resulting in a complete anesthesia of the right side of the body so severe that she was likely to cut or burn herself without being aware of it.

Nevertheless, she was able to point with her left hand to location on her right hand where she had been touched, even though she failed to report feeling the touch.

Anyhow, the PG areas are primarily visual.

The presence of a tactile analogue of blindsight is important because it suggests the existence of two tactile systems – one specialized for detection and an other for localization. Such specialization may be a general feature of sensory system organization (Kolb and Whishaw, 2003).

Object recognition

Warrington and Taylor (1973) described a common symptom of right-parietal-lobe lesion, in which patients having these lesions badly impaired at recognizing objects shown in unfamiliar view. They wrote that the deficit is not in forming a gestalt, or concept, but rather in perceptual classification.

Such allocation can be seen as a type of spatial matching in which the common view of an object must be rotated spatially to match the novel view.

Warrington and Taylor suggested that the focus for this deficit is roughly the right inferior parietal lobule, the same region proposed as the locus of contralateral neglect.

Pseudocerebellar syndrome

With anterior parietal lobe lesions there is often an associated hemiparesis, since the position of the parietal lobe contributes witch a considerable number of fibres to the corticospinal tract. Or, there is only a poverty of movement of the opposite side as part of the somatic neglect. The affected limbs, if weakened, tend to remain hypotonic and the musculature undergoes atrophy of a degree not explained by inactivity alone.

Exceptionally, at some phase in recovery from the hemisensory deficit, there is incoordination of movement and intention of tremor of the contralateral arm and leg, simulating a cerebellar deficit (pseudocerebellar syndrome) (Adams et al., 1997).

Somatosensory agnosias

There are two major types of somatosensory agnosias: astereognosis and asomatognosia.

Astereognosis

Astereognosis (Greek: a, priv.; + stereos, solid; + gnosis, knowledge) refers to the loss of the power of judging the form, shape and size of an object by touch, based on the impressions from deeper receptors.

Ahylognosia (Greek: a, priv.; + hyle, matter; + gnosis, recognition) is the inability to recognize differences of density, weight, texture and roughness of objects by touch. It depends mainly on cutaneous impressions.

The lack of recognition of texture, shape and form is frequently a manifestation of cortical disease but a similar clinical defect will occur if tracts that transmit tactile and proprioceptive sensation are interrupted by lesions of the spinal cord and brain stem (and, of course, of the peripheral nerves). The latter type of sensory defect is called stereoanesthesia and must be distinguished from astereognosis, which connotes an inability to identify an object by palpation, even though the primary sense data (touch, pain, temperature and vibration) are intact. In practice, a pure astereognosis is rarely encountered, and the term is employed when the impairment of superficial and vibratory sensation in the hand seems to be of insufficient severity to account for the defect. Defined in the way, astereognosis is either right- or left-sided, and, with the qualifications mentioned below, is the product of a lesion in the opposite hemisphere, involving the sensory cortex, particularly S 2, or the thalamoparietal projections.

Finally, there is a distinction to be made between astereognosis and tactile agnosia. Casselli (1991) defined tactile agnosia as a strictly unilateral disorder, right or left, in which the impairment of tactile object recognition is unencumbered by a disturbance of the primary sensory modalities. Such a disorder would be designated by other as a pure form of astereognosis. In accordance with Adams et al. (1997), tactile agnosia is a disturbance in which a one-sided lesion lying posterior to the postcentral gyrus of the dominant parietal lobe results in an inability to recognize an object by touch in both hands.

According to this view, tactile agnosia is a disorder of apperception of stimuli and of translating them into symbols akin to the defect in naming parts of the body, visualizing a plan or a route, or understanding the meaning of the printed or spoken words (visual or auditory verbal agnosia).

Asomatognosia

The idea that visual and tactile sensory information are synthesized during development into a body schema or image (perception of one's body and of the relations of bodily parts to one another) was first clearly formulated by Pick (1908) and extensively elaborated by Brain (1941).

The formation of the body schema is believed to be based on the constant influx and storage of sensations from our bodies as we move about; hence, motor activity is important in its development. Always, however, a sense of extrapersonal space is involved as well, and this dependents upon visual and labyrinthine impulses. The mechanisms upon which these perceptions depend are best appreciated by studying their derangements in the course of neurological disease (Adams et al., 1997).

Asomatognosia refers to the loss of knowledge or sense of one's own body and bodily condition. Unilateral asomatognosia (Anton-Babinsky syndrome) include: anosognosia (the unawareness or denial of illness); anosodiaphoria (indifference to illness); autotopagnosia (inability to localize and name body parts or inability to recognize any part of the body, a condition resulting from a lesion of the minor hemisphere); allocheiria (one-sided stimuli are felt on the other side); and asymbolia for pain (the absence of normal reaction to pain, such as reflexive withdrawal from a painful stimulus). These conditions resulting from a lesion of the minor hemisphere in which are included right parietal lobes. Anyhow, unilateral asomatognosia is seven times as frequent with right (nondominant) parietal lesions as with the left-sided ones, according to Hécaen's statistics (Hécaen, 1962). The apparent infrequency of right sided symptoms is attributable in part to their obscuration by an associated aphasia.

The observation that a patient with a dense left hemiplegia may be indifferent to, or unaware of the paralysis was first made by Anton. Babinsky named this disorder anosognosia. It may express itself in several ways: The patient may act as if nothing were the matter. If asked to raise the paralyzed arm, the patient may raise the intact one or do nothing at all. If asked whether the paralyzed arm has been moved, the patient may say yes. If the failure to do so is pointed out, the patient may admit that the arm is slightly weak. If told it is paralyzed, the patient may deny that this is so or offer an excuse: "My shoulder hurt" (Adams et al., 1997).

Some patients report that they feel as though their left side had disappeared, and when shown their paralyzed arm, they may deny it is theirs and assert that it belongs to someone else or even take hold of it and fling it aside.

This mental derangement, obviously includes a somatosensory defect, and loss of the stored engrams of the body schema as well as a conceptual negation and neglect of half of the body.

Anosognosia is usually associated with a blunted emotionality. The patient looks dull, is inattentative and apathetic, and shows varying degrees of general confusion. There may be an indifference to failure, a feeling that something is missing, visual and tactile illusions when sensing the paralyzed part, hallucinations of movement, and allocheiria (one sided stimuli are felt on the other side).

Weintraub and Mesulam (1987) indicated that patients with right parietal lesions show elements of ipsilateral neglect in addition to the striking degree of contralateral neglect, suggesting that, in respect to spatial attention, the right parietal lobe is truly dominant.

Neglect presents obstacles to understand. Heilman et al. (1993), examined 13 patients with neglect and noted that the area of lesions was the right inferior parietal lobule.

Anyhow, they wrote that contralateral neglect is occasionally observed subsequent to lesions to the frontal lobe and cingulate cortex, as well as to subcortical structures including the superior colliculus and lateral hypothalamus. Neglect is caused by either defective sensation or perception, or defective attention or orientation. The strongest argument favoring the theory of defective sensation or perception is that a lesion to the parietal lobes, which receive input from all the sensory regions, can disturb the integration of sensation into perception. Denny-Brown and Chambers (1976) termed this function morphosynthesis and its disruption amorphosynthesis. A current elaboration of this theory proposes that neglect follows a right parietal lesion because the integration of the spatial properties of stimuli becomes disturbed. As a result, although stimuli are perceived, their location is uncertain to the nervous system and they are consequently ignored.

In the absence of right hemisphere function, the left hemisphere is assumed to be capable of some rudimentary spatial synthesis that prevents neglect of the right side of the world. This rudimentary spatial ability cannot compensate, however, for the many other behavioral deficits resulting from right parietal lesions (Kolb and Whishaw, 2003).

Critchley (1953) and others suggested that neglect results from defective attention or orientation.

Heilman et al. (1993), propose that neglect is manifested by a defect in orienting to stimuli: the defect results from the disruption of a system whose function is to "arise" the person when new sensory stimulation is present.

The lesion responsible for the various forms of unilateral asomatognosia lies in the cortex and white matter of the superior parietal lobe but may extend variability into the postcentral gyrus, frontal motor areas, and temporal and occipital lobes, accounting for some of the associated abnormalities.

Rarely, a deep lesion of the ventrolateral thalamus and juxtaposed white matter of the parietal lobe will produce contralateral neglect.

Another aspect of parietal lobe physiology, revealed by human disease, is the loss of exploratory and orienting behavior with the contralateral arm and even a tendency to avoid tactile stimuli.

Mori and Yamadori (1989) call this "rejection behavior". Denny-Brown and Chambers (1976) attribute the released grasping and exploring that follow frontal lobe lesions to a disinhibition of parietal lobe automatism.

Left parietal syndrome

Generally, the dominance of the left hemisphere was amplified to encompass some important forms of nonverbal mental activity. Truly, the left hemisphere was, as the French neurologists characterized it, "the intellectual hemisphere", dominant in thought as well as in speech (Lhermitte, 1929).

In 1924 and 1927, Josef Gerstmann described finger agnosias as "a circumscribed disturbance of orientation towards one's body". Lange (1930) and Stengel (1944) suggested that this rather peculiar deficit as well as the other elements of the Gerstmann syndrome (right - left disorientation, agraphia, acalculia) should be considered as part of a more comprehensive syndrome of spatial disorientation involving external space and constructional praxis as well as the body schema.

Gerstmann and other argued that these symptoms accompany a circumscribed lesion in the left parietal lobe, roughly corresponding to the angular gyrus.

These four symptoms (fingeragnosia, right - left confusion; agraphia; and acalculia) became known as the Gerstmann syndrome, and the lesions could be localized in the angular gyrus. One or more of these manifestations may be associated with word blindness (alexia) and homonymous hemianopsia, or a lower quadrantanopsia, of which the patient is usually unaware.

Some authors believe that right - left confusion, digital agnosia, agraphia and acalculia have special significance, being linked through a unitary deficit in spatial orientation of finger, body sides, and numbers.

Apraxia and the parietal lobe

The term apraxia is applied to a state in which a clear-minded patient with no weakness, ataxia or other extrapyramidal derangement and no defect of the primary modes of sensation loses the ability to execute highly complex and previously learned skills and gestures.

In 1871, Heymann Steinthal first used the term "apraxia" for a loss of motor skills (cited by Heilman et al., 1997). Steinthal thought that apraxia was a defect in "the relationship between movements and the objects with which the movements were concerned". Afterwards, Liepmann (1900) described three forms of apraxia: limb kinetic, ideomotor and ideational. His anatomic data indicated that planned or commanded action is normally developed not in the frontal lobe, but in the parietal lobe of the dominant hemisphere, where visual, auditory, and somesthetic information is integrated. Presumably, the formation of engrams of skilled movements depends on the integrity of this part of the brain; if it is damaged, the engrams cannot be activated at all or the movements are faltering and inappropriate. On the other hand, we know that a significant portion of the pyramidal tract originates in neurons of the parietal cortex. Also, the parietal lobes are important sources of visual and tactile information necessary for the control of movement.

Paus et al. (1989), have described the motor disturbances due to the lesions of the parietal cortex. The patient is unable to maintain stable posture of the outstretched hand when his eyes are closed and cannot exert a steady contraction. Exploratory movements and manipulation of small objects are impaired, and the speed of tapping is diminished. Posterior parietal lesions (involving areas 5 and 7) are more detrimental in this respect than anterior ones (areas 1, 3, and 2), but with the most severe deficits both regions are affected.

To successful manipulate environmental stimuli the pyramidal motor neurons must be guided by movement programs. The programs must instruct the motor neurons how to position one's hand and arm to interact with a tool or object, to orient the limb toward the target of the limb's action, to move the limb in space, to determine the speed of the movement, to imitate a movement, to solve a mechanical problem and to order components of an act.

Disorders of these praxic systems are called apraxis. There are six major forms of limb apraxia: 1) ideomotor; 2) ideational; 3) conceptual; 4) limb kinetics; 5) dissociation; and 6) conduction. Each of these forms of apraxia is defined by the nature of errors made by the patient, and each of these disorders also has different mechanisms.

Ideomotor apraxia (IMA)

Failure to correctly position a limb, to move the limb correctly in space, and to properly orient the limb is called ideomotor apraxia.

IMA is probably the most common type of apraxia.

When patients with IMA perform learned skilled movements, including pantomimes, imitations, and use of actual objects, they make spatial and temporal errors.

In right-handed individuals, IMA is almost always associated with left hemisphere lesions, but, in left-handers, IMA is usually associated with right hemisphere lesions. IMA is associated with lesions in a variety of structures, including the corpus callosum, the inferior parietal lobe, the premotor areas, basal ganglia and white matter.

From sensory areas 5 and 7 in the dominant parietal lobe there are connections with the supplementary and premotor cortices of both cerebral hemispheres, wherein reside the innervatory mechanisms for patterned movement. The patient may know and remember the planned action, but because these connections are interrupted, he cannot execute it with either hand. This was Liepmann's concept of ideomotor apraxia.

Kimura (1977) showed that the patients with left posterior parietal lesions often present ideomotor apraxia. He also revealed that the deficits in such patients can be quantified by asking them to copy a series of arm movement. Patients with left-parietal lobe lesions are grossly impaired at this task, whereas people with right-parietal-lobe lesions perform the task normally.

Ideational apraxia

The inability to carry out a series of acts or sequence of action – an ideational plan that leads to goal – has been called ideational apraxia.

When performing a task that requires a series of acts, these patients have difficulty sequencing the acts in the proper orders. To determine its presence, patients should be tested for their ability to perform multistep sequential tasks. Failure to perform each step in the correct order suggests ideational apraxia.

Patients who select the wrong movement (content errors) have also been diagnosed as having ideational apraxia, but in order to avoid confusion these errors may be classified as conceptual apraxia (Heilman et al., 1997).

Ideational apraxia may occur with more diffuse brain diseases such as those associated with degenerative disorders or with focal lesions of the left hemisphere, particularly in the parietal lobe. In general, however, patients with frontal lesions have the most difficulty with sequencing.

Conceptual apraxia

To perform a skilled act, two types of knowledge are needed: conceptual knowledge and production knowledge.

Whereas dysfunction of praxis production system induces IMA, defects in the knowledge needed to successfully select and use the tools and objects are called conceptual apraxia.

Therefore, patients with IMA make production errors (e.g., spatial and temporal errors), and patients with conceptual apraxia make content and tool selection errors.

Patients with conceptual apraxia may not recall the type of actions associated with specific tools, utensils, or objects (tool-object action knowledge) and therefore make content errors (Heilman et al., 1997). For example, when asked to demonstrate the use of a screw driver by pantomiming as by using the tool, the patient with the loss of tool-object action knowledge may pantomime a hammering movement or use the screw driver as if it were a hammer.

Unfortunately, use of the term ideational apraxia has been confusing; with the term erroneously used to label other disorders (Heilman et al., 1997). The term ideational apraxia has been used to describe patients who make conceptual errors.

Patients with conceptual apraxia may be unable to recall which tool is associated with a specific object (tool-object association knowledge).

For example, when shown a partially driven nail, they may select a screw driver rather than a hammer from an array of tools. This conceptual defect also occurs in the verbal domain, which has these results (Heilman et al., 1997): when a tool is shown, the patient may be able to name it (e.g., hammer), but when the patient is asked to name or point to a tool when its function is described, he cannot. The patient may also be unable to describe the functions of tools.

Patients with conceptual apraxia may also have impaired mechanical knowledge (Heilman et al., 1997). Mechanical knowledge is also important for tool development, and patients with conceptual apraxia may be unable to correctly develop tools.

In 1920, Liepmann thought that conceptual knowledge was located in the caudal parietal lobe, but in 1989, Ochipa et al., placed it in the temporal-parietal junction.

Later, a patient was reported with left-handed and rendered conceptual apraxia by lesion in the right hemisphere, suggesting that both production and conceptual knowledge have lateralized representation and that such representations are contralateral to the preferred hand. Further evidence that these conceptual representations stored in the hemisphere that is contralateral to the preferred hand drives from the observations of a patient who had a callosal disconnection and demonstrated conceptual apraxia of the nonpreferred (left) hand (Ochipa et al., 1992).

Researchers studying right-handed patients who had either right or left hemisphere cerebral information found that conceptual apraxia was more commonly associated with left than right hemisphere injury (Heilman et al., 1997). However, they did not find any anatomic region that appeared to be critical, suggesting that mechanical knowledge may be widely disturbed in the left hemisphere of right-handed people. Although conceptual apraxia may be associated with focal brain damage, it is perhaps most commonly seen in degenerative dementia of the Alzheimer's type. It was also noted that the severity of conceptual and IMA did not always correlate.

The observation that patients with IMA may not demonstrate conceptual apraxia and patients with conceptual apraxia may not demonstrate IMA provides support for the postulate that the praxis production and praxis conceptual systems are independent. However, for normal function these two systems must interact (Heilman et al., 1997).

Limb kinetic apraxia

In 1920, Liepmann found that patients with limb kinetic apraxia have a loss of the ability to make finely graded, precise individual finger movements. Tasks such as finger tapping and pegboard may be impaired. The patient may have difficulty picking up a straight pin from the top of the deck using a pincer grasp of the thumb and forefinger.

Limb kinetic apraxia usually affects the hand that is contralateral to a hemispheric lesion.

Liepmann (1920) thought that limb kinetic apraxia was induced by lesions that injured the primary motor and sensory cortex. In 1986, it was demonstrated that monkeys with lesions confined to the corticospinal system show similar errors (Watson et al., 1986).

Conduction apraxia

Patients with IMA are generally able to imitate better than they can pantomime to command. However, one patient was reported who was more impaired when imitating than when pantomiming to command. Because this patient was similar to the conduction aphasic who repeats poorly, this disorder was termed conduction apraxia (Heilman and Rothi, 1985).

Whereas the lesions that induce conduction aphasia are usually in the supramarginal gyrus or Wernicke's area, the lesions that induce conduction apraxia are unknown.

The mechanism of conduction apraxia may be similar to that of conduction aphasia, such that there is a disconnection between the portion of the left hemisphere that contains the movement representation (input praxicon) and the part of the left hemisphere that are important for programming movements (output praxicon) (Heilman, 1997).

Dissociation apraxia

In 1973, Heilman described patients who, when asked to pantomime to command, looked at their hand but failed to perform any recognizable actions. Unlike patients with ideomotor and conduction apraxia, these patients' imitation and use of objects were flawless. In addition, when they saw the tool or object they were to pantomime, their performance was also flawless.

When asked to pantomime in response to visual or tactile stimuli, some patients were unable to do so, but these patients could pantomime to verbal command.

Patients with dissociation apraxia may have callosal lesions. In those patients with callosal lesions, it has been proposed that whereas language was mediated by their left hemisphere, the movement representations (praxicon) were stored bilaterally (Heilman, 1997). Therefore, their callosal lesion induced a dissociation apraxia only of the left hand because the verbal command could not get access to the right hemisphere's movement representations.

Not only can callosal lesions be associated with an IMA, but also callosal disconnection can cause dissociation apraxia. The subjects of Gazzaniga and associates (1967) and the patient described by Geschwind and Kaplan (1962) had disassociation apraxia of the left hand.

With the left hand, they could not gesture normally to command but performed well with imitation and actual tools, because these tasks do not need verbal mediation and the movement representations stored in their right hemisphere can be activated by tactile or visual input.

Right-handed patients who have both language and movement formulas represented in their left hemisphere may show combination of dissociation and IMA with callosal lesions.

When asked to pantomime with the left hand they perform no recognizable movement (dissociation apraxia), but when imitating or using actual tools, they may demonstrate the spatial and temporal errors seen with IMA (Heilman, 1997).

Not all callosal lesions cause IMA of the left hand, which suggests that not all right-handers have movement formulas entirely represented in their left hemisphere. Apraxia from right hemisphere lesions in a right-hander is rare but has been reported, suggesting that hand preference is not entirely determined by the laterality of movement representation and may be multifactorial (Heilman et al., 1997).

Left-handers may demonstrate an IMA without aphasia from a right hemisphere lesion. These left-handers are apraxic because their movement representations are stored in their right hemisphere and their lesions destroyed these representations. These left-handers were not aphasic because their left hemisphere mediated language (as in the majority of left-handers).

If these left-handers had callosal lesions, they may have demonstrated a dissociation apraxia of the left arm and on IMA of the right arm.

The dissociation apraxia from left hemisphere lesions that Heilman (1973) described was, unfortunately, incorrectly termed ideational apraxia. These patients probably had an intrahemispheric language-movement formula, visual-movement formula, or somesthetic-movement formula dissociation (Heilman, 1973). The location of lesions that cause intrahemispheric dissociation apraxia is not known.

Facial-oral apraxia

Facial-oral apraxia is probably the most common of all apraxias (Adams et al., 1997). It may occur with lesions that undercut the left supramarginal gyrus or the left motor association cortex and may be associated with apraxia of the limbs.

Such patients are unable to carry out facial movement to command (lick the lips, blow out a match, etc.), although they may do better when asked to imitate the examiner or when holding a lighted match.

With lesions that are restricted to the facial area of the left motor cortex, the apraxia will be limited to the facial musculature and may be associated with a verbal apraxia or cortical dysarthria.

Dressing apraxia

A particularly common group of parietal symptoms easily tested at the bedside, consists of neglect of one side of the body in dressing and grooming ("dressing apraxia"), recognition only on the intact side of bilaterally and simultaneously presented stimuli ("sensory extinction"), deviation of head and eyes to the side of the lesion and torsion of the body in the same direction (failure of directed attention to the body and to extrapersonal space on the side opposite the lesion).

The patient may fail to shave one side of the face, apply lipstick or comb the hair only on one side, or find it impossible to put on eyeglasses, insert denture, or put on a dressing gown when one of its sleeves has been turned inside out.

Unilateral spatial neglect is brought out by having the patient bisect a line, draw a daisy or a clock, or name all the objects in the room.

Homonymous hemianopsia and varying degrees of hemiparesis may or may not be present (Adams et al., 1997).

Constructional apraxia

Disturbance of the perception of space, other than language-related ones, are most evident in patients with lesions of the right, nondominant parietal lobe. These include disorders of topographic (extrapersonal) orientation and topographic and geographic memory, with resulting difficulties in route finding and an inability to reproduce geometric figures ("constructional apraxia").

A number of tests have been designed to elicit these disturbances, such as indicating the time by placement of the hands of a clock, drawing a map, spontaneous (free) drawing, copying a complex figure, reproducing stick-pattern constructions and block designs, three-dimensional constructions, and reconstructions of puzzles (Adams et al., 1997). In the majority of cases, as remarked above, the lesions responsible for these deficits prove to be in right hemisphere, though the unilateral dominance is not as striking as that of language and language-associated functions. In the most severe disturbances of visual-spatial perception, described by Holmes and Horrax in 1919, both parietal lobes were affected.

The terms dressing apraxia and constructional apraxia are sometimes used to describe certain symptoms of unilateral extinction or neglect (amorphosynthesis) that characterize parietal lobe lesions. These abnormalities are not apraxias in the strict sense as defined above but an imperception of the body.

In sum, from the above description it is evident that the left and right parietal lobes function differently. The most obvious difference, of course, is that language and arithmetical functions are centered in the left hemisphere. It is hardly surprising, therefore, that verbally mediated or verbally associated spatial functions are more affected with left-sided than with right-sided lesions. It must also be realized that language function involves cross-modal connections and is central to all cognitive functions.

Hence, cross-modal matching tasks (auditory-visual, visual-auditory, visual-tactile, tactile-visual, auditory-tactile, etc.) are most clearly impaired with lesions of the dominant hemisphere. Indeed, this is what Butters and Brody (1968) have found. Similarly, faults in what Luria (1973) has called logicogrammatical and syntactic aspects of language (which he considers to be quasispatial) occur with left parietal lesions. Such patients can read and understand spoken words, but cannot grasp the meaning of a sentence if it contains elements of relationship (e.g., "the mother's daughter" *versus* "the daughter's mother"; "the father's brother's son"). There are similar difficulties with calculation, as just described. The recognition and naming of parts of the body and the distinction of right from left and up from down are other learned, verbally mediated spatial concepts that are disturbed by lesions in the dominant parietal lobe.

Damage to the somatosensory regions of the parietal lobe produces deficits in tactile functions, ranging from simple somatosensation to the recognition of objects by touch.

Posterior parietal-lobe injury interferes with the visual guidance of hand and limb movements. Thus, effects of unilateral disease of the dominant parietal lobe (left hemisphere in right-handed patients) include: disorders of language (especially, alexia); Gerstmann syndrome; tactile agnosia (bimanual astereognosis); bilateral ideomotor, ideational, and limb apraxia; deficits in arithmetic and writing.

Effects of unilateral disease of the nondominant parietal lobe (right hemisphere in right-handed patients) includes: deficits in visual-spatial cognition topographic memory loss; Anton-Babinski syndrome, dressing and constructional apraxia; and contralateral neglect. These disorders may occur with lesions of either hemisphere but have been observed more frequently with lesions of the nondominant one.

Effects of unilateral disease of the parietal lobe, right or left, include: cortical sensory syndrome and sensory extinction (or total hemianesthesia with large acute lesions of white matter); mild hemiparesis; unilateral muscular atrophy in children; hypotonia; poverty of movement; hemiataxia; visual inattention; and sometimes anosognosia; neglect of one-half of the body and of extrapersonal space (observed more frequently with right than with left parietal lesions).

Effects of bilateral disease of the parietal lobes include: visual spatial imperception, optic ataxia, spatial disorientation, severe forms of constructional apraxia and confusion.

Generally, posterior parietal-lobe injury interferes with the visual guidance of hand and limb movements.

Localization and lateralization of language

Philosophers who argue that the mind controls behavior see "the mind" as indivisible. They suggest that the brain or mind does its work as a unified whole.

Thus, by the close of the first half of the nineteenth century there was still uncertainty about whether or not there was differentiation of function within the cerebral hemispheres of the human brain as opposed to the holistic concept that the hemispheres operated as a unit as envisioned by Flourens (1824). The influential physiologist Flourens insisted that the cerebral hemispheres operated as a unit, that each region subserved the same functions, and that the severity of behavioral impairment after brain insult was related to the quantity of tissue destroyed and not to its locus. Nevertheless, most victims of brain damage find that some behavior is lost and some survives, suggesting that different parts of the nervous system have different functions. For example, the physicians of the Salpêtrière and the Pitié pointed to the discretic deficits produced by stroke – e.g., monoplegia of an arm or of a leg, hemiplegia with or without sensory impairment, without paralysis – as evidence that specific cerebral centers governing those functions must exist. Postmortem examination did indeed disclose limited areas of hemorrhage or infarction in those patients. Nevertheless, it was not possible to achieve agreement about the precise location of the presumed centers.

Asymmetry in emotional system

Emotions are internal states of higher organisms that serve to regulate, by behavior and psychological changes, an organism's interaction with a definite object or its social environment. Evaluation has three main components: 1) the subjective experience; 2) the physiological response; and 3) the behavioral expression. On the other hand, emotions can be divided into three functionally distinct but interacting sets of processes: 1) the evaluation of a stimulus or event with respect to its value to the organism; 2) the subsequent triggering of an emotional reaction and behavior; and 3) the representation of 1 and 2 in the organism's brain, which constitutes emotional feeling. On the one hand, emotions are continuous with more basic motivational behaviors, such as responses to reward and punishment; on the other hand, emotions are continuous with complex social behavior. The former serves to regulate an organism's interaction and homeostasis with its physical environment, whereas the latter serves an analogous role in regard to the social environment (Le Doux, 1996).

Studies in animals have focused on the first of the two previously mentioned aspects of the emotion and have investigated the neuronal systems whereby behavior is guided by the reinforcing properties of stimuli. Structures such as the amygdala, orbitofrontal cortex, and ventral striatum have been shown to play critical roles in this regard.

In humans, these same structures have been shown to also participate in more complex aspects of social behavior; additionally, there are structures in the right hemisphere that may play a special role in the social aspects of emotion. Emotions influence nearly all aspects of cognition, including attention, memory, and reasoning (Adolphs, 2002).

Emotion refers to a variety of different aspects of nervous system function that relate representations of the external environment to the value and significance these have for the organism.

Such a value mapping encompasses several interrelated steps: evaluation of the external event or situation with which an organism is confronted, changes in the brain and body of the organism in response to the situation, behavior of the organism, and mapping of all the changes occurring in the organism that can generate a feeling of emotion (Rolls, 1999; Adolphs, 2002).

We can identify three components of emotion: 1) recognition / evaluation / appraisal of emotionally salient stimuli; 2) response / reaction / expression of the emotion (including endocrine, autonomic, and motor changes); 3) feeling (the conscious experience of emotion) (Davidson and Irwin, 1999; Adolphs, 2002).

Production of emotional facial expressions and other somatovisceral responses directly causes changes in emotional experience, brain activity, and autonomic state.

Although basic emotions may rely on largely innate factors, they do not appear immediately in infancy. Rather, like the development of language, emotions mature in a complex interplay between an infant's inborn urge to seek out and to learn certain things and the particular environment in which this learning takes place.

Brain structures studied in emotional behavior in humans

Natural structures that are important for emotional behavior in humans can be divided into: 1) structures important for homeostatic regulation and emotional reaction, such as the hypothalamus and the periaqueductal gray matter (PAG); and 2) structures for linking perceptual representation to regulation and reaction, such as the amygdala and orbitofrontal cortex (Le Doux, 1996; Rolls, 1999; Adolphs, 2002).

We will discuss the role of parietal and frontal regions in representing the organism's own changes in body state focusing on right fronto-parietal cortex right somatosensory-related cortices as well as other somatosensory structures such as the insula.

It is important to remember that all these structures are heavily interconnected, and that most play at least same role in multiple components of emotion.

The right hemisphere

Clinical and experimental studies have suggested that the right hemisphere is preferentially involved in processing emotion in humans.

The configurational processing of the right hemisphere lends itself most readily to the handling of the multidimensional and alogical stimuli that convey emotional tone, such as facial expressions (Benowitz et al., 1983; Moreno et al., 1990; Borod et al., 1997; Ivry and Lebby, 1998) and voice quality (Blumstein and Cooper, 1974; Ley and Bryden, 1982; Joanette et al., 1990).

Patients with right hemisphere damage tend to experience relative difficulty in discerning the emotional features of stimuli, whether visual or auditory, with corresponding diminution in their emotional responsivity (Cicone et al., 1980; Ruckdeschel-Hibbard et al., 1986; Van Lancker and Sidtis, 1992; Borod et al., 1998; Adolphs and Damasio, 2000).

While impairments in affective recognition appear to be supramodal, deficits in recognizing different kinds of affective communication (e.g., facial expressions, gestures, prosody) can occur independently of one another (Bowers et al., 1993). Patients with such deficits are limited in both their comprehension and their enjoyment of humor (Gardner et al., 1975; Gardner, 1994). Self-reference processing and self-evaluation appear to have mostly right hemisphere involvement (Keeman et al., 2000), although both hemispheres contribute to processing of aspects of personal information (Kircher et al., 2001).

Differences in emotional expression can also distinguish patients with lateralized lesions (Etcoff, 1986; Borod, 1993). Right hemisphere-lesioned patient's range and intensity of affective intonation are frequently inappropriate (Borod et al., 1985; Shapiro and Danly, 1985; Borod et al., 1990; Joanette et al., 1990). In the controversy over whether their facial behavior is less expressive than that of persons with left hemisphere damage or of normal control subjects, Brozgold and associated (1998) and Montreys and Borod (1998) say it is, while Pizzamiglio and Mammucari (1989) say it is not.

The preponderance of research on normal subjects indicates heightened expressiveness on the left side of the face (Sackeim et al., 1978; Dopson et al., 1984; Borod et al., 1998). These findings are generally interrupted as indicating right hemisphere superiority for affective expression.

Recognition of emotional facial expressions can be selectively impaired following damage to the right temporoparietal areas, and both PET and neuronal recordings corroborate the importance of this region for processing facial expressions of emotions.

For example, lesions restricted to right somatosensory cortex result in impaired recognition of emotion from visual presentation of face stimuli. These findings are consistent with a model that proposes that we internally stimulate body state in order to recognize emotions (Adolphs, 2002).

This is disagreement as to whether right hemisphere damaged patients experience emotions any less than other people. Same studies have found reduced autonomic responses to what would normally be an emotional stimulus (Gainotti, 2003).

Lezak and associates (2004) and others have observed strong – but not necessarily appropriate – emotional reactions in patients with right-lateralized damage, leading to the hypothesis that their experience of emotional communications and their capacity to transmit the nuances and subtleties of their own feeling states differ from normal affective processing (Barbizet, 1974; Morrow et al., 1981; Ross and Rush, 1981; Lezak, 1994), leaving them out of joint with those around them.

Patients whose injuries involve the right hemisphere are less likely to be dissatisfied with themselves or their performances than are those with left hemisphere lesions (Keppel and Crowe, 2000) and less likely to be aware of their mistakes (Mc Glynn and Schacter, 1989). They are more likely to be apathetic (Andersson et al., 1999), to be risk takers (Miller and Milner, 1985), and to have poorer social functioning (Brozgold et al., 1998).

At least in the acute or early stages of their condition, they may display an indifference reaction tending to deny or make light of the extent of their disabilities (Gainotti, 1972; Pimental and Kingsbury, 1989).

In extreme cases, patients are unaware of such seemingly obvious defects as crippling left-sided paralysis or slurred and poorly articulated speech. These patients tend to have difficulty making satisfactory psychological adaptations, with those whose lesions are anterior being most maladjusted in all areas of psychosocial functioning (Tellier et al., 1990).

Lesions in right temporal and parietal cortices have been shown to impair emotional experience, arousal, and imagery. It has been proposed that the right hemisphere contains systems specialized for computing effect from nonverbal information; these may have evolved to subserve aspects of social cognition.

Lesions and functional imaging studies have corroborated the role of the right hemisphere in emotion recognition from facial expressions and from prosody. There is currently controversy regarding the extent to which the right hemisphere participates in emotion: Is it specialized to process all emotions (the right hemisphere hypothesis), or is it specialized only for processing emotions of negative valence while the left hemisphere is specialized for processing emotions of positive valence (the valence hypothesis)? It may well be that an answer to this question will depend on more precise specification of which components of emotion are under consideration (Panksepp, 1998; Rolls, 1999; Adolphs, 2002).

In contrast to recognition of emotional stimuli, emotional experience appears to be lateralized in a pattern supporting the valence hypothesis, in which the left hemisphere is more involved in positive emotions and the right hemisphere is more involved in negative emotions.

So, is reported a higher incidence of depression in patients with anterior lesions 2-4 months poststroke (Kim and Choi-Kwan, 2000; Singh et al., 2000) and with right hemisphere lesions at six months poststroke (Mac Hale et al., 1998).

Gainotti (1993) suggests that the emotional processing tendencies of the two hemispheres are complementary: "The right hemisphere seems to be involved preferentially in functions of emotional arousal, intimately linked to the generation of the autonomic components of the emotional response, whereas the left hemisphere seems to play a more important role in functions of intentional control of the emotional expressive apparatus". These authors hypothesize that language development tends to override the left hemisphere's capacity for emotional immediacy, while, in contrast, the more spontaneous and pronounced affective display characteristic of right hemisphere emotionality gives that hemisphere the appearance of superior emotional endowment. As awareness of deficit is often muted or lacking with right hemisphere lesions (Carpenter et al., 1995; Meador et al., 2000), these patients tend to be spared of the agony of severe depression particularly early in the course of their condition.

When the lesion is on the right, the emotional disturbance does not seem to arise from awareness of defects so much as from the secondary effects of the patient's diminished self-awareness and social intensivity (Lezak et al., 2004). Patients with right hemisphere lesions who do not appreciate the nature or extent of their disability tend to set unrealistic goals for themselves or to maintain previous goals without taking their new limitations into account. As a result, they frequently fail to realize their expectations (Lezak et al., 2004). Depression in patients with right-sided cortical damage may take longer to develop than it does in patients with left hemisphere involvement since it is less likely to be an emotional response to immediately perceived disabilities than to a more slowly evolving reaction to their secondary consequences. When depression does develop in patients with right-sided disease, however, it can be more chronic, more debilitating, and more resistive to intervention (Lezak et al., 2004).

Inappropriate euphoria and self-satisfaction may accompany lesions involving other than right hemisphere areas of the cortex (Mc Glynn and Schacter, 1989). Further, premorbid personality colors the quality of patients' responses to their disabilities. Thus, the clinician should never be tempted to predict the site of damage from the patient's mood alone.

The left hemisphere

The analytic, bit-by-bit processing of the left hemisphere deals best with the words of emotion. Patients with left hemisphere lesions have less difficulty in appreciating facial expressions and voice intonation, and most are normally responsive to uncaptioned cartoons but do as poorly as right hemisphere patients when the stimulus is verbal (Heilman et al., 1995).

Hemispheric differences have been reported for the emotional and even personality changes that may accompany brain injury (Sackeim et al., 1982; Prigatano, 1987; Gainotti, 1993).

Patients with left hemisphere lesions can exhibit a catastrophic reaction (extreme and disruptive transient emotional disturbance). The catastrophic reaction may appear as acute – often disorganizing – anxiety, agitation, or tearfulness, disrupting the activity that provoked it. Typically, it occurs when patients are confronted with their limitations, as when taking a test (Prigatano, 1987; Robinson and Starkstein, 2002).

They tend to regain their composure as soon as the source of frustration is removed. Anxiety is also a common feature of left hemisphere involvement (Gainotti, 1972; Galin, 1974). It may show up as under cautiousness (Jones-Gotman and Milner, 1977) or oversensitivity to impairments and a tendency to exaggerate disabilities (Keppel and Crowe, 2000). Yet, despite tendencies to be overly sensitive to their disabilities, many patients with left hemisphere lesions ultimately compensate for them well enough to make a satisfactory adjustment to their disabilities and living situations (Tellier et al., 1990).

Davidson and Irwin (2002) and Davidson and Henriques (2000) posited an approach / withdrawal dimension, correlating increased right hemisphere activity with increases in withdrawal behaviors (including feelings such as fear or sadness, as well as depressive tendencies) and left hemisphere with increases in approach behaviors (including feelings such as happiness).

Patients whose left hemisphere has been inactivated from use of the Wada technique (intracarotid injections of sodium amytal for pharmacological inactivation of one side of the brain to evaluate lateralization of function before surgical treatment of epilepsy) (Wada and Rasmussen, 1960) are tearful and tell of feeling of depression more often than their right hemisphere counterparts, who are more apt to laugh and feel euphoric. In the same vein, Regard and Landis (1988) found that pictures exposed to the left visual field were disliked and those to the right were liked.

Since the emotional alterations seen with some stroke patients and in lateralized pharmacological inactivation have been interpreted as representing the tendencies of the disinhibited intact hemisphere, some investigators have hypothesized that each hemisphere is specialized for positive (the left) or negative (the right) emotions, suggesting a relationship between the lateralized affective phenomena and psychiatric disorders (Flor-Henry, 1986; Lee et al., 1990).

However, studies of depression in stroke patients have produced inconsistent results (Sato et al., 1999; Carson et al., 2000; Singh et al., 2000).

Shimoda and Robinson (1999) found that hospitalized stroke patients with the greatest incidence of depression were those with left anterior hemisphere lesions. At short-term follow-up (3-6 months), proximity of the lesion to the frontal pole and lesion volume correlated with depression in both right and left hemisphere stroke patients. At long-term follow-up (1-2 years), depression was significantly associated with right hemisphere lesion volume and proximity of the lesion to the occipital pole.

Moreover, the incidence of depression in patients with left hemisphere disease dropped over the course of the first year (Robinson and Manes, 2000).

Impaired social function was most evident in those patients who remained depressed.

Women are more likely to be depressed in the acute stages of left hemisphere stroke than men (Paradiso and Robinson, 1998). With left hemisphere damaged patients, depression seems to reflect awareness of deficit; the more severe the deficit and acute the patient's capacity for awareness, the more likely is that the patient will be depressed.

The occurrence of deviant emotional reaction in the course of disease is associated with lesions in some parts of the nervous system more regularly than in others. These have been grouped in the term limbic and are among the most complex and least understood parts of the nervous system. As defined by Broca (1878) and later by Papez (1937), the limbic system generally consists of the group of structures around the medical edge of the cerebral hemisphere.

These structures include the amygdala, the hippocampus, the parahipocampal gyrus, and related structures, such as the orbital / medial (orbitofrontal) cortex, cingulate cortex, anterior and mediodorsal thalamic nuclei, the ventromedial corpus striatum (i.e., the accumbens and medial caudate nucleus), and the nucleus basalis of Meynert. These structures have important roles in emotion, motivation, and memory.

Next we discuss those structures for which the most data are available from humans; the amygdala and the orbitofrontal cortex.

The human amygdala

The amygdala is a complex of several nuclei in the rostromedial part of the temporal lobe. There are several deep nuclei (lateral sulcus, basal sulcus and accessory basal nucleus) with differing input and output pathway with cerebral cortex, hippocampus, basal ganglia, thalamus, hypothalamus and brain stem nuclei.

The amygdala receives input from all the sensory systems (olfactory system, taste, visceral system, visual, and somatosensory systems). Functional imaging studies (e.g., positron emission tomography and functional magnetic resonance imaging) provided evidence that the amygdala responds to emotionally salient stimuli in the visual auditory, olfactory, and gustatory modalities.

In the dorsal part of the amygdala are the central nucleus and medial nucleus, which have connections with the hypothalamus and autonomic brain stem nuclei.

On the surface there are a number of modified cortical areas, many of which are interconnected with the olfactory system (olfactory bulbs) (Shepherd and Greer, 1998).

The outputs from the amygdala can be divided into three categories:

1. Return projections back to the sensory areas that project into the amygdala: In the case of the visual system, these return projections even extend back to the primary visual cortex.

2. Descending projections to the visceral control centers of hypothalamus and brain-stem: The central amygdaloid nucleus projects to a wide variety of autonomic related cell groups, including the lateral hypothalamus, the periaqueductal gray, the parabrachial nucleus, the nucleus of the solitary tract, the dorsal vagal sulcus, and the ventrolateral medulla. Through these projections, the amygdala can influence heart rate and blood pressure, and gut bowel function, respiratory function, bladder function, etc.

3. Interactions with the orbital and medial frontal cortex, both *via* direct amygdalocortical projections and *via* connections with the mediodorsal thalamic nucleus and the ventromedial parts of the basal ganglia: This circuit appears to be involved in determination of the affective "sign" of sensory stimuli (e.g., whether it is rewarding or aversive) and in setting mood.

Damage to the amygdala's interconnecting structures (e.g., the posterior septum lying between the hemispheres in front of the anterior commissure) has been associated with both hypersexuality and diminished aggressive capacity (Brodal, 1981; Gorman and Cummings, 1992).

The most prominent inputs are derived from higher order sensory association cortex, especially from the visual areas in the inferior temporal cortex (i.e., the temporal visual processing stream important for analysis of form and color and recognition of complex stimuli such as faces.

Seizure activity and experimental stimulation of the amygdala provoke visceral responses, particularly those concerned with feeding (e.g., chewing, salivating, licking, and gagging), with the visceral components of fear reactions, with facial expression of fear and with fright (Rolls, 1999).

Removal of the amygdala from both hemispheres can have a "taming" effect on humans and other animals alike, with loss of the ability to make emotionally meaningful discriminations between stimuli (Cahill and Mc Gaugh, 1998; Killcross, 2000; Pincus and Tucker, 2003). Amygdalectomized humans become apathetic showing little spontaneity, creativity, or affective expression (Lee et al., 1989; Aggleton, 1993).

In addition, the ability to make social interpretation of facial expressions is impaired in patients with bilateral amygdala lesions (Adolphs et al., 1998). Baron-Cohen et al. (2000), implicated dysfunction of amygdala in autism.

Bilateral destruction of the amygdala in humans does not produce a prominent amnestic disorder (Lee et al., 1988; Markowitsch et al., 1994), Material learned by amygdalectomized patients tends to be retained but they become more dependent on context and external structure for learning new material, for retrieval generally, and for maintaining directed attention and tracking than prior to surgery (Andersson, 1978).

Kluver-Bucy syndrome results from total bilateral temporal lobectomy (bilateral destruction of the uncus and amygdala) in adult rhesus monkeys. These animals were rather placid and lacked the ability to recognize objects visually (they could not distinguish edible from inedible objects), they had a striking tendency to examine everything orally, were unusually alert and responsive to visual stimuli (they touched or mouthed every object in their visual fields), became hypersexual, and increased their food intake.

This constellation of behavioral changes has been sought in human beings, but the complete syndrome has been described only infrequently (Marlowe et al., 1975). Pillieri (1967), has collected some of the cases that come closest to reproducing syndrome.

Orbitofrontal cortex

The importance of the frontal lobes in social and emotional behavior was demonstrated in the mid-1800s by the famous case of Phineas Gage. In 1850, Bigellow published this famous "crowbar case", originally described by Harlow (1848).

Gage, a railroad construction foreman, had sustained the passage of an iron bar (1.25 inches in diameter at the larger end, 3.5 feet in length and 13.5 pound in weight), which entered the left frontal lobe, emerged from the right frontal bone near the sagittal suture, leaving a circular opening of about 3.5 inches in diameter and destroying the left frontal lobe and anterior temporal pole, as well, in all probability, some right frontal tissue.

Phineas Gage did not appear to have suffered intellectual impairment in the narrow sense of the term. Four years after his injury, he went to South America where he worked for 8 years before returning to the United States, a year before his death. However, beginning about one month after his injury, he exhibited a remarkable change in personality.

Before the injury, Gage was considered a honest, reliable, polite, deliberate person and a good businessman.

Subsequently, he became uncaring, profane, childish, capricious, obstinate, showed poor judgment, used profane language, socially inappropriate in his conduct and was inconsiderate of others.

In short, he showed a distinctive type of personality change that later authors, such as Welt (1888), associated with prefrontal lobe disease.

The studies of Jastrowitz (1888), Welt (1888) and Oppenheim (1890) established that distinctive changes in personality and behavior could be related to disease of the prefrontal region, and Welt specifically implicated involvement of the orbital and mesial sectors of the region. The terms moria (turpidity) and Witzelsucht (addiction to joking) are linguistic residues of their observations.

In discussing frontal lobe symptomatology, Moritz Jastrowitz (1888) stated that he had seen a specific form of dementia, characterized by an oddly cheerful agitation, in patients with tumors of the frontal lobe, which he referred to as "so-called moria".

Leonore Welt (1888) wrote a paper in which she reported a personally observed case and presented a detailed review of earlier literature. Her patient, a 37-year-old man, had sustained a severe penetrating frontal fracture after a fall from a fourth storey window. Physical recovery was swift and uneventful after an operation for removal of bone from the brain. Beginning about 5 days after the traumatic event, the patient showed a remarkable change in personality. He was aggressive and malicious and given to making bad jokes. He teased other patients unmercyfully and played mean tricks on the hospital personnel. He showed no respect for the physicians and threatened to "expose" them in the daily press. He exhibited this objectionable behavior for about a month, at which time his behavior gradually improved.

1888

Some months later, he died from a pleuritic infection. Autopsy disclosed destruction of the gyrus rectus in both hemispheres as well as the mesial sector of the right inferior frontal gyrus.

Analyzing the eight autopsied cases showing personality change, she found that invariably there was involvement of the orbital gyri.

In 1890, Hermann Oppenheim wrote a comprehensive paper on the clinical manifestations of brain tumors. Four patients who exhibited Witzelsucht (addiction to joking) proved to have tumors of the right frontal lobe, three of which had invaded the mesial and basal area.

Extensive study of modern-day patients with similar anatomical profile (i.e., bilateral damage to ventromedial frontal lobe) has shed more light on this case. These patients show a severely impaired ability to function in society, even with normal IQ, language, perception, and memory.

Damasio (1994) and others have illuminated the importance of ventromedial frontal cortices in linking stimuli with their emotional and social significance.

So, orbitofrontal cortex plays a key role in impulse control and regulation and maintenance of set and of ongoing behavior (Stuss et al., 1983; Malloy et al., 1993). In healthy persons, this region is involved in the expression of aggressive behavior (Pietrini et al., 2000). Damage here can give rise to disinhibition and impulsivity, with such associated behavior problems as aggressive outbursts and sexual promiscuity (Grafman et al., 1996; Eslinger, 1999).

Lesions here also can disrupt a patient's ability to be guided by future consequences of their actions (Bechara et al., 1994) and lead to poor decisions (Bechara et al., 1999).

Left-sided traumatic damage to this area has been associated with prolonged unconsciousness (Salazar et al., 1987). Frontal lobe disturbances thus tend to have repercussions throughout the behavioral repertoire.

Emotional and social functions bear same resemblance to that of the amygdala, but with two important differences. First, it is clear that the ventromedial frontal cortices play an equally important role in processing stimuli with either rewarding or aversive contingencies, whereas the amygdala's role, at least in humans, is the clearest for aversive contingencies. Second, reward-related representations in ventromedial frontal cortex are less stimulus driven than in the amygdala and thus can play a role in more flexible computations regarding punishing or rewarding contingencies (Adolphs, 2002).

Temporal lobe connections to the orbitobasal forebrain are further implicated in cognitive functioning. Patients with lesions here are similar to patients with focal temporal lobe damage in displaying prominent modality, specific learning problems along with some less severe diminution in reasoning abilities (Salazar et al., 1986).

Because the structures involved in the primary processing of olfactory stimuli are situated at the base of the frontal lobe, odor discrimination is affected by orbitofrontal lesions – in both nostrils, when the lesions is on the right, but only in the left nostril, with left-sided lesions (Eslinger et al., 1982; Zatorre and Jones-Gotman, 1991).

Thus, impaired odor detection frequently accompanies the behavioral disorders associated with orbitofrontal damage (Malloy et al., 1993; Stuss, 1993; Varney and Menefee, 1993; Eslinger, 1999).

Diminished odor discrimination may also occur with lesions in the temporal lobes and with damage to temporal lobe pathways connecting these formations to the orbitofrontal olfactory centers. This effect appears with right but not left temporal pathway lesions (Martinez et al., 1993).

Anyhow, the amygdala and the orbitofrontal cortex function as components of neural system that can trigger emotional responses. The structure of such a physiological emotional response may also participate in attempts to reconstruct what it would feel like to be in a certain dispositional (emotional or social) state and hence to stimulate the internal state of another person (Adolphs, 2002).

As in the amygdala, single-neuron responses in the orbitofrontal cortex are modulated by the emotional significance of stimuli, such as their rewarding and punishing contingencies, although the role of the orbitofrontal cortex may be more general and less stimulus bound than that of the amygdala. Amygdala and orbitofrontal cortex are bidirectionally connected, and lesion studies have shown that disconnecting the two structures results in the impairments similar to those following lesions of either structure, providing further support that they function as components of a densely connected network.

REFERENCES

Aboitiz F, Scheibel AB, Zaidel E, Morphometry of the Sylvian fissure and the corpus callosum, with emphasis on sex differences. Brain 11; 1521-1541, 1992.

Abrahams S, Pickering A, Polkey CE, Morris RG, Spatial memory deficits in patients with unilateral damage to the right hippocampal formation. Neuropsychologia 35; 11-24, 1997.

Abu-Khalil A, Fu L, Grove EA, et al., Wnt genes define distinct boundaries in the developing human patterning. Journal of Comparative Neurology 474; 276-288, 2003.

Adams RD, Victor M, Ropper AA (eds), *Principles of Neurology*. Sixth Ed. Chapter 5, McGraw-Hill, New York etc., 84-93, 1997.

Adolphs R, Recognizing emotion from facial expressions: psychological and neurological mechanisms. Behav. Cogn. Neurosci. Rev. 1; 21-61, 2002.

Adolphs R, Damasio AR, Neurobiology of emotions at the systems level. In: JC Borod (ed) *The Neuropsychology of Emotion*. New York: Oxford University Press, 2000.

Adolphs R, Tranel D, Damasio AR, The human amygdala in social judgment. Nature 393; 470-474, 1998.

Aggleton JP, The contribution of the amygdala to normal and abnormal emotional states. Trends in Neurosciences 16; 328-333, 1993.

Alajouanine T, Lhermitte F, Non-verbal communication in aphasia. In: Reuck AVS, O'Conner M (eds), *Disorders of Language*. Boston: Little Brown and Co., 168-177, 1964.

Albanese E, Merlo A, Albanese A, Gomez E, Anterior speech region: Asymmetry and weight-surface correlation. Archives of Neurology 46; 307-310, 1989.

Albert ML, Goodglass H, Helm NA, et al., *Clinical Aspects of Dysphasia*. New York, Springer Verlag, 1981.

Alexander MP, Benson DF, The aphasias and related disturbances. In: RJ Joynt (ed): *Clinical Neurology*, Vol. 1, New York, Lippincott, Chap. 10, 1991.

Alexander MP, Naser MA, Palumbo C, Broca's area aphasias: Aphasia after lesions including the frontal operculum. Neurology 40; 353-362, 1990.

Alexopoulos DS, Sex differences and IQ. Personality and Individual Differences 20; 445-450, 1996.

Allen LS, Gorki RA, Sexual orientation and the size of the anterior commissure in the human brain. Journal of Comparative Neurology 312; 97-104, 1991.

Anderson B, Southern BD, Powers RE, Anatomic asymmetries of the posterior superior temporal lobes: A post-mortem study. Neuropsychiatry Neuropsychol Behav Neurol. 12; 247-254, 1999.

Andersson R, Cognitive changes after amygdalectomy. Neuropsychologia 16; 439-451, 1978.

Andersson S, Krogstad JM, Finset A, Apathy and depressed mood in acquired brain damage: Relationship to lesion localization and psychophysiological reactivity. Psychological Medicine 29, 447-456, 1999.

Andrianov OS, Structural basis for functional interhemispheric brain asymmetry. Human Physiology 5; 359-363, 1979.

Ankney CD, Sex differences in relative brain size: The mismeasure of woman, too? Intelligence, 16; 329-336, 1992.

Annett M, *Left, Right, Hand and Brain: The Right Shift Theory.* London: Erlbaum, 1985.

Annett MA, A classification of hand preference by association analysis. British Journal of Psychology 61; 303-321, 1970.

Anzola GP, Bertoloni G, Buchtel HA, Rizzolatti G, Spatial compatibility and anatomical factors in simple and choice reaction time. Neuropsychologia 15; 295-302, 1977.

Arato M, Frecska E, Tekes K, MacCrimmon DJ, Serotonergic inter-hemispheric asymmetry: Gender differences in the orbital cortex. Acta Psychiatr Scand. 84; 110-111, 1991

Aresu M, La superficie cerebrale nell uomo. Archives italiano di anatomia e di embriologia (Italian Journal of Anatomy and Embriology) 12; 380-433, 1914.

Babinski J, Contribution à l'étude des troubles mentaux dans l'hémiplégie organique cérébrale (anasognosie). Rev. Neurobiologique 22; 845-848, 1914.

Bakan P, Dibb G, Reed P, Handedness and birth stress. Neuropsychologia 11; 363-366, 1973.

Banich MT, Interhemispheric interaction: Mechanisms of unified processing. In: FL Kitterle (ed), *Hemispheric Communication. Mechanisms and Models.* Hillsdale, NJ, Erlbaum, 1995.

Banich MT, Heller W, Evolving perspectives on lateralization of function (Special issue). Current Directions in Psychological Science 7; 1-2, 1998.

Banich MT, Nicholas CD, Integration of processing between the hemispheres in word recognition. In: M Beeman and C Chiarello (eds), *Right Hemisphere Language Comprehension. Perspectives from Cognitive euroscience.* Mahwah, NJ, Erlbaum, 1998.

Banti G, *Afasia e sue forme.* Firenze (Florence): Tipografia Cenniniana, 1886.

Barbizet J, Role de l'hémisphère droit dans les perceptions auditives. In: Barbizet M, Ben Hamida and Ph Duizabo (eds), *Le monde de l'hémiplégique gauche.* Paris: Masson, 1972.

Barbizet J, Role de l'hémisphère droit dans les perceptions auditives. In: Barbizet M, Ben Hamida and Ph Duizabo (eds), *Le monde de l'hémiplégique gauche.* Paris: Masson, 1974.

Barbizet J, Duizabo P, Enos G, Fuchs D, Reconnaissance de messages sonores: bruits familiers et airs musicaux familiers lors des lésions cérébrales unilatérales. Rev. Neurol. 121; 624, 1969.

Baron-Cohen S, Ring HA, Bullmore ET, et al., The amygdala theory of autism. Neuroscience and Biobehavioral Reviews 24; 355-364, 2000.

Barris RW, Schuman HR, Bilateral anterior cingulate gyrus lesions: syndrome of the anterior cingulate gyri. Neurology 3; 44-52, 1953.

Basso A, De Renzi E, Faglioni P et al., Neurophysiological evidence for the existence of cerebral areas critical to the performance of intelligence tests. Brain 96, 715-728, 1973.

Batteman F, *On Aphasia or Loss of Speech.* London: John Churchill and Sons, 1870.

Baynes K, Gazzaniga MS, Callosal disconnection. In: TE Feinberg, and MJ Farah (eds), *Behavioral Neurology and Neuropsychology.* McGraw Hill. New York, St. Louis, San Francisco, etc, 419-425, 1997.

Baynes K, Eliassen JC, The visual lexicon: Its access and organization in commissurotomy patients. In: M Beeman and C Chiarello (eds), *Right Hemisphere Language Comprehension. Perspective from Cognitive Neuroscience.* Mahwah, NJ, Erlbaum, 1998.

Baynes HK and Gazzaniga MS, Consciousness, introspection, and the split brain: The two minds – one body problem. In: Gazzaniga (ed). *The Two Cognitive Neurosciences* (2nd ed). Cambridge, MA, MIT Press, 2000.

Bear D, Schiff D, Saver J, et al., Quantitative analysis of cerebral asymmetries: Fronto-occipital correlation, sexual dimorphism and association with handedness. Archives of Neurology 43; 598-603, 1986.

Beaton AA, The relationship of the planum temporale asymmetry and morphology of the corpus callosum to handedness, gender, and dyslexia: a review of the evidence. Brain and Language 60; 255-322, 1997.

Beaumont JG, Future research directions in laterality. Neuropsychology Review 7; 107-126, 1997.

Bechara A, Damasio AR, Damasio H, Anderson SW, Insensitivity to future consequences following damage to human prefrontal cortex. Cognition 50; 7-15, 1994.

Bechara A, Damasio H, Damasio AR, Lee GP, Different contributions of the human amygdala and ventromedial prefrontal cortex to decision making. Journal of Neuroscience 19; 5473-5481, 1999.

Beeman M, Coarse semantic coding and discourse comprehension. In: M Beeman and C Chiarello (eds), *Right Hemisphere Language Comprehension. Perspectives from Cognitive Neuroscience*. Mahwah, NJ, Erlbaum, 1998.

Beeman M, Chiarello C, *Right Hemisphere Language Comprehension. Perspectives from Cognitive Neuroscience*. Mahwah NJ, Erlbaum, 1998.

Bellugi U, Poizner H, Klima ES, Brain organization for language: Clues from sign aphasia. Human Neurobiology 2; 155-170, 1983.

Benbow CP, Stanley JC, Sex differences in mathematical ability: fact or artefact. Science 210; 1262-1264, 1980.

Benbow CP, Sex differences in mathematical reasoning ability in intellectually talented préadolescents: Their nature, effects, and possibble causes. Behavior and Brain Sciences 11; 169-232, 1988.

Bench CJ, Frith CD, Grasby PM et al., Investigations of the functional anatomy of attention using the stroop test. Neuropsychologia 31; 907-922, 1993.

Benowitz LJ, Bear DM, Rosenthal R, et al., Hemispheric specialization in nonverbal communication. Cortex 19; 5-11, 1983.

Benson DF, The third alexia. Archives of Neurology 34; 327-331, 1977.

Benson DF, Aphasia and the lateralization of language. Cortex 22; 71-86, 1986.

Benson DF, Stuss DT, *The Frontal Lobes*. New York: Raven, 1986.

Benton AL, The problem of cerebral dominance. Canad. Psychol. 6; 332, 1965.

Benton AL, The amusias. In: Critchley M and Henson RA (eds). *Music and the Brain*. London; William Heinemann, 1977.

Benton AL, Reflexions on the Gerstmann syndrome. Brain and Language 4; 45-62, 1977.

Benton AL, Focal brain damage and the concept of localization of function. In: C Loeb (ed), *Studies in Cerebrovascular Disease*. Milan: Masson Italia Editore, 1981; reprinted in: L Costa and O Spren (eds). *Studies in Neuropsychology*. New York: Oxford University Press, 1985.

Benton A, Aphasia (1800-1860). In: Benton A (ed). *Exploring the History of Neuropsychology. Selected Papers*. Oxford, University Press, 161-173, 2000.

Benton AL, Joynt RJ, Early descriptions of aphasia. Arch. Neurol. 3; 205-222, 1960.

Benton AL, Hecaen H, Stereoscopic vision in patients with unilateral cerebral disease. Neurology 20; 1084-1088, 1970.

Benton AL, Hamsher K, Sivan AB, *Multilingual Aphasia Examination* (3rd ed). Iowa City: AJA, 1994.

Berker EA, Berker AH, Smith A. Translation of Broca's 1865 report. Localization of speech in the third left frontal convolution. Arch Neurol. 43; 1065-1072, 1986.

Berridge CW, Espana RA, Stalnaker TA, Stress and coping: Asymmetry of dopamine efferents within the prefrontal cortex. In: K Hugdahl and RJ Davidson (eds) *The Asymmetrical Brain*. Cambridge, MA: MIT Press, 69-103, 2003.

Biemond A, The conduction of pain above the level of the thalamus opticus. Arch Neurol Psychiat 75; 231, 1956.

Bigellow HJ, Dr Harlow's case of recovery from the passage of an iron bar through the head. Am. J. Med. Sci 39; 13-22, 1850.

Binder JR, Rao SM, Hammeke TA, et al., Lateralized human brain language systems demonstrated by task subtraction functional magnetic resonance imaging. Archives of Neurology 52; 593-601, 1995.

Bishop DVM, Handedness and developmental disorder. Lippincott, Philadelphia, 1990.

Bisiach E, Gemineani G, Berti A, Rusconi ML, Perceptual and premotor factors in unilateral neglect. Neurology 40; 1278-1281, 1990.

Bisiach E, Tegner R, Ladavas E, at al., Dissociation of ophtalmokinetic and melokinetic attention in unilateral neglect. Cerebral Cortex 5; 439-447, 1995.

Blood AJ, Zatorre RJ, Intensely pleasurable responses to music correlate with activity in brain regions implicated in reward and emotion. Proc. Natl. Acad. Sci. USA 98; 11818-11823, 2001.

Blumstein S, Cooper WE, Hemispheric processing of intonation contours. Cortex 10; 146-158, 1974.

Boccardi E, Bruzzone MG, Vignola LA, Alexia in recent and late Broca's aphasia. Neuro-psychologia 22; 745-754, 1984.

Bogen JE, The other side of the brain. I. Disgraphia and dyscopia following cerebral commissurotomy. Bulletin of the Los Angeles Neurological Societies 34; 73-105, 1969 (a).

Bogen JE, The other side of the brain. II. An oppositional mind. Bulletin of the Los Angeles Neurological Societies 34; 135-162, 1969 (b).

Bogen JE, The callosal syndromes. In: Heilman KM, Valenstein E (eds): *Clinical Neuro-psychology,* 3rd ed, New York: Oxford University Press, 337-407, 1993.

Bogen JE, Memory: A neurosurgeon's perspective. In: MLJ Apuzzo (ed), *Surgery of the Third Ventricle* (2nd ed), Baltimore, MD: Williams and Wilkins, 1997.

Bogen JE, Gazzaniga MS, Cerebral commissurotomy in man: Minor hemisphere dominance for certain visuo-spatial functions. J Neurosurg 23; 394, 1965.

Boles DB, X-linkage of spatial ability: A critical review. Child Development 51; 625-635, 1980.

Borod JC, Carpenter M, Naeser M, Goodglass H, Left-handed and right-handed aphasics with left hemisphere lesions compared on nonverbal performance measures. Cortex 21; 81-90, 1985.

Borod JC, St. Clair J, Koff E, Alpert M, Perceive and poser asymmetries in processing facial emotion. Brain Cognition 13; 167-177, 1990.

Borod JC, Cerebral mechanisms underlying facial, prosodic and lexical emotional expression: A review of neuropsychological studies and methodological issue. Neuropsychology 7; 445-463, 1993.

Borod JC, Haywood CS, Koff E, Neuropsychological aspects of facial asymmetry during emotional expression: A review of the normal adult literature. Neuropsychology Review 7; 41-60, 1997.

Borod JC, Cicero BA, Obler LK, et al., Verbal aspects of emotional communication. In: M Beeman and Chiarello (eds), *Right Hemisphere Language Comprehension. Perspectives from Cognitive Neuroscience*. Mahwah NJ, Erlbaum,1998.

Borod J, Bloom RL, Santschi-Haywood C, Verbal aspects of emotional communication. In: M. Beeman and Chiarello (eds), *Right Hemisphere Language Comprehension. Perspectives from Cognitive Neuroscience*. Mahwah NJ, Erlbaum, 1998.

Botez MJ, Wertheim N, Expressive aphasia and amusia. Brain 82; 186, 1959.

Bottini G, Corcoran R, Sterzi R, et al., The role of the right hemisphere in the interpretation of figurative aspects of language. A positron emission tomography activation study. Brain 117; 1214-1253, 1994.

Bouillaud JB, Sur la faculté du langage articulé. Arch Gen Méd. 1; 575, 1865.

Bouma A, *Lateral Asymmetries and Hemispheric Specialization*. Amsterdam: Swets and Zeitlinger, 1990.

Bowers D, Bauer RM, Helman K, The nonverbal affect lexicon: Theoretical perspectives from neuropsychological studies of affect perception. Neuropsychology 71; 433-444, 1993.

Brain WR, Visual disorientation with special reference to lesions of the right cerebral hemisphere. Brain 64; 244-272, 1941.

Brinkman C, Porter R, Supplementary motor area in the monkey: Activity of neurons during performance of a learning motor task. J Psychol 42; 681-709, 1979.

Broadbend WM, A case of peculiar affection of speech. Brain 1; 484-503, 1878.

Broca P, Nouvelle observation d'aphémie produite par une lésion de la moitié posteriori des deuxième et troisième circonvolutions frontales gauches. Bull Soc Anat 36; 398-407, 1861 a.

Broca P, Perte de la parole: Ramollissement chronique et destruction partielle du lobe antérieur gauche du cerveau. Bull. Soc. Anthrop. 2; 235-238, 1861 b.

Broca P, Remarques sur le siège de la faculté du langage articulé suivies d'une observation d'aphémie. Bulletin de la Société d'anatomie 6 ; 350-357, 1861 c.

Broca P, Localisations des fonctions cérébrales: siége du langage articule. Bull. Soc Anthrop. 4; 2000-2004, 1863.

Broca P, Deux cas d'aphémie traumatique, produite par lésions du troisième circonvolution frontale gauche. Bull Soc Chir. 5; 51-54, 1864 a.

Broca P, *Sur* le siège du langage articulé : aphémie traumatique; lésion troisième circonvolutions frontale. Bull Soc Anthropol 5; 362-365, 1864 b.

Broca P, Sur le siège de la faculté du language articulé. Bull Soc Anthrop (Paris) 6; 377-393, 1865.

Broca P, Instructions craniologiques et craniométriques. Mémoires de la Société d'Anthropologie (Paris), 1875.

Broca P, Rapport sur un mémoir de M. Armand de Fleury intitule: De l'inégalité dynamique des deux hémisphères cérébraux. Bull Acad. Méd. (Paris) (Series 2) 6; 508-539, 1877.

Broca P, Anatomie comparée des circonvolutions cérébrales. Le grand lobe limbique et la scissure limbique dans la série des mammifères. Rev. Anthropol. 1; 385-398, 1878.

Broca P, Mémoires sur le cerveau de l'homme et des primates. Paris: Reinwald, 1888.

Brodal P, The corticopontine projection in the rhesus monkey: Origin and principles of organization. Brain 101; 251-283, 1978.

Brodal A, *Nerurological Anatomy* (3rd ed) New York: Oxford University Press, 1981.

Brookshire RH, *An Introduction to Aphasia* (2nd ed). Minneapolis: BRK, 1978.

Brozgold AZ, Borod JC, Martin CC, et al., Social functioning and emotional expression in neurological and psychiatric disorders. Applied Neuropsychology 5; 15-23, 1998.

Brownell H, Martino G, Deficits in inference and social cognition. In: M Beenman and C Chiarello (eds). *Right Hemisphere Language. Perspectives from Cognitive Neuroscience*. Mahwah NJ, Erlbaum, 1998.

Brunia CHM, Van Boxel GJM, Motor preparation. In: JT Cacciopo, LG Tassinary, and GG Berntson (eds), *Handbook of Psychophysiology (2nd ed)*. Cambridge, UK: Cambridge University Press, 2000.

Bryden MP, Strategy effects in the assessment of hemispheric asymmetry. In: G Underwood (ed), *Strategies of Information Processing*. New York: Academic Press, 1978.

Buckner RL, Koutstaal W, Schaster DL, et al., Functional anatomic study of episodic retrieval. II. Selective averaging of event-related fMRI trials to test the retrieval success hypothesis. Neuroimaging 7; 163-175, 1998.

Burgess C, Lund K, Modeling cerebral asymmetries in high-dimensional space. In: M Beeman and C Chiarello (eds), *Right Hemisphere Language. Perspectives from Cognitive Neuroscience* Mahwah, NJ, Erlbaum, 1998.

Burkland CW, Smith A, Language and the cerebral hemisphere. Neurology 27; 627-633, 1977.

Bradshaw J, Rogers L, The evolution of lateral asymmetries, language, tool-use, and intellect. New York: Academic Press, 1993.

Bryden MP, McManus IC, Bulman-Fleming MB, Evaluating the empirical support for the Geschwind-Behan-Galaburda model of cerebral lateralization. Brain and Cognition 26; 103-167, 1994.

Butters N, Brody BA, The role of the left parietal lobe in the meditation of intra- and cross-modal association. Cortex 4; 328-343, 1968.

Cahill L, Mc Gaugh JL, Mechanisms of emotional arousal and lasting declarative memory. Trends in Neurosciences 21; 294-299, 1998.

Caizergues R, Notes pour servir à l'histoire de l'aphasie. Montpellier Méd. 42; 178-180, 1879.

Campbell AW, *Histological Studies on the Localisation of Cerebral Function*. Cambridge University Press. New York; 360, 1905.

Cancelliere AE, Kertesz A, Lesion localization in acquired deficits of emotional expression and comprehension. Brain and Cognition 13; 133-147, 1990.

Caplan D, Neurolinguistics and linguistic aphasiology. Cambridge: Cambridge University Press, 1987.

Carlesimo GA, Caltagirone C, Components in the visual processing of known and unknown faces. Journal of Clinical and Experimental Neuropsychology 17; 691-705, 1995.

Carmon A, Disturbance of tactile sensitivity in patients with unilateral cerebral lesions. Cortex 7; 83, 1971.

Carmon A, Benton AL, Tactile perception of direction and number in patients with unilateral cerebral disease. Neurology 19; 525-532, 1969.

Carmon A, Harishanu Y, Lowinger E, Lavy S, Asymmetries in hemispheric blood volume and cerebral dominance. Behav. Biol. 7; 853-859, 1972.

Carosseli JS, Hiscock M, and Roebuck T, Asymmetric interference between concurrent tasks: An evaluation of competing explanatory models. Neuropsychologia 35; 457-469, 1997.

Carpenter K, Bert A, Oxbury S, et al., Awareness of and memory for arm weakness during intracarotid sodium amytal testing. Brain 118; 243-251, 1995.

Carson B, Javedan S, Freeman J, et al., Hemispherectomy: A hemidecortication approach and review of 52 cases. J Neurosurg 84; 903-911, 1996.

Carson AJ, Mac Hale S, Allen K, et al., Depression after stroke and lesion location: a systemic review: Lancet 336; 122-126, 2000.

Casseli RJ, Rediscovering tactile agnosia. Mayo Clin Proc 66; 129-142, 1991.

Cavada C, Goldman-Rakic PS, Posterior parietal cortex in rhesus monkey: II. Evidence for segregated corticocortical networks linking sensory and limbic areas with the frontal lobe. Journal of Comparative Neurology 287; 422-445, 1989.

Chao LL, Knight RT, Human prefrontal lesions increase distractibility to irrelevant sensory inputs. NeuroReport 6; 1605-1610, 1995.

Chelazzi L, Corbetta M, Cortical mechanisms of visuospatial attention in the primate brain. In: MS Gazzaniga (ed), *The Cognitive Neurosciences* (2nd ed) Cambridge, MA, MIT Press, 2000.

Chiarello C, Lateralization of lexical process in the normal brain; A review of visual half-field research. In: HA Whitaker (ed), *Contemporary Reviews in Neurophysiology*. New York: Springer-Verlag, 1988.

Chorover S, Cole M, Delayed alteration performance in patients with cerebral lesions. Neuropsychologia 4; 1-7, 1966.

Christman S, *Cerebral Asymmetries in Sensory and Perceptual Processing*. Elsevier, Amsterdam, 1997.

Cicone M, Wapner W, Gardner H, Sensitivity to emotional expressions and situations in organic patients. Cortex 16; 145-158, 1980.

Cohen JD, Botvinick M, Carter CS, Anterior cingulate and prefrontal cortex: Who's in control? Nature Neuroscience 3; 421-423, 2000.

Collins DW, Kimura D, A large sex difference on a two-dimensional mental rotation task. Behav Neurosci 111; 845-849, 1997.

Corballis MC, *The lopsided ape: Evolution of the generative mind*. Oxford: Oxford University Press, 1991.

Corballis MC, Can commissurotomized subjects compare digits between the visual fields? Neuropsychologia 32 (12); 1475-1486, 1994.

Corballis MC, The genetics and evolution of handedness. Psychol Rev. 104; 714-727, 1997.

Coren S, Left-handedness: Behavioral Implications and Anomalies. Advances in Psychology, No. 67. North-Holland, Amsterdam, 1990.

Coren S, *The Left-Hander Syndrome. The Causes and Consequences of Left-Handedness*. Random House, New York, 1993.

Coren S, Left-handedness. In: VS Ramachandran (ed.), *Encyclopedia of the Human Brain*. Vol. 2, Academic Press, An imprint of Elsevier Science. Amsterdam, Boston, London, New York, etc., 685-694, 2002.

Corkin S, Tactually guided maze learning in man: Effects of unilateral cortical excision and bilateral hippocampal lesions. Neuropsychologia 3; 339-351, 1965.

Corkin S, Milner B, Rasmussen T, Effects of different cortical excisions on sensory thresholds in man. Trans. Am Neurol Assoc. 89; 112-116, 1964.

Corkin S, Milner B, Rasmussen T, Somatosensory thresholds. Archives of Neurology 23; 41-58, 1970.

Corsi-Cabrera M, Arce C, Ramos J, Guevara MA, Effect of spatial ability and sex on inter- and intrahemispheric correlation of EEC activity. Neurophysiology 102; 5-11, 1997.

Coslett HB, Saffran EM, Reading and the right hemisphere: Evidence from acquired dyslexia. In: M Beeman and C Chiarello (eds), *Right Hemisphere Language Comprehension. Perspectives from Cognitive Neuroscience*. Mahwah NJ, Erlbaum, 1998.

Critchley M, *The Parietal Lobes*, London, 1953.

Critchley M, Personification of paralysed limbs in hemiplegics. Br Med J 30; 284-286, 1955.

Critchley M, Observations on anasodiaphoria. Encephale 46; 540-546, 1957.

Crossman AR, Cerebral hemisphere. In: Standring S (ed), *Gray's Anatomy. Fortieth edition*. Churchill, Livingstone, Elsevier. London, UK, Ch. 23; 335-359, 2008.

Cummings JL, *Clinical Neuropsychiatry*. Orlando, FL: Grune and Stratton, 1985.

Cummings JL, Frontal-subcortical circuits and human behavior. Arch Neurol 50; 873-880, 1993.

Cutting J, *The Right Cerebral Hemisphere and Psychiatric Disorders*. Oxford: University Press, 1990.

Dalin O, Berattelse om en dumbe, son Kan siunga. K Swenska Wetensk. Acad Handlingen Stockholm 6; 114-115, 1745.

Damasio HC, Neuroanatomy of frontal lobe in vivo: A comment on methodology. In: HS Levin, HM Eisenberg, and AL Benton (Eds.), *Frontal Lobe Function and Dysfunction. New York*: Oxford University Press, 1991.

Damasio AR, *Descartes' Error: Emotion, Reason and the Human Brain.* Grosset Putnam, New York, 1994.

Damasio AR, Geschwind N, *The Neural Basis of Language.* Annual Review of Neuroscience 7; 127-147, 1984.

Damasio AR, Tranel D, Nouns and verbs are retrieved with differently distributed neural systems. Proceedings of the National Academy of Sciences of the United States of America 90; 4957-4960, 1993.

Damasio AR, Anderson SW, The frontal lobes. In: KM Heilman and Valenstein (eds), *Clinical Neuropsychology* (4th ed). New York: Oxford University Press, 2003.

Danly M, Shapiro B, Speech prosody in Broca's aphasia. Brain and Language 16; 171-290, 1982.

Davidson RJ, Anterior cerebral asymmetry and the nature of emotion. Brain and Cognition 20; 125-151, 1992.

Davidson RJ, Sutton SK, Affective neuroscience: The emergence of a discipline. Current Opinion in Neurobiology 5; 217-224, 1995.

Davidson RJ, Irwin W, The functional neuroanatomy of emotion and affective style. Trends Cognitive Sci. 3; 11-22, 1999.

Davidson RJ, Irwin W, The functional neuroanatomy of emotion and affective style. In: JT Cacioppo et al., (eds). *Foundations in Social Neuroscience.* Cambridge MA: MIT Press, 2002.

Davidson RJ and Henriques J, Regional brain functions in sadness and depression. In: J Borod (ed), *The Neuropsychology of Emotion.* New York: Oxford University Press, 2000.

Dax G, Notes sur le même sujet. Gaz. Hebd. Méd. Chir. 2; 262, 1865.

Dax M, Lésions de la moitié gauche de l'encéphale coïncidant avec l'oubli des signes de la pensée. Gaz. Hebd. Méd. Chir. 2; 259- 262, 1865.

Dax G, Observations tendant à prouver la coïncidence constante de dérangements de la parole avec une lésion de l'hémisphère gauche du cerveau. Montpellier Méd, 1877.

Dănăilă L, Golu M, Role of the interaction of the two cerebral hemispheres in the integration of the language system. Rev. Roum. Sci. Sociales – Serie de Psychologie 31; 87-99, 1987.

Dănăilă L, Golu M, *Psychiatric Surgery. Posibilities and limbs.* Editura Academiei Republicii Socialiste România, Bucureşti; 270, 1988.

Dănăilă L, Golu M, *Tratat de Neuropsihologie*, Vol 2. Editura Medicală Bucureşti; 261-319, 2006.

Dănăilă L, Golu M, Iulia Iufu, The interaction of the two cerebral hemispheres in the integration of the language system. Rev. Roum. Neurol. Psychiat. 28; 97-107, 1990.

De Lacoste MC, Horvath DS, Woodward DJ, Possible sex differences in the developing of human fetal brain. Journal of Clinical and Experimental 13; 831-846, 1991.

De Renzi E, Faglioni P, The relationship between visuo-spatial impairment and constructional apraxia. Cortex 3; 327-342, 1967.

Direnfeld LK, Albert ML, Volicer L, et al., Parkinson's disease. The possible relationship of laterality to dementia and neurochemical findings. Archive of Neurology 41; 935-941, 1984.

Dehaene S, Cerebral bases of number processing and calculation. In: MS Gazzaniga (ed), *The New Cognitive Neurosciences* (2nd cd). Cambridge, MΛ: MIT Press, 2000.

Déjérine J, Contribution à l'étude anatomopathologique et clinique des différentes variétés de cécité verbale. Mém. Soc. Biol. 4; 61-90, 1892.

Delazer M, Bartha L, Transcoding and calculation in aphasia. Aphasiology 15; 64-679, 2001.

Delis DC, Wapner W, Gardner H, Moses JA, The contribution of the right hemisphere to the organization of paragraphs. Cortex 19; 43-50, 1983.

Delis DC, Robertson LC, Efron R, Hemispheric specialization of memory for visual hierarchical stimuli. Neuropsychology 30; 683-697, 1986.

Delis DC, Kramer J, Kaplan E, *California Proverb Test.* Lexington, MA: Boston Neuropsychological Foundation 1988.

Demonet JF, Price C, Wise R, Franckowiak RS, A PET study of cognitive strategies in normal subjects during language tasks: influence of phonetic ambiguity and sequence processing a phoneme monitoring. Brain 117; 671-682, 1994.

Denenberg VH, Hemispheric laterality in animals and the effects of early experience. Behavioral and Brain Sciences 4; 1-50, 1981.

Dennis M, Whitaker HA, Language acquisition following hemidecortication: Linguistic superiority of the left over the right hemisphere. Brain and Language 3; 404-433, 1976.

Dennis M, Capacity and strategy for syntactic comprehension after left or right hemidecortication. Brain and Language 10; 287-317, 1980.

Dennis M, Lovett M, Wiegel-Crump CA, Written language acquisition after left or right hemidecortication in infancy. Brain and Language 12; 54-91, 1981.

Denny-Brown D, Cerebral dominance. In: KJ Zulch, O Creutzfeldt, and GC Galbraith (eds), *Cerebral Localization.* New York: Springer-Verlag, 306-307, 1975.

Denny-Brown D, Chambers RA, Psychologic aspects of visual perception. 1. Functional aspects of visual cortex. Arch Neurol 33; 219, 1976.

Dewson JH, Preliminary evidence of hemispheric asymmetry of auditory function in monkeys. In: S Harnad, RW Doty, L Goldstein, J Jaynes, and G Krauthamer (eds), *Lateralization in the Nervous System.* New York: Academic Press, 1977.

Dolan RG, Paulescu E, Fletcher P, Human memory system. In: RSJ Franckowiak et al. (eds). *Human Brain Function.* San Diego, Academic, Press, 1997.

Dopson WG, Beckwith BF, Tucker DM, Bullard-Bates, Asymmetry of facial expression in spontaneous emotion. Cortex 20; 243-251, 1984.

Dordain M, Degos JD, Dordain G, Voice disorders in left hemiplegia. Revue de Laryngologie Otologie Rhinologie 92; 178-188, 1971.

Dorgeuille C, Introduction à l'Étude des Amusies. Thèse. Paris, 1966.

Dronkers NF, Redfern BB, Knight RT, The neural architecture of language disorder. In: MS Gazzaniga (ed), *The New Cognitive Neurosciences* (2nd ed), Cambridge, MA: The MIT Press, 2000.

Dubois B, Levy R, Verin M, et al., Experimental approach to prefrontal functions in humans. In: J Grafman, KJ Holyoak and F Boller (eds), *Structure and Functions of the Human Prefrontal Cortex.* New York, NY: New York Academy of Sciences, 41-60, 1995.

Duffy R, Duffy J, Pearson K, Pantomime recognition in aphasic patients. J. Speech Hear Res 18; 115-132, 1975.

Duncan J, Saitz RJ, Kolodny J, et al., A neural basis for general intelligence. Science 289; 457-460, 2000.

Esposito G, Van Horn JD, Weinberger DR, Berman KF, Gender differences in cerebral blood flow as a function of cognitive state with PET. Journal of Nuclear Medicine 37; 559-564, 1996.

Eacott MJ, Gaffan D, Interhemispheric transfer of visuomotor conditional learning *via* the anterior corpus callosum of monkeys. Behavioral Brain Research 38; 109-116, 1990.

Eslinger PJ, Orbital frontal cortex: Historical and contemporary views about its behavioral and physiological significance. Neurocase 5; 225-229, 1999.

Eslinger PJ, Geddes L, Behavioral and emotional changes after focal frontal lobe damage. In: J. Bogousslavsky and JL Cummings (eds), *Disorders of Behavior and Mood in Focal Brain Lesions*. New York: Cambridge University Press, 2001.

Eslinger PJ, Reichwein RK, Frontal lobe stroke syndromes. In: J Bogousslavsky and LR Caplan (eds), *Stroke Syndromes* (2nd ed). Cambridge UK: Cambridge University Press, 2001.

Eslinger PJ, Damasio AR, Van Hoesen GW, Olfactory dysfunction in man: Anatomical and behavioral aspects. Brain and Cognition 1; 259-285, 1982.

Etcoff NL, The neuropsychology of emotional expression. In: G Goldstein and RE Tarter (eds). Advances in Clinical Neuropsychology (Vol. 3). New York: Plenum Press, 1986.

Ethelberg S, Symptomatic "cataplexy" or callostic fits in cortical lesion of the frontal lobe. Brain 73; 499-512, 1950.

Eccles JC, Evolution of the brain in relation to the development of the self-conscious mind. Annals of the New York Academy of Sciences 299; 161-178, 1977.

Falzi G, Perrone P, Vignolo LA, Right-left asymmetry in anterior speech region. Archives of Neurology 39; 239-240, 1982.

Farah MJ, Gazzaniga MS, Holtzman JD, Kosslyn SM, A left hemisphere basis for visual imagery? Neuropsychologia, 23; 115-118, 1985.

Fedio P, Van Buren, Memory deficits during electrical stimulation of the speech cortex in conscious man. Brain and Language 1; 29-42, 1974.

Fendrich R, Gazzaniga MS, Evidence of foveal splitting in a commissurotomy patient. Neuropsychologia 27; 273-281, 1989.

Ferrier D, *The Functions of the Brain*. London: Smith Elder, 1876.

Filipek PA, Richelme C, Kennedy DN, Caviness VSJ, The young adult human brain: an MRI-based morphometric analysis. Cereb Cortex 4; 344-360, 1994.

Filley CM, *Neurobehavioral Anatomy*. Niwot, CO, University Press of Colorado, 1995.

Finkelnburg FC, Asymbolie. Berlin Klin Wschr 7; 449, 1870.

Fiore SM, Schooler JW, Right hemisphere contributions to creative problem solving: Converging evidence for divergent thinking. In: M Beenman and C Chiarello (eds). *Right Hemisphere Language Comprehension. Perspectives from cognitive neuroscience*. Mahwah, NJ, Erlbaum, 1998.

Flor-Henry P, Observations, reflexions and speculations on the cerebral determinants of mood and on the bilaterally asymmetrical distributions of the major neurotransmitter systems. Acta Neurol Scand 74 (Suppl 109); 75-89, 1986.

Flourens MJP, Recherches expérimentales sur les propriétés et les fonctions du système nerveux dans les animaux vertebrates. Paris, Ballière, 1824.

Fogassi L, Gallese V, Fadiga L, et al., Coding of peripersonal space in inferior premotor cortex. Journal of Neuropsychology 76; 144-157, 1996.

Fogassi L, Ferrari PF, Gesierich B, et al., Parietal lobe: From action organization to intention understanding. Science 308; 662 667, 2005.

Foundas AL, Leonard CM, Heilman KM, Morphologic cerebral asymmetry and handedness: The pars triangularis and planum temporale. Archives of Neurology 52; 501-508, 1995.

Foundas AL, Leonard CM, Gilmore RL, et al., Pars triangularis asymmetry and language dominance. Proceedings of the National Academy of Sciences of the United States of America 93; 719-722, 1996.

Franckowiak RSJ, Friston KJ, Frith CD, et al., *Human Brain Function*. San Diego Academic Press, 1997.

Freedman M, Alexander MP, Naeser MA, Anatomic basis of transcortical motor aphasia. Neurology 34; 409-417, 1984.

Freedman M, Oscar-Berman M, Bilateral frontal lobe disease and selective delayed response deficits in humans. Behav. Neurosci 100; 337-342, 1986.

Freedman JM Jr, Cuppernell C, Flannery K, Gabriel M, Cortex-specific multi-site cingulate cortical, limbic thalamic, and hippocampal neuronal activity during concurrent discriminative approach and avoidance training in rabbits. Journal of Neuroscience 16; 1538-1549, 1996.

Frisk V, Milner B, The relationship of working memory to the immediate recall stories following unilateral temporal or frontal lobectomy. Neuropsychologia 28; 121-135, 1990.

Frith CD, Friston KJ, Liddle PF, Franckowiak RS, A PET study of word finding. Neuropsychologia 29; 1137-1148, 1991.

Fritsch G, Hitzig E, Uber die elektrische Erregborkeit des Grosshirns. Arch. Anat. Physiol. 37; 300-332, 1870.

Frost JA, Binder JR, Springer JA, et al., Language processing is strongly left lateralized in both sexes. Evidence from functional MRI. Brain 122; 199-208, 1999.

Fujii N, Muskiake H, Tanji J, Rostrocaudal differentiation of dorsal premotor cortex with physiological criteria (Abstract). Society for Neuroscience 22; 2014, 1996.

Fukuda Y, Sawai H, Watanabe M, et al., Nasotemporal overlap of crossed and uncrossed retinal ganglion cell projections in the Japanese monkey (Macaca fuscata). J Neurosci 9; 2353-2373, 1989.

Funahashi S, Bruce CJ, Goldman-Rakic PS, Mnemonic coding of visual space in the monkey's dorsolateral prefrontal cortex. J. Neurophysiol 61; 331-349, 1989.

Funahashi S, Chafee MV, Goldman-Rakic PS, Prefrontal neuronal activity in Rhesus monkeys performing a delayed anti-saccade task. Nature 365; 753-756, 1993.

Fuster JM, Die Physiopathologie der Kataplexie. Confirm Neurol 15; 360-368, 1955.

Fuster JM, *Memory in the cerebral cortex*. Cambridge, MA: MIT Press, 1995.

Fuster JM, Cognitive functions of the frontal lobes. In: BL Miller and JL Cummings (eds), *The human frontal lobes: Functions and disorders*. New York, Guilford Press, 1999.

Fuster JM, *The Prefrontal Cortex*. Fourth Edition. Academic Press, Amsterdam, Boston, Heidelberg, etc., 185-186, 2009.

Gur RC, Gur RE, Obrist WD, et al., Sex and handedness differences in cerebral blood flow during rest and cognitive activity. Science 217; 659-661, 1982.

Gur RC, Turetsky BI, Yan M, et al., Sex differences in brain gray and white matter in healthy young adults: correlations with cognitive performance. Journal of Neuroscience 19; 4065-4072, 1999.

Goldstein JM, Seidman LJ, Horton NJ, et al., Normal sexual dimorphism of the adult human brain assessed by in vivo magnetic resonance imaging. Cerebral Cortex 11; 490-497, 2001.

Glick SD, Cox RD, Nocturnal rotation in normal rats: correlation with amphetamine-induced rotation and effects of nigrostriatal lesions. Brain Res 150; 149-161, 1978.

Glick SD, Ross DA, Lateralization of function in the rat brain: Basic mechanisms may be operative in humans. Trends Neurosci 4; 196-199, 1981.

Glick SD, Ross DA, Hough LB, Lateral asymmetry of neurotransmitters in human brain. Brain Research 234; 53-63, 1982.

Gualtieri T, Hicks RE, An immunoreactive theory of selective male affliction. Behavioural and Brain Sciences 8; 427-441, 1985.

Grimshaw GM, Bryden MP, Finegan JK, Relations between prenatal testosterone and cerebral lateralization at age 10. Journal of Clinical and Experimental Neuropsychology 15; 39-40, 1993.

Gabrieli JDE, Cognitive neuroscience of human memory. Annual Review of Psychology 49; 87-115, 1998.

Gaillard F, Converso G, Lecture et latéralisation. Le retour de L'homme calleux. Bulletin d'Audio-phonologie. Annales Scientifique de l'Université de Franche-Comté 4; 497-508, 1988.

Gainotti G, Emotional behavior and hemispheric side of one lesion. Cortex 8; 41-55, 1972.

Gainotti G, Emotional and psychosocial problems after brain injury. Neuropsychological Rehabilitation 3; 259-277, 1993.

Gainotti G, Emotional disorders in relation to unilateral brain disorders. In TE Feinberg and MJ Farah (eds), *Behavioral Neurology and Neuropsychology*. New York: McGraw-Hill, 2003.

Galaburda AM, Broca's region: Anatomic remarks made a century after the death of its discoverer. Revue Neurologique (Paris) 136; 609-616, 1980.

Galaburda AM, Asymmetries of cerebral neuroanatomy. In: Marsh J, Bock MJ (eds), *Biological Asymmetry and Handedness*, New York, Wiley, 219-226, 1991.

Galaburda AM, Rosen GD, Sherman GF, Individual variability in cortical organization: its relationship to brain laterality and implications it function. Neuropsychologia 28; 529-546, 1990.

Galin D, Implications for psychiatry of left and right cerebral specialization. Archives of General Psychiatry 31; 572-583, 1974.

Gardner H, Ling PK, Flamm L, Silverman J, Comprehension and appreciation of humorous material following brain damage. Brain 98; 399-412, 1975.

Gardner H, The stories of the right hemisphere. In: Spaulding (ed), *Forty-first Nebraska symposium on motivation*. Lincoln: University of Nebraska Press, 1994.

Gaymard B, Rivaud S, Pierrot-Deseilligny C, Role of the left and right supplementary motor areas in memory-guided saccade sequences. Annals of Neurology 34; 404-406, 1993.

Gazzaniga MS, *The bisected brain*. New York: Appleton-Century-Crofts, 1970.

Gazzaniga MS, Organization of the human brain. Science 245; 947-952, 1989.

Gazzaniga MS, Neuroscience. Regional differences in cortical organization. Science 289; 1887-1888, 2000.

Gazzaniga MS, Cerebral specialization and interhemispheric communication. Does the corpus callosum enable the human condition? Brain 123; 1293-1326, 2000.

Gazzaniga MS, The new cognitive neuroscience (2nd ed), Cambridge, MA: MIT Press, 2000.

Gazzaniga MS, Bogen J, Sperry R, Dyspraxia following diversion of the cerebral commissures. Arch Neurol. 16; 606-612, 1967.

Gazzaniga MS, *Consciousness and the Cerebral Hemispheres. The Cognitive Neurosciences*. Cambridge, MA: MIT Press, 1391-1400, 1995.

Gazzaniga MS, Principles of human brain organization derived from split-brain studies. Neuron 14; 217-228, 1995.

Gazzaniga MS, Smylie CS, Facial recognition and brain asymmetries: Clues to underlying mechanisms. Annals of Neurology 13; 536-540, 1983.

Gazzaniga MS, Smylie CS, Dissociation of language and cognition: a psychological profile of two disconnected right hemispheres. Brain 107; 145-153, 1984.

Gazzaniga MS, Smylie CS, Hemispheric mechanisms controlling voluntary and spontaneous facial expressions. Journal of Cognitive Neuroscience 2; 239-245, 1990.

Gehring WJ, Knight RT, Prefrontal-cingulate interactions in action monitoring. Nature Neuroscience 3; 516-520, 2000.

Gemba H, Miki N, and Sasaki K, Field potential change in the prefrontal cortex of the left hemisphere during learning processes of reaction time hand movement with complex tone in the monkey. Neuroscience Letters 190; 93-96, 1995.

George MS, Ketter TA, Parekh PJ, et al., Brain activity during transient sadness and happiness in healthy women. American Journal of Psychiatry 152; 341-351, 1995.

George MS, Parekh PJ, Rosinsky N, et al., Understanding emotional prosody activates right hemisphere regions. Archives of Neurology 53; 665-670, 1996.

Gerstmann J, Fingeragnosie: eine umschriebene Störungder Orientierung am eigenen Korper. Wien Klin Wschr 37; 1010-1012, 1924.

Gerstmann J, Fingeragnosie und isolierte Agraphie ein neues Syndrom. Z. Ges Neurol Psychiat 108; 152-177, 1927.

Geschwind N, Disconnection syndromes in animals and man. Brain 88; 237-294, 1965.

Geschwind DH, The organization of language and the brain. Sience 170; 940-944, 1970.

Geschwind N, Kaplan E, A Human cerebral disconnection syndromes. Neurology 12; 675-685, 1962.

Geschwind N, Galaburda A, Cerebral lateralization: biological mechanisms, associations, and pathology. Archives of Neurology 42; 428-458, 521-552, 1985.

Geschwind N, Galaburda AM, Cerebral Lateralization: biological mechanisms, associations and pathology. MIT Press: Cambridge, MA, 1987.

Geschwind DH, Iacoboni M. Structural and functional asymmetries of the human frontal lobes. In: Miller BL, Cummings JL, editors. *The human frontal lobes: functions and disorders.* New York, USA: Guilford Press, 45-70, 1999.

Geschwind DH, Iacoboni M, Structural and functional asymmetries of the human frontal lobes. In: BL Miller and JL Cummings (eds). *The Human Frontal Lobes Functions and Disorders.* Second Edition. The Guilford Press, New York, London, 68-91, 2007.

Geschwind DH, Iacoboni M, Mega MS, et al., Alien hand syndrome: Interhemispheric motor disconnection due to a lesion in the midbody of the corpus callosum. Neurology 45; 802-808, 1995.

Geyer S, Ledberg A, Schleicher A, et al., Two different areas within the primary motor cortex of man. Nature 389; 805-807, 1996.

Ghent L, Mishkin M, Teuber HL, Short-term memory after frontal lobe injury in man. J. Comp. Psychol 55; 705-709, 1962.

Gibson WC, Pioneers in localization of function in the brain. JAMA 180; 944-951, 1962.

Gibson C, Bryden MP, Dichaptic recognition of shapes and letters in children. Canadian Journal of Psychology 37; 132-142, 1983.

Glickson J, Myslobodsky MS, The representation of pattern of structural brain asymmetry in normal individuals. Neuropsychologia 31; 145-159, 1993.

Gloor R, Olivier A, Quesney LF, et al., The role of the limbic system in experimental phenomena of temporal lobe epilepsy. Annals of Neurology 12; 129-144, 1982.

Gold BT, Kertesz A, Right hemisphere semantic processing of visual words in an aphasic patient: An fMRI study. Brain and Language 73; 456-465, 2000.

Goldberg G, Supplementary motor area structure and function: Review and hypotheses. Behavioral and Brain Sciences 8; 567-616, 1985.

Goldberg E, Higher cortical functions in humans: The gradiental approach. In: E Goldberg (ed). *Contemporary Neuropsychology and the Legacy of Luria*. Hillsdale NJ, Erlbaum, 1990.

Goldberg E, Podell K, Lateralization in the frontal lobes. In: HH Jasper, S Riggio and P Goldman-Rakic (eds), *Epilepsy and the Functional Anatomy of the Frontal Lobe*. New York: Raven, 85-96, 1995.

Goldberg E, Costa LD, Hemisphere differences in the acquisition and use of descriptive system. Brain and Language 14; 144-173, 1981.

Goldman-Rakic PS, Circuitry of primate prefrontal cortex and regulation of behavior by representational memory. In: Mountcastle VB, (ed), *Handbook of Physiology – The Nervous System*, 373-417, 1987.

Gonzalez-Rothi LG, Raade AS, Heilman KM, Localization of lesions in limb and bucofacial apraxia. In: A. Kertesz (ed), *Localization and Neuroimaging in Neuropsychology*. San Diego, CA: Academic Press, 407-428, 1994.

Goodale MA, Perception and action in human visual system. In: MA Gazzaniga (ed) *The New Cognitive Neurosciences* (2nd. ed), Cambridge, MA, MIT Press, 2000.

Goodale MA, Milner AD, Separate visual pathways for perception and action. Trends in Neurosciences 15; 20-25, 1992.

Gordon DP, The influence of sex on the development of lateralization in speech. Neuropsychologia 21; 139-146, 1983.

Gorenstein EE, Frontal lobe functions in psychopaths. J. Abnormal Psychol 91; 368-379, 1982.

Gorman DG, Cummings JL, Hypersexuality following septal injury. Archives of Neurology 49; 308-310, 1992.

Grafman J, Rickard T, Acalculia. In: TE Feinberg and MJ Farah (eds). *Behavioral Neurology and Neuropsychology*. New York: McGraw-Hill, 1997.

Graham KS, Hodges JR, Differentiating the role of the hippocampal complex and the neocortex in long-term memory storage: Evidence from the study of semantic dementia and Alzheimer's disease. Neuropsychology 11, 77-89, 1997.

Grafman J, Schwab K, Warden D, et al., Frontal lobe injuries, violence and aggression: A report of the Vietnam Head Injury Study. Neurology 46; 1231-1238, 1996.

Grafton ST, Mapping memory systems in the human brain. Seminars in Neuroscience 7; 157-163, 1995.

Grafton ST, Arbib MA, Fadiga L, Rizzolatti G, Localization of grasp representations in humans by positron emission topography: Observation compared with imagination. Experimental Brain Research 112; 103-111, 1996.

Galaburda AM, Le May M, Kemper TL, Geschwind N, Right-left asymmetries in the brain. Science 199; 852-856, 1978.

Galaburda AM, Neurology of developmental dyslexia. Current Opinions in Neurobiology 3; 237-242, 1993.

Galuske RA, Schlote W, Bratzke H, Singer W, Interhemispheric asymmetries of the modular structure in human temporal cortex. Science 289; 1946-1949, 2000.

Garraghty PE, Kaas JH, Dynamic features of sensory and motor maps. Curr. Opin. Neurobiol 2; 522- 527, 1992.

Galaburda AM, Le May M, Kemper TL, Geschwind N, Right-left asymmetries in the brain. Science, 199; 852-856, 1978.

Galaburda AM, Neurology of developmental dyslexia. Current Opinions in Neurobiology 3, 237-242, 1993.

Habib M, Demonet JF, Franckowiak R, Cognitive neuroanatomy of language: contribution of functional cerebral imaging. Revue Neurologique (Paris) 152; 249-260, 1996.

Hadziselmovic H, Cus M, The appearance of internal structures of the brain in relation to configuration of the human skull. Acta Anatomica 63; 289-299, 1966.

Hall JA, *Non-verbal sex differences: Communication accuracy and expressive style.* Baltimore: John Hopkins University Press, 1984.

Hall JAY, Kimura D, Sexual orientation and performance on sexually dimorphic motor tasks. Archives of Sexual Behavior 24; 395-407, 1995.

Halligan P, Marshall J, Left neglect near but not for far space in man. Nature 350; 498-500, 1991.

Halpern DF, *Sex Differences in Cognitive Abilities.* Erlbaum, Mahwah, NJ, 2000.

Halsband U, Freud HJ, Premotor cortex and conditional motor learning in man. Brain 113; 207-222, 1990.

Halsband U, Ito N, Tonji J, Freud HJ, The role of premotor cortex and the supplementary motor area in the temporal control of movement in man. Brain 116; 243-266, 1993.

Hamilton D, *The monkey gland affair.* Chatto and Windus, London, 1986.

Hamilton CR, Vermeire BA, Complementary hemispheric specialization in monkeys. Science 242; 1691-1694, 1988.

Hamlin RM, Intellectual function 14 years after frontal lobe surgery. Cortex 6; 299-307, 1970.

Hampson E, Variations in sex-related cognitive abilities across the menstrual cycle. Brain and Cognition 14; 26-43, 1990.

Hampson E, Kimura D, Sex differences and hormonal influences on cognitive function in humans. In: Becker JB, Breedlove SM, Crews D (eds), *Behavioral endocrinology.* Cambridge MA: MIT Press, 1992.

Hamsher K, Levin HS, Benton AL, Facial recognition in patients with focal brain lesions. Arch Neurol. 36; 873-879, 1979.

Harasty J, Double KL, Halliday GM, Kril JJ, McRitchie DA, Language-associated cortical regions are proportionally larger in the female brain. Archives of Neurology 54; 171-175, 1997.

Hardyck C, Petrinovich LF, Left-handedness. Psychological Bulletin 84; 385-405, 1977.

Harlow JM, Passage of an iron bar through the head. Boston Medical and Surgical Journal 39; 389-393, 1848.

Harrington DL, Haalad KY, Motor sequencing with left hemisphere damage: Are some cognitive deficits to limb apraxia? Brain 115; 857-874, 1992.

Harris LJ, Sex differences in spatial ability: Possible environmental, genetic, and neurological factors. In: Kinsbourne M (ed), *Asymmetrical function of the brain* (405-521) London: Cambridge University Press, 1978.

Harshman RA, Hampson E, Berenbaum SA, Individual differences in cognitive abilities and brain organization, part 1: Sex and handedness differences in ability. Canadian Journal of Psychology 37; 144-192, 1983.

Hauser MD, Right-hemisphere dominance for the production of facial expression in monkeys. Science 261; 475-477, 1993.

Haverkort M, Stowe L, Wijers B, Paans A, Familial handedness and sex in language comprehension. Neuroimage 9; 12-18, 1999.

Haward D, Language in the Human Brain. In: MD Rugg (ed). *Cognitive Neuroscience.* Cambridge, MA: MIT Press, 1997.

Hayes TL, Lewis DA, Hemispheric differences in layer III pyramidal neurons of the anterior language area. Archives of Neurology 50; 501-505, 1993.

Hayes TL, Lewis DA, Anatomical specialization of the anterior motor speech area: Hemispheric differences in magnopyramidal neurons. Brain and Language 49; 289-308, 1995.

Head H, Holmes G, Sensory disturbances from cerebral lesions. Brain 34; 102, 1911.

Hebb DO, Intelligence in man after large removals of cerebral tissue: report of four left frontal lobe cases. Journal of General Psychology 21; 73-87, 1939.

Hécaen H, Clinical symptomatology in right and left hemispheric lesions. In: Mountcastle VB, (ed), *Interhemispheric Relations and Cerebral Dominance.* Baltimore, John Hopkins, Chap 10; 215-263, 1962.

Hécaen H, *Introduction à la Neuropsychologie.* Paris, Larousse, 1972.

Hécaen H, Angelergues R, *Le Cécité Psychique.* Masson: Paris, 1963.

Hécaen H, Sauguet J, Cerebral dominance in left-handed subjects. Cortex 7; 19-48, 1971.

Hécaen H, Consoli S, Analyse des troubles de language au cours des lésions de l'aire de Broca (Analysis of language disorders in lesions of Broca's area). Neuropsychologia 11; 377-388, 1973.

Hécaen H, De Agostini M, Monzon-Montes A, Cerebral organization in lefthanders. Brain Lang 12; 261-284, 1981.

Heffner HE, Heffner RS, Temporal lobe lesions and perception of species-specific vocalizations by macaques. Science 226; 75-76, 1984.

Heilman KM, Ideational apraxia – A redefinition. Brain 96; 861-864, 1973.

Heilman KM, The neurobiology of emotional experience. J. Neuropsychiatr. Clin Neurosci 9; 439-448, 1997.

Heilman KM, Valenstein E, Frontal lobe neglect in man. Neurology 22; 660-664, 1972.

Heilman KM, Van Den Abell T, Right hemisphere dominance for attention: The mechanism underlying hemispheric asymmetries of inattention (neglect). Neurology 30; 327-330, 1980.

Heilman KM, Rothi LJ, Apraxia. In: *Clinical Neuropsychology* (KM Heilman and E Valenstein (eds). Oxford University Press, New York, 1985.

Heilman KM, Maher LM, Greenwald ML, Rothi LJ, Conceptual apraxia from lateralized lesions. Neurology 49; 457-464, 1997.

Heilman KM, Watson RT, Valenstein E, Neglect and related disorders. In: KM Heilman and E Valenstein (eds). *Clinical Neuropsychology.* (3rd ed), New York, Oxford University Press, 1993.

Heilman KM, Chartter J, Doty LC, Hemispheric asymmetries of the near-far spatial attention. Neuropsychology 9; 58-61, 1995.

Heilman KM, Rothi LJ, Apraxia. In: KM Heilman and E Valenstein (eds). *Clinical Neuropsychology* (4th ed). New York: Oxford University Press, 2003.

Heiss WD, Kessler J, Thiel A, et al., Differential capacity of left and right hemispheric areas for comprehension of post-stroke aphasia. Annals of Neurology 45; 430-438, 1999.

Helliard RD, Hemispheric laterality effects on a facial recognition task in normal subjects. Cortex 9; 246-258, 1973.

Hellige JB, Hemispheric differences for processing spatial information: Categorization versus distance (abstract). Journal of Clinical and Experimental Neuropsychology 10; 330, 1988.

Hellige JB, Cerebral Hemispheric asymmetry: What's right and what's left. Harvard University Press, Cambridge, MA, 1993.

Hellige JB, Coordinating the different processing biases of the left and right cerebral hemispheres. In: FL Kitterle (ed), *Hemispheric Communication: Mechanisms and Models.* Hillsdale, NJ, Erlbaum, 1995.

Hellige JB, Cerebral hemispheric specialization in normal individuals: Experimental assessment. In: F Boiler and J Grafman (Eds), *Handbook of Neuropsychology*. Vol. 1, Elsevier Amsterdam, 2000.

Hellige JB, *Cerebral Hemisphere Asymmetry. What's Right and What's Left.* Harvard University Press, Cambridge MA, 2001.

Hellige JB, Laterality. In: VS Ramachandran (ed.), *Encyclopedia of the Human Brain*. Vol. 2, Academic, Press, An imprint of Elsevier Science, Amsterdam, Boston, London, New York, etc., 671-683, 2002.

Henschen SE, *Klinische und anatomische Beitrage zur Pathologie des Gehirns. Teil 5: Ueber Aphasie, Amusie und Akalkulie.* Stockholm: Nordiska Bakhandeln, 1920.

Herrick CJ, *Brain of rats and men.* University of Chicago Press, Chicago, 1926.

Hickock G, Bellugi U, Klima ES, Sign language in the brain. Scientific American 284; 58-65, 2001.

Hines M, Significance of the precentral motor cortex. In: PC Bucy (ed), *The Precentral Motor Cortex*. University Press. Urbana, Ch. 18; 461-494, 1949.

Hochberg FH, LeMay M, Arteriographic correlates of handedness. Neurology 25; 218-222, 1975.

Holloway V, Gadian DG, Vargha-Khadem F, et al., The reorganization of sensorimotor function in children after hemispherectomy. Brain 123; 2432-2444, 2000.

Holmes G, May WP, On the exact origin tract in man and other mammals. Brain 32; 1-43, 1909.

Holmes G, Horrax G, Disturbances of spatial orientation and visual attention with loss of stereoscopic vision. Arch. Neurol Psychiatry 1; 385-407, 1919.

Holtzman JD, Gazzaniga MS, Dual task interaction due exclusively to limits in processing resources. Science 218; 1325-1327, 1982.

Holtzman JD, Gazzaniga MS, Enhanced dual task performance following corpus commissurotomy in humans. Neuropsychologia 23; 315-321, 1985.

Holtzman JD, Sidtis JJ, Volpe BT, Wilson DH, Gazzaniga MS, Dissociation of spatial information for stimulus localization and the control of attention, Brain 104; 861-872, 1981.

Holtzman JD, Volpe BT, Gazzaniga MS, Spatial orientation following commissural section. In: Parasuraman R and Davies DR, eds. *Varieties of Attention.* New York: Academic Press, 375-394, 1984.

Horn G, Neural basis of recognition memory investigated through an analysis of imprinting. Philosophical Transaction of the Royal Society London B, 329; 133-142, 1990.

Hoster W, Ettlinger G, An association between hand preference and tactile discrimination performance in the rhesus monkey. Neuropsychologica 21; 411-413, 1985.

Huettner MS, Rosenthal BL, Hynd GW, Regional cerebral blood flow (fCBF) in normal readers: Bilateral activation with narrative text. Archives of Clinical Neuropsychology 4; 71-78, 1989.

Iacoboni M, Zaidel E, Channels of the corpus callosum: Evidence from simple reaction times to lateralized flashes in the normal and the split brain. Brain 118; 779-788, 1995.

Iacoboni M, and Zaidel E, Hemispheric independence in word recognition: Evidence from unilateral and bilateral presentations. Brain and Language, 121-140, 1996.

Iacoboni M, Woods RP, Mazziotta JC, Blood flow increases in left dorsal premotor cortex during sensorimotor integration learning. Society for Neuroscience. Abstract 22; 720, 1996 a.

Iacoboni M, Woods RP, Mazziotta JC, Brain-behavior relationships: Evidence from practice effects in spatial stimulus-response compatibility. Journal of Neuropsychology 76; 321-331, 1996 b.

Iacoboni M, Woods RP, Lenzi GL, Mazziotta JC, Miring of oculomotor and somatomotor space coding in the human right precentral gyrus. Brain 120; 1635-1645, 1997.

Incisa della Rocchetta AI, Classification and recall of pictures after unilateral frontal or temporal lobectomy. Cortex 22; 189-211, 1986.

Incisa della Rocchetta AI, and Milner B, Strategic search and retrieval inhibition: the role of frontal lobes. Neuropsychologia 31; 503-524, 1993.

Indefrey P, Levelt WJM, The neural correlates of language production. In: Gazzaniga (ed). *The Two Cognitive Neurosciences* (2nd ed). Cambridge, MA, MIT Press, 2000.

Inglis J, Lawson JS, A meta-analysis of sex differences in the effects of unilateral brain damage on intelligence test results. Canadian Journal of Psychology 36; 670-683, 1982.

Ivry RB, Lebby PC, The neurology of consonant perception: Specialized module or distributed processor? In: M Beeman and C Chiarello (eds), *Right hemisphere language comprehension*. Mahwah NJ, Erlbaum, 1998.

Iwatsubo T, et al., Corticofugal projections to the motor nuclei of the brain stem and spinal cord in humans. Neurology 40; 309-312, 1990.

Jackson JH, Deficit of intellectual expression (aphasia) with left hemiplegia. Lancet 1; 457, 1868.

Jackson JH, On aphasia, with left hemiplegia. Lancet 1; 637-638, 1880.

Jackson JH, Hughlings Jackson on aphasia and kindred affections of speech, together with a complete bibliography of his publications on speech and a reprint of some of the more important papers. Brain 38; 1-190, 1915.

Jäncke L, Steinmetz H, Anatomical brain asymmetries and their relevance for functional asymmetries. In: K Hugadahl and RJ Davidson (eds) *The Asymmetrical Brain*. Cambridge, MA:MIT Press, 187-230, 2003.

Jäncke L, Schlang G, Huang Y, Steinmetz H, Asymmetry of the planum parietale. Neuroreport 5; 1161-1163, 1994.

Janowsky JS, Shimura AP, Kritchevsky M, Squire LR, Cognitive impairment following frontal lobe damage and its relevance to human amnesia. Behav Neurosci 103; 548-560, 1989 a.

Janowsky JS, Oviatt SK, Orwoll ES, Testosterone influences spatial cognition in older men. Behav Neurosci 108; 325-332, 1994.

Jason GW, Studies of manual learning and performance after surgical excision for the control of epilepsy. In: J Enge Jr. (ed), *Fundamental Mechanisms of Human Brain Function*. New York: Raven Press, 1987.

Jastrowitz M, Beitrage zur Localisation im Grosshirn und uber deren praktische Verwerthung. Dtsch Med Wochenschr 14; 81-83, 1888.

Jeannerod M, Aribib MA, Rizzolatti G, Sakata H, Grasping objects: The cortical mechanisms of visuomotor transformation. Trends in Neurosciences 18; 314-320, 1995.

Jerison HJ, The theory of encephalization. Annals of the New York Academy of Sciences 299; 146-160, 1977.

Jinnai K, Matsuda Y, Neurons of the motor cortex projecting commonly in the caudate nucleus and the lower brain stem in the cat. Neurosci Lett 13; 121-126, 1979.

Jonas S, The supplementary motor region and speech. In: E Percman (ed), *The Frontal Lobe Revisited*. New York, IRBN Press, 1987.

Joanette Y, Goulet P, Hammequin D, *Right Hemisphere and Verbal Communication*. New York, Springer-Verlag, 1990.

Johanson SC, Saykin AJ, Flashman LA, et al., Brain activation on fMRI and verbal memory ability: Functional neuroanatomic correlates of CVLT performance. Journal of the International Neuropsychological Society 7; 55-62, 2001.

Jones-Gotman M, Milner B, Design fluency: The innervation of nonsense drawing after focal cortical lesions. Neuropsychologia 15; 653-674, 1977.

Jones-Gotman M, Right hippocampal excision impairs learning and recall of list of abstract designs. Neuropsychologia 24; 659-670, 1986.

Jones-Gotman M, Zatorre RJ, Olivier A, et al., Learning and retention of words and designs following excision from medial lateral temporal-lobe structures. Neuropsychologia 35; 963-973, 1997.

Jorge RE, Robinson RG, Starkstein SE, et al., Secondary mania following traumatic brain injury. American Journal of Psychiatry 150; 916-921, 1993.

Jossmann P, Motrische Amusie (Demonstration). Zbl. Neurol. Psychiat 44; 260, 1926.

Jossmann P, Die Beziehungen der motorischen Amusie zu den apraktischen Storungen Mschr. Psychiat Neurol. 63; 239, 1927.

Joynt RJ, Benton AL, The memoir of Marc Dax on aphasia. Neurology 14; 851-854, 1964.

Jurado MA, Junké C, Pujol J, et al., Impaired estimations of word occurrence frequency in frontal lobe patients. Neuropsychologia 35; 635-641, 1997.

Jurado MA, Junké C, Vendrell P, et al., Overestimation and unreliability in «feeling-of-doing judgments» about temporal ordering performance: impaired self-awareness following frontal lobe damage. J Clin Exp Neuropsychol 20; 353-364, 1998.

Juraska JM, Sex differences in developmental plasticity of behavior and the brain. In: Greenough WT, Juraska JM (eds), *Developmental Neuropsychobiology*, New York: Academic Press, 409-422, 1986.

Just MA, Carpenter PA, Keller TA, et al., Brain activation modulated by sentence comprehension. Science 274; 114-116, 1996.

Kaas JH, Stepniewska I, Motor cortex. In: VS Ramachandran (ed), *Encyclopedia of the Human Brain*. Volume 3. Academic Press, Amsterdam, Boston, London etc.; 159-169, 2002.

Kang DH, Davidson RJ, Coe CL. et al., Frontal brain asymmetry and immune function. Behavior Neuroscience 105; 860-869, 1991.

Kawashima R, Yamada K, Kinomura S, et al., Regional cerebral blood flow changes of cortical motor areas and prefrontal areas in humans related to ipsilateral and contralateral hand movement. Brain Research 623; 33-40, 1993.

Keeman JP, Wheeler MA, Gallup GG Jr., Pascual-Leone A, Self recognition and the right prefrontal cortex. Trends in Cognitive Sciences 4; 338-344, 2000.

Keppel CC, Crowe SF, Changes to body image and selfesteem following stroke in young adults. Neuropsychological Rehabilitation 10; 15-31, 2000.

Kertesz A, Lau WK, Palk M, The structural determinants of recovery in Wernicke's aphasia. Brain Long 44; 153-164, 1993.

Kesner RP, Hopkins RO, Fineman B, Item and order dissociation in humans with prefrontal cortex damage. Neuropsychologia 32; 881-891, 1994.

Kiehl KA, Liddle PF, Smith AM, et al., Neural pathways involved in the processing of concrete and abstract words. Human Brain Mapping 7; 225-233, 1999.

Killcross S, The amygdala, emotion, and learning. Psychologist 13; 502-507, 2000.

Kim JS, Choi-Kwan S, Post-stroke depression and emotional incontinence: Correlation with lesion location. Neurology 54; 1805-1810, 2000.

Kim Y, Morrow L, Passafiume D, Boller F, Visuoperceptual and visuomotor abilities and locus of lesion. Neuropsychologia 22; 177-185, 1984.

Kim SG, Ashe J, Hendrich K, Ellerman JM, Functional magnetic imaging of motor cortex: Hemispheric asymmetry and handedness. Science 261; 615-616, 1993.

Kim KHS, Relkin NR, Lee KM, Hirsch J, Distinct cortical areas associated with native and second languages, Nature 388; 171-174, 1997.

Kimura D, Sex differences in cerebral organization for speech and praxis functions. Canadian Journal of Psychology 37; 19-35, 1983.

Kimura D, *Sex and Cognition*. Cambridge, Massachusetts: The MIT Press, 1999.

Kimura D, Some effects of temporal lobe damage on auditory perception. Canadian Journal of Psychology 15; 156-165, 1961.

Kimura D, Left-right differences in the perception of melodies. Quarterly Journal of Experimental Psychology 16; 355-358, 1964.

Kimura D, Functional asymmetry of the brain in dichotic listening. Cortex 3; 163-178, 1967.

Kimura D, The asymmetry of the human brain. Scientific American 228; 70-78, 1973.

Kimura D, Acquisition of a motor skill after left hemisphere damage. Brain 100; 527-542, 1977.

Kimura D, Folb S, Neural processing of background sound. Science 161; 395-396, 1968.

Kingstone A and Gazzaniga MS, Subcortical transfer of higher-order information: More illusory than real? Neuropsychologia 9; 321-328, 1995.

Kircher TT, Senior C, Phillips ML, et al., Recognizing one's own face. Cognition 78; 1-15, 2001.

Kirshner HS, Language Disorders. Aphasia. In: Bradley WG, Daroff RB, Fenichel GM and Marsden CD (eds) *Neurology in Clinical Practice*. Vol. 1, Third Edition. Boston, Oxford, Singapore, Butterworth-Heinemann, 141-159, 2000.

Kirshner HS, Hughes T, Farkovarz T, Abou-Khalil B, Aphasia secondary to partial status epilepticus of the basal temporal language area. Neurology 45; 1616-1618, 1995.

Klebanoff SG, Psychological changes in organic brain lesions and ablations. Psychological Bulletin 42; 585-623, 1945.

Klein D, Milner B, Zatorre R, Meyer E, Evans A, The neural substrates underlying word generation: a bilingual functional-imaging study. Proceedings National Academy of Sciences USA 92; 2899-2903, 1995.

Klein D, Milner BA, Zatorre RJ, Zhao V, Nikelski EJ, Cerebral organization in bilinguals: A PET study of Chinese-English verb generation. NeuroReport 10; 2841-2846, 1999.

Kohn B, and Dennis M, Selective impairments of visuo-spatial abilities in infantile hemiplegies after right cerebral hemidecortication. Neuropsychologia 12; 505-512, 1974.

Kolb B, Stewart J, Sex-related differences in dendritic branching of cells in the prefrontal cortex of rats. J Neuroendocrinol 3; 95-99, 1991.

Kolb B, Whishaw IQ, Fundamentals of Human Neuropsychology. Fifth Edition. Worth Publishers USA, Chapter 11 and 12; 250-317, 2003.

Kolb B, Sutherland RJ, Nonneman AJ, Whishaw IQ, Asymmetry with cerebral hemisphere of the rat, mouse, rabbit and cat: The right hemisphere is larger. Experimental Neurology 78; 348-359, 1982.

Kolb B, Whishaw Q, *Fundamentals of Neuropsychology* (2nd ed). San Francisco: Freeman, 1985.

Kolb B, Whishaw Q, *Fundamentals of Neuropsychology* (4th ed). New York, Freeman, 1996.

Kolb B, Whishaw QI, *Fundamentals of Human Neuropsychology*. Fifth Edition. World Publishers, New York, 2003.

Kononova EP, Structural variability of the cortex cerebri. Inferior frontal gyrus in adults (Russian). In: "Annals of the Brain Research Institute". In: SA Sarkisov and IN Filimonov (eds), Vol. 1; 49-118, *State Press for Biological and Medical Literature*, Moscow, Leningrad, 1935.

Kononova EP, The frontal lobe (Russian). In: SA Sarkisov, IN Filimon and NS Preobrashenskaya (eds), *The Cytoarchitecture of the Human Cortex Cerebri.* Medgiz, Moscow, 309-343, 1949.

Konorski J, A new method of physiological investigation of recent memory in animals. Bull. Acad. Pol. Sci. 7; 115-117, 1959.

Kosslyn SM, *Image and Brain.* Cambridge, MA: MIT Press, 1996.

Kreindler A, Macovei M, Cardaş M, Dănăilă L, *Mutismul akinetic. Consideraţii anatomo-clinice.* St. Cert. Neurol. 11; 349-360, 1966.

Krynaw RA, Infantile hemiplegia treated by removing one's cerebral hemisphere. J Neurol Neurosurg Psychiatr. 13; 243-267, 1950.

Kuhl PK, Language, mind, and brain. Experience alters perception. In: MS Gazzaniga (ed), *The New Cognitive Neuroscience* (2nd ed), Cambridge, MA: MIT Press, 2000.

Kulynych JJ, Vladar K, Jones DW, Weinberger DR, Gender differences in the normal lateralization of the supratemporal cortex: MRI surface-rendering morphometry of Heschl's gyrus and planum temporale. Cerebral Cortex 4; 107-118, 1994.

Kushch A, Gross-Glenn K, Jallad B et al., Temporal lobe surface area measurements on MRI in normal and dyslexic readers. Neuropsychologia 31; 811-821, 1993.

Kussmaul A, *Die Stoerungen der Sprache.* Leipzig: Vogel, 1876.

Ladavas E, del Pesce M, Provinciali L, Unilateral attention deficits and hemispheric asymmetries. Neuropsychologia 27; 353-366, 1989.

Landis T, Regard M, Graves R, Goodglass H, Semantic paralexia: A release of right hemispheric from left hemispheric control? Neuropsychologia 21; 359-364, 1983.

Landis T, Regard M, The right hemisphere's access to lexical meaning: A function of its release from left-hemisphere control? In: Chiarello (ed). *Right Hemisphere Contribution to Lexical Semantics.* New York: Springer-Verlag, 1988.

Lange J, Fingernosie und Agraphie. Monatsschrift fuer Psychiatrie und Neurologie 76; 129-188, 1930.

Lapierre D, Braun CM, Hodgins S, Ventral frontal deficits in psychopathy: neuropsychological test findings. Neuropsychologia 33; 139-151, 1995.

Lashley KS, Studies of Cerebral Function in Learning. II. The Effects of Long Continued Practice Upon Cerebral Localization. Journal of Comparative Psychology 6; 453-468, 1921.

Lassek AM, The human pyramidal tract. II. A numerical investigation of the Betz cells of the motor area. Arch Neurol and Psychiatr. 44; 718-724, 1940.

Lassek AM, *The Pyramidal Tract: Its Status in Medicine.* Charles C Thomas, Publisher, Springfield, Ill; 166, 1954.

Le Doux J, *The Emotional Brain. The Mysterious Underpinning of Emotional Life.* New York: Simon and Schuster, 1996.

Le Doux JE, Gazzaniga MS, *The Integrated Mind.* New York, Plenum Press, 1978.

Le May M, Asymmetries of the skull and handedness: Phrenology revisited. Journal of Neurological Sciences 32; 243-253, 1977.

Le May M, Kido DK, Asymmetries of the cerebral hemispheres on computed tomograms. Journal of Computer Assisted Tomography 2; 471-476, 1978.

Lecours AR, Lhermitte F, *L'Aphasic.* Paris, Flammarion, 1970.

Lee GP, Meador KJ, Smith JR, et al., Preserved cross modal association following bilateral amygdalotomy in man. International Journal of Neuroscience 40; 47-55, 1988.

Lee GP, Loring DW, Thompson JL, Construct validity of material specific memory measures following unilateral temporal lobe ablations. Psychological Assessment 1; 192-197, 1989.

Lee GP, Loring DW, Meador KJ, Brooks BB, Hemispheric specialization for emotional expression: A reexamination of results from intracarotid administration of sodium amobarbital. Brain and Cognition 12; 267-280, 1990.

Lee AC, Rubins TW, Pickard JD, Owen AM, Asymmetric frontal activation during episodic memory: The effects of stimulus type on encoding and retrieval. Neuropsychologia 38; 677-692, 2000.

Levin PM, Bradford FK, The exact origin of the corticospinal tract in the monkey. J Comp Neurol 68; 411-422, 1938.

Levin M, Aggression, guilt, and cataplexy. Arch Neurol Psychiat 69; 224-235, 1953.

Levine SC, Individual differences in characteristics arousal asymmetry: Implications for cognitive functioning. In: FL Kitterle (ed). *Hemispheric Communication: Mechanisms and Models.* Hillsdale NJ, Erlbaum, 1995.

Levy J, Possible basis for the evolution of lateral specialization of the human brain. Nature 224; 164-165, 1969.

Levy J, Language, cognition, and the right hemisphere. A response to Gazzaniga. American Psychologist 38; 538-541, 1983.

Levy J, Trevarthen CB, Sperry RW, Perception of bilateral chimeric figures following hemispheric deconnection. Brain 95; 61-78, 1972.

Lewin J, Friedman L, Wu D, et al., Cortical localization of human sustained attention: Detection with functional MR using a visual vigilance paradigm. Journal of computer Assisted Tomography 20; 695-701, 1996.

Lewinsohn PM, Zieler RE, Libet J, et al., Short term memory: comparison between frontal and nonfrontal right- and left-hemisphere brain damage patients. J Comp. Psychol 81; 248-255, 1972.

Ley RG, Bryden MP, A dissociation of right and left hemispheric effects for recognizing emotional tone and verbal content. Brain and Cognition 1; 3-9, 1982.

Lezak MD, Domains of behavior from a neuropsychological perspective: The whole story. In: W Spaulding (ed), *41st Nebraska Symposium on Motivation, 1992-1993*. Lincoln: University of Nebraska Press, 1994.

Lezak MD, Newman SP, Verbosity and right hemisphere damage. Paper presented in the 2nd European Meeting of the International Neuropsychological Society Noordvijkerhout, Holland, 1979.

Lezak MD, Howieson DB, Loring DW, *Neuropsychological Assessment*. Forth Edition. Oxford University Press, Oxford, 76-77, 2004.

Lezak MD, Howieson DB, Loring DW, *Neuropsychological assessment*. Fourth Edition. Oxford University Press, 30-33, 2004.

Lezak MD, Howieson DB, Loring DW, The behavioral geography of the brain. In: MD Lezak, DB Howieson, DW Loring (eds) *Neuropsychological Assessment*. Fourth Edition. Oxford University Press, New York, 39-85, 2004.

Lhermitte J, Le lobe frontal. L'encéphale 24; 87-118, 1929.

Lhermitte F, Pillon B, Serdaru M, Human autonomy and the frontal lobes. Part I: Imitation and utilization behavior: a neuropsychological study of 75 patients. Ann Neurol 19; 236-334, 1986.

Liepmann H, Das Krankheitsbild der Apraxie. Mschr. Psychiat. Neurol 8; 15-44, 102-132, 182-197, 1900.

Liepmann H, Apraxia. Erbgn der ges Med 1; 516-543, 1920.

Liepmann H, Mass O, Fall von linksseitiger agraphie und apraxie bei techtsseitiger lahmung. Journal für Psychologie und Neurologie 10; 214-227, 1907.

Loring DW, Meador KJ, Neuropsychological aspects of temporal lobe epilepsy surgery. In: TE Feinberg and MJ Farah (eds), *Behavioral Neurology and Neuropsychiatry* (2nd ed), New York: McGraw-Hill, 2003.

Luck SJ, Hillyard SA, Mangun GR, Gazzaniga MS, Independent hemispheric attentional systems mediate visual search in split-brain patients. Nature 342; 543-545, 1989.

Luria AR, The frontal lobes and the regulation of behavior. In: KH Pribram and AR Luria (eds), *Psychology of the Frontal Lobes*. New York, Academic Press, 1973.

Luria AR, *Traumatic Aphasia*. The Hague: Mouton, 1970.

Luria AR, *The Working Brain*. Harmondworth, England, Penguin, 1973.

Lynn R, Sex differences in intelligence and brain size: A paradox resolved. Personality and Individual Differences 17; 257-271, 1994.

Mac Coby E, Jacklin C, *The psychology of Sex Differences*. Stanford, Calif: Stanford University Press, 1974.

Mac Hale SM, O'Rourke SJ, Wardlaw JM, Dennis MS, Depression and its relation to lesion location after stroke. Journal of Neurology, Neurosurgery, and Psychiatry 64; 371-374, 1998.

Mach E, *The Analysis of Sensations, and the Relation of the Physical to the Psychical*, 1st German edition, 1885.

MacNeilage P, The evolution of hemispheric specialization for manual function and language. In: SP Wise (ed.), *Higher Brain Functions*. New York: Wiley, 1987.

MacNeilage PF, Studdert-Kennedy MG, Lindblom B, Primate handedness reconsidered. The Behavioral and Brain Sciences 10; 247-263, 1987.

MacNeilage PF, Studdert-Kennedy MG, Lindblom B, Primate handedness: A foot in the door. The Behavioral and Brain Sciences, 11; 737-744, 1988.

Majeres RL, Sex differences in symbol-digit substitution and speeded matching. Intelligence 7; 313-327, 1983.

Malloy PF, Bihrale A, Duffy J, Cimino C, The orbitomedial frontal syndrome. Archives of Clinical Neuropsychology 8; 185-201, 1993.

Mangun GR, Luck SJ, Plager R, Loftus W, et al., Monitoring the visual world: Hemispheric asymmetries and subcortical processes in attention. Journal of Cognitive Neuroscience, 6; 267-275, 1994.

Mann L, Casuistische Betrage zur Hirnschirurgie und Hirnlokalisation. Mschr. Psychiat. Neurol. 4; 369, 1898.

Markowitsch HJ, Calabrese P, Wurker M, et al., The amygdala's contribution to memory – a study on two patients with Urbach-Wiethe disease. Neuroreport 5; 1349-1352, 1994.

Marlowe WB, Mancall EL, Thomas JJ, Complete Kluver-Bucy syndrome in man. Cortex 11; 53, 1975.

Marshuetz C, Order information in working memory: an integrative review of evidence from brain and behavior. Psychol Bull 131; 323-339, 2005.

Martin A, Wiggs CL, Weisberg J, Modulation of human medial temporal lobe activity by form, meaning, and experience. Hippocampus 7; 587-593, 1997.

Martinez BA, Cain WS, de Wiji RA et al., Olfactory functioning before and after temporal lobe resection for intractable seizures. Neuropsychology 7; 351-363, 1993.

Masdeu JC, Schoene WC, Funkenstein H, Aphasia following infarction of the left supplementary motor area: A clinicopathological study. Neurology 28; 1220-1223, 1978.

Matelli M, Luppino G, Rizzolatti G, Patterns of cytochrome oxidase activity in the frontal agranular cortex of the macaque monkey. Behavioral Brain research 18; 125-136, 1985.

Mazziota JC, Toga A, Evans P, et al., Brain maps: Linking the present to the future: In: RSJ Franckowiak et al. (eds.), *Human Brain Function*. San Diego, Academic Press, 1997.

Mc Carthy RA, Warrington EK, *Cognitive Neuropsychology: A Clinical Introduction*. San Diego: Academic Press, 1990.

Mc Carthy G, Blamire AM, Rothman DL, et al., Echo-planar magnetic resonance imaging studies of frontal cortex activation during word generation in humans. Proceedings of the National Academy of Sciences of the United States of America 90; 4952-4956, 1993.

Mc Dermott KB, Ojemann JG, Petersen SE, et al., Direct comparison of episodic encoding and retrieval of words: An event-related fMRI study. Memory 7; 661-678, 1999.

Mc Glynn, Schacter DL, Unawareness of deficit in neuropsychological syndrome. Journal of Clinical and Experimental Neuropsychology 11; 143-205, 1989.

McGlone J, Sex differences in the cerebral organization of verbal functions in patients with unilateral brain lesions. Brain 100; 775-793, 1977.

McGlone J, Sex differences in human brain asymmetry: a critical survey. Behavioural and Brain Sciences 3; 215-27, 1980.

Meador KJ, Watson RT, Bowers D, Heilman KM, Hypometria with hemispatial and limbic motor neglect. Brain 109; 293-305, 1986.

Meador KJ, Loring DW, Lee GP, et al., Right cerebral specialization for tactile attention as evidenced by intracarotid sodium amytal. Neurological 38; 1763-1766, 1988.

Meador KJ, Loring DW, Ray PG, et al., Differential cognitive effects of carbamezepine and gabapentin. Epilepsia 40; 1279-1285, 1999.

Meador KJ, Loring DW, Feinberg TE, et al., Anosognosia and asomatognosia during intracarotid amobarbital inactivation. Neurology 55; 816-820, 2000.

Mehta Z, Newcombe F, Dissociable contributions of the two cerebral hemispheres to judgments of line orientation. Journal of the International Neuropsychological Society 2; 335-339, 1996.

Mehta Z, Newcombe F, Ratecliff G, Patterns of hemispheric asymmetry set against clinical evidence. In JR Crawford and DM Parker (eds). *Developments in Clinical and Experimental Neuropsychology*. New York, Plenum Press, 1989.

Mesulam MM, From sensation to cognition. Brain 121; 1913-1952, 1998.

Mesulam MM, Aging, Alzheimer's disease, and dementia. Clinical and neurobiological perspectives. In MM Mesulam (ed). *Principles of Behavioral and Cognitive Neurology* (2nd ed). New York: Oxford University Press, 2000.

Metter EJ, Brain-behavior relationship in aphasia studied by positron emission tomography. Annals of the New York Academy of Science 620; 153-164, 1991.

Middleton FA, Strick PL, Basal ganglia output and cognition: Evidence from anatomical, behavioral, and clinical studies. Brain and Cognition 42; 183-200, 2000.

Miller L, Milner B, Cognitive risk-taking after frontal or temporal lobectomy – II. Neuropsychologia 23; 371-379, 1985.

Milles CK, Mc Connell JW, The naming centre, with the report of a case indicating its location in the temporal lobe. J. Nerv. Ment. Dis. 22; 1-7, 1895.

Milner B, Some effects of frontal lobectomy in man. In: JM Waren and K Akert (eds), *The Frontal Granular Cortex and Behavior*. New York, NY: McGraw-Hill, 313-334, 1964.

Milner B, Visual recognition and recall after right temporal lobe excision in man. Neuropsychologia 6; 191-209, 1968.

Milner B, Memory and the medial temporal regions of the brain. In: KH Pribram and DE Broadlent (eds). *Biology of memory* New York: Academic Press, 1970.

Milner B, Interhemispheric differences in the localization of psychological processes in man. Br Med. Bull 27; 272-277, 1971.

Milner B, Disorders of learning and memory after temporal lobe lesions in man. Clinical Neurosurgery 19; 421-446, 1972.

Milner B, Some cognitive effects of frontal lobe lesions in man. Phil Trans R Soc Lond B 298; 211-226, 1982.

Milner B, Aspects of human frontal lobe function. Advances in Neurology 66; 67-81, 1995.

Milner B, and Teuber HL, Alteration of perception and memory in man: reflections on methods. In: L Weiskrantz (ed), *Analysis of Behavioral Change*. New York, NY: Harper and Row; 268-275, 1968.

Milner B, Taylor L, Right hemisphere superiority in tactile pattern recognition after cerebral comissurotomy. Neuropsychologia 10; 1-15, 1972.

Milner B, Petrides M, Behavioral effects of frontal-lobe lesions in man. Journal of Neuroscience 7; 403-407, 1984.

Milner AD, Goodale MA, *The visual brain in action.* New York: Oxford University Press, 1995.

Milner B, Petrides M, Smith ML, Frontal lobes and the temporal organization of memory. Human Neurobiol 4; 137-142, 1985.

Milner B, Carey DP, Harvey M, Visuality guided action and the "need to know". Behavioral and Brain Sciences 17; 213-214, 1994.

Milles CK, Mc Connell JW, The naming centre, with the report of a case indicating its location in the temporal lobe. J. Nerv. Ment. Dis. 22; 1-7, 1895.

Mirsky AF, The neuropsychology of attention: Elements of a complex behavior. In: E Perecman (ed), *Integrating theory and practice in clinical neuropsychology.* Hillsdale NJ, Erbaum, 1989.

Mohr JP, Pessin MS, Finkelstein S, et al., Broca aphasia: Pathologic and clinical. Neurology 28; 311-324, 1978.

Molfese DL, Molfese VJ, Right hemisphere responses from preschool children to temporal cues contained in speech and nonspeech materials: Electrophysiological correlates. Brain and Language 33; 245-259, 1988.

Monrad-Krohn GH, Dysprosody or attention in "melody of language". Brain 70; 405-415, 1947.

Montreys CR, Borod JC, A preliminary evaluation of emotional experience and expression following unilateral brain damage. International Journal of Science 96; 269-283, 1998.

Moreno CR, Borod JC, Welkowitz I, Alpert M, Lateralization for the expression and perception of facial emotion as a function of age. Neuropsychologia 28; 199-209, 1990.

Morgan M, Embryology and inheritance of asymmetry. In: S Harnad, RW Doty, L Goldstein, J Jaynes, G Krauthamer (Eds.), *Lateralization in the Nervous System.* New York, Academic Press, 1977.

Mori E, Yamadori A, Rejection behavior: A human analogue of the abnormal behavior of Denny-Brown and Chambers' monkey with bilateral parietal ablation. J. Neurol Neurosurg Psychiatry 52; 1260, 1989.

Morris RG, Abrahams S, Polkey CE, Recognition memory for words and faces following unilateral temporal lobectomy. British Journal of Clinical Psychology 34; 571-576, 1995.

Morrow LA, Vertunski PB, Kim Y, Boller F, Arousal responses to emotional stimuli and laterality of lesions. Neuropsychologia 19; 65-71, 1981.

Moscovitch M, The development of lateralization of language functions and its relation to cognitive and linguistic development: A review and some theoretical speculations. In: SJ Segalowitz and FA Gruber (eds). *Language Development and Neurological Theory*. New York: Academic Press, 1977.

Mottaghy FM, Gangitano M, Sparing R, et al., Segregation of areas related to visual working memory in the prefrontal cortex revealed by rTMS. Cerebral Cortex 12; 369-375, 2002.

Muakkassa KF and Strick PL, Frontal lobe inputs to primate motor cortex: evidence for four somatotopically organized "premotor" areas. Brain Res. 177; 176-182, 1979.

Müller NG, Knight RT, The functional neuroanatomy of working memory: contributions of human brain lesion studies. Neuroscience 139; 51-58, 2006.

Müller NG, Machado L, Knight RT, Contributions of subregions of the prefrontal cortex to working memory: evidence from brain lesions in humans. J Cogn Neurosci 14; 673-686, 2002.

Murdoch GE, *Acquired speech and language disorders: A neuroanatomical and functional neurological approach.* New York: Chapman and Hall, 1990.

Murphy DG, DeCarli C, McIntosh AR, et al., Sex differences in human brain morphometry and metabolism: an in vivo quantitative magnetic resonance imaging and positron emission tomography study on the effect of aging. Archives of General Psychiatry 53; 585-598, 1996.

Murphy K, Peters M, Right-handers and left-handers show differences and important similarities in task integration when performing manual and vocal tasks concurrently. Neuropsychologia 32; 663-674, 1994.

Nauta WJH, Some brain structures and functions related to memory. Neurosciences Research Progress Bulletin II; 1-20, 1964.

Netley C, Dichotic listening of callosal agenesis and Turner's syndrome patients. In: SJ Segalowitz and FA Gruber (eds), *Language Development and Neurological Theory*, New York, Academic Press, 376, 1977.

Neville H, Electroencephalographs testing of cerebral specialization in normal and congenitally deaf children: A preliminary report. In: Segalowitz SJ, Gruber FA (eds) *Language development and neurological theory*. New York, Acad. Press, 122-134, 1977.

Nichelli P, Grafman J, Pietrini P, et al., Where the brain appreciates the moral of a story. Neuro Report 6; 2309-2313, 1995.

Nielsen JM, Jacobs LL, Bilateral lesions of the anterior cingulate gyri: report of case. Bull LA Neurol Soc 16; 231-234, 1951.

Nilsson LG, Nyberg L, Klingberg T, et. al., Activity in motor areas while remembering action events. Neuroreport 11; 2199-2201, 2000.

Nothnagel H, Experimentelle Untersuchungen über die Funktionen DES Gehirns. Archiv für pathologische Anatomie und Physiologie und für Clinische Medizin 57; 184-214, 1873.

Nottebohm F, Origins and mechanisms in the establishment of cerebral dominance. In: MS Gazzaniga (ed), *Handbook of Behavioral Neurobiology*. Neuropsychology (Vol. 2). New York: Plenum Press, 1979.

Nottebohm F, Brain pathways for vocal learning in birds: a review of the first 10 years, Prog. Psychobiol. Physiol. Psychol. 9; 85-124, 1981.

Novelly RA, Augustine EA, Mattson RH, et al., Selective memory improvement and impairment in temporal lobectomy for epilepsy. Annals of Neurology 15; 64-67, 1984.

Obler LK, Zatorre RJ, Galloway L, Vaid J, Cerebral lateralization in bilinguals: methodological issues. Brain and Language 15; 40-54, 1982.

Ochipa C, Rothi LJG, Heilman KM, Ideational apraxia: A deficit in tool selection and use Ann Neurol 25; 190-193, 1989.

Ochipa C, Rothi LJG, Heilman KM, Conceptual apraxia in Alzheimer's disease. Brain 114; 2593-2603, 1992.

Ojemann GA, Organization of short-term verbal memory in language areas of human cortex: Evidence from electrical stimulation. Brain and Language 5; 331-340, 1978.

Ojemann GA, Individual variability in cortical localization of language. Journal of Neurosurgery 50; 164-169, 1979.

Ojemann GA, Mateer C, Human language cortex: Localization of memory, syntax, and sequential motor-phoneme identification systems. Science 205; 1401-1403, 1979.

Ornstein R, Herron J, Johnstone J, Swencionis C, Differential right hemisphere involvement in two reading tasks. Psychology 16; 398-401, 1979.

Oppenheim H, *Lehrbuch der Nervenkrankheiten für Aerzte und Studirende*, II Aufl, Berlin, Karger, 1898.

Oppenheim H, Zur Pathologie der Gehirngeschwulste. Archiv für Psychiatrie 21; 560-578, 1890.

Oscar-Berman M, McNamara P, Freedman M, Delayed-response tasks: Parallels between experimental ablation studies and findings in patients with frontal lesions. In: HS Levin, HM Eisenberg and AL Benton (eds), *Frontal Lobe Function and Dysfunction*. New York, NY: Oxford University Press, 230-255, 1991.

Owen AM, Evans AC, Petrides M, Evidence for a two stage model of spatial working memory processing within the lateral frontal cortex: A positron emission tomography study. Cerebral Cortex 6; 31-38, 1996.

Paillard J, Michel F, Stelmach G, Localization without content: A tactile analogue of "blindsight". Archives of Neurology 40, 548-551, 1983.

Pakkenberg B, Gundersen HJ, Neocortical neuron number in humans: effect of sex and age. J Comp Neurol. 384; 312-320, 1997.

Pandya DN, Barnes CL, Architecture and connections of the frontal lobe. In: Perecman E, *The Frontal Lobes Revised*. New York: IRBN Press, 1987.

Pandya DN, Yeterian EH, Comparison of prefrontal architecture and connections. In: Roberts AC, Robbins TW, Weiskrantz L, (eds) *The Prefrontal Cortex. Executive and Cognitive Functions*. New York: Oxford University Press, 1998.

Panksepp J, *Affective Neuroscience: The Foundation of Human and Animal Emotions*. Oxford Univ. Press, New York, 1998.

Papanicolaou AC, Moore BD, Deutsch G, et al., Evidence for right-hemisphere involvement in recovery from aphasia. Archives of Neurology 45; 1025-1029, 1988.

Papcun G, Krashen D, Terbeek R, et al., Is the left hemisphere organized for speech, language and / or something else? Journal of the Acoustical Society of America 55; 319-327, 1974.

Papez JW, A proposed mechanism of emotion. Arch Neurol Psychiatry 38; 725-743, 1937.

Paradiso S, Robinson RG, Gender differences in post-stroke depression. Journal of Neuro-psychiatry and Clinical Neuroscience 10; 41-47, 1998.

Pardo JV, Fox PT, Raichle ME, Localization of a human system for sustained attention by positron emission tomography. Nature 34; 61-64, 1991.

Pardo JV, Pardo TP, Raichle ME, Natural correlates of self-induced dysphoria. American Journal of Psychiatry 150; 713-719, 1993.

Pascual-Leone A, Dang N, Cohen LG, et al., Modulation of muscle responses evoked by transcranial magnetic stimulation during the acquisition of new fine motor skills. J. Neurophysiol 74; 1037-1045, 1995.

Pascual-Leone A, Catala MD, Pascual-Leone P, Lateralized effect of rapid-rate transcranial magnetic stimulation of the prefrontal cortex on mood. Neurology 46; 499-502, 1996.

Passingham RE, *The Frontal Lobes and Voluntary Action*. New York: Oxford University Press, 1993.

Passingham R, Functional organization of the motor system. In: RSJ Franckowiak et al. (eds), *Human Brain Function*. San Diego: Academic Press, 1997.

Paulescu E, Frith CD, Franckowiak RS, The neural correlates of the verbal component of working memory. Nature 362; 342-345, 1993.

Paus M, Kunesch E, Bincofski F, et al., Sensorimotor disturbances in patients with lesions of the parietal cortex. Brain 112; 159, 1989.

Paus T, Petrides M, Evans A, Meyer E, Role of the human anterior cingulate cortex in the control oculomotor, manual, and speech responses. A positron emission tomography study. Neurophysiology 70; 453-469, 1993.

Paus T, Otaky N, Caramanos Z, et al., In vivo morphometry of the intrasulcal gray matter in the human cingulate, paracingulate, and superior-rostral sulci: Hemispheric asymmetries, gender differences and probability maps. Journal of Comparative Neurology 376; 664-673, 1996.

Paus T, Tomaiuola F, Otaki N, et al., Human cingulate and paracingulate sulci: Pattern, variability, asymmetry, and probabilistic map. Cerebral Cortex 6; 207-214, 1996.

Pelet S, Gudbjartsson H, Westin CF, Kikinis R, Jolesz FA, Magnetic resonance imaging shows orientation and asymmetry of white matter fiber tracts. Brain Research 780; 27-33, 1998.

Penfield W, Functional localization in temporal and deep sylvian areas. Research Publication, Association for Nervous and Mental Disease 36; 210-227, 1958.

Penfield W, Welch K, The supplementary motor area of the cerebral cortex. A clinical and experimental study. Neurol and Psychiat 66; 289-317, 1951.

Penfield W, Boldrey E, Somatic motor and sensory representation in the cerebral cortex as studied by electrical stimulation. Brain 60; 389-443, 1958.

Penfield W, Roberts L, *Speech and Brain Mechanisms*. Princeton, NY: Princeton University Press, 1959.

Perry DW, Zatorre RJ, Petrides M, et al., Localization of cerebral activity during simple singing. Neuroreport 10; 3453-3458, 1999.

Petersen Jr SE, Fox PT, Posner MI, et al., Positron emission tomographic studies of the cortical anatomy of single-word processing. Nature 331; 585-589, 1988.

Petersen MR, Beecher MD, Zoloth SR, et al., Neural lateralization of species-specific vocalizations by Japanese macaques (Macaca fuscata). Science 202; 324-327, 1978.

Petrides M, Frontal lobes and working memory: evidence from investigations of the effects of cortical excitations in nonhuman primates. In: F Boller and J. Grafman (eds), *Handbook of Neuropsychology* (Vol. 9). Amsterdam: Elsevier, Handbook Neuropsychol, 59-82, 1994.

Petrides M, Alivisatos B, Mayer E, Evans AC, Functional activation of the human frontal cortex during the performance of verbal working memory tasks. Proceedings of the National Academy of Sciences of the United States of America 90; 878-882, 1993.

Petrides M, Deficits on conditional associative-learning tasks after frontal- and temporal-lobe lesions in man. Neuropsychologia 23; 601-614, 1985.

Picard N, Strick PL, Motor areas of the medial wall. A review of their localization and functional activation. Cerebral Cortex 6; 342-353, 1996.

Pick A, *Über Störungen der Orientierung am einigen Körper*. Berlin, Karger, 1908.

Pierrot-Deseilligny C, Rivaud S, Gaymard B, Agid Y, Corectal control of memory-guided saccades in man. Exp Brain Res 83; 607-617, 1991.

Pietrini P, Guazzelli M, Gasso G, et al., Neural correlates of imaginal aggressive behavior assessed by positron emission tomography in healthy subjects. American Journal of Psychiatry 157; 1772-1781, 2000.

Pilcher WH, Ojemann GA, Presurgical evaluation and epilepsy surgery. In: Apuzzo MLJ (ed) *Brain Surgery: Complications, Avoidance and Management*. New York, Raven Press, 417-424, 1993.

Pillieri G, The Kluver-Bucy syndrome in man. Psychiatr, Neurol 152; 65, 1967.

Pillon B, Bazin B, Deweer B, et al., Specificity of memory deficits after right or left temporal lobectomy. Cortex 35; 561-571, 1999.

Pimental PA, Kingsbury NA, The injured right hemisphere: Classification of related disorders. In: *Neuropsychological aspects of right brain injury*. Austin TX: Pro-Ed, 1989.

Pincus JH, Tucker GJ, *Behavioral Neurology* (4th ed). New York: Oxford University Press, 2003.

Pizzamiglio L, Mammucari A, Disturbance of facial emotional expression in brain-damaged subjects. In: G Gainotti and C Caltagirone (eds), *Emotions and the Dual Brain.* Berlin: Springer-Verlag, 1989.

Ploner CJ, Rivaud-Pechoux S, Gaymard BM, et al., Errors of memory-guided saccades in humans with lesions of the frontal eye field and the dorsolateral prefrontal cortex. J. Neuropsychol 82; 1986-1090, 1999.

Poizner H, Bellugi U, Klima ES, Biological foundations of language. Clue from sign language. annual Review in Neuroscience 13; 283-307, 1990.Poppel D, Some remaining questions about studying phonological processing with PET: Response to Demonet, Fiez, Paulescu, Patersen, and Zatorre. Brain and Language 55; 380-385, 1996.

Posner MI, Dehaene S, Attentional networks. Trend in Neuroscience 2; 75-79, 1994.

Posner MI, Hierarchical distributed networks in the neuropsychology of selective attention. In: Caramazza (ed), *Cognitive Neuropsychology and Neurolinguistics: Advances in Models of Cognitive Function and Impairment*. Hillsdale, NJ, Erlbaum, 1990.

Pötzl O, Uiberall H, Zur Pathologie der Amusie. Wiener Klin Wschr 50; 770, 1937.

Pötzl O, Zur Pathologie der Amusie. Z. Neurol. Psychiat. 165; 187, 1939.

Pötzl O, Bemerkungen zum Problem der Kortikalen Vorgänge bei der akustisken Wahrnehmung. Mschr. Ohrenhlk 77; 422, 1943.

Prather P, Jarmulowicz L, Barwnell H, Gardner H, Selective attention and the right hemisphere: A failure in integration, not detection (abstract). Journal of clinical and Experimental Neuropsychology 14, 35, 1992.

Preuss TM, Caceres M, Oldham MC, Geschwind DH, Human brain evolution: Insight from microscopy. Nature Reviews: Genetics 5; 850-860, 2004.

Price CJ, Functional anatomy of reading. In: RSJ Franckowiak et al., (eds), *Human Brain Function.* San Diego: Academic Press, 1997.

Prigatano GP, Personality and psychosocial consequences after brain injury. In: MJ Meier et al. (eds) *Neuropsychological Rehabilitation.* Edinburgh: Churchill Livingstone, 1987.

Proust A, Arch Gen Méd. Cited by Ballet (1866) and Henschen (1920).

Proust A, *De l'Aphasie*. Arch. Gen. Méd. 1, 147, 1872.

Provins KA, Handedness and speech: A critical reappraisal of the role of genetic and environmental factors in the cerebral lateralization of function. Psycholo Rev 104; 554-571, 1997.

Ptito A, Crane J, Leonard G, et al, Visual-spatial localization by patients with frontal lobe lesions invading or sparing area 46. NeuroReport 6; 1781-1784, 1995.

Pugh KR, Shaywitz BA, Shaywitz SE, et al. Cerebral organization of component processes in reading. Brain 119; 1221-1238, 1996.

Raichle ME, Fiez JA, Videen TO et al., Practice-related changes in human brain functional anatomy during nonmotor learning. Cerebral Cortex 4; 8-26, 1994.

Rajkowska G, Goldman-Rakic P, Cytoarchitectonic definition of prefrontal areas in the normal human cortex: II. Variability in locations of areas 9 and 46 and relationship to the Talairach coordinate system. Cerebral Cortex 5; 323-337, 1995.

Rapport RL, Tan CT, Whitaker HA, Language function and dysfunction among Chinese- and English-speaking polyglots: cortical stimulation, Wada testing and clinical studies. Brain and Language 18; 342-366, 1983.

Rasmussen T, Surgery of frontal lobe epilepsy. In: Purpura DP, Penry JK, Walter RD, (eds) *Advances in Neurology*, Vol. 8. New York: Raven Press, 1975.

Rasmussen T, Commentary: Extratemporal cortical excisions and hemispherectomy. In: Engel J Jr (ed): *Surgical Treatment of the Epilepsies*. New York: Raven Press, 417-424, 1987.

Rasmussen T, Milner B, The role of early left-brain injury in determining lateralization of cerebral speech functions. Annals of the New York Academy of Science 299; 355-369, 1977.

Ratcliff G, Dila C, Taylor L, Milner B, The morphological asymmetry of the hemispheres and cerebral dominance for speech: A possible relationship. Brain and Language 11; 87-98, 1980.

Regard M, and Landis, The Procedure vs. content learning: effects of emotionality and repetition in a new clinical memory test (Abstract. Journal of Clinical and Experimental Neuro-psychology 10; 86, 1988.

Reite M, Sheeder J, Teale P, et al., MEG based brain laterality: sex differences in normal adults. Neuropsychologia 33; 1607-1617, 1995.

Rivers DL, Love RL, Language performance on visual processing tasks in right hemisphere lesion cases. Brain and Language 10; 348-366, 1980.

Rizzolatti G, Matelli M, Pavesi G, Deficits in attention and movement following the removal of postarcuate (area 6) and prearcuate (area 8) cortex in macaque monkeys. Brain 106; 655-673, 1983.

Rizzolatti G, Fadiga L, Matelli M, et al., Localization of grasp representations in humans by PET: 1. Observation *versus* execution. Experimental Brain Research 111; 246-252, 1996 a.

Rizzolatti G, Fadiga L, Gallese V, Fogassi L, Premotor cortex and the recognition of motor actions. Cognitive Brain Research 3; 131-141, 1996 b.

Robertson LC, Rafal R, Disorders of visual attention. In: Gazzaniga (ed), *The New Cognitive Neuroscience* (2nd ed), 633-649. Cambridge: MIT Press, 2000.

Robinson RG, Neuropsychiatric consequences of stroke. Ann Rev Med 48; 217-229, 1997.

Robinson RG, Manes F, Elation, mania, and mood disorders. Evidence from neurological disease. In: JC Borod (ed), *The Neuropsychology of Emotion*. New York: Oxford, University Press, 2000.

Robinson RG, Starkstein SE, Neuropsychiatric aspects of cerebrovascular disorders. In: SC Yudofsky and RE Hales (eds). *Essentials of Neuropsychiatry and Clinical Neurosciences*. Washington DC: American Psychiatric Press, 2002.

Robinson RG, Kubas KL, Starr LB, et al., Mood disorders in stroke patients : Importance of location of lesion. Brain 107; 81-93, 1984.

Rogers LJ, Early experimental effects on laterality: Research on chicks has relevance to other species. Laterality 2; 199-219, 1997.

Roland PE, Metabolic measurements of the working frontal cortex in man. Trends Neurosci. 7; 430-435, 1984.

Rolls ET, *The Brain and Emotion.* Oxford Univ. Press, New York, 1999.

Ross DA, Glick SD, Right-sided population bias and lateralization of activity in normal rats. Brain Res. 205; 222-225, 1981.

Rossor M, Fahrenkrug J, Emson P, et al., Reduced cortical choline acetyltransferase activity in senile dementia of Alzheimer type is not accompanied by changes in vasoactive intestinal polypeptide. Brain Res 201; 249-253, 1980.

Ross DA, Affective prosody and the aprosodias. In: MM Mesulam (ed), *Principles of Behavioral and Cognitive Neurology.* New York, Oxford University Press, 2000.

Ross ED, The aprosodias. In: TE Feinberg and MJ Farah (eds), *Behavioral Neurology and Neuropsychology* (2nd ed). New York: McGraw-Hill, 2003.

Ross ED, Mesulam MM, Dominant language functions of the right hemisphere? Prosody and emotional gesturing. Archives of Neurology 36; 144-148, 1979.

Ross ED, Rush AJ, Diagnosis and neuroanatomical correlates of depression in brain damaged patients. Archives of General Psychiatry 38; 1344-1354, 1981.

Rossion B, Dicot L, Devolder A, et al., Hemispheric asymmetries for whole-based and part-based face processing in the human fusiform gyrus. Journal of Cognitive Neuroscience 12; 793-802, 2000.

Ruckdeschel-Hibbard M, Gordon WA, Diller L, Affective disturbances associated with brain damage. In: SB Filskov and TJ Boll (eds), Handbook of clinical neuropsychology (Vol. 2). New York: Wiley, 1986.

Rudel RG, Denckla MB, Spalten E, The functional asymmetry of Braille letter learning in normal sighted children. Neurology 24; 733-738, 1974.

Sackeim HA, Gur RC, Saucy MC, Emotions are expressed more intensely on the left side of the face. Science 202; 434-436, 1978.

Sackeim HA, Greenberg MS, Weiman AL, et al., Hemisphere asymmetry in the expression of positive and negative emotions. Archives of Neurology 39; 210-218, 1982.

Salazar AM, Grafman J, Jabbari B, et al., Epilepsy and cognitive loss after penetrating head injury. Advances in Epidemiology 16; 627-631, 1987.

Salazar AM, Grafman J, Schlesselman S, et al., Penetrating war injuries of the basal forebrain: Neurology and Cognition. Neurology 36; 459-465, 1986.

Sass KJ, Buchanan CP, Kraemer S, et al., Verbal memory impairment resulting from hippocampal neuron loss among epileptic patients with structure lesions. Neurology 45; 2154-2158, 1995.

Sato R, Bryan RN, Fried LP, Neuroanatomic and functional correlates of depresses of depressed mood: The Cardiovascular Health Study. American Journal of Epidemiology 150; 919-929, 1999.

Scheibel AB, Paul LA, Fried J, et al., Dendritic organization of the anterior speech area. Experimental Neurobiology 87; 109-117, 1985.

Schilder P, *The Image and Appearance of the Human Body.* K Paul, London, 1935.

Schlaepfer TE, Harris GJ, Tien AY, et al., Structural differences in the cerebral cortex of healthy female and male subjects: A magnetic resonance imaging study. Psychiatry Research 61; 129-135, 1995.

Schluter ND, Krams M, Rushorth MF, Passingham RE, Cerebral dominance for action in the human brain: the selection of action. Neuropsychologia 39; 105-113, 2001.

Schramm J, Behrens E, Entzian W, Hemispherical deafferentation: An alternative to functional hemispherectomy. Neurosurgery 36; 509-516, 1995.

Schramm J, Kral T, Clusmann H, Transsylvian keyhole functional hemispherectomy. Neurosurgery 49; 891-901, 2001.

Schuster P, Taterka H, Beitrag zur Anatomie und Klinik der reinen worttaubheit. Z. Neurol Psychiat 105; 494, 1926.

Schwartz J, Tallal P, Rate of acoustic change may underlie hemispheric specialization for speech perception. Science 207; 1380-1381, 1980.

Searleman A, A review of right hemisphere linguistic capabilities. Psychological Bulletin 84; 503-528, 1977.

Seidenberg M, Hermann B, Wyler AR, et al., Neuropsychological outcome following anterior temporal lobectomy in patients with and without the syndrome of musical temporal lobe epilepsy. Neuropsychology 12; 303-316, 1998.

Seidenwurm D, Bird CR, Enzmann DR, Marshall WH, Left-right temporal region asymmetry in infants and children. AJNR 6; 777-779, 1985.

Semmes J, Weinstein L, Ghent L, Teuber HL, *Somatosensory changes after penetrating brain wounds in man*. Cambridge, MA, Harvard University Press, 1960.

Semmes J, Weinstein L, Ghent L, Teuber HL, Correlates of impaired orientation in personal and extrapersonal space. Brain 86; 747-772, 1963.

Semmes J, Turner B, Effects of cortical lesions on somatosensory task. Journal of Investigations in Dermatology 69; 181-189, 1977.

Sergent J, Unified response to bilateral hemispheric stimulation by a split-brain patient. Nature 305; 800-802, 1983.

Sergent J, Inferences from unilateral brain damage about normal hemispheric functions in visual pattern recognition. Psychological Bulletin 96; 99-115, 1984.

Sergent J, Face perception and the right hemisphere. In: L Weiskrantz (ed), *Through without Language*. Oxford Clarendon Press, 1988.

Sergent J, Furtive incursions into bicameral minds. Brain 113; 537-568, 1990.

Sergent J, Processing of spatial relations within and between the disconnected cerebral hemispheres. Brain 114; 1025-1043, 1991.

Sergent J, Judgment of relative position and distance on representations of spatial relations. Journal of Exp. Psychol: Human Perception and Performance 91; 762-780, 1991.

Seymour SE, Reuter-Lorenz PA, Gazzaniga MS, The disconnection syndrome: Basic findings reaffirmed. Brain 117; 105-115, 1994.

Shapiro BE, Danly M, The role of the right hemisphere in the control of speech prosody in positional and affective contents. Brain and Language 25; 19-36, 1985.

Shapiro BE, Grossman M, Gardner H, Selective musical processing deficits in brain damage populations. Neuropsychologia 19; 161-169, 1981.

Shaywitz BA, Shaywitz SE, Pugh KR, et al., Sex differences in the functional organization of the brain for language. Nature 373; 607-609, 1995.

Shepherd GM, and Green CA, Olfactory bulb. In: GM, Shepherd (ed), *The Synaptic Organization of the Brain* (4th ed). New York: Oxford University Press, 1998.

Shimamura AP, Janowsky JS, Squire LR, Memory for the temporal order of events in patients with frontal lobe lesions and amnestic patients. Neuropsychologia 28; 803-813, 1990.

Shimizu T, Nariai T, Maehara T, et al., Enhanced motor cortical excitability in the unaffected hemisphere after hemispherectomy. Neuroreport 11; 3077-3084, 2000.

Shimoda K, Robinson RG, The relationship between poststroke depression and lesion location on long-term follow-up. Radiological Psychiatry 45; 187-192, 1999.

Simonds RJ, Scheibel AB, The postnatal development of the motor speech area: A preliminary study. Brain and Language 37; 42-58, 1989.

Singh A, Blake SE, Herrman N, et al., Functional and neuroanatomic correlation in poststroke depression. The Sunnybrook Stroke study. Stroke 31; 637-644, 2000.

Smith EE, Jonides J, Koeppe RA, Dissociating verbal and spatial working memory using PET. Cortex Cerebral 6; 11-20, 1996.

Smith ML, Memory disorders associated with temporal-lobe lesions. In: F. Boller and J Grafman (eds). *Handbook of Neuropsychology,* Vol. 3, Amsterdam, Elsevier, 1989.

Smith WK, The functional significance of the rostral cingular cortex by its response to electrical excitation. J Neurophisiol 8; 241-255, 1945.

Sowell ER, Trauner DA, Gamst A, Jernigan TL, Development of cortical and subcortical brain structures in childhood and adolescence: a structural MRI study. Dev. Med. Child. Neurol. 44; 4-16, 2002 a.

Sowell ER, Thompson PM, Rex D, et al., Mapping sulcal pattern asymmetry and local cortical surface gray matter distribution in vivo: maturation in perisylvian cortices. Cerebral Cortex 12; 17-26, 2002 b.

Sperry RW, Consciousness, personal identity and the divided brain. In: Lepore, F, Ptito, M., and Jasper, H (Eds), *Two Hemispheres: One Brain.* New York, Alen Liss; 3-20, 1986.

Spreen O, Benton AL., and Fincham RW, Auditory agnosia without aphasia. Arch. Neurol. 13, 84, 1965.

Springer SP, Deutch G, *Left Brain, Right brain.* Freeman, New York, 1995

Springer SP, Deutsch G, *Left Brain / Right Brain; Perceptives from Cognitive Neuroscience.* Freeman, New York 1998.

St. John RC, Lateral asymmetry in face perception. Can J, Psychol 35; 213-223, 1981.

Starkstein SE, Bryer JB, Bethier ML, et al., Depression after stroke: The importance of cerebral hemisphere asymmetries. Journal of Neuropsychiatry and Clinical Neurosciences 3; 276-285, 1991.

Starkstein SE, Federoff JP, Price TR, et al., Neuropsychological and neuroradiologic correlates of emotional prosody comprehension. Neurology 44; 515-522, 1994.

Starkstein SE, Robinson RG, Mechanism of disinhibition after brain lesions. Journal of Nervous and Mental Diseases 185, 108-114, 1997.

Starkstein SE, Pearlson GD, Boston J, Robinson RG, Mania after brain injury: A controlled study of causative factors. Archives of Neurology 44; 1069-1973, 1987.

Starkstein SE, Robinson RG, Honing MA, et al., Mood changes after right-hemisphere lesions. British Journal of Psychiatry 155; 79-85, 1989.

Stelmach GE, Motor learning: Toward understanding acquired representations. In: JR Bloedel, TJ Ebner and SP Wise (eds), *The Acquisition of Motor Behavior in Vertebrates.* Cambridge, MA: MIT Press, 391-408, 1996.

Stemmer B, Joanette Y, The interpretation of narrative discourse of brain-damaged individuals within the framework of multilevel discourse model. In: M Beeman and C Chiarello (eds), *Right Hemisphere Language Comprehension. Perspectives from Cognitive Neuroscience.* Mahwah NJ, Erlbaum, 1998.

Stengel E, Loss of spatial orientation, constructional apraxia and Gerstmann's syndrome. J Ment. Sci. 90; 753-760, 1944.

Stepniewska I, Preuss TM, Kaas JH, Architectonics, somatotopic organization, and ipsilateral cortical connections of the primary motor area (M1) of owl monkey. Journal of Comparative Neurology. 330; 238-271, 1993.

Stewart J, Kolb B, The effects of neonatal gonadectomy and prenatal stress on cortical thickness and asymmetry in rats. Behav. Neural Biol. 49; 344-360, 1988.

Stewart J, Kolb B, Dendritic branching in cortical pyramidal cells in response to ovariectomy in adult female rats: suppression by neonatal exposure to testosterone. Brain Research 654; 149-154, 1994.

Stone J, The naso-temporal division of the cat's retina. J. Comp. Neur. 126; 585-600, 1966.

Strauss E, Lapointe JS, Wada JA, et al., Language dominance: correlation of radiological and functional data. Neuropsychologia 23; 415-420, 1985.

Strauss E, Wada J, Hunter M, Sex-related differences in the cognitive consequences of early left-hemisphere lesions. J Clin Exp Neuropsychol 14; 738–748, 1992.

Stuss DT, Assessment of neuropsychological dysfunction in frontal lobe degeneration. Dementia 4; 220-225, 1993.

Stuss DT, Interference effects on memory functions in postleukotomy patients: an attentional perspective. In: HS Levin, HM Eisenberg and AL Benton (eds), *Frontal Lobe Function and Dysfunction.* New York, NY: Oxford University Press, pp. 157-172, 1991.

Stuss DT, Benson DF, *The frontal lobes.* New York: Raven Press, 1986.

Stuss DT, Benson DF, The frontal lobes and language. In: E Goldberg (ed). *Contemporary Neuropsychology and the Legacy of Luria.* Hillsdale NJ, Erlbaum, 1990.

Stuss DT, Benson DF, Kaplan EF, et al., The involvement of orbitofrontal cerebrum in cognitive tasks. Neuropsychologia 21; 235-248, 1983.

Stuss DT, Eskes GA, Foater JK, Experimental neuropsychological studies of frontal functions. In: F Boller and J Grafman (eds), *Handbook of Neuropsychology* (Vol. 9), Amsterdam: Elsevier, 1994.

Subirana A, Handedness and cerebral dominance. In: PJ Vinken, GW Bruyn, M Critchley and JAM Frederiks (eds), *Handbook of Clincal Neurology*, Vol. 4, Amsterdam; North-Holland Publishing Co., 1969.

Sun T, Patione C, Abu-Khalil A, et al., Early asymmetry of gene transcription in embryonic human left and right cerebral cortex. Science 308; 1794-1798, 2005.

Swaab DF, Fliers E, A sexually dimorphic nucleus in the human brain. Science 228; 1112-1115, 1995.

Swithenby SJ, Bailey AJ, Brautigam S, et al., Neural processing of human faces: A magneto-encephalographic study. Experimental Brain Research 118; 501-510, 1998.

Tanji J, The supplementary motor area in the cerebral cortex. Neurosci Res 19; 251-268, 1994.

Tanji J, Shima K, Role for supplementary motor area cells in planning several movements ahead. Nature 371; 413-416, 1994.

Tellier A, Adams KM, Walker AE, Rourke BP, Long-term effects of severe penetrating head injury on psychosocial adjustment. Journal of Consulting and Clinical Psychology 58; 531-537, 1990.

Thompson PM, Cannon TD, Narr KL, et al., Genetic influences on brain structure. Nature Neuroscience 4; 1253-1258, 2001.

Thomas H, Jamison W, Hummel DD, Observation is insufficient for discovering that the surface of still water is invariantly horizontal. Science 191; 173-174, 1973.

Thurnam J, On the weight of the brain and the circumstances affecting it. Journal of mental science, 1866.

Tinley F, The brain of prehistoric man. Archives of Neurology and Psychiatry 17; 289-299, 1927.

Toga AW, Thompson PM, Mori S, Amunts K, Zilles K, Towards multimodal atlases of the human brain. Nature Reviews Neuroscience 7; 952-966, 2006.

Tognola G, Vignola LA, Brain lesions associated with oral apraxia in stroke patients: A clinico-neuroradiological investigation with the CT scan. Neuropsychologia 18; 257-272, 1980.

Tonkonogy J and Goodglass H, Language function, foot of the third frontal gyrus, and Rolandic operculum. Archives of Neurology 38; 486-490, 1981.

Ungerleider LG, Mishkin M, Two cortical visual system. In: DJ Ingle and RJF Mansfield (eds), *Analysis of Visual Behavior.* Cambridge, MA: MIT Press, 1982.

Uyehara JM, Cooper WC, Hemispheric differences for verbal and nonverbal stimuli in Japanese- and English-speaking subjects assessed by Tsunoda's method. Brain and Language 10; 405-417, 1980.

Valdes JJ, Mactutus CF, Cory RN, Cameron WR. Lateralization of norepinephrine, serotonin and choline uptake into hippocampal synaptosomes of sinistral rats. Physiol Behav 27; 381-383, 1981.

Vallortigara G, Comparative neuropsychology of the dural brain: A stroll through animals' left and right perceptual worlds. Brain and Language 73, 189-219, 2000.

Van Lancker D, Nicklay CKH, Comprehension of personally relevant (PERL) versus novel language in two globally aphasic patients. Aphasiology 6; 37-61, 1992.

Van Lancker DR, Sidtis JJ, The identification of affective-prosodic stimuli by left- and right-hemisphere-damaged subjects: all errors are not created equal. J. Speech and Hearing Research 35 (5); 963-970, 1992.

Van Lancker DR, Kreiman J, Cummings J, Voice perception deficits: Neuroanatomical correlates of phonoagnosia. Journal of Clinical and Experimental Neuropsychology 11; 665-674, 1989.

Varfaellie M, Heilman KM, Response preparation and response inhibition after lesions of the medial frontal lobe. Archives of Neurology 44; 1265-1271, 1987.

Varney NR, Linguistic correlates of pantomime recognition. J. Neurol. Neurosurg. Psychiatry 41; 564-568, 1978.

Varney NR, Benton AL, Qualitative aspects of pantomime recognition defects in aphasia. Brain Cogn. 1; 132-139, 1982.

Varney NR, Menefee L, Psychosocial and executive deficits following closed head injury: Implications for orbital frontal cortex. Journal of Head Trauma Rehabilitation 8; 32-44, 1993.

Vendrell P, Junque C, Pujol J, et al., The role of prefrontal regions in the Strop task. Neuropsychologia 33; 341-352, 1995.

Verin M, Partiot A, Pillon B, et al., Delayed response tasks and prefrontal lesions in man-evidence for self-generated patterns of behavior with poor environmental modulation. Neuropsychologia 31; 1379-1396, 1993.

Vidor M, Personality changes following prefrontal leucotomy as referred by the Minnesota Multiphasic Personality Inventory and the resulty of psychometric testing. J Ment Sci 97; 159-173, 1951.

Vignolo LA, Auditory agnosia: a review and report of recent evidence. In: Benton AL (ed), *Contributions to Clinical Neuropsychology.* Chicago: Aldine Publishing Co., Ch. 7; 172-208, 1969.

Villemure JG, Mascott CR: Peri-insular hemispherotomy: surgical principles and anatomy. Neurosurgery 37; 975-981, 1995.

Von Bonin G, Anatomical asymmetries of the cerebral hemispheres. In: VB Mountcastle (ed), *Interhemispheric Relations and Cerebral Dominance*. Baltimore: Johns Hopkins University Press, 1-6, 1962.

Wada J, Rasmussen T, Intra-carotid injection of sodium amytal for the lateralization of cerebral speech dominance. Journal of Neurosurgery 17; 266-282, 1960.

Wada JA, Clarke R, Hamm A, Cerebral hemispheric asymmetry in humans. Archives of Neurology 32; 239-246, 1975.

Wagner AD, Poldrack RA, Eldridge LL, et al., Material-specific lateralization of prefrontal activation during episodic encoding and retrieval. Neuroreport 9; 3711-3717, 1998.

Warburton E, Wise RJ, Price CJ, Weiller C, et al., Noun and verb retrieval by normal subjects. Studies with PET. Brain 119, 159-179, 1996.

Warren JM, Functional Lateralization of the Brain. In: *Evolution and the Lateralization of the Brain*. Annals of the New York Academy of Sciences. 299; 273-280, 1977.

Warrington EK, Taylor AM, The contribution of the right parietal lobe to object recognition. Cortex 9; 152-164, 1973.

Wasserstein J, Zappulla R, Rosen J, et al., In search of closure: Subjective contour illusions, gestalt completion tests, and implications. Brain and Cognition 6; 1-14, 1987.

Watson RT, Shepherd Fleet W, Gonzales-Rothi L, Heilman KM, Apraxia and supplementary motor area. Arch. Neurol 43; 787-792, 1986.

Weber DP, Sex differences in cognition: A function of the maturation rate? Science 192; 572-574, 1976.

Webster WG, Thurber AD, "Problem-solving strategies and manifest brain asymmetry". Cortex 14; 474-484, 1978.

Weintraub S, Mesulam M-M, Right cerebral dominance in spatial attention. Arch Neurol 44; 621, 1987.

Weintraub S, Mesulam M-M, and Kramer L, Disturbances in prosody: a right-hemisphere contribution to language. Archves of Neurology 38; 742-744, 1981.

Welt L, Über Charakterveranderungen des Menschen infolge von Läsionen des Stirnhirns, Deutsche Archiv für Kliniche Medizin 42; 339-390, 1888.

Wernicke C, *Der aphasische Symptomencomplex*: Breslau, Cohn and Weigert, Breslau, 1874.

Wilson SAK, An experimental research into the anatomy and physiology of the corpus striatum. Brain 36; 427-492, 1914.

Wilson FA, Scalaidhe SP, Goldman-Rakic PS, Dissociation of object and spatial processing domains in primate prefrontal cortex. Science 260; 1955-1958, 1993.

Witelson SF, Early hemisphere specialization and interhemispheric plasticity: An empirical and theoretical review. In: SJ Segalowitz and FA Gruber (eds), *Language Development and Neurological Theory*. New York: Academic Press, 1977.

Witelson SF, Anatomic asymmetry in the temporal lobes: its documentation, phylogenesis, and relationship to functional asymmetry. Annals of the New York Academy of Sciences 299; 328-354, 1977.

Witelson SF, The brain connection: The corpus callosum is larger in left-handers. Science 229; 665-668, 1985.

Witelson SF, Hand and sex differences in the isthmus and genu of the human corpus callosum: A postmortem morphological study. Brain 112; 799-835, 1989.

Witelson SF, Cognitive neuroanatomy: a new era. *Neurology* 42 (4); 709-13, 1992.

Witelson SF, Neuroanatomical bases of hemispheric functional specialization in the human brain: Possible developmental factors. In: FL Kitterle (ed), *Hemispheric Communication: Mechanisms and Models Hillsdale* NJ, Elbaum, 1995.

Witelson SF, Goldsmith CH, The relationship of hand preference to anatomy of the corpus callosum in men. Brain Research 545; 175-182, 1991.

Witelson SF, Kigar DL, Sylvian fissure morphology and asymmetry in men and women: bilateral differences in relation to handedness in men. Journal of Comparative Neurology 323; 326-340, 1992.

Witelson SF, Lezner II, Kigar DL, Women have greater density of neurons in posterior temporal cortex. Journal of Neuroscience 15; 3418–3428, 1995.

Wolf ME, and Goodale MA, Oral asymmetries during verbal and non-verbal movements of the mouth. Neuropsychologia 25; 375-396, 1987.

Woolley CS, Gould E, Frankfurt M, McEwen BS, Naturally occurring fluctuations in dendritic spine density on adult hippocampal pyramidal neurons. J Neurosci; 10; 4035-4039, 1990.

Woolsey CN, Settlage PH, Meyer DR, et al., Patterns of localization in precentral and "supplementary" motor areas and their relation to the concept of a premotor area. Res Publ Ass Nerv Ment Dis 30; 238-262, 1952.

Yakovlev PL, Rakic P, Patterns of decussation of bulbar pyramids and distribution of pyramidal tracts on two sides of the spinal cord. Trans American Neurological Association 91; 366-367, 1966.

Yamadori A, Osumi Y, Masuhara S, Okubo M, Preservation of singing in Broca's aphasia. Journal of Neurology Neurosurgery and Psychiatry 40; 221-224, 1977.

Yamadori A, Mori E, Tabuchi M, et al., Hypergraphia: a right hemisphere syndrome. Journal of Neurology, Neurosurgery and Psychiatry 49, 1160-1164, 1986.

Zaidel E, Lexical organization in the right hemisphere. In: PA Buser and Rougeul-Buser (eds). *Cerebral Correlates of Conscious Experience.* INSERM Symposium 6. Amsterdam Elsevier / North-Holland, 1978.

Zaidel E, Language functions in the two hemispheres following cerebral commissurotomy and hemispherectomy. In F. Boller & J. Grafman (eds) *Handbook of Neuropsychology.* New York Elsevier. Vol. 4; 115-150, 1990.

Zaidel E, Iacobini M, *The parallel brain.* Cambridge: Mit Press, 2002.

Zaidel E, Aboitiz F, Clarke J et al., Sex differences in interhemispheric relation for language. In: FL Kitterle (ed), *Hemispheric Communication: Mechanisms and Models.* Hillsdale NJ, Erlbaum, 1995.

Zangwill OL, Intelligence in aphasia. In: Reuck AVS, O'Conner M (eds), *Disorders of Language.* Boston: Little Brown and Co.; 261-274, 1964.

Zatorre RJ, Jones-Gotman M, Human olfactory discrimination after unilateral frontal or temporal lobectomy. Brain 114; 71-84, 1991.

Zatorre RJ, Binder RJ, Functional and structural imaging of the human auditory system. In: *Brain Mapping: The Systems.* A Toga and J Mazziotta (eds). Academic Press, San Diego; 365-402, 2000.

Zatorre RJ, Peretz I (eds), The biological foundations of music. Ann. NY Acad. Sci. 930; 2001.

Zatorre RJ, Meyer E, Gjedde A, Evans AC, PET studies of phonetic processing of speech: Review, replication, and reanalysis. Cerebral Cortex 6; 21-30, 1996.

Zimmerberg B, Glick SD, Serussi TP, Neurochemical correlate of a spatial preference in rats. Science 185; 623-625, 1974.

Zimmerberg B, Strumpf AJ, Glick SD, Cerebral asymmetry and left-right discrimination, Brain Research 140; 194-196, 1978.

Chapter 24

THE NEURAL BASIS
OF CONSCIOUSNESS

Introduction

Consciousness is an universal set of neurologic and mental or spiritual processes produced by the brain in awake state, which allows people to understand the mind of others (mind reading); it also allows an optimal social living to perform any kind of high normal behavior activity (social, political, professional, moral, ethic, religious, etc.) related to the self and the environment (family, society).

So, the two separate forms of consciousness are neurologic and mental or spiritual. The neurologic form of consciousness is based on interactions between the brain stem, midbrain, diencephalon, limbic system and the cerebral cortex. There is the idea of being conscious versus unconscious.

Consciousness may be also defined as our awareness of our environment, our bodies and ourselves (Hobson, 2007). Awareness of ourselves implies an awareness of awareness, that is the conscious recognition that we are a conscious being. Awareness of ourselves implies meta-cognition (Hobson, 2007).

Although many theorists treat consciousness as single, all-or-nothing phenomenon, others distinguish between first-order consciousness and a meta-level of consciousness. For example, they may distinguish between consciousness and metaconsciousness (Schooler, 2002), primary consciousness and higher-order consciousness (Edelman and Tononi, 2000), or core consciousness and extended consciousness (Damasio, 1999). Animals possess primary (core) consciousness which comprises sensory awareness, attention, perception, memory (or learning), emotion and action (Edelman, 1992). According to Hobson (2007), what differentiates humans from their fellow mammals and gives humans what Edelman defines as secondary consciousness, depends upon language and the associated enrichment of cognition that allow humans to develop and to use verbal and numeric abstraction. Spoken and written language are human specializations. These mental capacities contribute to our sense of self as agents and as creative beings. It also determines the awareness of awareness that we assume our animal "collaborators" do not possess (Hobson, 2007).

Many factors are involved in the establishing levels of consciousness commonly referred to as wakefulness and sleep. Such factors include the enormous driving of the cerebral cortex over the ascending activating and inhibiting systems and the influence of cyclic limbic activation of cerebral cortical areas. There are complex interconnections between these areas of the nervous system: the hypothalamus, thalamus and hippocampal formation. Our state of consciousness includes accompanying autonomic responses such as changes in respiration, heart rate, or body temperature. Injuries that involve a considerable part of tegmentum of the midbrain result in a profound coma because of the interruption of ascending multisynaptic activating system (AAS) as well as descending hypothalamotegmental and dorsal longitudinal fasciculus path.

In humans, the complex system of mental and spiritual processes depends on and is produced by the highest psychical activities, i.e., it depends on and is produced by the brain, making people: use symbolic representation and language; reflect on the past and anticipate and plan for the future; transform thought into speech and action; logically record the personal experience and transmit it orally by writing and / or by drawing; participate in the progress and civilization; read through other people's thoughts, judge correctly their intentions and act consequently; use abstractization and generalization to make new discoveries; know, spread and protect the ethical, moral and religious standards in order to live an optimal social life; organize behavior and extrapolate it in time; deal with cognitive novelty.

The prediction and comprehension of others' behavior are evidently very important aspects of social functioning.

The consciousness processes belong, in essence, to people who act by control mechanisms of psychological activities, generalization and abstractization mechanisms, exploring and handling of mental images to solve all the problems man is facing with.

In humans, the level of consciousness depends on the complexity of the brain ontogenetic evolution; the human brain makes culture and technology possible. We believe that the cerebral cortex is absolutely necessary for this function; machines that are responsive to sensory events and are capable of complex movements are not conscious. According to this view, the brain stem occupies the bottom of the totem pole, providing the basic arousal mechanism without which the higher brain regions cannot operate.

On the other hand, consciousness must be a function of numerous interacting systems. The major structures supposed to play a key role in the neural correlates of consciousness are: **the brain stem, the midbrain, the diencephalon** (especially the hypothalamus and thalamus), **the limbic system**, and **the cerebral cortex**.

Thus, the brain "language" can be conceptualized as the transmission of neural signals (Yamazaki and Tanaka, 2007). The "grammar" of the brain's language system concerns the proper timing of neuronal impulses. Neuronal impulse timing is based upon proper integration and balance of excitatory and inhibitory processes (Hatta et al., 2004).

Patients and method

In our attempt to demonstrate the presence of the ascending inhibitory system, of the consciousness disorders and its modular aspect, a group of nine patients has been subject to evaluation and surgery within the Neurosurgery department of the National Institute of Neurology and Neurological Diseases in Bucharest. Eight of the patients have been diagnosed with brain tumors, and one patient with encephalitis; patient mean age was 42,88 years, the youngest being 21 and the oldest 73 years.

Six (66,66%) of the patients were males and three (33,33) females. In 8 patients, the main examination was computed tomography (CT) and magnetic resonance imaging (MRI). In the patient presenting multiple brain metastases, the brain was subject to examination after death.

In this section we will present the clinical symptomatology of the above patients.

Case 1. A 21-year-old man presented with a history of sudden onset of coma. MRI-scan revealed a bilateral ponto-mesencephalic hemorrhage triggered by a cavernoma. After total resection of the cavernoma and hematoma, patient's status has improved significantly, presenting only a remaining minimal right side weakness and hemisensory deficit. Now the patient is a student, and has an excellent state.

Case 2. A 38-year-old woman presented with logorrhea syndrome, with hyper-kinesia, hyperwakefulness and hyperprosexia. The patient could sleep for only a short time, and then awake and was unable to fall back asleep. MRI-scan revealed a petroclival meningioma which significantly compresses the superior part of the brain stem.

Case 3. A 36-year-old man presented with intermittent increased intracranial pressure, paralysis of the conjugate upward gaze (Parinaud's sign) and pseudo-Argyll Robertson pupil. A contrast-enhanced CT-scan revealed a tumor of the pineal area. Only 15% of the patients with tumors of the pineal area, which are compressing the dorsal area of the mesencephalon, also experience arousal disorders.

Case 4. A 29-year-old woman presented with left hemiparesis by compression of the adjacent internal capsule, palsies of vertical and lateral gaze, absence of convergence, retraction nystagmus, and mild sensory deficit in the opposite side of the body, including the trunk. Pain and thermal sensation was more affected than touch, vibration and position.

Involvement of ventral posterolateral and posteromedial nuclei of the thalamus causes loss or diminution of all forms of sensation on the opposite side of the body.

Contrast medium-enhanced coronal and axial MRI shows a big right thalamic tumor.

The tumor was fully resected and after the surgery the patient remained with a mild sensory deficit and a hemiparesis, but she returned to an independent life.

Case 5. A 56-year-old man presented with a sudden onset of coma and fever.

Coronal and axial Tl-weighted MRI-scans revealed edematous, demyelination symmetrical changes infra- and supratentorial which involved the entire midbrain, both thalamic formations, bilateral basal ganglia, two-side temporo-occipital convolution and hippocampus, determined by encephalitis (limbic encephalitis). After 9 days of coma the patient died.

Case 6. A 56-year-old man with a history of severe headaches, presented with taste and smell disorder, excessive euphoria accompanied by peculiar kind of compulsive, shallow and childish humor (moria), irritability, hypomania and puerilism.

The patient also shows disorders of attention and motility, distractibility, hyper-reactivity, hyperkinesia, perseveration, emotional lability, cognitive dysfunction that impede the initiation and temporal organization of actions and lacks of initiative, wrong decision and instinctual disinhibition.

Contrast enhanced computed tomography (CT) scan shows a giant size olfactory groove meningioma and displacement of anterior brain.

Post surgery, after complete resection of the tumor, the orbitofrontal syndrome disappeared almost completely.

Case 7. A 35-year-old woman was admitted to our department of neurosurgery with a bilateral meningioma of the anterior falx who compressed dorsolateral premotor and prefrontal cortex (Brodmann's areas 6, 8, 9, 10, and 46).

As symptoms, she had attention disorder directed to a particular item of sensorium or inner experience and incapacity to suppress from inner experience items that can interfere with what is currently on focus.

She was apathetic, disinterested in herself and the world around her. Visuospatial neglect along with gaze abnormalities were also present because the lesion encroaches on area 8. According to our experience, the apathy is present in all lateral-damage conditions, and is mostly apparent after large bilateral lesions of the frontal convexity.

Perseveration, dysexecutive syndrome with attention, working-memory and planning disorders were among the symptoms. Language disorders were directly linked to failure of temporal integration.

In this patient, depression was secondary to cognitive disorder.

Case 8. A 46-year-old man was admitted to our department of neurosurgery with olfactory hallucination ("uncinate fit") often accompanied by a dreamy state of mind, auditory elementary hallucination, when the patient heard the sound of running water, impaired recognition of melodies in the absence of words, the usual tendency for the patient to report the current date as an earlier one and prosopagnosia.

Coronal Tl-weighted, gadolinium-enhanced MRI prior to surgery showed a large right-sided temporobasal tumor (a).

Post surgery coronal Tl-weighted, gadolinium-enhanced MRI (b) obtained after complete removal of the tumor (astrocytoma). The patient improved very much and was discharged after 2 weeks.

Case 9. Patient, aged 73, was admitted to our neurosurgery department with a coma and deceased within 18 hours. On autopsy, more than 110 bilateral cortical and intracerebral metastases have been discovered, originating from a melanocarcinoma situated in the right abdominal area, previously subject to surgery 7 months earlier.

Results

Starting from clinical neuropsychology, we present our results, along with the comments made on the main cerebral formation, which play an important role in understanding this extremely complex problem, which is the consciousness.

BRAINSTEM

The brain stem is the portion of the central nervous system rostral to the spinal cord and caudal to the cerebral hemispheres.

The net-like appearance of the brain stem neurons led to the designation "reticular formation", a term that was originally used in a purely descriptive anatomical sense.

The reticular formation

The reticular formation (RF), beginning in the medulla and extending to the midbrain, plays a major role in the sleep-wakefulness cycles of animals and humans. It occupies a significant portion of the dorsal brain stem and forms a network of reticular fibres that synapse with and modulate many ascending and descending fibre tracts.

Nuclei of RF receive afferent information from all sensory (visual, auditory, etc.) and motor systems as well as from other major structures of the brain, and project their axons upwards and downwards to virtually all parts of the nervous system. Through their connections with the thalamus, hypothalamus and directly to the cerebral cortex they can send information to, and receive it from all areas of the cortex. There are ascending (or forward) and descending (or backward) connections between them.

The RF is also known as the reticular activating system and the reticular inhibitory system (Dănăilă, 1972; Arseni and Dănăilă, 1977; Dănăilă and Pascu, 2009).

The role of reticular formation is to awake or to get to sleep the cerebral cortex.

After waking, the cortex allows all modes of sensory processing (sight, hearing, touch, etc.) to combine with conscious thought and experience in order to focus on some inputs and suppress others.

Neuroscientists now recognize that the various nuclei within the brain stem serve many functions and that only a few take part in waking and sleeping.

Instead of being used in a descriptive analogical way, the reticular formation was promoted to a functional concept, a brain stem system which, by virtue of its nonspecific connectivity, could act as a kind of volume control for the degree of conscious arousal and sleeping and as a homeostatic system.

Ascending (reticular) activating system (AAS)

In 1929, Hans Berger reported a technologic innovation, the electroencephalogram (EEG) which is correlated closely with the level of consciousness of the patients. Since Berger's first observation, the various ongoing brain oscillations have been used successfully to characterize mental status such as sleep, the waking state or vigilance and mental pathologies such as epilepsy. Sensory evoked potentials (EEG signals triggered by an external stimulation) have demonstrated that such mental factors as sensation, attention, intellectual activity, and planning of movement, all have distinctive electrical correlates at the surface of the skull (Zeman, 2001). Afterwards, in 1935 and 1936, Bremer examined the EEG waveforms in cats into which he had placed lesions of the brain stem. He found that after a transection between the medulla and the spinal cord, a preparation that he called the encephale isolé, or isolated brain, animals showed a desynchronized (low-voltage, fast-wave) EEG pattern and appeared to be fully awake. When he transected the neuraxis between the superior and inferior colliculus, a preparation he called the cerveau isolé, or isolated cerebrum, the EEG showed a synchronized, or high-voltage, slow-wave pattern indicative of deep sleep and the animals were behaviorally unresponsive. Bremer concluded that the forebrain fell asleep due to the lack of somatosensory and auditory sensory inputs.

The reticular activating system obtained this designation in 1949, when Moruzzi and Magoun stimulated it electrically in anesthetized cats and found that the stimulation produced a waking pattern of electrical activity in cat's cortex. When Moruzzi and Magoun placed lesions in the paramedian reticular formation of the midbrain, the animals showed cortical-evoked responses to somatosensory or auditory stimuli, but the background EEG was synchronized and the animals were behaviorally unresponsive. These observations emphasized the midbrain reticular core as relaying important arousing influences to the cerebral cortex and this pathway was labeled the ascending reticular activating system (initially called ARAS, but today named AAS).

The most important reticular nuclei for arousal and consciousness are the raphe nuclei and the central nuclei. These groups receive significant converging sensory input from all sensory modalities and project to the thalamus (i.e., intralaminar nuclei), cholinergic basal forebrain nuclei, and the entire cerebral cortex. An important component of the central reticular activating system is thought to be the noradrenergic nuclei, particularly the locus ceruleus, at the pontomesencephalic junction.

The centromedian and parafascicular nuclei, two of the intralaminar nuclei of the thalamus representing the rostral extent of the AAS receive inputs from the spinothalamic, trigeminothalamic and multisynaptic ascending pathways (of the reticular formation) relaying pain sensation. As a result of their diffuse cortical connections, they are involved in the maintenance of arousal.

The neurons of the locus ceruleus project to the thalamus, hypothalamus, basal cholinergic nuclei, and the neocortex (Moore and Bloom, 1979).

Immediate coma results from the destruction of the central reticular nuclei at or above the upper pontine level (Fig. 24.1, case 1).

Anyhow, AAS acts on the cerebral cortex through the thalamus, directly, and through the arousal caudal hypothalamic neurons (tuberomammillary nucleus) which are connected with suprachiasmatic nuclei (Fig. 24.2).

As a result, the reticular formation comes to be known as the reticular activating system to maintain general arousal, and as the reticular inhibitory system for sleeping.

However, an exact physiologic role of the reticular activating system in consciousness is unclear. The awake condition like the sleep has many phases: a quick short phase which is determined by the direct action of AAS on the cerebral cortex, a longer phase during the 24 hours, determined by indirect action of AAS on the cortex through the thalamus; and a rhythmical phase determined by the AAS action on the cerebral cortex through the hypothalamus awaking system under the influence of the suprachiasmatic nucleus. These nuclei are serially interconnected with AAS not only in the forward, but also in the reverse direction (backward).

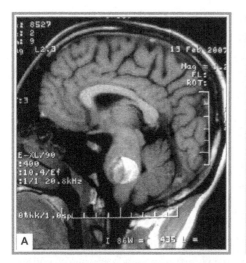
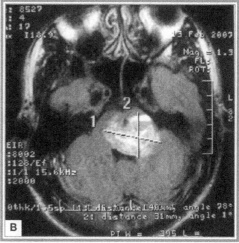
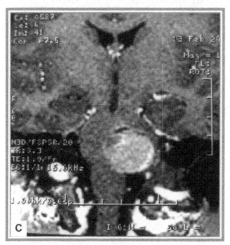
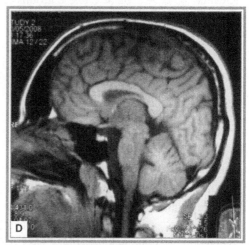
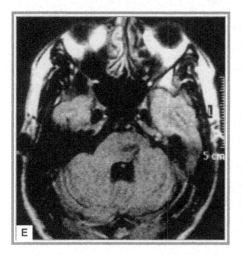
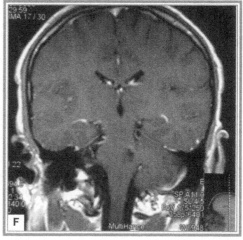

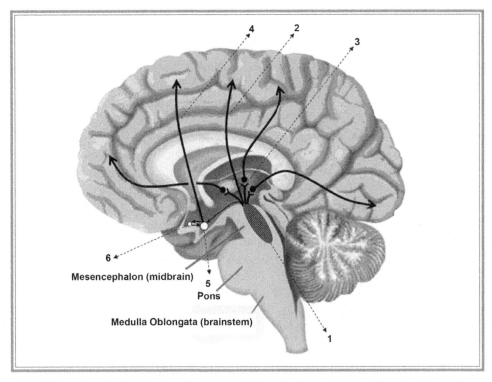

Fig. 24.2. The Ascending Reticular Activating System (ARAS) is found in the brain stem (1), and sends projections throughout the cortex: directly (2), through the thalamus (3), or through the hypothalamus (4), tuberomammillary neurons (5), which receive influence from suprachiasmatic nucleus (6).

It is generally agreed that a key component of the reticular activating system is a group of cholinergic nuclei near the pons-midbrain junction that project to thalamocortical neurons. The relevant neurons in the nuclei are characterized by high discharge rates during the waking. When stimulated, these nuclei cause "desynchronization" of the electroencephalogram (that is, a shift of EEG activity from high-amplitude, synchronized waves to lower amplitude, higher-frequency, desynchronized ones).

In 1980, McGuiness and Krauthamer have concluded that the intralaminar nuclei acted not only as a thalamic pacemaker and as a relay for cortical arousal but was characterized also by the presence of cells responding to visual auditory and somesthetic stimuli. Schiff and Plum (1999) wrote "cortical and subcortical innervations of the intralaminar nuclei place them in a central position to influence distributed networks

◀ **Fig. 24.1.** A 21-year old man who presented with a history of sudden onset of coma.
Sagittal (A), axial (B) and coronal (C) T1-weighted magnetic resonance imaging (MRI) scans revealed a gross pontine hemorrhage (1.9 cm) from a cavernous malformation that reached the surface of the floor of the fourth ventricle and in the cerebelopontine angle.
The lesion was resected through a suboccipital approach. Sagittal (D), axial (E), and coronal (F) MRI scans, one year later, reveal no recurrence. Two months after surgery, the patient presented with minimal right sided weakness and hemisensory deficits. Now the patient is a student, and has an excellent state.

underlying arousal, attention, intention, working memory and sensorimotor integration, including gaze control". Thus, there are three main types of thalamic projections: the specific (for vision, audition), the diffuse and the projection to striatum (essentially, all, from intralaminar nuclei). Diffuse intralaminar nuclei efferents are widely, though sparsely, distributed to most of neocortex: it is this diffuse projection that has to do with consciousness. One can understand how intralaminar nuclei could directly influence ideation, as ideation is a function of cortex (Bogen, 2007).

Activity of these neurons is not, however, the only neuronal basis of wakefulness: there are also involved, the noradrenergic neurons of the locus ceruleus; the serotonergic neurons of the raphe nuclei; and histamine-containing neurons in the tuberomammillary nucleus (TMN) of the hypothalamus. The locus ceruleus and raphe nuclei are modulated by the TMN neurons located near the tuberal region that synthesize the peptide orexin (also called hypercretin). Orexin promotes waking, and thus may have useful applications in jobs where operators need to stay alert. On the other hand, antihistamines inhibit the histamine-containing TMN network, and thus tend to make people drowsy (Willie et al., 2003).

Arousal systems are regulated not only by external stimuli, but also by control systems of the brain. For example, the frontal cortex, particularly the orbitofrontal area, regulates the thalamic reticular nucleus and the cholinergic, basal forebrain structures. Patients with lesions in this area show deficits in arousal (Marrocco and Field, 2002). Cortical control is not limited to cholinergic modulation. In a work on the norepinephrine system, Minzenberg et al. (2008) demonstrated the role of locus ceruleus-norepinephrine system in the prefrontal cortex function and cognitive control.

The frontal cortex also exerts an influence on the limbic system, which regulates emotional arousal. The anterior cingulate region is important in the self-regulation of arousal through its connections with the cholinergic basal forebrain (Marrocco and Field, 2002).

In sum, AAS can exert both direct and indirect action on the cerebral cortex. However, the reticular formation which appears to be responsible for maintaining cortical arousal is not the same with consciousness.

Ascending (reticular) inhibitory system (AIS)

According to case 2, it is impossible that the two important functions of the central nervous system, arousal and sleep, or activation and inhibition, depend only on AAS. The two compulsory conditions (arousal and sleep) cannot be determined or explained by the AAS activity or inactivity only.

Dănăilă (1972), Arseni and Dănăilă (1977) and Dănăilă and Pascu (2009) have clinically demonstrated that, besides the AAS, there is an ascending reticular inhibitory system (AIS) as well, of which lesion leads to the appearance of the logorrhea syndrome with hyperkinesia, hyperwakefulness, and hyperprosexia.

Normally, during the 24 daily hours, after arousal follows sleep, which is based on AIS. The two reticular systems (AAS and AIS) are under the influence of the suprachiasmatic nucleus and of the awake and sleep centers in the hypothalamus.

As much as awake is determined by AAS, sleep, considered the most profound natural alteration of consciousness, is determined by AIS. It acts on the cerebral cortex directly, through the thalamus, through the ventrolateral preoptic (VLPO) nucleus of the hypothalamus, which in its turn is under the influence of the suprachiasmatic nucleus, and through the basal ganglia.

The lateral group of the reticular formation, localized in the pons and rostral part of the brain stem, gives origin to AIS. When AIS is activated, the cerebral cortex becomes inactive and the person asleep. This system receives inhibitory signals from the cerebellum and sends output signals to the thalamus, to the hypothalamic sleeping center, and directly to the cerebral cortex (Fig. 24.3).

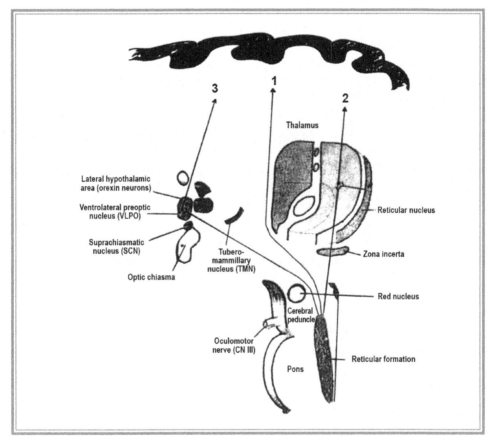

Fig. 24.3. The Ascending Reticular Inhibitory System (ARIS) is found in the brain stem, and sends projections throughout the cortex: directly (1), through the thalamus (2), or through the hypothalamus; ventrolateral preoptic nucleus-VLPO, (3), which receives influence from suprachiasmatic nucleus.

The raphe nuclei, in the midline of the brain stem, use serotonin as their primary neurotransmitter and have diffuse connections to the cerebral cortex and subcortical gray matter (Moore et al., 1978).

Thus, the correlated activity between reticular neurons leads to a strengthened connection, both excitatory and inhibitory. In the absence of inhibition, any external input, weak or strong, would generate more or less the same one-way pattern, an avalanche of excitatory stimuli involving the whole population (Hopfield and Tank, 1986). Cortical networks gain their nonlinearity and functional complexity primarily from the inhibitory interneuronal system (Pouille and Scanziani, 2001). The specific firing patterns of principal cells in a network depend on the temporal and spatial distribution of inhibition. Without inhibition and dedicated neural formation, excitatory circuits cannot accomplish anything useful (Buzsaki, 2006). Fast coupling of the excitatory and inhibitory influences can bring about a submillisecond precision of spike timing (Pouille and Scanziani, 2001).

Anyhow, reticular nucleus efferents terminate in the immediately underlying thalamic nuclei and the reticular nuclei efferents are GABA-ergic (the neurons in reticular nuclei are exclusively inhibitory, using GABA as their transmitter) (Bogen, 1997, 2001). Thus, thalamocortical communication can be simultaneously inhibited by this reticular nucleus efferents that terminate in the underlying thalamic nuclei. In the brain and particularly in the cerebral cortex, there are multiple influences, both inhibitory and facilitatory. When a performance has been lost because the competence has lost some facilitation, re-emergence of the performance can result simply from the subsidence of inhibition (Sherrington, 1932). The same suggestion was made by von Monakow in 1911. The main point is that a loss of performance is not necessarily the result of damage to the competence for that performance; it may result from unbalanced or excessive inhibition of the competence (Bogen, 2001).

Generally, the reticular formation of the brain stem is, in turn, influenced by circadian clocks located in the suprachiasmatic nuclei and the arousal (tuberomammillary nucleus) and sleeping (ventrolateral preoptic nucleus) centers of the hypothalamus. The clock adjusts periods of sleep and wakefulness to appropriate duration during the 24-hours cycle of light and darkness. So, in all structures of the nervous system, inhibition plays a pivotal role.

Thus, brain uses not only excitation, but also inhibition during its normal operations and behaviors. With no inhibitory cells in a network, depending on the temporal and spatial distribution and dedicated interneurons, excitatory circuits cannot accomplish anything useful (Buzsaki, 2006). Excitatory potentials dominate on the dendrites of principal cells, whereas only inhibitory postsynaptic potentials impinge upon the cell body (soma). Interneurons provide autonomy and independence to neighboring principal cells but they offer, at the same time, useful temporal coordination. The functional diversity of principal cells is enhanced by the domain-specific actions of GABA-ergic interneurons which can dynamically alter the qualities of the principal cells (Buzsaki, 2006). The separation of inputs in a network with only excitatory connections and circuits is not possible. Like all somatic functions at all levels of the system, executive functions, beginning with attention, make use of inhibition for focus, contrast suppression of interference, order, and timeliness (Fuster, 2009). Inhibition enhance saliency and contrast. Inhibition appears essential for the control of impulsivity and a wide array of instinctual drives.

So, there are two opposing active processes that could summate, algebraically, a control excitatory reticular system and a control inhibitory one. Thus, the brain uses not only excitation, but also inhibition during its normal function.

Ascending output of the brain stem reticular formation not only subserves arousal and sleep but also contains information about other bodily states and other neural formation outside the reticular formation. This is why ARAS and ARIS might be named ascending activatory system (AAS) and, respectively, ascending inhibitory system (AIS).

Clinical aspects

It is important to distinguish between alertness and impairment of the wakeful state. It is possible to be awake and not conscious, but it is impossible to be conscious and not awake. A combination of clinical lesion studies and animal data has identified the following major mechanisms through which alterations in consciousness are produced: disturbance of the ascending reticular system; bilateral lesions of the midbrain and diencephalon; and bilateral involvement of the cerebral cortex (hemispheres). To what degree same damage will render unconsciousness of a person remains to be clarified.

Coma

Destructive lesions of the brain stem may occur as a result of vascular disease, tumor, infection, or trauma. Unlike compressive lesions, which can often be reversed by removing a mass, destructive lesions cannot be reversed. Between the conscious state of mind and coma there are multiple intermediary stages that manifest through: confusion or lethargy, drowsiness, stupor, semicoma (light coma), locked-in syndrome persistent vegetative state, loss of conscious in concussion (diffuse axonal injury). We will shortly discuss below the most important of them.

Persistent vegetative state

The term persistent vegetative state was introduced by Jannet and Plum in 1972, to describe the state of preservation of autonomic function and primitive reflexes, without the ability to interact meaningfully with external environment.

The vegetative state has been differentiated from the newly introduced category of **minimally conscious state** (MCS; Giacino et al., 2002). MC patients may show islands of relatively preserved brain response (Schiff et al., 2002; Bly et al., 2004), as well as fragments of behaviors interpretable as signs of perception and voluntary movement that preclude the diagnosis of vegetative state (Zeman, 2001). Both, the vegetative and minimally conscious state need to be distinguished from the locked-in syndrome in which the patient is fully conscious but, due to a circumscribed brain stem lesion, is unable to communicate in any way other than by lid closure and vertical eye movements. Overall, brain metabolism is less reduced in locked-in patients (Levy et al., 1987).

Diffuse axonal injury (loss of consciousness in concussion)

The mechanism of loss of consciousness with a blow to the head is not completely understood.

Brief loss of consciousness, which in humans is usually not associated with any changes in CT and MRI scan, may be due to the shearing forces transiently applied to the ascending arousal system at the mesodiencephalic junction. Physiologically, the concussion causes abrupt neural depolarization and promotes release of excitatory neurotransmitters. There is an efflux of potassium from cells with calcium influx into cells and sequestration in mitochondria leading to impaired oxidative metabolism. There are also alterations in cerebral blood flow and glucose metabolism, all of which impair neuronal and axonal function (Giza and Hovda, 2001).

Concussion or hemorrhage into the dorsolateral mesopontine tegmentum may be visible on MRI, but diffuse axonal injury is generally not. Magnetic resonance spectroscopy may be useful in evaluating patients with diffuse axonal injury, who typically have a reduction in N-acetylaspartate as well as elevation of glutamate / glutamine and choline / creatinine ratio (Adams et al., 2000; Brooks et al., 2001; Schutter et al., 2004).

Logorrhea syndrome with hyperkinesia

The activity in the reticular formation is the mechanism that induces the sleep and awakens you from sleep and brings you back to full consciousness.

Thus, damage in the reticular formation typically sends a person into coma because this is an on / off switch for all higher brain centers or determines the logorrhea syndrome with hyperkinesia (Dănăilă, 1972; Arseni and Dănăilă, 1977; Dănăilă and Pascu, 2009). In a study on the behavior of patients with brain stem tumors and another neurosurgical condition, Dănăilă (1972), Arseni and Dănăilă (1977) observed that, apart from the locked-in syndrome, persistent vegetative state or coma, the patients may also manifest various other aspects, especially logorrhea syndrome with hyperkinesia, hyperwakefulness and hyperprosexia (Fig. 24.4, case 2). In our opinion, the logorrhea syndrome

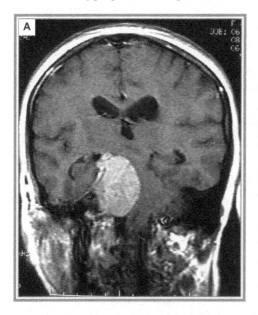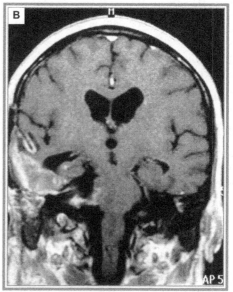

Fig. 24.4. MRI studies of a petroclival meningioma (A) which compresses from outside the brain stem provoke logorrhea syndrome with hyperkinesia and hyperwakefulness. Postsurgery (B) this syndrome disappears.

with hyperkinesia, hyperwakefulness and hyperprosexia reflect a hyperconsciousness or, in other words, a super-arousal determined by eliberation of the AAS from the influence of AIS which is damaged.

Thus, the logorrhea syndrome with hyperkinesia is produced by the lesion of the AIS and is an argument in favor of the existence of AIS.

The lesions found in our cases (pons, rostral part of the brain stem) mark the location of the AIS. Trillet et al. (1995) have described a syndrome of hemiballisme and logorrhea determined by a hematome of the left subthalamic nucleus. The right hemiballisme is explained by the influence on the subthalamic nucleus, but not the logorrhea. In our opinion, the image given in Fig. 1 of theirs article shows multiple subthalamic lesions which affect zona incerta; one knows that zona incerta has an inhibitory role (Jones, 2007).

In conclusion, we think that the logorrhea syndrome is, in this case, given by the lesion produced to the zona incerta which is located in the immediate neighborhood of the subthalamic nucleus. AIS passes through zona incerta.

In sum, besides the other homeostatic systems, the reticular system (AAS and AIS) represents an actual regulator system of the entire neuraxis, as proven by its participation in the regulation of all the psychical processes (attention, memory, reasoning, behavior, etc.), speech, muscular tonus, and the physiognomy of movement.

MIDBRAIN (Mesencephalon)

The midbrain is the short portion of the brain between the pons and the cerebral hemispheres. It consists of tectum, contains the four corpora quadrigemina and two cerebral peduncles with tegmentum and crus cerebri.

The cerebral aqueduct, surrounded by the central gray matter, separates the tectum from the tegmentum. The cerebral peduncle consists of two parts: 1) a dorsal part, the tegmentum; and 2) a ventral part, the crus cerebri. These two parts are separated from each other by substantia nigra.

The midbrain tegmentum contains the trochlear and oculomotor nuclei, neural structures concerned with ocular and visual reflexes, the mesencephalic reticular formation, the red nuclei and many scattered collections of cells.

Dorsal midbrain syndrome

The midbrain may be forced downward through the tentorial opening by a mass lesion impinging upon it from the dorsal surface (Fig. 24.5, case 3).

The most common causes are masses in the pineal gland, in the posterior thalamus, or in upward transtentorial herniation which kinks the midbrain.

Primary midbrain hemorrhages, which may be of either type, are rare. Most of such patients present acutely with headache, alteration of consciousness and abnormal eye signs. Most of them recover completely from bleeds from cavernous angiomas, but some remain with mild neurologic deficit.

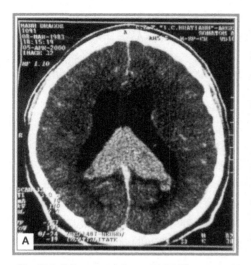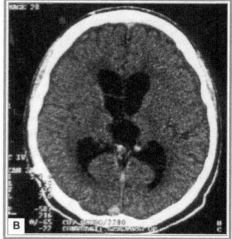

Fig. 24.5. A) A contrast-enhanced axial CT-scan of a 36-year-old man with hydrocephalus and a large pineal region tumor, that was totally resected. Postsurgery, the patient remains clinically intact. B) Axial CT-scan, 3 months postsurgery confirming total removal of the tumor (germinoma).

Pressure from this direction produces the characteristic dorsal midbrain syndrome, manifested first by limited upgaze. In severe cases, the eyes may be fixed in forced, downward position. There may also be a deficit of convergent eye movements and associated pupilloconstriction. The presence of retractory nystagmus, in which all of the eye muscle contracts simultaneously to pull the globe back into the orbit, is characteristic. Motor responses are difficult to obtain or result in extensor posturing. Motor tone and tendon reflexes may be heightened, and plantar responses are in extension.

If the cerebral aqueduct is compressed sufficiently to cause acute hydrocephalus, however, an acute increase in supratentorial pressure may ensue.

This may cause an acute increase in downward pressure on the midbrain, resulting in sudden lapse into deep coma (Posner et al., 2007).

Most patients in whom the herniation can be reversed suffer chronic neurologic disability (Brendler and Selverstone, 1970; Zervas and Hedley-Whyte, 1972).

After the midbrain stage becomes complete, it is rare for patients to recover fully.

DIENCEPHALON

The diencephalon contains the hypothalamus, thalamus, subthalamus (substantia nigra, the zona incerta, the nucleus of the tegmental fields of Forel, ansa lenticularis, Forel's field H1 – thalamic fasciculus – Forel's field H2 – lenticular fasciculus-, and subthalamic fasciculus), metathalamus (medial geniculate body and lateral geniculate body), and epithalamus (pineal body, habenular trigones, stria medullaris, and roof of the third ventricle).

In the following, we study only the role of the hypothalamus and thalamus in sleep, arousal, and circadian rhythm.

The hypothalamus

The hypothalamus is composed of about 22 small nuclei, the fibre system that passes through it and the pituitary gland. Although the hypothalamus comprises only about 0.3% of the brain weight, it takes part in nearly all aspects of motivated behavior, including sleeping, arousal, temperature regulation, emotional behavior, endocrine function, metabolism, sexual behavior, and movement.

From our point of view, the ventrolateral preoptic nucleus (sleeping system), the tubero-mammillary nucleus (arousal system), and the suprachiasmstic nucleus (day - night cycle system) are important.

The sleep is a circadian function, and although the suprachiasmatic nuclei are not essential for its generation, they are responsible for consolidation of sleep in cycles that occur within a circadian framework.

According to Hobson (2007), when humans go to sleep they rapidly become less conscious. The initial loss of awareness of the external world that may occur when we are reading in bed is associated with the slowing of the EEG that is called Stage I. At sleep onset, although awareness of the outside world is lost, subject may continue to have visual imagery and associated reflective consciousness. Even in the depths of stage IV non-REM sleep, when consciousness appears to be largely obliterated, the brain remains highly active and it is still capable of processing its own information. From PET and single neuron studies, it can safely be concluded that the brain remains about 80% active in the depths of sleep. Most of the brain activity is not associated with consciousness. Non-REM, Stage IV is characterized by low-frequency, high-amplitude EEG in which subjects may report not only some thought-like mentation but also movie-like dreams (Bosinelli, 1995).

The circuitry through which AIS influences the sleep, being localized in the upper pons and rostral parts of the brain stem, includes the hypothalamic ventrolateral preoptic nuclei, suprachiasmatic nuclei, the thalamus, and the cerebral cortex. Saper et al. (2005) provide very good arguments regarding the sleep and arousal. Nevertheless, in our opinion, the explanation of the sleep / wakefulness given by them as due to a flip-flop switch, to the influence of suprachiasmatic nucleus, to the homeostatic mechanism and to the allostatic mechanism is not enough. It is our opinion that the explanation should also include the existence of the AAS and AIS which are working also under the influence of the suprachiasmatic nucleus, homeostatic mechanisms and allostatic mechanism and which control the sleep.

The arousal, like sleep, exhibits more steps: a rapid one, which has a short lifetime and which is determined by the direct action of the ascending activating system on the cerebral cortex; another, with a longer lifetime, within the 24 hours, which is caused by indirect action of AAS on the cerebral cortex *via* thalamus; and the third, which is rhythmic and it is determined by the AAS action on the cerebral cortex *via* the hypothalamic arousal system which, in its turn, is found under the influence of the suprachiasmatic nucleus.

Some studies have demonstrated that the influence of the hypothalamus on arousal is not restricted to the tuberomammillary neurons in caudal hypothalamus. In particular, a prominent group of neurons confined to the lateral hypothalamus has been implicated in the sleep disorder known as narcolepsy (Card et al., 1999).

These neurons express novel neuropeptides known as hypocretins or orexins and are differentially concentrated within the perifornical nucleus that surrounds the fornix in the tuberal hypothalamus. Mapping studies have shown that hypocretin (orexin) neurons are similar to tuberomammillary neurons in that they are confined to the hypothalamus and give rise to extensive projections throughout the neuraxis (Parent, 1997).

Human sleep occurs with circadian periodicity. Thus, humans have an internal "free-running clock" that operates even in the absence of information about the period of 24 hours (Aschoff, 1965; Hobson, 1989; Colwell and Michel, 2003). This clock is controlled by the suprachiasmatic nucleus.

So, circadian rhythms provide temporal organization and coordination for physiological, biochemical, and behavioral variables in all eukaryotic organisms and in some prokaryotes. Circadian rhythms that are genetically determined, not learned (Hall, 1990, Rosato et al., 1997; von Schantz and Archer, 2003), are generated by an endogenous self-sustained pacemaker.

The pineal body synthesizes the sleep-promoting neurohormone melatonin and secretes it into the bloodstream where it modulates the sleep.

The thalamus

The physiological understanding of the human thalamus is limited. The fundamental function of the thalamus is that of relay and it modulates peripheral information to the cerebral cortex and to the basal ganglia, keeping the somatosensory, mental, and emotional activity of a living individual in harmony.

With the exception of the thalamic reticular nucleus, all thalamic subnuclei possess thalamic projection neurons that relay processed information to the cerebral cortex. In addition, the thalamic subnuclei also have inhibitory GABA-ergic interneurons whose cell bodies and processes are confined to a single subnucleus. The reticular nucleus of the thalamus is a continuation into the diencephalon of the reticular formation of the brain stem. It receive inputs from the cerebral cortex and thalamic nuclei. The former are collaterals of corticothalamic projections and the latter are collateral of thalamocortical projections. The reticular nucleus projects to other thalamic nuclei. The inhibitory neurotransmitter of this projection is GABA. The reticular nucleus is unique amongst the thalamic nuclei because its axons do not leave the thalamus. Based on its connections, the reticular nucleus plays a role in integrating and gating activities of the thalamic nuclei.

As the termination site for the reticular ascending system is considered, it is not surprising that the thalamus has an important arousal and sleep-producing function (Green 1987; Steriade et al., 1990; La Berge, 2000; Jones, 2007) and that it alerts, activates or inhibits a specific processing and response system. Its involvement in attention shows up in diminished awareness of stimuli impinging on the side opposite to the lesion (unilateral inattention) (Dănăilă, 1972; Arseni and Dănăilă, 1977; Ojemann, 1984; Posner, 1988; Heilman et al., 2003).

The ascending input to intralaminar nuclei can help explain consciousness of primitive percepts (non-cognitive component). So, ascending output of the brain stem reticular formation not only subserves arousal but also contains information about other states. Thus, other input to reticular formation comes from the spinothalamic system, and trigeminal complex, and from dentate nuclei in the cerebellum conveying proprioceptive signals. There are also ascending inputs to intralaminar nuclei from deep layers of the periaqueductal gray, substantia nigra and amygdala with affective information, and from the vestibular nuclei with information about body position (McGuiness and Krauthamer, 1980; Kaufman and Rosenquist, 1985; Royce et al., 1991; Jones, 2007).

Intralaminar nuclei. These nuclei, embedded in the internal medullary lamina, consist of centralis, lateralis, paracentralis, central medial nuclei (anterior group), and centromedial and parafascicular nuclei (posterior group) (Ohye, 2002). The latter are often called the centromedian-parafascicular complex.

The anterior group receives different projections from the spinothalamic tract, deep cerebellar nucleus, brain stem reticular formation, etc.

The posterior group has a reciprocal connection with the basal ganglia. The efferent connection with the cerebral cortex is very wide and was thought to be a diffuse projection. The intralaminar nuclei were classified as representatives of the "nonspecific system" rather than of the "specific system", such as the thalamic station for the visual, auditory, or somatosensory system with definite modality-specific peripheral input.

Reticular nucleus. This nucleus is considered to be related to arousal, attention, cognitive function, etc. As discussed later, it plays a role in maintaining cortical activity in a disease state of epilepsy (Ohye, 1990; Ohye, 1998; Jones, 2007).

Ohye (2002) studied the human thalamus using microrecordings during stereotactic thalamotomy for dyskinesia and found verbal command neurons in this nucleus and adjacent area.

Surround-type inhibition mediated by thalamic reticular nuclei may selectively gate out extraneous stimuli while allowing focused relay important sensory data to the thalamocortical circuits, which endow a given neural activity pattern with the property of conscious perception (Ames and Marshall, 2003). But how is this neurophysiologic activity coordinated in time to produce a somewhat unified conscious stream? Data suggest the answer may lie in the acquisition of gamma synchrony, most commonly at approximately 40 Hz (Gray and Viana di Prisco, 1997).

Gamma synchrony has also been hypothesized to "bind" disparate features of a given object, such as color, size, texture, and motion, into a temporally unified sensory stimulus (Singer and Gray, 1995).

On the other hand, thalamocortical neurons receive ascending projections from the locus ceruleus (noradrenergic), raphe nuclei (serotonergic), reticular junction (cholinergic), TMN (histaminergic) and project to cortical pyramidal cells.

In the tonic firing state, thalamocortical neurons transmit information to the cortex that is correlated with the spike trains encoding peripheral stimuli (Steriade, 1992, 1999).

In brief, the control of sleep and wakefulness depends on the brain stem and hypothalamic modulation of the thalamus and cortex.

The epithalamus

The function of the epithalamus is not well understood.

Production of the pineal hormone melatonin is cyclic, with high levels of synthesis occurring at night and low levels during the day.

A destructive disease of the diencephalon

Unilateral thalamic or diencephalic lesions (tumors, hemorrhage, etc.) do not determine coma.

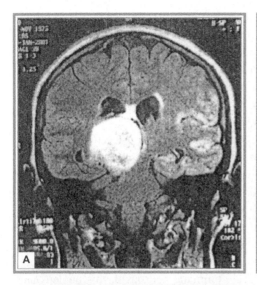
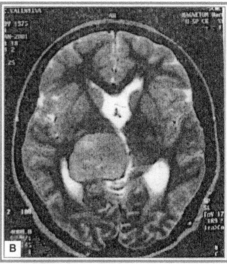
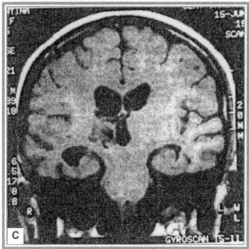
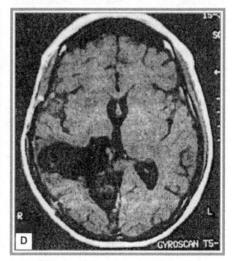

Fig. 24.6. Contrast medium-enhanced coronal (A) and axial (B) magnetic resonance imaging showing a big right thalamic tumor that proved to be an astrocytoma. Thirteen months following resection and radiotherapy, coronal (C) and axial (D) magnetic resonance imaging demonstrates the absence of tumor.
The patient was conscious and in good state.

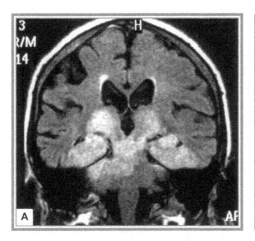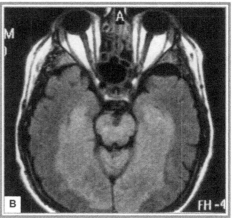

Fig. 24.7. A 56-year-old man who presented with a sudden onset of coma and fever. Coronal (A) and axial (B) T1-weighted magnetic resonance imaging (MRI) scans revealed edematous, demyelination symmetrical changes infra- and supratentorial, which involve entire midbrain, both thalamic formations, bilateral basal ganglia, two-side temporooccipital convolution and hippocampus, determined by encephalitis. After 9 days of coma, the patient died.

We had the case of a 29-year-old woman whose CT demonstrated a spontaneous hypodense tumor, located in the right thalamus. On MRI the tumor appeared hypointense in T1-weighted image and hyperintense in T2-weighted image, surrounded by a moderate edema (Fig. 24.6, case 4). At the operation, the tumor was totally resected. The histological exam showed an astrocytic cell population. Thirty-five days after surgery, the patient started radiation therapy using a 10 MeV photons energy linear accelerator. The clinical examination, performed thirteen months after surgery, demonstrated a very good health condition of the patient. Control cerebral MRI showed the absence of any intracerebral tumor mass and reduced hydrocephalus.

Bilateral destructive lesions of the diencephalic region result in deep coma and death, despite an intact cortex.

Occasional inflammatory and infectious disorders may have a predilection for the diencephalon (Fig. 24.7, case 5). Fatal familial insomnia, a prior disorder, is reported to affect the thalamus selectively, and this has been proposed as a cause of the sleep disorder, although this produces hyperwakefulness, not coma (Della Porta et al., 1964). Humans with bilateral damage to the region of the dorsal pons, midbrain, and thalamus (by trauma, brain tumor, viral or bacterial infection, ischemic or hemorrhagic stroke) may exhibit an impaired state of alertness, possibly becoming stuporose or comatose.

LIMBIC SYSTEM AND HIPPOCAMPUS

Broca (1878) first described and named the limbic lobe. In a subsequent phase in speculation on the limbic lobe by observers such as Papez (1937) and Brodal (1947), it was suggested that, in humans, this lobe is partially olfactory and is mainly concerned with emotional behavior. In addition, the amygdala was seen as part of limbic lobe. Finally, Papez showed that the hippocampus projects, *via* the fornix, back to the hypothalamus. Nauta (1958) developed this concept further, insisting on the functional importance of certain regions of the neural axis, such as the septum, cingulate gyrus, orbitofrontal cortex, preoptic area, "limbic striatum" (including the nucleus accumbens, mesolimbic dopaminergic tract), nonspecific thalamic nuclei, hypothalamus and midbrain tegmental area, regions closely related to the amygdala and hippocampus. These regions form a ring, or "limbus", around the base of the brain. Anterior cingulate cortex (ACC) is part of a neural circuit that mediates outcome-contingent changes in behavior (Ito et al., 2003; Kerns et al., 2004; Kennerley et al., 2006) and processes fictive information in human (Chiu et al., 2008). The ACC is interconnected with the orbitofrontal cortex which mediates fictive thinking in humans (Camille et al., 2004; Ursu and Carter, 2005).

Hayden et al. (2009) hypothesized that neurons in the ACC, which monitors the consequences of actions and mediates subsequent changes in behavior, would respond to fictive reward information.

Generally, the hypothalamus makes a link between the limbic and endocrine system reasonable. The limbic system is now considered to be a functional unit. Areas around the limbic system are called paralimbic and have a more complex histologic structure. Anyhow, the limbic system makes a link between external and internal world.

The Hippocampus. The hippocampus occupies the medial part of the floor of the temporal horn and is divided into three parts: head, body and tail.

Structure. The hippocampus is bilaminar, consisting of the cornu Ammonis (or hippocampus proper) and the gyrus dentatus (or fascia dentata), with one lamina rolled up inside the other.

Functions and connections: the possible functions of the hippocampus are divided into four categories: (1) learning and memory, (2) regulation of emotional behavior, (3) certain aspects of motor control; and (4) regulation of hypothalamic functions (Duvernoy, 2005). The hippocampus and related diencephalic structures form and consolidate declarative memories that are ultimately stored elsewhere.

The hippocampus is also involved in the regulation of the hypothalamo-hypophysial axis. Through its projections to the paraventricular hypothalamic nucleus, it may inhibit the hypophysial secretion of adrenocorticotrophic hormone (ACTH) (Jacobs et al., 1979; Teyler et al., 1980; Herman et al., 1989; Diamond et al., 1996).

The amygdala: amygdala is a complex mass of gray matter buried in the anterior-medial portion of the temporal lobe, just rostral to the hippocampus.

The amygdala and its interconnections with an array of neocortical areas in the prefrontal cortex and anterior temporal lobe, as well as several subcortical structures, appear to be especially important in the higher order processing of emotion.

The amygdala links cortical regions that process sensory information with hypothalamic and brain stem effector systems. In a review of the role of the amygdala in emotional processing, Phelps and Le Doux (2005) identified five areas in which there is evidence from studies of cognition-emotion interactions involving the amygdala:

1) implicit emotional learning and memory;
2) emotional modulation of memory;

3) emotional influences on perception and attention;
4) emotion and social behavior;
5) emotion, inhibition and regulation.

CEREBRAL CORTEX

The cerebral cortex of the cerebral hemispheres, the convoluted outer layer of gray matter composed of tens billions of neurons and their synaptic connections, is the most highly organized correlation center of the brain, but the specific of cortical structures in mediating behavior is neither clear-cut nor circumscribed (Collins, 1990; Franckowiak et al., 1997). This multitude of neurons send a large number of axons in all directions, covered by supportive myelin. This forms the white matter of the cortex which fills the large subcortical space.

The cerebral cortex receives sensory information from internal / external environment of the organism, processes this information and then decides on and carries out the response to it.

Generally, the hemispheres supply much of the content and registration function of consciousness, including language, abstract reasoning, somatosensory visual and spatial abilities, map of the physical dimensions of the self, executive function, complex emotion, feelings, memory and ability to read other's mind.

While the cortex is vital for cognitive functions, it interacts constantly with major satellite organs, notably the thalamus, basal ganglia, hypothalamus, cerebellum, brainstem and limbic regions, among others.

In order to be conscious, to operate at normal parameters, to record and potentiate the internal and external sensory data, and to correctly process them based on the previous individual experience, and to answer adequately, it is necessary that the cerebral cortex should be integer and aroused by the ascending activating system.

These considerations suggest that there might be multiple conscious awareness systems, each supporting conscious awareness in different mental domains.

Unilateral and diffuse, bilateral cortical destruction

Different regions of the cerebral cortex have modular specific functions (somatic sensory and motor, visceral sensory and motor, integrative cognitive functions, speech functions, etc.) responsible for the high-order cognitive processing or conscious mind. These correspond to the Brodmann areas, as well to each of the four cerebral lobes.

Being aware of the somatic and visceral ego refers to the ability of being conscious of the components of one's body, concrete activities and their status. Thus, a lesion of the parietal lobe leads to a destruction of the ego, which manifests through agnosia, such as asomatognosia (denial of one's own body part), finger agnosia, tactile agnosia, hemiasomatognosia.

The ideational consciousness refers to the ability of one person to be aware of their concrete activities, ideas and thoughts that are expressed through spoken or written words. A lesion of the frontal, parietal, occipital, temporal lobe and the callous body leads to apraxia, Gerstmann's syndrome, Balint's syndrome, akinetic mutism, aphasia and agraphia. Emotional consciousness refers to the ability of being aware of emotions. The frontal lobe and the left parietal lobe coordinate positive emotions, whereas ones on the right side coordinate negative emotions.

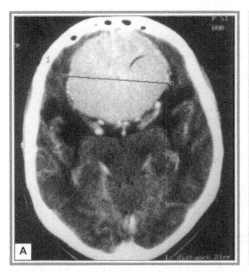
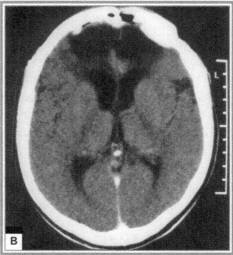

Fig. 24.8. A presurgery contrast enhanced computed tomographic (CT) scan of a 56-year-old man shows a giant size olfactory groove meningioma and displacement of anterior brain (A). The patient presents an orbitofrontal syndrome. Postsurgery contrast-enhanced CT scan showing no residual tumor (B) and orbitofrontal syndrome disappeared.

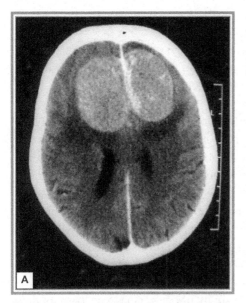
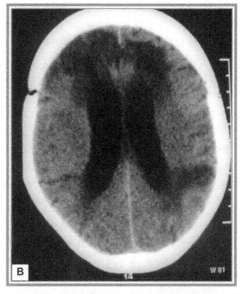

Fig. 24.9. A presurgery contrast enhanced computed tomographic (CT) scan of a 35-year-old woman shows a bilobed meningioma of the anterior falx. She has a dorsolateral frontal syndrome (A). Postsurgery contrast-enhanced computed tomography scan showing no residual tumor (B) and frontal syndrome disappeared.

We want to stress the existence of the same discrete modules in the brain for each possible neuropsychological capacity. Adjacent modules communicate with each other more than do non-adjacent modules. So, the term of modular or functional localization of consciousness is used to indicate that certain functions can be localized to particular areas of the cerebral cortex. The mapping of cortical function began with inference made from the deficits produced by cortical lesions in humans.

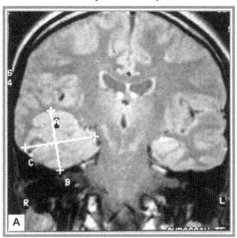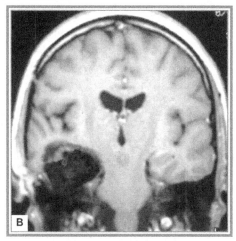

Fig. 24.10. (A) Preoperative coronal T1-weighted, gadolinium-enhanced magnetic resonance images obtained for a 46-year-old man who presented prosopagnosia and memory disturbance. It demonstrated a large right-sided temporo-basal astrocytoma. (B) Image was obtained after complete removal of the tumor. After two months the symptoms disappeared.

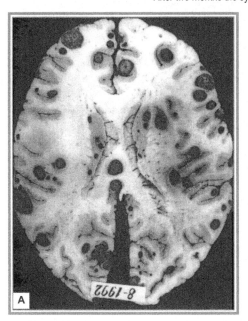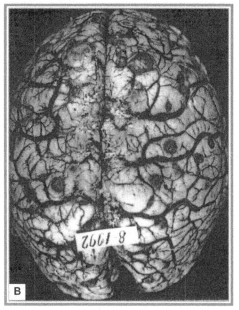

Fig. 24.11. Bilateral, cortical and subcortical, more than 110 cerebral metastases (A and B). The primitive tumor was a melanocarcinoma.

1951

As we have noticed, partial lesion of some Brodmann specialized areas or of one of the lobes leads to the modular loss of consciousness (Fig. 24.8, case 6), (Fig. 24.9, case 7), (Fig. 24.10, case 8). When all the cerebral cortex is destroyed as well as the white matter of the two hemispheres that globally depress neuronal activity, the consciousness level decreases and coma is produced. These causes of diseases include cortical and subcortical tumors (Fig. 24.11, case 9), hypoxia, sedatives, hypnotics, neurotransmitter receptor antagonists, neural toxins, infectious disease and metabolic disease. Careful studies of split-brain patients make it clear that the right hemisphere has a consciousness of its own, even if it lacks the ability to communicate its experiences verbally.

Discussion

The consciousness processes belong to people who act by control mechanisms of psychological activities, generalization and abstractization mechanisms, as well as by exploring and handling of mental images to solve all the problems man is facing with. The consciousness level depends on the complexity of the brain ontogenetic evolution. It must be a function of numerous interacting systems. Data based on our experience support this statement.

According to Tononi and Laureys, consciousness can be dissociated from other brain function, such as responsiveness to sensorial inputs, motor control, attention, language, memory, reflection, spatial frames of reference, the body and perhaps even the self (Tononi and Laureys, 2009). We consider this point of view to be incorrect because consciousness cannot appear without these function. It cannot be dissociated from them. The respective functions represent modules of the consciousness. The consciousness results from the respective cerebral activities. Lesions of some functions lead to modular disorder of the consciousness.

The major structures supposed to play a key role in the neural correlates of consciousness are: the brain stem, the diencephalon (the hypothalamus and thalamus), the limbic system (especially the hippocampus and amygdala), basal ganglia, cerebellum, and the cerebral cortex. The brain stem is the source of massive reticular formation pathways that activate or inhibit higher and lower brain centers. They are the core of the basic arousal and sleeping cycle.

The hypothalamus, the thalamus and the cerebral cortex are likely closely intertwined with RF which plays a key role in consciousness. Generally, there are an ascending activating system (AAS) and an ascending inhibitory system (AIS).

However, AAS which appears to be responsible for maintaining cortical arousal is not the same with consciousness.

Sleep is based on ascending reticular inhibitory system. The two reticular systems (AAS and AIS) are under the influence of the suprachiasmatic nucleus and of the awake and sleep centers in the hypothalamus. So, as much as awake is determined by AAS, sleep, considered the most profound natural alteration of consciousness, is determined by AIS. AAS and AIS are not neurological basis of consciousness but they rather constitute the necessary substrate for consciousness to emerge.

Lesions of the ascending reticular inhibitory system produced the logorrhea syndrome with hyperkinesia, hyperwakefulness and hyperprosexia.

Bilateral lesions / destructions of the neurological formations (brain stem, midbrain, diencephalon, limbic system and cerebral cortex) lead to the loss of consciousness.

The ascending inhibitory system is important in explaining the sleep and many other behaviors.

On the other side, the cerebral cortex and consciousness have a modular structure. AAS and AIS reach the cerebral cortex directly, through the thalamus and the hypothalamus. In order to be conscious, it is necessary that the cerebral cortex should be integer and aroused.

Thus, to be conscious is equivalent of having access to information about the self and the environment and to have the capacity to read another individual's intention. The consciousness is the most developed form of expressing the personality. The self similar to the ego, the spirit, the soul is the main expert or primary knower. So, consciousness is not equal to the awakened state of mind, as it involves functions of almost the entire brain. But different brain structures and functions have a certain role in generating consciousness. Consciousness, as a result of functions from almost entire brain, is composed by modules which have different important values and features.

Injuring one module only leads to partial modification of the conscious state. Thus, attention, memory, sensorial input, motor output, language, introspection / reflection, space, body and self, perception, imagination, gnosias etc. are necessary prerequisite of consciousness. The measurement scale of the (actual) level of consciousness of a current person in the awakened state of mind and under ordinary life condition is composed of several modules such as: being aware of the somatic, visceral, cognitive, emotional and spiritual ego, and being aware of the physical, spatial, social, socio-relational extra ego.

Conclusions

– Bilateral destruction of the reticular activating nuclei at the rostral pons and midbrain lead to loss of consciousness and the induction of coma.

– The damage of the ascending reticular inhibitory system lead to the appearance of the logorrhea syndrome with hyperkinesia, hyperwakefulness, and hyperprosexia.

– The ascending inhibitory system is very important in explaining the sleep and many other behaviors.

– AAS and AIS reach the cerebral cortex by three distinct ways: directly, through the thalamus and through the hypothalamus.

– The sleep is controlled by action of the AAS-AIS dipole.

– With respect to its functioning, the cerebral cortex may be compared to a continuous chess game between of the two systems, AAS and AIS, which act in perfect equilibrium in order to perform all functions and behaviors of the individual.

– The cerebral cortex and consciousness have a modular structure.

REFERENCES

Adams JH, Graham D, Jennett B, The neuropathology of the vegetative state after an acute brain insult. Brain 123; 1327-1338, 2000.

Ames C, Marshall L, Differential diagnosis of altered states of consciousness. In: HR Winn (ed), *Youmans Neurological Surgery*. Vol. 1. Fifth Edition. Saunders, Philadelphia. Pennsylvania, 277-299, 2003.

Arseni C, Dănăilă L, Logorrhea syndrome with hyperkinesia. Eur Neurol 15; 183-187, 1977.

Aschoff J, Circadian rhythms in man. Science 148; 1427-1432, 1965.

Berger H, Ueber das electroenkephalogramm des menschen. Arch. Psychiatr. Nervenkr. 87; 527-570, 1929.

Bly M, Faymonville ME, Peigneux P, Auditory processing in severely brain injured patient: differences between the minimally conscious state and the persistent vegetative state. Archives of Neurology 61; 233-238, 2004.

Bogen JE, Some neurophysiologic aspects of consciousness. Semin Neurol. 17; 95-103, 1997.

Bogen JE, The thalamic intralaminar nuclei and the property of consciousness. In: P.D. Zelazov, M Moscovitch, E Thompson (eds), *The Cambridge Handbook of Consciousness*, Cambridge Univ Press, 775-807, 2001.

Bosinelli M, Mind and consciousness during sleep. Behavioural Brain Research 69; 195-201, 1995.

Bremer F, Cerveau isolé et physiologie du sommeil. Comp. Rend. Soc. Biol 118; 1235-1242, 1935.

Bremer F, Nouvelles recherches sur le mécanisme du sommeil. Comp. Rend. Soc. Biol. 122; 460-464, 1936.

Brendler SJ, Selverstone B, Recovery from decerebration. Brain 93; 381-392, 1970.

Broca P, Anatomie comparée des circonvolutions cérébrales. Le grand lobe limbique et la scissure limbique dans la série des mammifères. Rev Anthropol 1; 385-398, 1878.

Brodal A, The hippocampus and the sense of smell. A review. Brain 70; 179- 222, 1947.

Brooks WM, Friedman SD, Gasparovic C, Magnetic resonance spectroscopy in traumatic brain injury. J. Head Trauma Rehabil 16; 149-164, 2001.

Buzsaki G, Diversity of cortical functions is provided by inhibition. In: G. Buzsaki (ed), *Rhythms of the Brain*, Oxford University Press, Cycle 3; 61-79, 2006.

Camille N, Coricelli G, Sallet J, Pradat-Diehl P, Duhamel JR, Sirigu A, The involvement of the orbitofrontal cortex in the experience of regret. Science, 1167-1170, 2004.

Card JP, Swanson LW, Moore RY,. The hypothalamus: An overview of regulatory system. In: *Fundamental Neuroscience* (M. Zigmond, FE Bloom, SC Landis, L Roberts, LR Squire, Eds), Academic Press, San Diego, 1013-1026, 1999.

Chiu PH, Lohrent TM, Montague PR, Smokers' brains compute, but ignore, a fictive error signal in a sequential investment task. Nature Neuroscience 11; 514-520, 2008

Collins RC, Cerebral Cortex. In: AL Pearlman and RC Collins (eds.), *Neurobiology of disease*, New York: Oxford University Press, 1990.

Colwell CS, Michel S, Sleep and circadian rhythms: Do sleep centers talk to the clock?, Nature Neurosci 10; 1005-1006, 2003.

Damasio AR, *Descartes' error: Emotion, reason, and the human brain*. New York: Putnam, 1994.

Damasio AR, *The feeling of what happens*. New York: Harcourt Press, 1999.

Dănăilă L, Clinical and experimental study on the reticular substance psychopathology (in Romanian language), 110 pp. Graduating thesis, Faculty of Philosophy, University of Bucharest, 1972.

Dănăilă L, Pascu ML, *Lasers in Neurosurgery*. Ed. Acad. Române, 2001.

Dănăilă L, Pascu ML, Second International Symposium on Coma and Consciousness: Clinical, Social and Ethical Implications, Berlin, 4-5 June. Abst. 21, 2009.

Della Porta P, Maiolo AT, Negri VU, Cerebral blood flow and metabolism in therapeutic insulin coma. Metabolism 13; 131-140, 1964.

Denes-Ray V, Epstein S, Conflict between intuitive and rational processing: When people behave against their bitter judgment. Journal Personality and Social Psychology 66; 819-829, 1994.

Diamond DM, Fleshner M, Ingersoll N, Rose GM, Psychological stress impairs spatial working memory: relevance to electronophysiological studies of hippocampal function. Behav. Neurosci 110; 661-672, 1996.

Duvernoy HM, *The Human Hippocampus*. Third Ed., Springer Verlag, Berlin, Heidelberg, 2005.

Edelman GM, *Bright air, brilliant fire: On the matter of the mind*. New York: Basic Books, 1992.

Edelman GM, Tononi G, *A universe of consciousness*. New York: Basic Books, 2000.

Franckowiak RSJ, Friston KJ, Frith CD, Dolan RJ, Mazziota JC, Human brain function. San Diego, Academic Press, 1997.

Fuster JM, *The Prefrontal Cortex*. Fourth Edition. Amsterdam, Boston, Heidelberg, etc. Academic Press Elsevier, 2009.

Gaus SE, Strecker RE, Tate BA, Parker RA, Saper CB, Ventrolateral preoptic nucleus contains sleep-active, galaninergic neurons in multiple mammallian species. Neuroscience 115; 285-294, 2002.

Giza CC, Hovda DA, The neurometabolic cascade of concussion. J. Athl. Train 36; 228-235, 2001.

Gray CM, Viana di Prisco G, Stimulus dependent neuronal oscillations and local synchronization in striate cortex of the alert cat. J. Neurosci 17; 3239-3253, 1997.

Green S, *Physiological psychology*. New York, Routledge and Kegan Paul, 1987.

Hall JC, Genetics of circadian rhythms. Ann. Rev Genet 24; 659-694, 1990.

Hatta T, Masui T, Ito E, Hasegawa Y, Matsuyama Y, Relation between the prefrontal cortex and cerebro-cerebellar functions: evidence from the results of stabilometrical indexes. Apply. Neuropsychology 11; 153-160, 2004.

Hayden BY, Pearson JM, Platt ML, Fictive reward signals in the anterior cingulate cortex. Science 324; 948-950, 2009.

Heilman KM, Watson RT, Valenstein E, Neglect and related disorders. In: KM Heilman and E Valenstein (eds.), *Clinical neuropsychology* (4th ed). New York University Press, 2003.

Herman JP, Schäfer MKH, Young EA, Thompson R, Douglass J, Akil H, Watson SJ, Evidence for hippocampal regulation of neuroendocrine neurons of the hypothalamo-pituitary-adrenocortical axis. J. Neurosci. 9; 3072-3082, 1989.

Hobson JA, *Sleep*. New York: Scientific American Library, 1989.

Hobson JA, State of consciousness: normal and abnormal variation. In: PD Zelazov, M. Marcovitch and E Thompson (eds), *The Cambridge Handbook of Consciousness*, Chapter 16. Cambridge University Press, Cambridge, New York; 435-444, 2007.

Hopfield, JJ, Tank DW, Computing with neural circuits: A model. Science 233; 625-633, 1986.

Ito S, Stuphorn V, Brown JW, Schall JD, Performance monitoring the anterior cingulate cortex during saccade countermanding. Science 303; 120, 2003.

Jannett B, Plum F, Persistent vegetative state after brain damage: A syndrome in research of a name. Lancet 1; 734-737, 1972.

Jacobs MS, Mc Farland WL, Morgane PJ, The anatomy of the brain of the bottlenose dolphin (Tursiops truncatus). Rhinic lobe (rhinencephalon): the archicortex. Brain Res Bull 4 (Suppl.1); 1-108, 1979.

Jones GJE, *The Thalamus*. Second edition. Vol. I and II. Cambridge, New York, Melbourne etc., Cambridge University Press, 2007.

Kagan J, *The second year: The emergence of self-awareness*. Cambridge, MA: Harvard University Press, 1981.

Kennerley SW, Walton ME, Behrens EJ, Buckley M., Rushworth MSF, Optimal decision making and the anterior cingulate cortex. Nature Neuroscience 9; 940-947, 2006.

Kerns JG, Cohen JD, MacDonald AW, Cho YR, Stenger AV, Carter SC, Anterior cingulate conflict monitoring and adjustments in control. Science 303; 1023-1026, 2004.

La Berge D, Networks of attention. In: MS Gazzaniga (ed). *The new cognitive neuroscience* (2nd ed). Cambridge MA, MIT Press, 2000.

Levy DE, Sidtis JJ, Rottenberg DA, Jarden JO, Differences in cerebral blood flow and glucose utilization in vegetative versus locked-in patients, 1987. Annals of Neurology 22; 673-682, 1987.

Lewis M, The development of self-consciousness. In: J Roessler and N. Eilan (eds). *Agency and self-awareness*. Oxford: Oxford University Press, 275-295, 2003.

Marrocco RT, Field BA, Arousal. In: V.S. Ramachandran (ed.), *Encyclopedia of the Human Brain*. Amsterdam, Boston, London etc., Academic Press, 223-236, 2002.

McGuiness CM, Krauthamer GM, The afferent projections to the centrum medianum of the cat as demonstrated by retrograde transport of horseradish peroxidase. Brain Research 184; 255-269, 1980.

Minzenberg MJ, Watrous AJ, Yoon JH, Ursu S, Carter C, Modafinil shifts human locus ceruleus to low-tonic, high-phasic activity during functional MRI. Science 322; 1700-1702, 2008.

Moore RY, Bloom FE, Central catecholamine system: Anatomy and physiology of the norepinephrine and epinephrine systems. Ann. Rev Neurosci 2; 113-168, 1979.

Moore RY, Halaris AE, Jones BE, Serotonin neurons of the midbrain raphe: Ascending projections. J. Comp. Neurol. 180; 417-438, 1978.

Moruzzi G, Magoun WH, Brain stem reticular formation and activation of the EEG. Electroencephalography and Clinical Neurophysiology 1; 455-473, 1949.

Nauta WJH, Hippocampal projections and related neural pathways to the midbrain in the cat. Brain 81; 319-340, 1958.

Ohye C, Thalamus. In: *The Human Nervous System* (G. Paxinos ed.) Academic Press, San Diego, 439-468, 1990.

Ohye C, Thalamotomy for Parkinson's disease and other types of tumor. Part 1: Historical background and technique. In: *Textbook of Stereotactic and Functional Neurosurgery* (PL Gildenberg and RR Tasker Eds), 1167-1178, McGraw-Hill, New York, 1998.

Ohye C, Thalamus and thalamic damage. In: V.S. Ramachandran (ed), *Encyclopedia of the human brain* Vol. 4. Academic Press, Amsterdam, Boston, London; 575-597, 2002.

Ojemann GA,. Common cortical and thalamic mechanisms for language and motor functions. American Journal of Physiology 246; 901-903, 1984.

Papez JW, A proposed mechanism of emotion. Arch Neurol Psychiatry 38; 725-743, 1937.

Parent A, *Hypothalamus. In: Carpenter's Human Neuroanatomy*, 9th ed, Williams and Wilkins, Baltimore, 706-743, 1997.

Phelps EA, Le Doux JE, Contributions of the amygdala to emotion processing from animal models to human behavior. Neuron 48; 175-187, 2005.

Posner MI, Structures and functions of selective attention. In: Boll and B.K. Bryant (eds), *Clinical neuropsychology and brain function: Research, measurement, and practice.* Washington DC, American Psychological Association, 1988.

Posner JB, Saper CB, Schiff ND, Plum F, *Plum and Posner's Diagnosis of Stupor and Coma.* Fourth Edition, Oxford University Press, 110-112, 2007.

Posner JB, Saper CB, Schiff ND, Plum F, (eds). *Plum and Posner's Diagnosis of Stupor and Coma.* Chapter 3. Structural causes of stupor and coma. Oxford University Press, 88-118, 2007.

Pouille F, Scanziani M, Enforcement of temporal fidelity in pyramidal cells by somatic feed-forward inhibition. Science 293; 1159-1163, 2001.

Rosato E, Piccin A, Kyriacou CP, Molecular analysis of circadian behavior. Bioassays 19; 1075-1082, 1997.

Saper CB, Scammell TE, Lu J,. Hypothalamic regulation of sleep and circadian rhythms. Nature 437; 1257-1263, 2005.

Schiff ND, Plum F, Web forum: The neurology of impaired consciousness: Global disorder and implied models. http://athena.english.vt.edu/egi-bin/netforum, 1999.

Schiff ND, Ribary U, Moreno DR, Residual cerebral activity and behavioural fragments can remain in the persistently vegetative brain. Brain, 215; 1210-1234, 2002.

Schooler JW,.Re-presenting consciousness: dissociations between experience and meta-consciousness. Trends in Cognitive sciences 6; 339-344, 2002.

Schutter L, Tang KA, Holshouser BA, Proton MRS in acute traumatic brain injury: role for gluta-mate / glutamine and choline for outcome prediction. J. Neurotrauma 21; 1693-1705, 2004.

Sherin JE, Elmquist JK, Torrealba F, Saper CB, Innervation of histaminergic tuberomammillary neurons by GABAergic and galaninergic neurons in the ventrolateral preoptic nucleus of the rat. J. Neurosci. 18; 4705-4721, 1998.

Sherrington CS, *Inhibition as a coordinative factor*. Elsevier, Amsterdam, 1932.

Singer W, Gray CM, Visual feature integration and the temporal correlation hypothesis. Ann. Rev Neurosci 18; 555-586, 1995.

Steriade M, Basic mechanisms of sleep generation. Neurol 42; 9-18, 1992.

Steriade M, Coherent oscillations and short-term plasticity in corticothalamic networks. TINS 22; 337-345, 1999.

Steriade M, Jones EG, Llinas RR, *Thalamic oscillations and signaling*. New York, Wiley, 1990.

Szymusiak R, Alam N, Steininger TL, McGinty D, Sleep-waking discharge patterns of ventrolateral preoptic / anterior hypothalamic neurons in rats, Brain Res. 803; 178-188, 1998.

Teyler TJ, Vardaris RM, Lewis D, Rawitech AB, Gonadal steroid: effects of excitability of hippocampal pyramidal cells. Science 209; 1017-1019, 1980.

Tononi G, Edelman G, Consciousness and complexity. Science 282; 1846-1851, 1998.

Tononi G, Laureys S, The neurology of consciousness: an overview. In: S Laureys and G Tononi (eds), *The Neurology of Consciousness: Cognitive Neuroscience and Neuropathology*. Academic Press, Amsterdam, Boston, Heidelberg, 375-412, 2009.

Trillet M, Vighetto A, Croisile N, et al., Hémiballisme avec libération thymo-affective et logorrhée par hématome du noyau sous-thalamique gauche. Rev. Neurol. (Paris) 151; 416-419, 1995.

Ursu S, Carter CS, Outcome representations, counterfactual comparisons and the human orbitofrontal cortex: implications for neuroimaging studies of decision-making. Cognitive brain research 23 (1); 51-60, 2005.

Von Monakow C, (ed),. *Localization of brain functions*. Springfield, IL: CC Thomas, 1911.

Von Schantz M, Archer SN, Clocks, genes and sleep. J. Roy Soc Med 96; 486-489, 2003.

Weyhenmeyer JA, Gallman EA, *Rapid Review Neuroscience*. MOSBY, Elsevier, 2007.

Willie JT, Chemelli RM, Sinton CM, et al., Distinct narcolepsy syndromes in orexin receptor-2 and orexin null mice: Molecular genetic dissection of non-REM and REM sleep regulatory processes. Neuron 38; 715-730, 2003.

Yamazaki T, Tanaka S, The cerebellum as a liquid state machine. Neural Networks 20; 290-297, 2007.

Zeman A, Consciousness. Brain, 124 (Pt. 7); 1263-1269, 2001.

Zervas NT, Hedley-Whyte J, Successful treatment of cerebral herniation in five patients. N Engl J Med 286; 1075-1077, 1972.

INDEX

Made in United States
Orlando, FL
15 August 2022

21053016R00337